Feature Reviews in
Pharmaceutical Technology

Feature Reviews in Pharmaceutical Technology

Editors

Silviya Petrova Zustiak
Era Jain

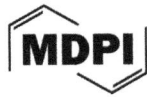

Basel • Beijing • Wuhan • Barcelona • Belgrade • Novi Sad • Cluj • Manchester

Editors

Silviya Petrova Zustiak
Biomedical Engineering
Saint Louis University
Saint Louis
United States

Era Jain
Biomedical and Chemical Engineering
Syracuse University
Syracuse
United States

Editorial Office
MDPI
St. Alban-Anlage 66
4052 Basel, Switzerland

This is a reprint of articles from the Special Issue published online in the open access journal *Pharmaceuticals* (ISSN 1424-8247) (available at: www.mdpi.com/journal/pharmaceuticals/special_issues/6Z9TCK5683).

For citation purposes, cite each article independently as indicated on the article page online and as indicated below:

Lastname, A.A.; Lastname, B.B. Article Title. *Journal Name* **Year**, *Volume Number*, Page Range.

ISBN 978-3-7258-0038-4 (Hbk)
ISBN 978-3-7258-0037-7 (PDF)
doi.org/10.3390/books978-3-7258-0037-7

© 2024 by the authors. Articles in this book are Open Access and distributed under the Creative Commons Attribution (CC BY) license. The book as a whole is distributed by MDPI under the terms and conditions of the Creative Commons Attribution-NonCommercial-NoDerivs (CC BY-NC-ND) license.

Contents

About the Editors vii

Preface ix

Silviya Petrova Zustiak and Era Jain
Feature Reviews in Pharmaceutical Technology
Reprinted from: *Pharmaceuticals* 2023, 16, 1336, doi:10.3390/ph16101336 1

Samuel T. Stealey, Akhilesh K. Gaharwar and Silviya Petrova Zustiak
Laponite-Based Nanocomposite Hydrogels for Drug Delivery Applications
Reprinted from: *Pharmaceuticals* 2023, 16, 821, doi:10.3390/ph16060821 4

Rita Oliveira and Isabel F. Almeida
Patient-Centric Design of Topical Dermatological Medicines
Reprinted from: *Pharmaceuticals* 2023, 16, 617, doi:10.3390/ph16040617 23

Qi Wang, Keerthi Atluri, Amit K. Tiwari and R. Jayachandra Babu
Exploring the Application of Micellar Drug Delivery Systems in Cancer Nanomedicine
Reprinted from: *Pharmaceuticals* 2023, 16, 433, doi:10.3390/ph16030433 41

Aleš Franc, David Vetchý and Nicole Fülöpová
Commercially Available Enteric Empty Hard Capsules, Production Technology and Application
Reprinted from: *Pharmaceuticals* 2022, 15, 1398, doi:10.3390/ph15111398 83

Olena Litvinova, Elisabeth Klager, Nikolay T. Tzvetkov, Oliver Kimberger, Maria Kletecka-Pulker and Harald Willschke et al.
Digital Pills with Ingestible Sensors: Patent Landscape Analysis
Reprinted from: *Pharmaceuticals* 2022, 15, 1025, doi:10.3390/ph15081025 102

Chien-Ming Hsieh, Ting-Lun Yang, Athika Darumas Putri and Chin-Tin Chen
Application of Design of Experiments in the Development of Self-Microemulsifying Drug Delivery Systems
Reprinted from: *Pharmaceuticals* 2023, 16, 283, doi:10.3390/ph16020283 121

Jae Cheon Kim, Eun Ji Park and Dong Hee Na
Gastrointestinal Permeation Enhancers for the Development of Oral Peptide Pharmaceuticals
Reprinted from: *Pharmaceuticals* 2022, 15, 1585, doi:10.3390/ph15121585 148

Ayushi Nair, Alosh Greeny, Rajalakshmi Rajendran, Mohamed A. Abdelgawad, Mohammed M. Ghoneim and Roshni Pushpa Raghavan et al.
KIF1A-Associated Neurological Disorder: An Overview of a Rare Mutational Disease
Reprinted from: *Pharmaceuticals* 2023, 16, 147, doi:10.3390/ph16020147 183

Hao Li, Wenni Dai, Zhiwen Liu and Liyu He
Renal Proximal Tubular Cells: A New Site for Targeted Delivery Therapy of Diabetic Kidney Disease
Reprinted from: *Pharmaceuticals* 2022, 15, 1494, doi:10.3390/ph15121494 200

Jihoon Lee, Min-Koo Choi and Im-Sook Song
Recent Advances in Doxorubicin Formulation to Enhance Pharmacokinetics and Tumor Targeting
Reprinted from: *Pharmaceuticals* 2023, 16, 802, doi:10.3390/ph16060802 214

Angela Bonaccorso, Anna Privitera, Margherita Grasso, Sonya Salamone, Claudia Carbone and Rosario Pignatello et al.
The Therapeutic Potential of Novel Carnosine Formulations: Perspectives for Drug Development
Reprinted from: *Pharmaceuticals* **2023**, *16*, 778, doi:10.3390/ph16060778 . . . . **246**

Jessica Lee Aldrich, Arjun Panicker, Robert Ovalle and Blanka Sharma
Drug Delivery Strategies and Nanozyme Technologies to Overcome Limitations for Targeting Oxidative Stress in Osteoarthritis
Reprinted from: *Pharmaceuticals* **2023**, *16*, 1044, doi:10.3390/ph16071044 . . . . **272**

About the Editors

Silviya Petrova Zustiak

Dr. Zustiak has a diverse academic background with a bachelor's degree in bioelectrical engineering, a doctoral degree in biochemical engineering and a postdoctoral training in biophysics. She is currently a Professor and Associate Chair in Biomedical Engineering at Saint Louis University, St Louis, MO, where she also co-directs two large institutes: the Institute for Drug and Biotherapeutic Innovation and the Institute for Translational Neuroscience. Dr. Zustiak has editorial roles in several journals, including *Pharmaceuticals* and is an active member of several professional societies, including the Society for Biomaterials and Biomedical Engineering Society. Dr. Zustiak has received multiple professional awards, including the NIH Fellows Award for Research Excellence during her postdoctoral fellowship, Outstanding Parks Graduate Faculty Award, Scholarly Works Award, and Woman of the Year Award at Saint Louis University. Dr. Zustiak's research is focused on developing hydrogel biomaterials as cell scaffolds, drug screening platforms and drug delivery devices, and is highly multidisciplinary. Her work has been funded by various government agencies such as the National Institutes of Health and the National Science Foundation, private foundations, and industry, and has resulted in over 70 peer-reviewed publications, over 250 conference presentations, four awarded patents and multiple provisional patent applications.

Era Jain

Dr. Era Jain is an Assistant Professor in the Biomedical and Chemical Engineering Department at the College of Engineering and Computer Science, Syracuse University. Before joining Syracuse University, Dr. Jain was a research scientist at Washington University in Saint Louis, where she developed sustained drug delivery systems for the treatment of osteoarthritis. Prior to Washington University, she was a postdoctoral fellow at Saint Louis University where she developed biodegradable hydrogels for the controlled delivery of therapeutic proteins. Dr. Jain earned her Ph.D. at the Indian Institute of Technology, Kanpur, India. Dr. Jain's research focuses on engineering immunomodulatory biomaterials and drug delivery systems for advancing the treatment of musculoskeletal disorders and related inflammatory disorders. She is a member of the Society for Biomaterials, the Biomedical Engineering Society, and the Orthopaedics Research Society. She has contributed to 25 publications and three patents. She recently received the Discovery Award from the Department of Defense for her work targeting activated macrophages for developing immunomodulatory therapies for osteoarthritis.

Preface

The reprint "Feature Reviews in Pharmaceutical Technology" aims to highlight exciting developments in pharmaceutical technologies. With the continuous discovery of a plethora of new drug candidates, both small-molecule drugs and large biomolecules, such technologies are becoming essential for the advancement of patient treatments. This issue features twelve review papers broadly classified into formulation development and drug delivery devices. These technologies address important issues of improving drug bioavailability, decreasing treatment toxicity and side effects, and enhancing treatment efficacy to both cure patients and improve their quality of life.

Silviya Petrova Zustiak and Era Jain
Editors

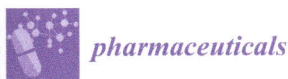

Editorial

Feature Reviews in Pharmaceutical Technology

Silviya Petrova Zustiak [1,*] and Era Jain [2,*]

1. Department of Biomedical Engineering, Saint Louis University, St. Louis, MO 60103, USA
2. Department of Biomedical and Chemical Engineering, Syracuse University, Syracuse, NY 13244, USA
* Correspondence: silviya.zustiak@slu.edu (S.P.Z.); erjain@syr.edu (E.J.)

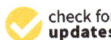

Citation: Zustiak, S.P.; Jain, E. Feature Reviews in Pharmaceutical Technology. *Pharmaceuticals* **2023**, *16*, 1336. https://doi.org/10.3390/ph16101336

Received: 25 July 2023
Accepted: 19 September 2023
Published: 22 September 2023

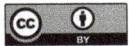

Copyright: © 2023 by the authors. Licensee MDPI, Basel, Switzerland. This article is an open access article distributed under the terms and conditions of the Creative Commons Attribution (CC BY) license (https://creativecommons.org/licenses/by/4.0/).

We are excited to present the Special Issue, "Feature Reviews in Pharmaceutical Technology", aiming to highlight exciting developments in pharmaceutical technologies. With the continual discovery of a plethora of new drug candidates, both small-molecule drugs and large biomolecules, such technologies are becoming essential for the advancement of patient treatments. This issue features eleven review papers broadly classified into formulation development and drug delivery devices. These technologies address important issues of improving drug bioavailability, decreasing treatment toxicity and side effects, and enhancing treatment efficacy to both cure patients and improve their quality of life.

Several reviews focus on formulation and drug delivery devices with a focus on the delivery device. A review by Stealey et al. [1] describes the use of nanosilicates and nanosilicate–hydrogel composites for the sustained and localized delivery of small-molecule drugs as well as large biomolecules. The charged nanosilicate faces allow for drug adsorption via electrostatic interactions and subsequent sustained release, while preserving therapeutic structure and bioactivity [1]. A paper by Oliveira et al. [2] describes a patient-centric design of topical dermatological medicines to improve patient compliance. In a patient-centered approach, the needs and preferences of the patient as well as the needs associated with the disease are all taken into account when designing new topical vehicles meant to improve patient satisfaction and adherence [2]. Yet, another review by Wang et al. [3] describes polymeric micellar formulations used in cancer therapy, which can target specific tissues and prolong therapeutic bioavailability. The review describes polymers used in micelle formulations, tailoring them to be responsive to stimuli for drug delivery applications [3]. Another review by Franc et al. [4] focuses on Enteric Capsule Drug Delivery Technology, which is used to prepare hard enteric capsules meant to survive the acidic stomach environment and slowly erode when passing through the digestive tract. Such capsules could be used for individual therapy or the clinical evaluation of therapeutic substances such as fecal material or probiotics, when administered orally [4]. Lastly, a review from Litvinova et al. [5] offers a patent landscape analysis for pills with digital sensors, showing an increase in patents for applications such as mobile clinical monitoring, smart drug delivery, and endoscopy diagnostics. Such pills have been used to treat various diseases, such as mental health issues, HIV/AIDS, pain, cardiovascular diseases, diabetes, cancer, tuberculosis, etc. [5].

Other feature reviews focus on the co-formulants and process parameters used to design drug delivery devices which influence their performance. For example, a review by Hsieh et al. [6] focuses on oral delivery via self-microemulsifying systems, which improve drug solubility and absorption by enabling drug self-emulsification in a combination of oil, surfactant, and co-surfactant. The authors highlight the use of "design of experiments" systematic approaches for formulation optimization for drugs in different excipients [6]. Another review by Kim et al. [7] focuses on gastrointestinal permeation enhancers for the development of oral peptide products, particularly semaglutide and octreotide, where an oral dosage form of semaglutide is used for the treatment of type 2 diabetes and octreotide capsule is used for the treatment of acromegaly. The article discusses the permeation properties of sodium salcaprozate and medium-chain fatty acids, sodium caprate and sodium caprylate, focusing on transient permeation enhancer technology and gastrointestinal permeation enhancement technology [7].

Some reviews focus on delivery devices for specific diseases and take a disease-centered approach. For example, a paper by Nair et al. [8] focuses on KIF1A-associated neurological diseases, which are caused by changes in the KIF1A microtubule motor protein as a result of gene mutations. While there is no treatment for this class of diseases, the review discusses the promise of experimental gene therapy approaches, such as gene replacement, gene knockdown, symptomatic gene therapy, and cell suicide gene therapy [8]. Another example by Li et al. [9] focuses on diabetic kidney disease, which is a leading cause of end-stage kidney disease in the world. Specifically, the paper discusses proximal tubule cell-targeted drug delivery strategies, such as prodrugs, large molecule carriers and nanoparticles; the proximal tubule is critical for disease progression, and hence, is a worthy target [9].

Several papers focus on formulation development for specific therapeutics, where the focus is on some critical therapeutics. For example, a review by Lee et al. [10] focuses on formulations and drug delivery devices meant to improve the efficacy and reduce the toxicity of the chemotherapeutic doxorubicin. The discussed technologies, such as liposomes, polymeric micelles, polymeric nanoparticles, and polymer–drug conjugates, are currently in clinical use or clinical trials [10]. Another paper by Bonaccorso et al. [11] focuses on the therapeutic potential of formulations for carnosine, which is an endogenous dipeptide with anti-oxidant and ant-inflammatory properties and is found in tissues with a high metabolic rate. Because this dipeptide is rapidly hydrolyzed in plasma, drug modifications and drug delivery systems have been employed to improve its bioavailability as well as to enhance other pharmacological properties, such as blood–brain barrier transport, biological activity, or transport to different tissues [11].

In summary, the papers in this Special Issue highlight the diversity of approaches in formulations and drug delivery device development as well as the diversity of applications that benefit from the advancement of such pharmaceutical technologies. The common goal for such technologies is to improve drug bioavailability, which translates to better efficacy and patient outcomes. In certain instances, as exemplified above, formulations and drug delivery devices can be used to provide targeted treatment, which reduces side effects. They can also be used to provide sustained release, which reduces the treatment frequency and improves patient compliance, ultimately improving the patient's quality of life. With the discovery of newer biotherapeutics, such as the peptides highlighted above, formulations and drug delivery devices have become essential for countering the usually unfavorable pharmacokinetic drug profiles. Hence, innovation in the realm of formulations and drug delivery devices will expand therapy options for patients and has the potential to cure previously incurable diseases.

Author Contributions: Conceptualization, S.P.Z. and E.J.; writing—original draft preparation, S.P.Z.; writing—review and editing, S.P.Z. and E.J. All authors have read and agreed to the published version of the manuscript.

Conflicts of Interest: The authors declare no conflict of interest.

References

1. Stealey, S.T.; Gaharwar, A.K.; Zustiak, S.P. Laponite-Based Nanocomposite Hydrogels for Drug Delivery Applications. *Pharmaceuticals* **2023**, *16*, 821. [CrossRef] [PubMed]
2. Oliveira, R.; Almeida, I.F. Patient-Centric Design of Topical Dermatological Medicines. *Pharmaceuticals* **2023**, *16*, 617. [CrossRef] [PubMed]
3. Wang, Q.; Atluri, K.; Tiwari, A.K.; Babu, R.J. Exploring the Application of Micellar Drug Delivery Systems in Cancer Nanomedicine. *Pharmaceuticals* **2023**, *16*, 433. [CrossRef] [PubMed]
4. Franc, A.; Vetchý, D.; Fülöpová, N. Commercially Available Enteric Empty Hard Capsules, Production Technology and Application. *Pharmaceuticals* **2022**, *15*, 1398. [CrossRef] [PubMed]

5. Litvinova, O.; Klager, E.; Tzvetkov, N.T.; Kimberger, O.; Kletecka-Pulker, M.; Willschke, H.; Atanasov, A.G. Digital pills with ingestible sensors: Patent landscape analysis. *Pharmaceuticals* **2022**, *15*, 1025. [CrossRef] [PubMed]
6. Hsieh, C.-M.; Yang, T.-L.; Putri, A.D.; Chen, C.-T. Application of Design of Experiments in the Development of Self-Microemulsifying Drug Delivery Systems. *Pharmaceuticals* **2023**, *16*, 283. [CrossRef] [PubMed]
7. Kim, J.C.; Park, E.J.; Na, D.H. Gastrointestinal Permeation Enhancers for the Development of Oral Peptide Pharmaceuticals. *Pharmaceuticals* **2022**, *15*, 1585. [CrossRef] [PubMed]
8. Nair, A.; Greeny, A.; Rajendran, R.; Abdelgawad, M.A.; Ghoneim, M.M.; Raghavan, R.P.; Sudevan, S.T.; Mathew, B.; Kim, H. KIF1A-Associated Neurological Disorder: An Overview of a Rare Mutational Disease. *Pharmaceuticals* **2023**, *16*, 147. [CrossRef] [PubMed]
9. Li, H.; Dai, W.; Liu, Z.; He, L. Renal Proximal Tubular Cells: A New Site for Targeted Delivery Therapy of Diabetic Kidney Disease. *Pharmaceuticals* **2022**, *15*, 1494. [CrossRef] [PubMed]
10. Lee, J.; Choi, M.-K.; Song, I.-S. Recent Advances in Doxorubicin Formulation to Enhance Pharmacokinetics and Tumor Targeting. *Pharmaceuticals* **2023**, *16*, 802. [CrossRef] [PubMed]
11. Bonaccorso, A.; Privitera, A.; Grasso, M.; Salamone, S.; Carbone, C.; Pignatello, R.; Musumeci, T.; Caraci, F.; Caruso, G. The Therapeutic Potential of Novel Carnosine Formulations: Perspectives for Drug Development. *Pharmaceuticals* **2023**, *16*, 778. [CrossRef] [PubMed]

Disclaimer/Publisher's Note: The statements, opinions and data contained in all publications are solely those of the individual author(s) and contributor(s) and not of MDPI and/or the editor(s). MDPI and/or the editor(s) disclaim responsibility for any injury to people or property resulting from any ideas, methods, instructions or products referred to in the content.

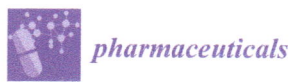

Review

Laponite-Based Nanocomposite Hydrogels for Drug Delivery Applications

Samuel T. Stealey [1], Akhilesh K. Gaharwar [2] and Silviya Petrova Zustiak [1,*]

[1] Department of Biomedical Engineering, Saint Louis University, Saint Louis, MO 63103, USA; samuel.stealey@slu.edu

[2] Department of Biomedical Engineering, Texas A&M University, College Station, TX 77843, USA; gaharwar@tamu.edu

* Correspondence: siliviya.zustiak@slu.edu; Tel.: +314-977-8331; Fax: 314-977-8403

Abstract: Hydrogels are widely used for therapeutic delivery applications due to their biocompatibility, biodegradability, and ability to control release kinetics by tuning swelling and mechanical properties. However, their clinical utility is hampered by unfavorable pharmacokinetic properties, including high initial burst release and difficulty in achieving prolonged release, especially for small molecules (<500 Da). The incorporation of nanomaterials within hydrogels has emerged as viable option as a method to trap therapeutics within the hydrogel and sustain release kinetics. Specifically, two-dimensional nanosilicate particles offer a plethora of beneficial characteristics, including dually charged surfaces, degradability, and enhanced mechanical properties within hydrogels. The nanosilicate–hydrogel composite system offers benefits not obtainable by just one component, highlighting the need for detail characterization of these nanocomposite hydrogels. This review focuses on Laponite, a disc-shaped nanosilicate with diameter of 30 nm and thickness of 1 nm. The benefits of using Laponite within hydrogels are explored, as well as examples of Laponite–hydrogel composites currently being investigated for their ability to prolong the release of small molecules and macromolecules such as proteins. Future work will further characterize the interplay between nanosilicates, hydrogel polymer, and encapsulated therapeutics, and how each of these components affect release kinetics and mechanical properties.

Keywords: nanosilicate; nanoclay; nanocomposite; hydrogel; Laponite; drug delivery

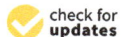

Citation: Stealey, S.T.; Gaharwar, A.K.; Zustiak, S.P. Laponite-Based Nanocomposite Hydrogels for Drug Delivery Applications. *Pharmaceuticals* **2023**, *16*, 821. https://doi.org/10.3390/ph16060821

Academic Editor: Dimitris Tsiourvas

Received: 5 May 2023
Revised: 26 May 2023
Accepted: 29 May 2023
Published: 31 May 2023

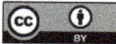

Copyright: © 2023 by the authors. Licensee MDPI, Basel, Switzerland. This article is an open access article distributed under the terms and conditions of the Creative Commons Attribution (CC BY) license (https://creativecommons.org/licenses/by/4.0/).

1. Introduction

Hydrogels are widely used for drug delivery applications due to their potential for localized delivery of a variety of therapeutics while preserving drug bioactivity. However, a notable challenge with hydrogels is their susceptibility to the initial burst release of loaded therapeutics [1]. This is mostly attributed to a highly porous and hydrated network, which facilitates the diffusion of encapsulated drug molecules. To address this issue, several techniques have been employed to minimize this burst release and achieve sustained drug release kinetics [2]. These techniques include the utilization of stimuli-responsive polymers, the attachment of drugs to the polymer network, and the incorporation of nanomaterials into the polymeric network.

The use of nanoparticles in reinforcing hydrogels and enhancing drug delivery is attractive due to their ability to improve mechanical properties, increase drug loading capacity, enable controlled and sustained drug release, and facilitate targeted delivery. Extensive research is being conducted on a wide range of nanoparticles, including polymeric, carbon-based, metal, metal oxides, and ceramic nanoparticles, to reinforce hydrogel networks for drug delivery applications [3]. Among the various nanomaterials being explored for nanocomposite hydrogel drug delivery devices, Laponite (nanosilicates) stands out as a particularly promising and emerging nanomaterial [4]. Laponite is a synthetic two-dimensional (2D) nanosilicate particle that has garnered significant attention in the field [5]. Laponite exhibits a unique shape and surface charge that makes it well-suited for drug delivery applications. Its structure consists of disc-shaped particles with a high aspect ratio, allowing for the efficient loading of therapeutic molecules. Due to discotic charge characteristics, Laponite also enhances interactions with cationic, anionic, or neutral molecules [6]. The combination of high surface area and charge also results in the sustained release of loaded therapeutics [7]. Interestingly, a range of therapeutics, including small molecule drugs, peptides, and large proteins, can be easily loaded and delivered using Laponite.

As Laponite is highly hydrophilic, it can easily interact with a range of polymeric hydrogels. The addition of Laponite to the polymeric network has been shown to improve shear-thinning characteristics, which is important for the minimally invasive and localized delivery of therapeutics [8]. Moreover, Laponite addition has also been shown to improve the mechanical strength as well as physiological stability of polymeric hydrogels. A range of studies have demonstrated the high biocompatibility of Laponite, establishing its widespread application in biomedical applications. More recently, Laponite-loaded polymeric hydrogels received 510k approval from the US Food and Drug Administration (FDA) establishing their clinical potential [9].

In this review, we critically evaluate the use of Laponite-based nanocomposite hydrogels for drug delivery applications. Specifically, we focus on unique characteristics of Laponite, such as the shape, size, and charge, that make it attractive for drug delivery applications. Then, we examine the interactions of Laponite with various polymers to design nanocomposite hydrogels and explore its unique and beneficial properties. The ability of Laponite-based nanocomposite hydrogels for sustained and controlled release of small molecules and macromolecules such as proteins, is examined. In addition, we discuss the structure and stoichiometry of Laponite–therapeutics complexes, which can represent the next frontier in harnessing the utility of Laponite–hydrogel nanocomposites for drug delivery applications.

2. Hydrogels in Drug Delivery Applications

Hydrogels are water-swollen polymer networks that have been extensively characterized and widely utilized for drug delivery applications [2]. Hydrogels can be fabricated from a wide variety of natural polymers (gelatin, collagen, hyaluronic acid, etc.) and/or synthetic polymers (polylactic acid, polyglycolic acid, polyethylene glycol, etc.). Hydrogels are attractive for drug delivery applications due to their highly biocompatible, ability to mimic the physical properties of most soft tissues, and capability to maintain the bioactivity of encapsulated therapeutics [10,11].

Furthermore, the mesh size and degradation profiles of hydrogels can be tunable based on polymer structure, molecular weight, crosslinking mechanism, and degradability [12]. For example, some hydrogels may undergo hydrolytic or enzymatic cleaving, leading to the release of entrapped therapeutics [13]. Slow-degrading hydrogels can release encapsulated cargo and then be degraded or resorbed, eliminating the need for device removal following release [14]. In most hydrogels, the release is controlled by diffusion, which is governed by the relative size ratio of the solute and the mesh size of hydrogels [15]. Small-molecule therapeutics (<500 Da) are typically rapidly released from hydrogels, where hydrogel mesh size is typically much larger than the small molecules [2]. Conversely, larger molecules of therapeutics (>10 kDa), such as proteins, will diffuse slowly [16]. This diffusion-controlled release by hydrogels can lead to high initial burst release, where a significant amount of the encapsulated cargo is rapidly release before achieving a stable sustained release profile [17,18]. While some applications such as wound healing may desire initial burst dosing, in some cases such a burst release can lead to undesirable pharmacokinetic properties [19,20]. A high concentration of the drug may lead to toxicity, while a low plasma concentration of the drug will prevent the desired therapeutic effect [21]. Undesired burst release can be economically wasteful, as significant quantities of drugs are rapidly cleared by the body [17].

It is desirable to design hydrogels with controlled and sustained release strategies that have been implemented to prolong the release of encapsulated therapeutics from hydrogels. For example, encapsulated therapeutics may be tethered to the polymer matrix, preventing rapid diffusion until linkages are cleaved [22,23]. Cleaving of these tethers offers good tunability, but may alter the structure of the drug, reducing its activity [24]. Stimuli-responsive hydrogels may have variable swelling properties based on local environmental pH, salinity, or temperature, thereby altering the release rate [25–28]. Drug release kinetics are, therefore, altered based on the swollen hydrogel mesh size, in which higher swelling leads to faster release. While stimuli-responsive hydrogels offer the potential for delayed and controlled release, swelling may be difficult to predict in a translational setting and may vary from patient to patient, thereby causing variance in release rates [29]. In another strategy, the incorporation of nanomaterials into hydrogels allows for physical or chemical entrapment of encapsulated cargo to allow for sustained release, which is the focus of this review.

3. Nanocomposite Hydrogels in Drug Delivery

Nanomaterials, which are defined as materials that have at least one dimension in the range of 1–100 nm, exist in a wide variety of shapes and compositions, thereby leading to a range of interactions with therapeutic molecules [30]. For example, gold and silver nanoparticles have been widely explored as tethering agents [31–33]. These nanoparticles offer benefits, such as high drug loading, prolonged drug stability, and targeted delivery [34]. Therapeutics have also been entrapped within liposomes, preventing drug diffusion out of the hydrogel until the dissolution of the liposomal structure [35,36]. Mesoporous silica nanoparticles have been entrapped within hydrogels to provide a tortuous path for encapsulated cargo to diffuse, leading to sustained release [37,38]. Two-dimensional (2D) charged nanosilicates have also recently been incorporated into hydrogels to electrostatically adsorb drugs and prolong release kinetics [39–41] and are the main focus of this review.

The incorporation of nanomaterials into hydrogel structures offers a variety of benefits, including augmented hydrogel physical and mechanical properties, adsorption/intercalation of drugs to mitigate burst release, physical crosslinking of polymers, and localization of therapeutic release. The nanocomposite hydrogels offer advantages not afforded by the individual components by themselves. For example, hydrogels may slow drug release, but are susceptible to diffusion-controlled burst release and difficulty in achieving sustained release. On the other hand, nanomaterials by themselves can offer sustained release, but these particles may be rapidly cleared, which is undesirable for localized delivery applications.

4. Two-Dimensional (2D) Nanosilicates

Silicate minerals, which are the largest group of minerals and consist of subunits with the formula $[SiO_{2+n}]^{2n-}$ balanced by metallic anionics, exist in a variety of naturally occurring and synthetic structures that can be utilized in a plethora of biomedical applications. Major types of silicates include nesosilicates, cyclosilicates, sorosilicates, inosilicates, tectosilicates, and phyllosilicates. These phyllosilicates typically form sheet structures made of hydrated aluminosilicates in a Si_2O_5 ratio [42]. Cations such as Mg, K, Na, Ca, and Fe may be naturally substituted into the structures, giving rise to desirable charge characteristics that may be used to interact with drugs for delivery applications. Phyllosilicate sheets are formed by stacked tetrahedral and octahedral sheets in a 1:1 or 2:1 ratio. The tetrahedral layers are formed by Si cations coordinated to O atoms in a hexagonal pattern, while the octahedral layer is formed by the coordination of metal cations with O, OH^-, or F^- of the tetrahedral layer [43]. Phyllosilicates, also known as nanoclays, may exist in a layered or tubular structure.

In 2:1 tetrahedral:octahedral nanoclays, the cationic substitution of aluminum is possible, leading to nanoclays containing magnesium, iron, lithium, and iron. These substitutions lead to a charge unbalance, giving rise to nanoclays with a varying net charge, surface reactivity, cationic exchange capacity, and swelling behaviors [44]. Nanoclays without cationic aluminum substitution (known as prophyllites) exhibit similar properties to 1:1 nanoclays, with low reactivity and low swelling behavior, making them less appropriate for delivery applications. Other 2:1 clay minerals are talc, illites, smectites, chlorites, and vermiculites. Illites and chlorites have low cationic exchange capacity and water retention, limiting their utility for drug delivery [45,46]. In a study by Lima et al., talc was loaded into chitosan-based hydrogels and exhibited high loading capacities and prolonged release of the anti-diuretic amiloride [47]. Interestingly, X-ray diffractograms revealed mostly surface adsorption of the drug as opposed to intercalation. Vermiculite has also been used in hydrogel composite delivery devices to deliver antibacterial compounds due to its relatively high cation exchange capacity [48,49].

Of these 2:1 nanoclays, smectites are the class with high swelling potential, making them the most investigated phyllosilicates for biomedical applications [50]. The various groups of smectites are listed in Table 1. The swelling behaviors of smectites make them attractive for biomedical applications, allowing for electrostatic adsorption of molecules as well as intercalation of molecules into the interlayer space, which is typically made of sodium or calcium ions and water molecules [51,52].

Table 1. Chemical formula and diameter of smectite nanoclays [53–59].

Silicate Nanoclay	Chemical Formula	Cationic Exchange Capacity [meq/g]
Montmorillonite	$(Na,Ca)_{0.33}(Al,Mg)_2(Si_4O_{10})(OH)_2 \cdot nH_2O$	1.2
Hectorite	$Na_{0.3}(Mg,Li)_3(Si_4O_{10})(F,OH)_2$	0.6
Saponite	$Ca_{0.25}(Mg,Fe)_3((Si,Al)_4O_{10})(OH)_2 \cdot nH_2O$	0.1
Nontronite	$Na_{0.3}Fe_2((Si,Al)_4O_{10})(OH)_2 \cdot nH_2O$	0.5
Beidellite	$(Na,Ca_{0.5})_{0.3}Al_2((Si,Al)_4O_{10})(OH)_2 \cdot nH_2O$	0.7
Laponite	$Na_{0.7}Si_8Mg_{5.5}Li_{0.3}O_{20}(OH)_4$	0.5

Of the smectites, montmorillonite is by far the most well-studied nanoclay for delivery applications due to its abundance in nature and high cationic exchange capacity. Montmorillonite has been incorporated into numerous hydrogel systems for the delivery of both small molecules and macromolecules [44,60–63]. Hectorite was used in an alginate hydrogel system developed by Joshi et al. to deliver quinine, a small-molecule antimalarial drug [64]. Similarly, saponite was also used to adsorb and deliver quinine by Kumeresan et al. [65]. Nontronite hydrogel composites have been shown to have variable swelling behavior based on local pH and salinity, offering the potential for release applications [66], but no delivery studies were found in the literature. Chitosan–beidellite composites were fabricated by Cheikh et al. and exhibited sustained release of diclofenac sodium, a model drug [67]. Recently, a burst of interest has been dedicated to studying Laponite for biomedical applications, including drug delivery.

5. Laponite

Laponite is a synthetic hectorite with an octahedral layer consisting of magnesium and lithium cations with a diameter of ~30 nm and a layer thickness of ~1 nm. This high aspect ratio and surface area lends itself to a variety of biomedical applications, as Laponite is known to impart beneficial mechanical properties to hydrogels, such as stiffness and shear-thinning behavior (Figure 1) [68]. Laponite has a dual-charged nature, where particle edges are positively charged due to the charge imbalance caused by magnesium and/or lithium of octahedral aluminum, while the faces (top and bottom surfaces) are negatively charged as a result of the silicate tetrahedral layers. As such, both negatively charged and positively charged molecules may be electrostatically adsorbed to the surface of Laponite particles [7]. Neutral molecules may still interact with Laponite particles if their charge is anisotropically distributed [69]. Additionally, the high swelling behavior of Laponite particles allows for interlayer intercalation of molecules [70]. Thus, the charged nature of Laponite easily lends itself to drug delivery applications in which drug molecules may electrostatically interact with Laponite particles to slow diffusion and subsequent release.

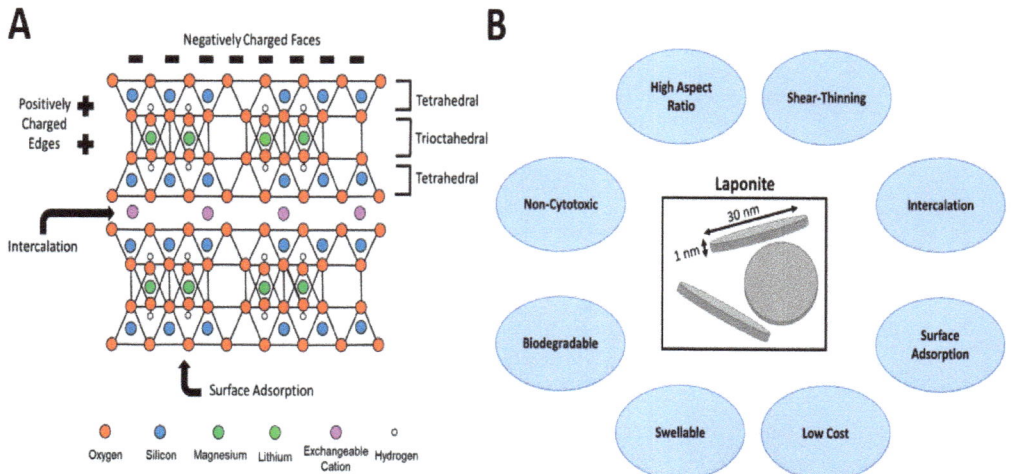

Figure 1. (**A**). Structure of Laponite with 2:1 tetrahedral:trioctahedral layering, allowing for intercalation and adsorption of drug molecules. (**B**). Properties of Laponite particles making them beneficial for use in drug delivery applications.

Laponite has been used for a variety of other applications as well. It has been shown to impart osteogenic and angiogenic potential in the absence of therapeutics [71,72]. The shear-thinning behavior of Laponite makes it attractive for bioprinting applications, as well as injectable biomaterials [4,73,74]. Outside of biomedical applications, Laponite has been used for wastewater treatment and a variety of industrial applications, such as a rheological modifier in cosmetics, cleaning products, and polymer films [75–78].

The synthesis of Laponite and synthetic hectorites has been well established, with a common procedure of crystallizing an aqueous mixture of LiF, $Mg(OH)_2$, and SiO_2 at high temperature [79,80]. Modification of the reactant molar ratios, heating method, and temperature can affect final product purity and size [81]. The review by Zhang et al. provides a deeper dive into how different synthetic hectorite fabrication methods can produce a variety of closely related structures. However, Laponite is typically produced and used commercially, with the brand name Laponite first introduced by Laporte Industries (now BYK) in the early 1960s [82].

6. Degradation and Cytotoxicity of Laponite

Laponite particles naturally dissociate into their constituent ions (Li^+, Mg^+, and $Si(OH)$) in environments where the local pH is less than that of the isoelectric point of Laponite (pH ~10) [83]. It has been hypothesized that in these lower pH environments, H^+ ions react with the nanoclay and leach Mg^+ and Li^+ ions, thereby degrading the nanosilicate particles in about 20–50 days [55,84]. In vivo, Laponite particles are thought to be internalized by clathrin-mediated endocytosis and subsequently degraded within the low pH environment of endosomes (Figure 2) [83,85,86].

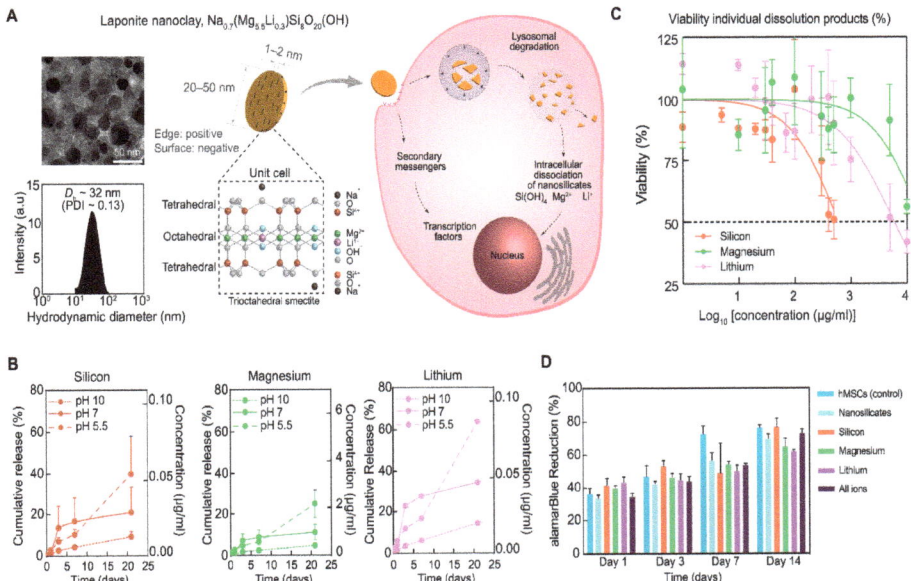

Figure 2. Structure, physiological stability, and cellular compatibility of Laponite. (**A**) Laponite (nanosilicates, nSi) are plate-like poly-ions composed of simple or complex salts of silicic acids with a heterogeneous charge distribution and patchy interactions. Transmission electron microscopy (TEM) images show the size of Laponite to be between 20 and 50 nm in diameter. Dynamic light scattering (DLS) shows the hydrodynamic diameter (D_h) of Laponite to be ~32 nm in aqueous conditions, with a polydispersity index (PDI) of ~0.13. The schematic shows the potential interactions of Laponite with cells. Laponite dissociates into individual ions once introduced to a physiological microenvironment (pH < 9). a.u., arbitrary units. (**B**) The dissolution of Laponite was monitored using inductively coupled plasma mass spectrometry (ICP-MS) at different pH to mimic the extracellular (pH~7.4) and intracellular (pH~5.5) microenvironments. Laponite is expected to be stable at pH~10, and thus, pH 10 was used as control. (**C**) The effect of Laponite and its ionic dissolution products (silicon, magnesium, and lithium) on cellular viability was evaluated using an MTT assay. Three technical replicates were used for each condition. Half-maximal inhibitory concentration (IC50) is labeled at 50% viability. Concentrations of released ions from Laponite fall well below the IC50 value. (**D**) Long-term cellular viability after treatment with nanoparticles and its ionic dissolution products was assessed using an alamarBlue assay to detect metabolically active cells (n = 3). Adapted with permission from Ref. [83]. 2022. Science.

When used for therapeutic delivery applications, the delivery vehicle itself must not induce significant adverse effects. Gaharwar et al. demonstrated individual Laponite particles are non-cytotoxic beneath a critical concentration, with an IC50 of 4 mg/mL Laponite [71]. A study by Veernala et al. claimed an IC50 of 2.2 mg/mL Laponite [87]. Becher et al. showed IC50 values of approximately 0.5–1.5 mg/mL Laponite when incubated with HeLa or MCF-7 cells [88]. Li et al. reported Laponite concentrations of up to 10% w/v (100 mg/mL) showed insignificant changes in the cellular viability of pre-osteoblastic MC3T3-E1 cells [89]. Therefore, the range of IC50 values of Laponite varies rather considerably. The concentration of Laponite in the nanocomposite hydrogel delivery devices discussed in this review varies considerably—from 0.05 to 50 mg/mL. However, encapsulation of Laponite within a hydrogel network may reduce the plasma concentration of Laponite particles as the nanoclays are embedded within the hydrogel structure. Laponite particles have been shown to naturally degrade in ~30 days on average (~20–50 days), so a hydrogel with a residence time of >30 days allows for complete Laponite particles to not escape the hydrogel, thereby preventing adverse cytotoxicity [83].

Hemolysis and coagulation induced by clay particles is yet another consideration for the use of these nanocomposite systems in vivo. Luo et al. demonstrated that the incorporation of Laponite into a Dextran-based hydrogel did not significantly alter hemolysis [90]. Li et al. showed that the incorporation of Laponite into a gelatin hydrogel improved antithrombogenicity and hemocompatibility [91]. Wang et al. demonstrated Laponite particles showed <5% hemolysis, which could be improved by sintering Laponite particles at high heat [92]. Hence, hemolysis and coagulation should not be a major concern for Laponite–hydrogel composites.

7. Laponite–Polymer Composite Hydrogels

Laponite and other nanoclays have been widely shown to improve the mechanical properties of hydrogels when incorporated into the polymer matrix as nanofillers. The nanoclay particles increase the excluded volume within hydrogels, leading to higher stiffness and toughness [93,94]. This toughness can prevent undesired mechanical degradation of hydrogels during or after implantation [95,96]. Furthermore, the addition of Laponite can improve the shear-thinning behavior of hydrogels, which is highly desirable for injectable hydrogel devices where encapsulated drugs and/or cell activity must be preserved during the high shear stress experienced in the injection process [8].

Polymers and Laponite particles may interact with each other in several ways [8]. First, nanoclay particles may persist in their stacked, tactoid structure and be effectively phase-separated from the surrounding polymer if affinity between the two species is low, rarely leading to improved mechanical properties [97,98]. Second, polymer chains may be partially intercalated within the inter-particle space of the nanoclays in a "swollen" or more disordered manner. The extent of these interactions depends on the affinity between the polymer chains and Laponite faces [99,100]. Third, Laponite particles may be fully exfoliated into individual sheets with random orientation, surrounded by polymer chains. It is with this third case that hydrogel mechanical properties may be most improved following the addition of Laponite [98,100,101]. The nature of the Laponite particle dispersion within the hydrogel matrix can lead to changes in encapsulation efficiency and drug release kinetics and is, therefore, an important parameter that must be considered when deciding what fabrication method would be used for nanocomposite hydrogels. For example, when Laponite particles were dispersed and interacted with a model small molecule prior to encapsulation within a polyethylene glycol (PEG)-based hydrogel, release was significantly slower than when Laponite particles were embedded within the hydrogel and then subsequently exposed to the small molecule [102].

Laponite particles may also be used as physical or chemical crosslinkers to form hydrogel structures. The charged nature of Laponite lends itself to weak interactions between its negatively charged faces or positively charged edges and ionizable moieties of polymers through van der Waals forces or hydrogen bonding [103]. Laponite particles may also be chemically modified to form covalent linkages between polymers to act as a primary or secondary crosslinker [104]. A study by Batista et al. revealed Laponite could enhance photopolymerization conversion for a UV-crosslinked polystyrenesulfonate nanocomposite hydrogel [105]. Modulation of Laponite concentration can also be used to tune the Laponite–polymer interactions, allowing for control of nanocomposite hydrogel mechanical properties [106]. Thus, Laponite–hydrogel composites may exist in a variety of structures and crosslinking mechanisms [105].

In addition to forming nanocomposite hydrogel structures with polymers, Laponite particles may self-aggregate into a weak gel above a critical concentration (~20 mg/mL) [107]. Edge-face particle interactions lead to the self-assembly of a "house-of-cards" structure that forms the gel structure [108,109]. These hydrogels are typically much softer than their polymer counterparts and are heavily dependent on local salinity and pH, which can affect their stability [55,110]. Wang et al. demonstrated the loading of the chemotherapeutic doxorubicin into the interlayer space of Laponite particle gels, demonstrating the utility of these nanoclay-only gels for delivery applications [111]. Becher et al. developed Laponite nanogels using inverse mini-emulsion to successfully deliver therapeutics into cancer cells, showing the potential benefits of a Laponite-only nanogel for cellular targeting [88].

8. Laponite–Hydrogel Nanocomposites for Delivery of Small Molecules

Laponite particles have been widely used in recent years as delivery vehicles for a variety of small molecules and macromolecules due to the benefits of adsorption and/or intercalation on release kinetics. Such examples can be found in reviews by Davis et al. and Kiaee et al. [7,112]. This review specifically focuses on hydrogels containing Laponite.

Many examples in the literature describe Laponite–hydrogel composites used for the delivery of small molecules (<1000 Da) (Table 2). The large surface area and charge characteristics of Laponite lend to its effectiveness as a delivery vehicle for small molecules. Surface adsorption onto either the faces or edges of Laponite particles provides a facile way to load drugs and therapeutics into hydrogels for subsequent sustained release [113]. Small molecules may also be intercalated into the interlayer space between Laponite particles via cationic exchange [70,114]. Such intercalation is easily determined as the interlayer spacing increases, as observed via X-ray diffraction [102,115]. Following adsorption and/or intercalation of small molecules onto or into Laponite particles, they may be reversibly released due to local salinity, pH, temperature, or Laponite degradation [116]. For example, increased local salinity can cause a cationic exchange of sodium or calcium ions with the intercalated small molecules, thereby leading to release [117]. Charge shielding may also occur at high salt concentrations, leading to an electrostatic double layer that prevents small molecule adsorption [118].

Table 2. Examples of Laponite–polymer composite hydrogels for the delivery of small molecules (<1000 Da), including the application of the encapsulated molecule, the polymer used for hydrogel fabrication, the small molecule delivered, and whether the study included in vivo experiments.

Application	Polymer	Small Molecule Delivered	In Vivo Studies	References
Anti-Cancer	Alginate	Doxorubicin	Yes	[119,120]
	PEG	Acridine Orange, Doxorubicin, Alexa 546	No	[102,117]
	PPO-PEO	β-Lapachone	No	[121]
	Hyaluronic Acid	Methotrexate	Yes	[122]
	None	Cisplatin, 4-fluorouracil, cyclophosphamide	Yes	[88]
	Hyaluronic Acid	Doxorubicin	No	[123]
Anti-Bacterial	Chitosan	Ofloxacin	No	[124]
	Dextran	Ciprofloxacin	No	[90]
Anti-Inflammatory	Gellan Gum	Theophylline, vitamin B12	No	[125]

A variety of clinically relevant therapeutics have been loaded into Laponite–polymer composite hydrogels. Goncalves et al. described an alginate–Laponite composite hydrogel for the delivery of doxorubicin (Figure 3) [119,120]. Release of the small molecule was significantly slower from nanocomposite hydrogels compared to alginate-only samples, and the release kinetics were contingent on environmental pH. Cancer cells showed reduced viability in the presence of the doxorubicin-loaded nanocomposite hydrogel compared to a bolus drug dose, which was attributed to Laponite particles serving as nanocarriers across the cellular membrane. In another study, β-Lapachone was released from a poly(propylene oxide)-poly(ethylene oxide) (PPO-PEO) block copolymer hydrogel device [121]. The chemotherapeutics' solubility was increased 40-fold in the presence of Laponite and the delivery device demonstrated cytotoxicity towards cancer cells.

These studies, among many others, demonstrate the significantly slowed release of small molecules when interacted with Laponite within composite hydrogels.

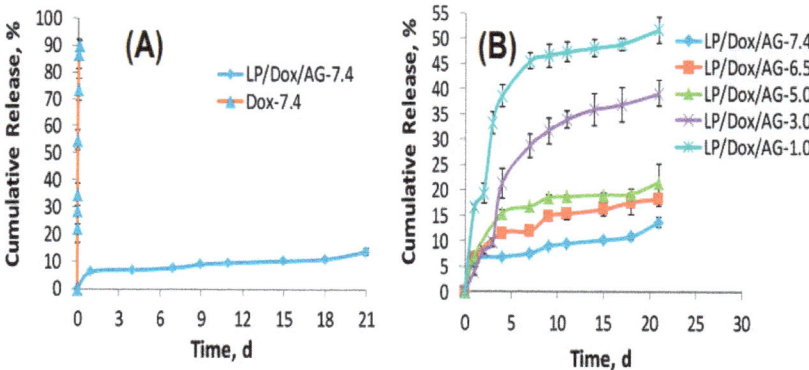

Figure 3. Release of free Doxorubicin (DOX) and DOX from Alginate (AG)/Laponite (LP) nanocomposite hydrogels at pH 7.4 (**A**) and at different pH values in PBS (**B**). Reprinted with permission from Ref. [119]. 2014, Elsevier.

Small-molecule net charge plays a key role in governing release kinetics due to the surface area and charge characteristics of Laponite. Net negative guest molecules are primarily limited to interaction with the edge of Laponite particles, which represents a much smaller surface area than the negatively charged faces of Laponite. Therefore, positively charged molecules (higher pKa) are expected to interact more substantially with Laponite particles. Such trends have been observed in the literature, further corroborating the electrostatic nature of Laponite–small molecule interactions [88,102,117,126].

The use of the Laponite–polymer composite system allows for localized delivery and the opportunity for targeted delivery, which is more difficult to achieve with Laponite particles only. Depending on the geometry and size of the bulk hydrogel, Laponite nanocomposite hydrogels may remain at the desired location longer than when individualized [127], since Laponite particles may be rapidly cleared due to their small size. For example, Jiang et al. developed a hyaluronic acid-based device that allowed for specific targeting of CD44-positive cells, improving the efficacy of doxorubicin delivery [123].

In addition to the response of Laponite–small molecule interactions to local salinity and pH, encapsulation of Laponite particles allows for the complete nanocomposite hydrogel to exhibit stimuli-responsive properties. A dextran-based hydrogel containing Laponite exhibited stimuli-responsiveness to near-infrared stimulation, providing a tuned release of ciprofloxacin [90]. Gharaie et al. developed a pH-responsive gelatin-based hydrogel that incorporated Laponite, providing varying release kinetics of rhodamine B, a model small molecule [128]. Such stimuli-responsive delivery devices allow for another lever by which release can be modulated in addition to Laponite–drug interactions.

9. Laponite Composite Hydrogels for Delivery of Macromolecules

While 2D silicate nanoclays have been widely used for the adsorption and delivery of small molecules, much less research has been devoted to macromolecules such as proteins and nucleic acids. The larger size of these macromolecules may lead to varying interactions with nanoclays compared to small molecules [129]. Proteins have been shown to form relatively large complexes with Laponite, with the size of these complexes being contingent on protein charge and nanoclay concentration [39,69]. Positively charged proteins form larger complexes with Laponite than do negatively charged proteins, which can be attributed to the positively charged proteins having a larger nanoclay surface area on which to bind than the negatively charged proteins, which are primarily limited to adsorption on the relatively small nanoclay edges. However, macromolecules such as proteins may exhibit surface-patch binding onto Laponite particles, in which proteins "bind across their pH" [69]. For example, a positively charged region on an overall negatively charged protein may interact with the Laponite particle face. Therefore, protein and other macromolecules can form complex interactions with Laponite particles and are not limited to face-only or edge-only interactions.

Similarly, Kim et al. adsorbed albumin and lysozyme to Laponite in a hyaluronic acid hydrogel that was physically crosslinked by modified Laponite particles [104]. In this system, Laponite served a dual purpose: Laponite edges served as physical crosslinking sites to interact with the polymer to form a hydrogel; Laponite faces were uninvolved with the polymer to remain available for adsorption of proteins. As expected, negatively charged albumin was released faster than positively charged lysozyme. Importantly, the release was shown in a mouse model, demonstrating in vivo release kinetics and retention of protein bioactivity to induce osteogenic effects. In another example, Koshy et al. demonstrated protein adsorption and sustained release of five clinically relevant proteins with varying sizes and charges from a Laponite-containing alginate click hydrogel [130]. Proteins were incubated with Laponite and then encapsulated within the hydrogel. Burst release was mitigated for all proteins and release kinetics were demonstrated to be contingent on Laponite concentration, allowing for tunable release times. A study by Li et al. utilized an alginate/Laponite nanocomposite hydrogel device in which Laponite particles were complexed with insulin-like growth factor-1 mimetic protein (ILGF-1) and subsequently entrapped within an alginate hydrogel [131]. ILGF-1 release kinetics were dependent on Laponite concentration and showed release up to 4 weeks in a rat model. While these studies demonstrated successful electrostatic interactions between Laponite and protein, as well as slowed release kinetics, there are few studies elaborating the stability and structure of Laponite–protein intermediaries.

In a paper by Stealey et al., Laponite was incubated with three model proteins of varying size and charge (Figure 4) to investigate Laponite–protein interactions. Laponite–protein complex size increased with increasing Laponite concentration due to the increase in surface area available for adsorption. Importantly, the buffer in which Laponite was dispersed played a key role in determining Laponite–protein complex size, with high osmotic buffers triethanolamine and phosphate buffered saline showing little particle exfoliation or Laponite–protein complex formation. Conversely, deionized water allowed for facile exfoliation and interaction with proteins, thereby resulting in large Laponite–protein complexes.

The formation of these nanoclay–protein complexes also showed a significantly slowed release of three model proteins from PEG–nanoclay composite hydrogels in vitro. Positively charged ribonuclease A (RNase) and lysozyme (Lys) were released up to 23 times slower following complexation with Laponite, compared to PEG-only hydrogels. Negatively charged bovine serum albumin (BSA) was also released significantly slower in the PEG–nanosilicate hydrogels, though this effect was less profound than for the positively charged proteins. This can once again be attributed to the formation of smaller Laponite–protein complexes for negatively charged proteins. While this research gave more insight into the formation of Laponite–protein complexes, the stoichiometry, structure, reversibility, and stability of the complexes remain unresolved.

Because of the importance of protein secondary and tertiary structure on bioactivity, protein structure must be preserved following interaction and release from Laponite. Cross et al. demonstrated the binding of human bone morphogenetic protein 2 (rhBMP2) and transforming growth factor-β3 (TGF-β3) with Laponite particles [132]. Proteins exhibited sustained release following adsorption onto Laponite particles in the absence of a polymeric hydrogel. Importantly, osteogenic effects were observed in a 2D cell culture model following the release of proteins, demonstrating that released proteins remained bioactive following interaction with Laponite. In another example of proteins preserving their bioactivity, gelatin methacrylate–Laponite nanocomposite hydrogels were fabricated by Waters et al. that incorporated human mesenchymal stem cell-derived growth factors [133]. Sustained release of vascular endothelial growth factor (VEGF) and fibroblast growth factor 2 (FGF2) was demonstrated in vitro. The secretome-loaded nanocomposite hydrogel demonstrated the potential to enhance angiogenesis and cardio-protection. In another study that demonstrated the utility of Laponite composite hydrogels, Liu et al. developed an alginate/gelatin/Laponite nanocomposite hydrogel system that was shown to be noncytotoxic and could successfully deliver bone marrow mesenchymal stem cells in a critical-size rat bone calvarial defect [134]. The degradation products of Laponite were shown to enhance the osteogenic potential compared to hydrogels without Laponite. The authors suggested that this nanocomposite hydrogel system could also be loaded with drugs to further enhance bone regeneration. Together, these studies show proteins retain at least a portion of their bioactivity following release from Laponite–hydrogel composites and can achieve desired physiological outcomes.

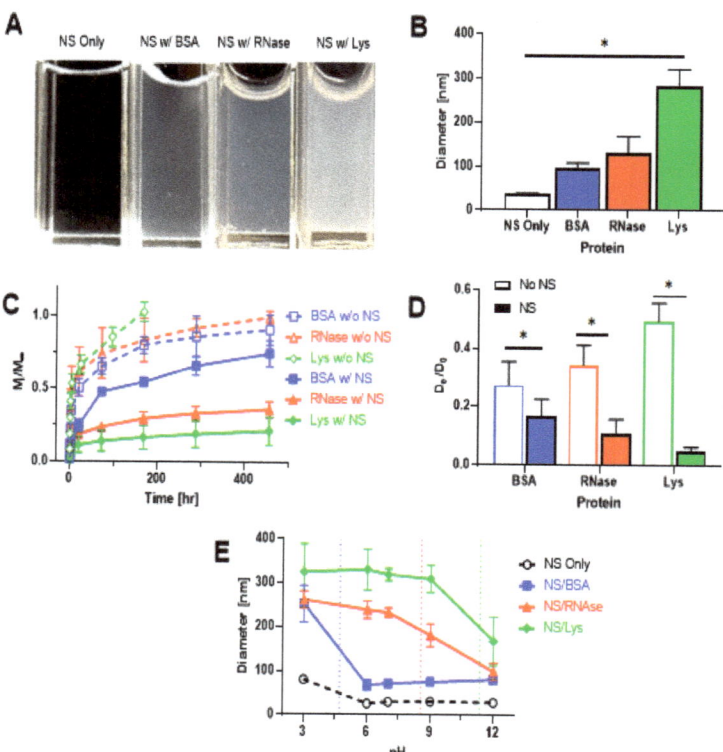

Figure 4. (**A**). Visual observation of complexation of nanosilicates (NS; 10 mg/mL) with Lys, BSA, and RNase (2 mg/mL). (**B**). Diameter of NS only (no protein) and NS–protein complexes measured via dynamic light scattering. NS concentration was 1 mg/mL and protein concentration was 1 mg/mL. * Indicates significant difference (N = 6, $p < 0.05$). (**C**). Release profiles of BSA, RNase, and Lys from PEG-only (dashed lines) and NS–PEG (10 mg/mL NS, solid lines) hydrogels. (**D**). Normalized diffusivity of proteins in PEG-only (No NS) compared to NS–PEG hydrogels. * indicates statistically significant difference (N = 6, $p < 0.05$). (**E**). Diameter of NS only (no protein) and NS–protein complexes as a function of pH. NS (100 µg/mL) and protein (50 µg/mL) were incubated for 30 min before measurements. Vertical dashed lines represent isoelectric points of BSA (blue; pI = 4.7), RNase (red; pI = 8.54), and Lys (green; pI = 11.35). Republished with permission from Ref. [39]. 2021. American Chemical Society.

In a unique hydrogel fabrication method, Dawson et al. fabricated self-assembling Laponite hydrogels for protein delivery [135]. Laponite was added dropwise above a critical Laponite concentration to varying concentrations of NaCl to form microcapsules. These Laponite microcapsules showed sustained release of albumin and lysozyme compared to bolus dose and control alginate hydrogels. VEGF was then loaded into the Laponite microcapsules and demonstrated enhanced angiogenesis in 2D cell culture, thereby demonstrating retention of protein bioactivity following interaction with Laponite particles. A collagen scaffold was then used to subencapsulate the Laponite microcapsules to release VEGF and BMP2 in a rat model, which showed enhanced angiogenesis in vivo. This group further demonstrated these Laponite gel capsules could successfully localize the release of BMP2 to achieve ectopic bone formation in a rat model due to the release and preservation of protein bioactivity [136]. Therefore, Laponite may be used as a gel-forming agent in the absence of polymers, while still achieving sustained release and retained bioactivity.

The surface of Laponite particles may also be modified via interactions with proteins to promote more specific or effective binding of another target protein. Wang et al. designed a blended hydrogel system with heparin and Laponite to deliver fibroblast growth factor 4 (FGF4) for the treatment of spinal cord injury [137]. Heparin was first reacted with FGF4 to form a heparin protein complex, which was then adsorbed onto Laponite particles. The system exhibited sustained release of over 35 days and enhanced the recovery process in a rat model.

Together, these studies reveal the utility of Laponite–hydrogel composites for the delivery of macromolecules where release kinetics are slowed and molecular bioactivity is maintained. However, more research must be conducted to determine the stoichiometry, geometry, and stability of the formed Laponite–protein complexes. Additionally, an understanding of protein activity while adsorbed to Laponite is also desired to determine whether bioactivity is retained throughout the adsorption and subsequent release, or if a temporary (or permanent) unfolding of protein occurs during interaction with Laponite. Without knowledge of the processes that govern the Laponite–protein interactions, the use and tunability of Laponite nanocomposite hydrogels as drug delivery devices may not be fully realized.

10. Potential Challenges and Drawbacks of Laponite Composite Hydrogels

While the incorporation of Laponite within hydrogels offers a plethora of benefits, some challenges may persist that may delay or hinder their clinical use. Because of the prolonged release profiles of drugs afforded by electrostatic interaction with Laponite, release may be too slow for some applications. For example, the use of a Laponite hydrogel composite may not be appropriate for applications where a relatively high drug plasma concentration is needed for only a short time. Laponite may delay delivery of the drug and result in ineffective dosing. Furthermore, Laponite–drug interactions may last longer than the typical degradation time of the hydrogel and or Laponite particle itself. This may result in a pseudo burst release or at least steep increase in release kinetics due to escape and/or degradation of Laponite particles, thereby releasing adsorbed cargo. However, such a secondary burst release does not appear in the literature to our knowledge. Consideration must also be given to optimization of Laponite concentration within hydrogels. While increasing Laponite concentration may lead to slower release kinetics, too high of a Laponite concentration may adversely affect hydrogel mechanical properties due to hinderance of desired crosslinking. When used for protein delivery, Laponite composite hydrogels must not irreversibly denature or unfold proteins, rendering them inactive. Examples in the literature seemingly indicate that released proteins retain their bioactivity, but further characterization and understanding of the Laponite–protein complex structure is necessary. Another potential complication would be the behavior of Laponite–drug complexes in physiological fluids, which are rich with a variety of small molecules and proteins. Understanding how these other molecules affect Laponite–drug interactions and stability is paramount to achieving controllable release profiles [138].

11. Conclusions and Future Directions

Laponite–hydrogel composites offer great potential for use as devices for the delivery of both small molecules and macromolecules because of the unique benefits of the nanocomposite system that cannot be achieved with just a hydrogel or just Laponite. Drugs may be adsorbed or intercalated onto or into Laponite particles, significantly reducing burst release and lengthening the duration of sustained release. For both small molecules and proteins, guest molecule net charge plays a key role in determining release kinetics due to the unique charge and surface area characteristics of Laponite. Release kinetics may also be governed by Laponite concentration and environmental pH and/or salinity. Importantly, release drugs have been shown to retain their bioactivity to achieve desired in vivo responses. In addition to the benefits of controlling release, the incorporation of Laponite particles can positively affect hydrogel mechanical and physical properties, making them even more suitable as injectable delivery devices. Encapsulating Laponite within hydrogels also allows for tunable, localized release, with the nanocomposite hydrogel serving as a depot for drug release.

Going forward, more in-depth research must be conducted on the nature of Laponite–macromolecule complexes to fully harness the power of these nanocomposite hydrogel delivery devices. An understanding of how macromolecules of varying sizes and charges interact with Laponite will allow for enhanced tunability of release profiles for specific applications. Currently, a significant gap in the literature exists in determining the stability, reversibility, and stoichiometry of Laponite–protein complexes. Knowledge of potential protein unfolding or denaturation when adsorbed to Laponite is crucial to ensure effective protein delivery. Furthermore, the delivery of macromolecules other than proteins should be explored, such as that of nucleic acids and immunoglobulins, which each represent their challenges.

In the future, Laponite-based nanocomposite hydrogels are anticipated to have widespread applications in tissue engineering and regenerative medicine. They may be utilized in personalized medicine, enabling patient-specific hydrogels, as well as in the development of smart hydrogels with stimuli-responsive drug release. Integration with bioelectronics and sensors could facilitate real-time monitoring, while bioprinting techniques could allow for the creation of complex tissue constructs. Combination therapies, bioactive coatings for implants, and integration with AI for predictive modeling are also potential advancements. Additionally, these nanocomposite hydrogels show promise in additive biomanufacturing, particularly in extrusion-based bioprinting, where the inclusion of Laponite enables shear-thinning behavior. Therapeutics can be incorporated into printed structures to guide cellular functions, allowing for the creation of heterogeneous tissue architectures. This approach has the potential to revolutionize drug testing and accelerate the clinical translation of therapeutics.

As more hydrogel–Laponite composite delivery devices emerge, we will obtain a better knowledge of how the devices perform in vivo and interact with cells and blood in physiological environments. While Laponite-containing devices have shown great promise so far, we must be able to translate the beneficial release kinetics in a physiological environment where numerous other molecules will compete for interactions with Laponite particles.

Author Contributions: S.T.S., A.K.G. and S.P.Z. all contributed to the writing, editing, and proofing of the manuscript. All authors have read and agreed to the published version of the manuscript.

Funding: This research was funded by the Institute for Drug and Biotherapeutic Innovation seed grant, Saint Louis University awarded to S.P.Z. and Parks College of Engineering, Aviation, and Technology Graduate Assistantship awarded to S.T.S.

Institutional Review Board Statement: Not applicable.

Informed Consent Statement: Not applicable.

Data Availability Statement: No new data were created or analyzed in this study. Data sharing is not applicable to this article.

Conflicts of Interest: The authors declare no conflict of interest.

References

1. Vigata, M.; Meinert, C.; Hutmacher, D.W.; Bock, N. Hydrogels as Drug Delivery Systems: A Review of Current Characterization and Evaluation Techniques. *Pharmaceutics* **2020**, *12*, 1188. [CrossRef] [PubMed]
2. Li, J.; Mooney, D.J. Designing hydrogels for controlled drug delivery. *Nat. Rev. Mater.* **2016**, *1*, 16071. [CrossRef] [PubMed]
3. Mitchell, M.J.; Billingsley, M.M.; Haley, R.M.; Wechsler, M.E.; Peppas, N.A.; Langer, R. Engineering precision nanoparticles for drug delivery. *Nat. Rev. Drug Discov.* **2021**, *20*, 101–124. [CrossRef]
4. Chimene, D.; Miller, L.; Cross, L.M.; Jaiswal, M.K.; Singh, I.; Gaharwar, A.K. Nanoengineered Osteoinductive Bioink for 3D Bioprinting Bone Tissue. *ACS Appl. Mater. Interfaces* **2020**, *12*, 15976–15988. [CrossRef] [PubMed]
5. Gaharwar, A.K.; Cross, L.M.; Peak, C.W.; Gold, K.; Carrow, J.K.; Brokesh, A.; Singh, K.A. 2D Nanoclay for Biomedical Applications: Regenerative Medicine, Therapeutic Delivery, and Additive Manufacturing. *Adv. Mater.* **2019**, *31*, 1900332. [CrossRef]
6. Jansson, M.; Belić, D.; Forsman, J.; Skepö, M. Nanoplatelet interactions in the presence of multivalent ions: The effect of overcharging and stability. *J. Colloid Interface Sci.* **2020**, *579*, 573–581. [CrossRef]
7. Davis, R.; Urbanowski, R.A.; Gaharwar, A.K. 2D layered nanomaterials for therapeutics delivery. *Curr. Opin. Biomed. Eng.* **2021**, *20*, 100319. [CrossRef]
8. Samimi Gharaie, S.; Dabiri, S.M.H.; Akbari, M. Smart Shear-Thinning Hydrogels as Injectable Drug Delivery Systems. *Polymers* **2018**, *10*, 1317. [CrossRef]
9. U.S. Food & Drug Administration. Obsidio 510(k) Approval Letter. June 2022. Available online: https://www.accessdata.fda.gov/cdrh_docs/pdf21/K213385.pdf (accessed on 5 May 2023).
10. Ghassemi, Z.; Ruesing, S.; Leach, J.B.; Zustiak, S.P. Stability of proteins encapsulated in Michael-type addition polyethylene glycol hydrogels. *Biotechnol. Bioeng.* **2021**, *118*, 4840–4853. [CrossRef]
11. Raza, F.; Zafar, H.; Zhu, Y.; Ren, Y.; Ullah, A.; Khan, A.U.; He, X.; Han, H.; Aquib, M.; Boakye-Yiadom, K.O.; et al. A Review on Recent Advances in Stabilizing Peptides/Proteins upon Fabrication in Hydrogels from Biodegradable Polymers. *Pharmaceutics* **2018**, *10*, 16. [CrossRef]
12. Zustiak, S.P.; Leach, J.B. Hydrolytically Degradable Poly(Ethylene Glycol) Hydrogel Scaffolds with Tunable Degradation and Mechanical Properties. *Biomacromolecules* **2010**, *11*, 1348–1357. [CrossRef] [PubMed]
13. Chen, W.; Zhou, Z.; Chen, D.; Li, Y.; Zhang, Q.; Su, J. Bone Regeneration Using MMP-Cleavable Peptides-Based Hydrogels. *Gels* **2021**, *7*, 199. [CrossRef] [PubMed]
14. Wang, Y.; Xi, L.; Zhang, B.; Zhu, Q.; Su, F.; Jelonek, K.; Orchel, A.; Kasperczyk, J.; Li, S. Bioresorbable hydrogels prepared by photo-initiated crosslinking of diacrylated PTMC-PEG-PTMC triblock copolymers as potential carrier of antitumor drugs. *Saudi Pharm. J.* **2020**, *28*, 290–299. [CrossRef] [PubMed]
15. Axpe, E.; Chan, D.; Offeddu, G.S.; Chang, Y.; Merida, D.; Hernandez, H.L.; Appel, E.A. A Multiscale Model for Solute Diffusion in Hydrogels. *Macromolecules* **2019**, *52*, 6889–6897. [CrossRef]
16. Peppas, N.A.; Keys, K.B.; Torres-Lugo, M.; Lowman, A.M. Poly(ethylene glycol)-containing hydrogels in drug delivery. *J. Control. Release* **1999**, *62*, 81–87. [CrossRef] [PubMed]
17. Huang, X.; Brazel, C.S. On the importance and mechanisms of burst release in matrix-controlled drug delivery systems. *J. Control. Release* **2001**, *73*, 121–136. [CrossRef]
18. Bhattacharjee, S. Understanding the burst release phenomenon: Toward designing effective nanoparticulate drug-delivery systems. *Ther. Deliv.* **2021**, *12*, 21–36. [CrossRef]
19. Hu, B.; Gao, M.; Boakye-Yiadom, K.O.; Ho, W.; Yu, W.; Xu, X.; Zhang, X.Q. An intrinsically bioactive hydrogel with on-demand drug release behaviors for diabetic wound healing. *Bioact. Mater.* **2021**, *6*, 4592–4606. [CrossRef]
20. Adepu, S.; Ramakrishna, S. Controlled Drug Delivery Systems: Current Status and Future Directions. *Molecules* **2021**, *26*, 5905. [CrossRef]
21. Cam, M.E.; Yildiz, S.; Alenezi, H.; Cesur, S.; Ozcan, G.S.; Erdemir, G.; Edirisinghe, U.; Akakin, D.; Kuruca, D.S.; Kabasakal, L.; et al. Evaluation of burst release and sustained release of pioglitazone-loaded fibrous mats on diabetic wound healing: An in vitro and in vivo comparison study. *J. R. Soc. Interface* **2020**, *17*, 20190712. [CrossRef]
22. Brandl, F.; Hammer, N.; Blunk, T.; Tessmar, J.; Goepferich, A. Biodegradable hydrogels for time-controlled release of tethered peptides or proteins. *Biomacromolecules* **2010**, *11*, 496–504. [CrossRef] [PubMed]
23. Rajkumar, M.; Sakthivel, M.; Senthilkumar, K.; Thangaraj, R.; Kannan, S. Galantamine tethered hydrogel as a novel therapeutic target for streptozotocin-induced Alzheimer's disease in Wistar rats. *Curr. Res. Pharmacol. Drug Discov.* **2022**, *3*, 100100. [CrossRef] [PubMed]
24. Correa, S.; Grosskopf, A.K.; Lopez Hernandez, H.; Chan, D.; Yu, A.C.; Stapleton, L.M.; Appel, E.A. Translational Applications of Hydrogels. *Chem. Rev.* **2021**, *121*, 11385–11457. [CrossRef] [PubMed]
25. Sood, N.; Bhardwaj, A.; Mehta, S.; Mehta, A. Stimuli-responsive hydrogels in drug delivery and tissue engineering. *Drug Deliv.* **2016**, *23*, 748–770. [CrossRef] [PubMed]

26. Rizwan, M.; Yahya, R.; Hassan, A.; Yar, M.; Azzahari, A.D.; Selvanathan, V.; Sonsudin, F.; Abouloula, C.N. pH Sensitive Hydrogels in Drug Delivery: Brief History, Properties, Swelling, and Release Mechanism, Material Selection and Applications. *Polymers* **2017**, *9*, 137. [CrossRef] [PubMed]
27. HaqAsif, A.; Karnakar, R.R.; Sreeharsha, N.; Gite, V.V.; Borane, N.; Al-Dhubiab, B.E.; Kaliyadan, F.; Rasool, T.; Nanjappa, S.H.; Meravanige, G. pH and Salt Responsive Hydrogel based on Guar Gum as a Renewable Material for Delivery of Curcumin: A Natural Anti-Cancer Drug. *J. Polym. Environ.* **2021**, *29*, 1978–1989. [CrossRef]
28. Huang, H.; Qi, X.; Chen, Y.; Wu, Z. Thermo-sensitive hydrogels for delivering biotherapeutic molecules: A review. *Saudi Pharm. J.* **2019**, *27*, 990–999. [CrossRef]
29. Li, Z.; Zhou, Y.; Li, T.; Zhang, J.; Tian, H. Stimuli-responsive hydrogels: Fabrication and biomedical applications. *VIEW* **2022**, *3*, 20200112. [CrossRef]
30. Baig, N.; Kammakakam, I.; Falath, W. Nanomaterials: A review of synthesis methods, properties, recent progress, and challenges. *Mater. Adv.* **2021**, *2*, 1821–1871. [CrossRef]
31. Gao, W.; Zhang, Y.; Zhang, Q.; Zhang, L. Nanoparticle-Hydrogel: A Hybrid Biomaterial System for Localized Drug Delivery. *Ann. Biomed. Eng.* **2016**, *44*, 2049–2061. [CrossRef]
32. Ko, W.-K.; Lee, S.J.; Kim, S.J.; Han, G.H.; Han, I.-B.; Hong, J.B.; Sheen, S.H.; Sohn, S. Direct Injection of Hydrogels Embedding Gold Nanoparticles for Local Therapy after Spinal Cord Injury. *Biomacromolecules* **2021**, *22*, 2887–2901. [CrossRef]
33. Pangli, H.; Vatanpour, S.; Hortamani, S.; Jalili, R.; Ghahary, A. Incorporation of Silver Nanoparticles in Hydrogel Matrices for Controlling Wound Infection. *J. Burn Care Res.* **2021**, *42*, 785–793. [CrossRef] [PubMed]
34. Merino, S.; Martín, C.; Kostarelos, K.; Prato, M.; Vázquez, E. Nanocomposite Hydrogels: 3D Polymer–Nanoparticle Synergies for On-Demand Drug Delivery. *ACS Nano* **2015**, *9*, 4686–4697. [CrossRef] [PubMed]
35. Jøraholmen, M.W.; Johannessen, M.; Gravningen, K.; Puolakkainen, M.; Acharya, G.; Basnet, P.; Škalko-Basnet, N. Liposomes-In-Hydrogel Delivery System Enhances the Potential of Resveratrol in Combating Vaginal Chlamydia Infection. *Pharmaceutics* **2020**, *12*, 1203. [CrossRef] [PubMed]
36. Li, D.; An, X.; Mu, Y. A liposomal hydrogel with enzyme triggered release for infected wound. *Chem. Phys. Lipids* **2019**, *223*, 104783. [CrossRef]
37. Gerstenberg, M.; Stürzel, C.M.; Weil, T.; Kirchhoff, F.; Lindén, M. Modular Hydrogel–Mesoporous Silica Nanoparticle Constructs for Therapy and Diagnostics. *Adv. NanoBiomed Res.* **2022**, *2*, 2100125. [CrossRef]
38. Hu, Y.; Dong, X.; Ke, L.; Zhang, S.; Zhao, D.; Chen, H.; Xiao, X. Polysaccharides/mesoporous silica nanoparticles hybrid composite hydrogel beads for sustained drug delivery. *J. Mater. Sci.* **2017**, *52*, 3095–3109. [CrossRef]
39. Stealey, S.T.; Gaharwar, A.K.; Pozzi, N.; Zustiak, S.P. Development of Nanosilicate–Hydrogel Composites for Sustained Delivery of Charged Biopharmaceutics. *ACS Appl. Mater. Interfaces* **2021**, *13*, 27880–27894. [CrossRef]
40. Giri, A.; Ghosh, T.; Panda, A.B.; Pal, S.; Bandyopdhyay, A. Tailoring carboxymethyl guargum hydrogel with nanosilica for sustained transdermal release of diclofenac sodium. *Carbohydr. Polym.* **2012**, *87*, 1532–1538. [CrossRef]
41. Zhang, S.; Guo, Y.; Dong, Y.; Wu, Y.; Cheng, L.; Wang, Y.; Xing, M.; Yuan, Q. A novel nanosilver/nanosilica hydrogel for bone regeneration in infected bone defects. *ACS Appl. Mater. Interfaces* **2016**, *8*, 13242–13250. [CrossRef]
42. Constantinescu, F.; Boiu Sicuia, O.A. Chapter 13—Phytonanotechnology and plant protection. In *Phytonanotechnology*; Thajuddin, N., Mathew, S., Eds.; Elsevier: Amsterdam, The Netherlands, 2020; pp. 245–287. [CrossRef]
43. García-Villén, F.; Ruiz-Alonso, S.; Lafuente-Merchan, M.; Gallego, I.; Sainz-Ramos, M.; Saenz-Del-Burgo, L.; Pedraz, J.L. Clay Minerals as Bioink Ingredients for 3D Printing and 3D Bioprinting: Application in Tissue Engineering and Regenerative Medicine. *Pharmaceutics* **2021**, *13*, 1806. [CrossRef]
44. Tipa, C.; Cidade, M.T.; Borges, J.P.; Costa, L.C.; Silva, J.C.; Soares, P.I.P. Clay-Based Nanocomposite Hydrogels for Biomedical Applications: A Review. *Nanomaterials* **2022**, *12*, 3308. [CrossRef] [PubMed]
45. Hughes, R.E.; DeMaris, P.J.; White, W.A.; Cowin, D.K.; Schultz, L.G.; Olphen, H.v.; Mumpton, F.A. Origin of Clay Minerals in Pennsylvanian Strata of the Illinois Basin. In *Proceedings of the International Clay Conference, Denver, 1985*; Clay Minerals Society: Chantilly, VA, USA, 1985. [CrossRef]
46. Khatoon, N.; Chu, M.Q.; Zhou, C.H. Nanoclay-based drug delivery systems and their therapeutic potentials. *J. Mater. Chem. B* **2020**, *8*, 7335–7351. [CrossRef] [PubMed]
47. Lima, L.C.B.; Coelho, C.C.; Silva, F.C.; Meneguin, A.B.; Barud, H.S.; Bezerra, R.D.S.; Viseras, C.; Osajima, J.A.; Silva-Filho, E.C. Hybrid Systems Based on Talc and Chitosan for Controlled Drug Release. *Materials* **2019**, *12*, 3634. [CrossRef] [PubMed]
48. Soleimanpour Moghadam, N.; Azadmehr, A.; Hezarkhani, A. Improving the 6-Aminopenicillanic acid release process using vermiculite-alginate biocomposite bead on drug delivery system. *Drug. Dev. Ind. Pharm.* **2021**, *47*, 1489–1501. [CrossRef]
49. Hundáková, M.; Tokarský, J.; Valášková, M.; Slobodian, P.; Pazdziora, E.; Kimmer, D. Structure and antibacterial properties of polyethylene/organo-vermiculite composites. *Solid State Sci.* **2015**, *48*, 197–204. [CrossRef]
50. Neeraj, K.; Chandra, M. Basics of Clay Minerals and Their Characteristic Properties. In *Clay and Clay Minerals*; Do Nascimento, G.M., Ed.; IntechOpen: Rijeka, Croatia, 2021; Chapter 2. [CrossRef]
51. Ghadiri, M.; Chrzanowski, W.; Rohanizadeh, R. Biomedical applications of cationic clay minerals. *RSC Adv.* **2015**, *5*, 29467–29481. [CrossRef]
52. Viseras, C.; Cerezo, P.; Sanchez, R.; Salcedo, I.; Aguzzi, C. Current challenges in clay minerals for drug delivery. *Appl. Clay Sci.* **2010**, *48*, 291–295. [CrossRef]

53. Smectite Group. *Mindat.org*. Available online: https://www.mindat.org/min-11119.html (accessed on 8 February 2023).
54. Delavernhe, L.; Pilavtepe, M.; Emmerich, K. Cation exchange capacity of natural and synthetic hectorite. *Appl. Clay Sci.* **2018**, *151*, 175–180. [CrossRef]
55. Jatav, S.; Joshi, Y.M. Chemical stability of Laponite in aqueous media. *Appl. Clay Sci.* **2014**, *97–98*, 72–77. [CrossRef]
56. Zeyen, N.; Wang, B.; Wilson, S.A.; Paulo, C.; Stubbs, A.R.; Power, I.M.; Steele-Maclnnis, M.; Lanzirotti, A.; Newville, M.; Paterson, D.J.; et al. Cation Exchange in Smectites as a New Approach to Mineral Carbonation. *Front. Clim.* **2022**, *4*, 913632. [CrossRef]
57. Yu, B.-S.; Hung, W.-H.; Fang, J.-N.; Yu, Y.-T. Synthesis of Zn-Saponite Using a Microwave Circulating Reflux Method under Atmospheric Pressure. *Minerals* **2020**, *10*, 45. [CrossRef]
58. Kapoor, B.S. Acid character of nontronite: Permanent and pH-dependent charge components of cation exchange capacity. *Clay Miner.* **1972**, *9*, 425–433. [CrossRef]
59. Belhanafi, H.; Bakhti, A.; Benderdouche, N. Study of interactions between rhodamine B and a beidellite-rich clay fraction. *Clay Miner.* **2020**, *55*, 194–202. [CrossRef]
60. Jayrajsinh, S.; Shankar, G.; Agrawal, Y.K.; Bakre, L. Montmorillonite nanoclay as a multifaceted drug-delivery carrier: A review. *J. Drug Deliv. Sci. Technol.* **2017**, *39*, 200–209. [CrossRef]
61. Kouser, R.; Vashist, A.; Zafaryab, M.; Rizvi, M.A.; Ahmad, S. Na-Montmorillonite-Dispersed Sustainable Polymer Nanocomposite Hydrogel Films for Anticancer Drug Delivery. *ACS Omega* **2018**, *3*, 15809–15820. [CrossRef]
62. Sharifzadeh, G.; Hezaveh, H.; Muhamad, I.I.; Hashim, S.; Khairuddin, N. Montmorillonite-based polyacrylamide hydrogel rings for controlled vaginal drug delivery. *Mater. Sci. Eng. C* **2020**, *110*, 110609. [CrossRef]
63. Park, J.H.; Shin, H.J.; Kim, M.H.; Kim, J.S.; Kang, N.; Lee, J.Y.; Kim, K.T.; Lee, J.I.; Kim, D.D. Application of montmorillonite in bentonite as a pharmaceutical excipient in drug delivery systems. *J. Pharm. Investig.* **2016**, *46*, 363–375. [CrossRef]
64. Joshi, G.V.; Pawar, R.R.; Kevadiya, B.D.; Bajaj, H.C. Mesoporous synthetic hectorites: A versatile layered host with drug delivery application. *Microporous Mesoporous Mater.* **2011**, *142*, 542–548. [CrossRef]
65. Kumaresan, S.; Pawar, R.R.; Kevadiya, B.D.; Bajaj, H.C. Synthesis of Saponite Based Nanocomposites to Improve the Controlled Oral Drug Release of Model Drug Quinine Hydrochloride Dihydrate. *Pharmaceuticals* **2019**, *12*, 105. [CrossRef]
66. Rodrigues, F.H.A.; Pereira, A.G.B.; Fajardo, A.R.; Muniz, E.C. Synthesis and characterization of chitosan-graft-poly(acrylic acid)/nontronite hydrogel composites based on a design of experiments. *J. Appl. Polym. Sci.* **2013**, *128*, 3480–3489. [CrossRef]
67. Cheikh, D.; García-Villén, F.; Majdoub, M.; Viseras, C.; Zayani, M.B. Chitosan/beidellite nanocomposite as diclofenac carrier. *Int. J. Biol. Macromol.* **2019**, *126*, 44–53. [CrossRef]
68. Das, S.S.; Neelam; Hussain, K.; Singh, S.; Hussain, A.; Faruk, A.; Tebyetekerwa, M. Laponite-based Nanomaterials for Biomedical Applications: A Review. *Curr. Pharm. Des.* **2019**, *25*, 424–443. [CrossRef] [PubMed]
69. Das, K.; Rawat, K.; Bohidar, H.B. Surface patch binding induced interaction of anisotropic nanoclays with globular plasma proteins. *RSC Adv.* **2016**, *6*, 104117–104125. [CrossRef]
70. Jiang, W.-T.; Tsai, Y.; Wang, X.; Tangen, H.J.; Baker, J.; Allen, L.; Li, Z. Sorption of Acridine Orange on Non-Swelling and Swelling Clay Minerals. *Crystals* **2022**, *12*, 118. [CrossRef]
71. Gaharwar, A.K.; Mihaila, S.M.; Swami, A.; Patel, A.; Sant, S.; Reis, R.L.; Marques, A.P.; Gomes, M.E.; Khademhosseini, A. Bioactive Silicate Nanoplatelets for Osteogenic Differentiation of Human Mesenchymal Stem Cells. *Adv. Mater.* **2013**, *25*, 3329–3336. [CrossRef]
72. Cidonio, G.; Alcala-Orozco, C.R.; Lim, K.S.; Glinka, M.; Mutreja, I.; Kim, Y.H.; Dawson, J.I.; Woodfield, T.B.F.; Oreffo, R.O.C. Osteogenic and angiogenic tissue formation in high fidelity nanocomposite Laponite-gelatin bioinks. *Biofabrication* **2019**, *11*, 035027. [CrossRef]
73. Afghah, F.; Altunbek, M.; Dikyol, C.; Koc, B. Preparation and characterization of nanoclay-hydrogel composite support-bath for bioprinting of complex structures. *Sci. Rep.* **2020**, *10*, 5257. [CrossRef]
74. Rajput, S.; Deo, K.A.; Mathur, T.; Lokhande, G.; Singh, K.A.; Sun, Y.; Alge, D.L.; Jain, A.; Sarkar, T.R.; Gaharwar, A.K. 2D Nanosilicate for additive manufacturing: Rheological modifier, sacrificial ink and support bath. *Bioprinting* **2022**, *25*, e00187. [CrossRef]
75. Prasannan, A.; Udomsin, J.; Tsai, H.-C.; Wang, C.-F.; Lai, J.-Y. Robust underwater superoleophobic membranes with bio-inspired carrageenan/laponite multilayers for the effective removal of emulsions, metal ions, and organic dyes from wastewater. *Chem. Eng. J.* **2020**, *391*, 123585. [CrossRef]
76. Lull, M.A.; Howell, A.L.; Novack, C.D. *Laponite Clay in Cosmetic and Personal Care Products*; Avon Products Inc.: New York, NY, USA, 2015.
77. Bott, J.; Franz, R. Investigation into the Potential Migration of Nanoparticles from Laponite-Polymer Nanocomposites. *Nanomaterials* **2018**, *8*, 723. [CrossRef] [PubMed]
78. Lee, W.P.; Martinez, A.; Xu, D.; Brooker, A.; York, D.W.; Ding, Y. Effects of laponite and silica nanoparticles on the cleaning performance of amylase towards starch soils. *Particuology* **2009**, *7*, 459–465. [CrossRef]
79. Zhang, J.; Zhou, C.H.; Petit, S.; Zhang, H. Hectorite: Synthesis, modification, assembly and applications. *Appl. Clay Sci.* **2019**, *177*, 114–138. [CrossRef]
80. Decarreau, A.; Vigier, N.; Pálková, H.; Petit, S.; Vieillard, P.; Fontaine, C. Partitioning of lithium between smectite and solution: An experimental approach. *Geochim. Cosmochim. Acta* **2012**, *85*, 314–325. [CrossRef]

81. Vicente, I.; Salagre, P.; Cesteros, Y.; Guirado, F.; Medina, F.; Sueiras, J.E. Fast microwave synthesis of hectorite. *Appl. Clay Sci.* **2009**, *43*, 103–107. [CrossRef]
82. Shafran, K.; Jeans, C.; Kemp, S.J.; Murphy, K. Dr Barbara S. Neumann: Clay scientist and industrial pioneer; creator of Laponite®. *Clay Miner.* **2020**, *55*, 256–260. [CrossRef]
83. Brokesh, A.M.; Cross, L.M.; Kersey, A.L.; Murali, A.; Richter, C.; Gregory, C.A.; Singh, I.; Gaharwar, A.K. Dissociation of nanosilicates induces downstream endochondral differentiation gene expression program. *Sci. Adv.* **2022**, *8*, eabl9404. [CrossRef]
84. Mohanty, R.P.; Joshi, Y.M. Chemical stability phase diagram of aqueous Laponite dispersions. *Appl. Clay Sci.* **2016**, *119*, 243–248. [CrossRef]
85. Carrow, J.K.; Cross, L.M.; Reese, R.W.; Jaiswal, M.K.; Gregory, C.A.; Kaunas, R.; Singh, I.; Gaharwar, A.K. Widespread changes in transcriptome profile of human mesenchymal stem cells induced by two-dimensional nanosilicates. *Proc. Natl. Acad. Sci. USA* **2018**, *115*, e3905–e3913. [CrossRef]
86. Iturrioz-Rodríguez, N.; Martín-Rodríguez, R.; Renero-Lecuna, C.; Aguado, F.; González-Legarreta, L.; González, J.; Fanarraga, M.L.; Perdigón, A.C. Free-labeled nanoclay intracellular uptake tracking by confocal Raman imaging. *Appl. Surf. Sci.* **2021**, *537*, 147870. [CrossRef]
87. Veernala, I.; Giri, J.; Pradhan, A.; Polley, P.; Singh, R.; Yadava, S.K. Effect of Fluoride Doping in Laponite Nanoplatelets on Osteogenic Differentiation of Human Dental Follicle Stem Cells (hDFSCs). *Sci. Rep.* **2019**, *9*, 915. [CrossRef] [PubMed]
88. Becher, T.B.; Mendonça, M.C.P.; de Farias, M.A.; Portugal, R.V.; de Jesus, M.B.; Ornelas, C. Soft Nanohydrogels Based on Laponite Nanodiscs: A Versatile Drug Delivery Platform for Theranostics and Drug Cocktails. *ACS Appl. Mater. Interfaces* **2018**, *10*, 21891–21900. [CrossRef] [PubMed]
89. Li, J.; Tian, Z.; Yang, H.; Duan, L.; Liu, Y. Infiltration of laponite: An effective approach to improve the mechanical properties and thermostability of collagen hydrogel. *J. Appl. Polym. Sci.* **2023**, *140*, e53366. [CrossRef]
90. Luo, J.; Ma, Z.; Yang, F.; Wu, T.; Wen, S.; Zhang, J.; Huang, L.; Deng, S.; Tan, S. Fabrication of Laponite-Reinforced Dextran-Based Hydrogels for NIR-Responsive Controlled Drug Release. *ACS Biomater. Sci. Eng.* **2022**, *8*, 1554–1565. [CrossRef] [PubMed]
91. Li, C.; Mu, C.; Lin, W.; Ngai, T. Gelatin Effects on the Physicochemical and Hemocompatible Properties of Gelatin/PAAm/Laponite Nanocomposite Hydrogels. *ACS Appl. Mater. Interfaces* **2015**, *7*, 18732–18741. [CrossRef]
92. Wang, S.; Wang, S.; Li, K.; Ju, Y.; Li, J.; Zhang, Y.; Li, J.; Liu, X.; Shi, X.; Zhao, Q. Preparation of laponite bioceramics for potential bone tissue engineering applications. *PLoS ONE* **2014**, *9*, e99585. [CrossRef]
93. Wu, C.-J.; Gaharwar, A.K.; Chan, B.K.; Schmidt, G. Mechanically Tough Pluronic F127/Laponite Nanocomposite Hydrogels from Covalently and Physically Cross-Linked Networks. *Macromolecules* **2011**, *44*, 8215–8224. [CrossRef]
94. Lee, J.H.; Han, W.J.; Jang, H.S.; Choi, H.J. Highly Tough, Biocompatible, and Magneto-Responsive Fe_3O_4/Laponite/PDMAAm Nanocomposite Hydrogels. *Sci. Rep.* **2019**, *9*, 15024. [CrossRef]
95. Chen, Y.; Kang, S.; Yu, J.; Wang, Y.; Zhu, J.; Hu, Z. Tough robust dual responsive nanocomposite hydrogel as controlled drug delivery carrier of asprin. *J. Mech. Behav. Biomed. Mater.* **2019**, *92*, 179–187. [CrossRef]
96. Balavigneswaran, C.K.; Jaiswal, S.; Venkatesan, R.; Karuppiah, P.S.; Sundaram, M.K.; Vasudha, T.K.; Aadinath, W.; Ravikumar, A.; Saravanan, H.V.; Muthuvijayan, V. Mussel-Inspired Adhesive Hydrogels Based on Laponite-Confined Dopamine Polymerization as a Transdermal Patch. *Biomacromolecules* **2023**, *24*, 724–738. [CrossRef]
97. Babu Valapa, R.; Loganathan, S.; Pugazhenthi, G.; Thomas, S.; Varghese, T.O. Chapter 2—An Overview of Polymer–Clay Nanocomposites. In *Clay-Polymer Nanocomposites*; Jlassi, K., Chehimi, M.M., Thomas, S., Eds.; Elsevier: Amsterdam, The Netherlands, 2017; pp. 29–81. [CrossRef]
98. Raquez, J.-M.; Habibi, Y.; Murariu, M.; Dubois, P. Polylactide (PLA)-based nanocomposites. *Prog. Polym. Sci.* **2013**, *38*, 1504–1542. [CrossRef]
99. Persenaire, O.; Raquez, J.-M.; Bonnaud, L.; Dubois, P. Tailoring of Co-Continuous Polymer Blend Morphology: Joint Action of Nanoclays and Compatibilizers. *Macromol. Chem. Phys.* **2010**, *211*, 1433–1440. [CrossRef]
100. Chen, B.; Evans, J.R.G.; Greenwell, H.C.; Boulet, P.; Coveney, P.V.; Bowden, A.A.; Whiting, A. A critical appraisal of polymer–clay nanocomposites. *Chem. Soc. Rev.* **2008**, *37*, 568–594. [CrossRef]
101. Tolle, T.B.; Anderson, D.P. Morphology development in layered silicate thermoset nanocomposites. *Compos. Sci. Technol.* **2002**, *62*, 1033–1041. [CrossRef]
102. Tsai, T.-Y.; Lu, S.-T.; Li, C.-H.; Huang, C.-J.; Liu, J.-X.; Chen, L.-C. Effect of bifunctional modifiers of the clay on the morphology of novolac cured epoxy resin/clay nanocomposites. *Polym. Compos.* **2008**, *29*, 1098–1105. [CrossRef]
103. Stealey, S.; Khachani, M.; Zustiak, S.P. Adsorption and Sustained Delivery of Small Molecules from Nanosilicate Hydrogel Composites. *Pharmaceuticals* **2022**, *15*, 56. [CrossRef]
104. Xie, F.; Boyer, C.; Gaborit, V.; Rouillon, T.; Guicheux, J.; Tassin, J.F.; Geoffroy, V.; Réthoré, G.; Weiss, P. A Cellulose/Laponite Interpenetrated Polymer Network (IPN) Hydrogel: Controllable Double-Network Structure with High Modulus. *Polymers* **2018**, *10*, 634. [CrossRef]
105. Kim, Y.-H.; Yang, X.; Shi, L.; Lanham, S.A.; Hilborn, J.; Oreffo, R.O.C.; Ossipov, D.; Dawson, J.I. Bisphosphonate nanoclay edge-site interactions facilitate hydrogel self-assembly and sustained growth factor localization. *Nat. Commun.* **2020**, *11*, 1365. [CrossRef]
106. Batista, T.; Chiorcea-Paquim, A.-M.; Brett, A.M.O.; Schmitt, C.C.; Neumann, M.G. Laponite RD/polystyrenesulfonate nanocomposites obtained by photopolymerization. *Appl. Clay Sci.* **2011**, *53*, 27–32. [CrossRef]

107. Sällström, N.; Capel, A.; Lewis, M.P.; Engstrøm, D.S.; Martin, S. 3D-printable zwitterionic nano-composite hydrogel system for biomedical applications. *J. Tissue Eng.* **2020**, *11*, 2041731420967294. [CrossRef]
108. Mourchid, A.; Lécolier, E.; Van Damme, H.; Levitz, P. On viscoelastic, birefringent, and swelling properties of laponite clay suspensions: Revisited phase diagram. *Langmuir* **1998**, *14*, 4718–4723. [CrossRef]
109. Au, P.-I.; Hassan, S.; Liu, J.; Leong, Y.-K. Behaviour of LAPONITE® gels: Rheology, ageing, pH effect and phase state in the presence of dispersant. *Chem. Eng. Res. Des.* **2015**, *101*, 65–73. [CrossRef]
110. Afewerki, S.; Magalhães, L.S.S.M.; Silva, A.D.R.; Stocco, T.D.; Silva Filho, E.C.; Marciano, F.R.; Lobo, A.O. Bioprinting a Synthetic Smectic Clay for Orthopedic Applications. *Adv. Healthc. Mater.* **2019**, *8*, 1900158. [CrossRef] [PubMed]
111. Suman, K.; Joshi, Y.M. Microstructure and Soft Glassy Dynamics of an Aqueous Laponite Dispersion. *Langmuir* **2018**, *34*, 13079–13103. [CrossRef] [PubMed]
112. Wang, S.; Wu, Y.; Guo, R.; Huang, Y.; Wen, S.; Shen, M.; Wang, J.; Shi, X. Laponite Nanodisks as an Efficient Platform for Doxorubicin Delivery to Cancer Cells. *Langmuir* **2013**, *29*, 5030–5036. [CrossRef] [PubMed]
113. Kiaee, G.; Dimitrakakis, N.; Sharifzadeh, S.; Kim, H.-J.; Avery, R.K.; Moghaddam, K.M.; Haghniaz, R.; Yalcintas, E.P.; Barros, N.R.d.; Karamikamkar, S.; et al. Laponite-Based Nanomaterials for Drug Delivery. *Adv. Healthc. Mater.* **2022**, *11*, 2102054. [CrossRef]
114. Ghadiri, M.; Chrzanowski, W.; Lee, W.H.; Rohanizadeh, R. Layered silicate clay functionalized with amino acids: Wound healing application. *RSC Adv.* **2014**, *4*, 35332–35343. [CrossRef]
115. Lv, G.; Li, Z.; Jiang, W.-T.; Chang, P.-H.; Jean, J.-S.; Lin, K.-H. Mechanism of acridine orange removal from water by low-charge swelling clays. *Chem. Eng. J.* **2011**, *174*, 603–611. [CrossRef]
116. Adeyemo, A.A.; Adeoye, I.O.; Bello, O.S. Adsorption of dyes using different types of clay: A review. *Appl. Water Sci.* **2017**, *7*, 543–568. [CrossRef]
117. Xiao, S.; Castro, R.; Maciel, D.; Gonçalves, M.; Shi, X.; Rodrigues, J.; Tomás, H. Fine tuning of the pH-sensitivity of laponite-doxorubicin nanohybrids by polyelectrolyte multilayer coating. *Mater. Sci. Eng. C Mater. Biol. Appl.* **2016**, *60*, 348–356. [CrossRef]
118. Khachani, M.; Stealey, S.; Dharmesh, E.; Kader, M.S.; Buckner, S.W.; Jelliss, P.A.; Zustiak, S.P. Silicate Clay-Hydrogel Nanoscale Composites for Sustained Delivery of Small Molecules. *ACS Appl. Nano Mater.* **2022**, *5*, 18940–18954. [CrossRef]
119. Sheikhi, A.; Afewerki, S.; Oklu, R.; Gaharwar, A.K.; Khademhosseini, A. Effect of ionic strength on shear-thinning nanoclay–polymer composite hydrogels. *Biomater. Sci.* **2018**, *6*, 2073–2083. [CrossRef] [PubMed]
120. Gonçalves, M.; Figueira, P.; Maciel, D.; Rodrigues, J.; Qu, X.; Liu, C.; Tomás, H.; Li, Y. pH-sensitive Laponite®/doxorubicin/alginate nanohybrids with improved anticancer efficacy. *Acta Biomater.* **2014**, *10*, 300–307. [CrossRef] [PubMed]
121. Gonçalves, M.; Figueira, P.; Maciel, D.; Rodrigues, J.; Shi, X.; Tomás, H.; Li, Y. Antitumor Efficacy of Doxorubicin-Loaded Laponite/Alginate Hybrid Hydrogels. *Macromol. Biosci.* **2014**, *14*, 110–120. [CrossRef] [PubMed]
122. Câmara, G.B.M.; Barbosa, R.d.M.; García-Villén, F.; Viseras, C.; Almeida Júnior, R.F.d.; Machado, P.R.L.; Câmara, C.A.; Farias, K.J.S.; de Lima e Moura, T.F.A.; Dreiss, C.A.; et al. Nanocomposite gels of poloxamine and Laponite for β-Lapachone release in anticancer therapy. *Eur. J. Pharm. Sci.* **2021**, *163*, 105861. [CrossRef]
123. Li, J.; Yang, Y.; Yu, Y.; Li, Q.; Tan, G.; Wang, Y.; Liu, W.; Pan, W. LAPONITE® nanoplatform functionalized with histidine modified oligomeric hyaluronic acid as an effective vehicle for the anticancer drug methotrexate. *J. Mater. Chem. B* **2018**, *6*, 5011–5020. [CrossRef]
124. Jiang, T.; Chen, G.; Shi, X.; Guo, R. Hyaluronic Acid-Decorated Laponite® Nanocomposites for Targeted Anticancer Drug Delivery. *Polymers* **2019**, *11*, 137. [CrossRef] [PubMed]
125. Yang, H.; Hua, S.; Wang, W.; Wang, A. Composite hydrogel beads based on chitosan and laponite: Preparation, swelling, and drug release behaviour. *Iran. Polym. J.* **2011**, *20*, 479–490.
126. Adrover, A.; Paolicelli, P.; Petralito, S.; Di Muzio, L.; Trilli, J.; Cesa, S.; Tho, I.; Casadei, M.A. Gellan Gum/Laponite Beads for the Modified Release of Drugs: Experimental and Modeling Study of Gastrointestinal Release. *Pharmaceutics* **2019**, *11*, 187. [CrossRef]
127. Dharmesh, E.; Stealey, S.; Salazar, M.A.; Elbert, D.; Zustiak, S.P. Nanosilicate-hydrogel microspheres formed by aqueous two-phase separation for sustained release of small molecules. *Front. Biomater. Sci.* **2023**, *2*, 1157554. [CrossRef]
128. Petit, L.; Barentin, C.; Colombani, J.; Ybert, C.; Bocquet, L. Size Dependence of Tracer Diffusion in a Laponite Colloidal Gel. *Langmuir* **2009**, *25*, 12048–12055. [CrossRef] [PubMed]
129. Jaber, M.; Lambert, J.-F.; Balme, S. 8—Protein adsorption on clay minerals. In *Developments in Clay Science*; Schoonheydt, R., Johnston, C.T., Bergaya, F., Eds.; Elsevier: Amsterdam, The Netherlands, 2018; Volume 9, pp. 255–288.
130. Koshy, S.T.; Zhang, D.K.Y.; Grolman, J.M.; Stafford, A.G.; Mooney, D.J. Injectable nanocomposite cryogels for versatile protein drug delivery. *Acta Biomater.* **2018**, *65*, 36–43. [CrossRef] [PubMed]
131. Li, J.; Weber, E.; Guth-Gundel, S.; Schuleit, M.; Kuttler, A.; Halleux, C.; Accart, N.; Doelemeyer, A.; Basler, A.; Tigani, B.; et al. Tough Composite Hydrogels with High Loading and Local Release of Biological Drugs. *Adv. Healthc. Mater.* **2018**, *7*, 1701393. [CrossRef]
132. Cross, L.M.; Carrow, J.K.; Ding, X.; Singh, K.A.; Gaharwar, A.K. Sustained and Prolonged Delivery of Protein Therapeutics from Two-Dimensional Nanosilicates. *ACS Appl Mater Interfaces* **2019**, *11*, 6741–6750. [CrossRef]
133. Waters, R.; Pacelli, S.; Maloney, R.; Medhi, I.; Ahmed, R.P.H.; Paul, A. Stem cell secretome-rich nanoclay hydrogel: A dual action therapy for cardiovascular regeneration. *Nanoscale* **2016**, *8*, 7371–7376. [CrossRef]

134. Liu, B.; Li, J.; Lei, X.; Miao, S.; Zhang, S.; Cheng, P.; Song, Y.; Wu, H.; Gao, Y.; Bi, L.; et al. Cell-loaded injectable gelatin/alginate/LAPONITE® nanocomposite hydrogel promotes bone healing in a critical-size rat calvarial defect model. *RSC Adv.* **2020**, *10*, 25652–25661. [CrossRef] [PubMed]
135. Dawson, J.I.; Kanczler, J.M.; Yang, X.B.; Attard, G.S.; Oreffo, R.O. Clay gels for the delivery of regenerative microenvironments. *Adv. Mater.* **2011**, *23*, 3304–3308. [CrossRef] [PubMed]
136. Gibbs, D.M.; Black, C.R.; Hulsart-Billstrom, G.; Shi, P.; Scarpa, E.; Oreffo, R.O.; Dawson, J.I. Bone induction at physiological doses of BMP through localization by clay nanoparticle gels. *Biomaterials* **2016**, *99*, 16–23. [CrossRef]
137. Wang, C.; Gong, Z.; Huang, X.; Wang, J.; Xia, K.; Ying, L.; Shu, J.; Yu, C.; Zhou, X.; Li, F.; et al. An injectable heparin-Laponite hydrogel bridge FGF4 for spinal cord injury by stabilizing microtubule and improving mitochondrial function. *Theranostics* **2019**, *9*, 7016–7032. [CrossRef]
138. Shi, P.; Kim, Y.-H.; Mousa, M.; Sanchez, R.R.; Oreffo, R.O.C.; Dawson, J.I. Self-Assembling Nanoclay Diffusion Gels for Bioactive Osteogenic Microenvironments. *Adv. Healthc. Mater.* **2018**, *7*, 1800331. [CrossRef]

Disclaimer/Publisher's Note: The statements, opinions and data contained in all publications are solely those of the individual author(s) and contributor(s) and not of MDPI and/or the editor(s). MDPI and/or the editor(s) disclaim responsibility for any injury to people or property resulting from any ideas, methods, instructions or products referred to in the content.

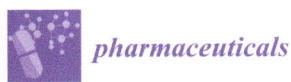

Review

Patient-Centric Design of Topical Dermatological Medicines

Rita Oliveira [1,2,3] and Isabel F. Almeida [2,3,*]

[1] FP-BHS—Biomedical and Health Sciences Research Unit, FFP-I3ID—Instituto de Investigação, Inovação e Desenvolvimento, Faculdade de Ciências da Saúde, Universidade Fernando Pessoa, Rua Carlos da Maia 296, 4200-150 Porto, Portugal; ritao@ufp.edu.pt

[2] UCIBIO—Applied Molecular Biosciences Unit, MedTech, Laboratory of Pharmaceutical Technology, Department of Drug Sciences, Faculty of Pharmacy, University of Porto, Rua Jorge Viterbo de Ferreira 228, 4050-313 Porto, Portugal

[3] Associate Laboratory i4HB—Institute for Health and Bioeconomy, Faculty of Pharmacy, University of Porto, Rua Jorge Viterbo de Ferreira 228, 4050-313 Porto, Portugal

* Correspondence: ifalmeida@ff.up.pt

Abstract: Topical treatments are essential approaches to skin diseases but are associated with poor adherence. Topical vehicles have the primary purpose of ensuring drug effectiveness (by modulating drug stability and delivery, as well as skin properties) but have a marked impact on treatment outcomes as they influence patient satisfaction and, consequently, adherence to topical treatments. There is also a wide variety of vehicles available for topical formulations, which can complicate the decisions of clinicians regarding the most appropriate treatments for specific skin disorders. One of the possible strategies to improve topical-treatment adherence is the implementation of patient-centric drug-product design. In this process, the patient's needs (e.g., those related to motor impairment), the needs associated with the disease (according to the skin lesions' characteristics), and the patient's preferences are taken into consideration and translated into a target product profile (TPP). Herein, an overview of topical vehicles and their properties is presented, along with a discussion of the patient-centric design of topical dermatological medicines and the proposal of TPPs for some of the most common skin diseases.

Keywords: patient-centric; drug-product design; topical medicines; adherence; vehicles

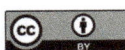

Citation: Oliveira, R.; Almeida, I.F. Patient-Centric Design of Topical Dermatological Medicines. *Pharmaceuticals* 2023, 16, 617. https://doi.org/10.3390/ph16040617

Academic Editors: Silviya Petrova Zustiak and Era Jain

Received: 2 March 2023
Revised: 10 April 2023
Accepted: 13 April 2023
Published: 19 April 2023

Copyright: © 2023 by the authors. Licensee MDPI, Basel, Switzerland. This article is an open access article distributed under the terms and conditions of the Creative Commons Attribution (CC BY) license (https://creativecommons.org/licenses/by/4.0/).

1. Introduction

Non-adherence to treatment is universally recognized as a public health problem. Non-adherence leads to suboptimal health outcomes, lower quality of life, and higher healthcare costs [1]. Poor adherence has been reported for several dermatological conditions [2–5]. The World Health Organization (WHO) recommends that the determinants of non-adherence are classified into five main dimensions: socioeconomic factors, health-care and system-related factors, therapy-related factors, condition-related factors, and patient-related factors. Topical treatments are widely used in dermatology and are the most commonly used therapeutic approaches [6]. However, several reports suggested low satisfaction with topical treatments. For instance, patients with psoriasis consider topical therapy to be one of the most negative aspects of the disease. Their satisfaction is significantly lower with this treatment compared to systemic treatments [7]. The rates of adherence to topical treatments are relatively low (50–70%) and have been related to poor cosmetic acceptability [8–10]. Satisfaction with topical treatment seems to be a key determinant of adherence [11], and this is the rationale for prioritizing these formulations for inclusion in patient-centric drug-product-design processes, thus contributing to the maximization of adherence. Iversen et al. suggested that the improvement of the vehicles through which topical treatments are applied has the potential to result in significant clinical and patient benefits [12]. Despite technological advances, commercial drug products and clinical prescriptions of compounding formulations are focused on a reduced number of vehicles.

This review aims to address a variety of topical vehicles, the process of patient-centric topical dermatological medicines' design, and its relevance in dermatological treatments.

2. Vehicles/Bases Used in Topical Dermatological Treatments

Vehicles are mixtures of excipients that carry the drug to the administration site. Although the term vehicle is commonly used for any dosage form, according to the European Pharmacopoeia, it refers only to liquid formulations, while for semisolid dosage forms, the official designation is base [13].

Topical vehicles/bases, i.e., products intended for application on the skin, scalp, or nails, include solutions, emulsions, suspensions, ointments, creams, pastes, gels, foams, sticks, and powders. They are designed to be inert and cosmetically acceptable, and most have emollient and moisturizing properties. Creams and ointments are the commonly most used bases in the treatment of skin disorders [10,14].

Liquid vehicles include solutions, suspensions, and emulsions, with variable viscosity (Table 1) [15,16], and when they are applied topically, they are also known as lotions. Solutions are defined as liquid formulations, in which a solute (or solutes) is (or are) dispersed in a solvent at the molecular level. Solutions can be applied in several anatomic areas, such as the body skin, scalp, or nails. Shampoos are liquid preparations that are composed of a surfactant dispersion, suitable for scalp application.

Table 1. Characteristics of liquid vehicles [15,16].

Vehicle	Composition	Characteristics	Examples
Solutions	Solute (or solutes) dissolved in a liquid solvent such as water, alcohol, glycols, or oil	Clear and transparent	Urea aqueous solution
Suspensions	Insoluble powders dispersed in a liquid phase	Translucent or opaque; with time, the suspended solids tend to settle	Aqueous zinc suspension
Emulsions	Homogeneous two-phase liquid systems of water, liquid oils, and emulsifying agents	Opaque and homogeneous	Lanette lotion

Suspensions are liquid formulations in which insoluble solid particles are dispersed. Usually, the particles tend to settle, and agitation before use is required.

Emulsions are homogeneous two-phase liquid systems, obtained from the dispersion of immiscible liquids, wherein the internal phase is dispersed in droplets in the outer phase. Depending on the composition of the internal and external phases, they are classified as W/O emulsions (with oil as the outer and continuous phase) or O/W emulsions (with water as the outer and continuous phase). The water- and oil-phase components and the emulsifying system determine the type of emulsion and its occlusive properties. When they are semisolid, they are called creams.

Semisolid bases allow drug retention at the application site and are usually easily spread on the skin; most have lubricating and emollient properties. They consist of different types of bases that vary according to consistency and hydrophilicity/lipophilicity, namely, hydrophobic, absorption, emulsions, hydrophilic, hydrogels, pastes, and foams (Table 2) [15,16].

Table 2. Characteristics of semisolid bases [15,16].

Base	Composition	Characteristics	Examples
Hydrophobic	Solid and liquid paraffin, petrolatum, waxes, triglycerides, vegetable oils, silicone oils	Emollients, occlusive, greasy, and difficult to remove; high retention on the skin; form an occlusive layer that prevents water loss; rapid delivery of hydrophilic drugs; very low water absorption (<5%)	Coal-tar-paraffin ointment
Absorption	Water-absorbent components: lanolin; lanolin alcohols; cholesterol; bees wax; emulsifying agents	Emollient, occlusive, and greasy, albeit less than hydrophobic bases; make emulsions by adding water;	Hydrophilic ointment (USP) or Cetylic ointment (PPh)
Water-in-oil (W/O) cream	Water, hydrocarbons, waxes, polyethylene glycols, and emulsifying agents	Water-in-oil two-phase system; occlusive properties; when applied to the skin, they leave an oily film on the surface of the skin	Cold cream (USP) Cooling ointment (FNA)
Oil-in-water (O/W) cream	Water, hydrocarbons, waxes, polyethylene glycols, and emulsifying agents	Oil-in-water two-phase system; non-occlusive; non-greasy; moisturizing and emollient effect	Lanette cream (BP)
Anhydrous hydrophilic	PEGs of different molecular weights	Non-occlusive, non-oily, and easily removable; exudate miscibility but hyperosmotic miscible; low water absorption	Macrogol ointment
Hydrogels	Organic macromolecules or polymers dispersed in water: natural (xanthan gum, alginate); semi-synthetics (cellulose derivatives); synthetics (carbomer)	Transparent aqueous formulations with no grease; easy to apply and remove; refreshing properties; little moisturizing or emollient effect; may contain alcohol, so they are likely to cause irritation and have drying ability; the aqueous medium is susceptible to degradation	Carbomer gel Carboxymethylcellulose gel
Oleogels	Organic macromolecules or polymers dispersed in a lipophilic oil	Moisturizing or emollient effect; leave an oily film on the surface of the skin	12-hydroxystearic acid Oleogel
Pastes	Insoluble drug in an ointment or a hydrophilic base	High content of insoluble powders; protective effect; drying effect; varied consistency and solubility	Zinc-oxide paste Darier paste
Foams	Nonpolar hydrocarbons as propellants; Solvents include water, oils, ethanol, acetone, hexadecyl alcohol, glycol ethers, and polyglycols	Pressurized solutions or fluid emulsions mixed with a propellant; no need to spread the product and quick-drying; low skin residue low hydration or occlusive effect	Coal-tar foam (Scytera®)

USP, United States Pharmacopoeia; PPh, Portuguese Pharmacopoeia; PEG, Polyoxyethylene glycol; FNA, Nederland Formulary (Formularium der Nederlandse Apothekers); BP, British Pharmacopoeia.

Ointments are one-phase preparations that comprise hydrophobic, absorption (or water-emulsifying), and anhydrous hydrophilic bases, with the common property of low water miscibility and an occlusive effect that varies with their composition. They have high viscosity and low spreadability, and are difficult to wash off. Furthermore, W/O creams are made of a lipophilic outer phase that incorporates water with the presence of W/O-type emulsifying agents. They are emollient and slightly occlusive, and their greasiness depends on the amount of oil phase (20–50%), which allows good absorption of liposoluble drugs, such as corticosteroids, retinoids, and hormones. Additionally, O/W creams are composed of an external water phase and O/W-type emulsifying agents. They are non-occlusive and non-oily, easily applied, and removable (from the skin and hair). Based on the type of surfactant, they can be divided into anionic and nonionic emulsions. Anionic emulsions are reproducible and stable but can be also irritants due to their components (e.g., sodium lauryl sulfate), and they may present some incompatibilities with the drugs incorporated. Four classic emulsions, presented in ascending order of fat content, are Lanette lotion, Beeler base cream, Lanette base cream, and hydrophilic ointment. Nonionic emulsions are suitable for sensitive skin, since they are composed of non-irritating emulgents with low fat contents and, therefore, exert milder effects on the skin.

Emerging emulsified vehicles/bases tend to be more compatible with the skin and less aggressive than the more frequently prescribed anionic emulsions/creams. Thus, the aims of current emulsions are to reduce of the number of ingredients, ensure the high quality and purity of ingredients, avoid irritating or photosensitizing substances, perfumes, and colorants, reduce the amount of preservatives, and ensure compatibility with the physiological pH of the skin. Glycoside emulsions/creams have a low fat content and include non-ionic and non-ethoxylated emulsifying agents that are compatible with the skin, such as sugar-based emulsifying agents (esters of glucose or sucrose; polyglyceryl stearates), which are better-tolerated [17]. They present very good organoleptic properties and they are moisturizing, fluid, and suitable for facial areas and sensitive or reactive skin [18]. Cream gels or emulgels also have very good skin tolerance, as they are composed mainly of water, a low-fat phase, and well-tolerated polymers (such as polyacrylate polymers) [19]. Water-in-silicon emulsions/creams have an outer phase composed of silicones instead of fats. They form a water-repellent film with no oily residue, present good cosmetic properties, and constitute non-comedogenic oil-free emulsions [20,21].

Gels are usually composed of a matrix of colloidal organic polymers that entrap the solvent (if they are water-based, they are called hydrogels) and drug. Inorganic polymers can also originate hydrogels with a semisolid consistency. Oleogels can be obtained through the jellification of liquid oils with a bivalent soap or another organogelator. Recently, several new organogelators were studied [22–24].

Pastes contain large amounts of insoluble powders in hydrophobic bases (the most common) or hydrophilic bases. Both present drying and absorbent effects.

Foams are liquids or semisolids in special pressurized packages with a propellant hydrocarbon, delivering the product through an actuated valve. They are easy to use on all skin surfaces without spreading and, in general, leave no residue on the skin. Continuous innovations have taken place in foam technology, which has moved from hydroethanolic-based formulations to aqueous or emulsion-based foams [25,26].

Solid vehicles are probably the least commonly used vehicles in topical applications. Powders are dry and fine solids and are frequently used for their drying and astringent effects [15,16]. Solid sticks are prepared by molding and can have different compositions, such as hydrophobic (a combination of waxes and oils), high-molecular-weight PEGs, or soaps (sodium stearate). All solid sticks have the advantage of high drug stability and sliding application of the drug.

Several authors have classified topical vehicles/bases according to their ingredients and properties [27–31] but, in general, they do not relate them to skin disorders or patient preferences. A patient-centric approach is crucial for obtaining maximum therapeutic effectiveness and is further discussed in the context of dermatological medicines.

3. Patient-Centric Topical-Medicine Design

Regulatory authorities are increasingly placing patients at the center of pharmaceutical development. The European Medicines Agency (EMA, Amsterdam, Netherlands) has issued guideline/reflection papers for pediatric [32,33] and older populations [34], while the United States Food and Drug Administration (FDA, Silver Spring, MD, USA) has developed a series of guidance documents on patient-focused drug development, with the primary goal of incorporating the patient's voice in drug development and evaluation [35], as well as other research [36–38]. The International Council for Harmonization of Technical Requirements for Pharmaceuticals for Human Use (ICH, Geneva, Switzerland) also published a guideline to advance patient-focused drug development [39]. Patient-centric drug-product design (PCDPD, Wanchai, Hong Kong) can be defined as the process of identifying the comprehensive needs of individuals or target patient populations and utilizing the identified needs to design pharmaceutical drug products that provide the best overall benefit-to-risk profile for specific target patient populations for the intended duration of treatment [40]. Patient-centric drug-product design is a stepwise approach (Figure 1) that starts with the evaluation of patient preferences and needs to obtain the necessary patient input to define the target product profile (TPP) [41,42]. It has been applied to the design of oral pediatric formulations [43], solid dosage forms [44,45], and medications for the elderly, as well as topical formulations, such as an emulgel for psoriasis [46]. Although PCDPD can be applied at any stage of the drug-development lifecycle, this paper focuses on the definition of TPP for topical formulations. Since topical medicines are often associated with poor satisfaction, they are an obvious choice for the application of the PCDPD process. Target product profiles are defined according to insights into patients, drugs, and drug products collected with questionnaires or based on scientific research. The drug product is then designed, prepared, and characterized concerning relevant features from the patient's perspective. At this point, the matching of its features to the TPP is evaluated and reformulation takes place, if necessary. After obtaining the optimized formulations, the translation into a higher level of patient satisfaction with the topical treatment in comparison with standard treatment should be verified in a sample population (Figure 1). The putative advantages include the satisfaction of unmet needs and higher satisfaction with treatment, which in turn encourages better medication adherence and therapeutic outcomes [41].

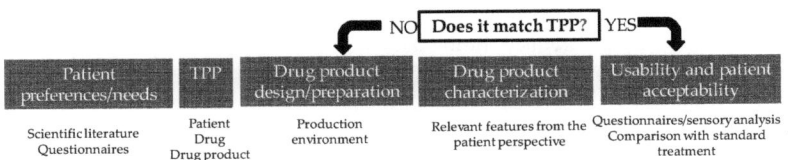

Figure 1. Patient-centric drug-product-design stepwise approach.

In a PCDPD approach, the patient's perspective can be included in product development at various stages, such as defining outcomes in clinical evaluation by establishing the most significant symptoms, the tolerability of adverse effects, risk–benefit assessment, or preferences for improving acceptability and adherence [39]. Even in the early development phases, communication between multiple stakeholders during the product development chain would help to meet patients' needs, improving their quality of life [47].

When describing a drug product and its attributes for pharmaceutical development, several dimensions must be taken into account to obtain a medicine that complies with quality, efficacy, and safety requirements. The definition and prioritization of critical attributes are performed through risk management, establishing the greatest impact on the final product. The acceptability and usability assessment of the product is the main key to patient-centric drug-design approaches. Stegemann et al. developed a roadmap to achieve the TPP, which can be further integrated into the Quality-by-Design process during the development phase, re-formulation, or other life-cycle phases of the drug product [48].

Providing a TPP suitable for some groups of skin disorders, adverse effects, adherence, usability, and acceptability represent the patient's preferences and needs, which may also affect the course of the disease.

3.1. Patient Preferences and Needs Regarding Topical Medicines

3.1.1. Patient- and Disease-Related Needs in Dermatology

The selection of vehicles/bases for dermatological treatments should consider the type of skin lesion. Very dry lesions are lichenified (with thickening, darkening, pleating of the skin) and xerotic. They require very occlusive vehicles to soften the skin. Dry lesions (with scaling) represent a large proportion of skin pathologies and also require occlusive vehicles, reducing the fat content, especially in the face and capillary zones. Subacute lesions present intermediate characteristics between those of dry and wet lesions: scaling, excoriations, and crusts. Vehicles/bases should be emollient but not overly occlusive to reduce macerated skin. Wet lesions present erythema and edema, but are not exudative. In these cases, vehicles/bases should not be occlusive, in order to avoid edema (with low or no fat content). Furthermore, W/O emulsions are recommended for wet and interdigital lesions and pastes present drying effect. For exudative lesions, drying vehicles/bases are used (often containing antiseptics) and when they stop exuding, they are treated as wet lesions. Solutions or hydrogels are the vehicles of choice [31].

The anatomic site determines the skin properties, namely the thickness, and vehicles need to be customized [30]. The palmoplantar region presents thicker skin, while facial and pleated areas are more permeable and, therefore, need different fat contents. Glabrous areas, such as the trunk and limbs (when little hair-bearing) are considered intermediate in terms of thickness. For nail pathologies, nail varnishes allow the easy application and high retention of drugs. For hairy sites, the vehicles should facilitate the application and removal of the product with reduced consistency and lipophilicity. The most common vehicles are hydroalcoholic solutions, shampoos, hydrogels, and light and volatile oils. In hyperkeratotic lesions with crust formation (as in psoriasis or seborrheic dermatitis) due to the dry effects of solutions and when emulsions are not easily applied to the scalp, heavy-oily solutions are applied overnight. In skin conditions, such as ichthyosis, psoriasis, and atopic dermatitis, in which the epidermal barrier is damaged, excessive friction should be avoided during the application of topical treatments. Topical preparations in these cases should present specific attributes, such as ease of spread, and high pressure should not be applied during their application [49].

Table 3 summarizes the recommended vehicles/bases according to anatomic site.

Table 3. Vehicle/base selection according to the type of lesion and body area.

	Palmoplantar	Glabrous	Hairy	Facial or Intertrigital
Very dry	Hydrophobic ointments Absorption ointments	Hydrophobic ointments Absorption ointments W/O emulsions	Oil solutions W/O emulsions	W/O emulsions O/W emulsions W/S emulsions
Dry	Hydrophobic ointments Absorption ointments W/O emulsions	Absorption ointments W/O emulsions O/W emulsions	Oil solutions O/W emulsions	W/O emulsions O/W emulsions W/S emulsions
Subacute	Hydrophobic ointments W/O emulsions O/W emulsions	W/O emulsions O/W emulsions Hydrophobic pastes	Oil solutions Shampoos	W/O emulsions O/W emulsions W/S emulsions
Wet	W/O emulsions O/W emulsions	O/W emulsions	O/W emulsions Hydrogels Aqueous solutions	O/W emulsions Hydrogels Hydrophilic pastes
Exudative	Hydrogels Aqueous solutions Hydrophilic pastes	Hydrogels Aqueous solutions Hydrophilic pastes	Hydrogels Aqueous solutions	Hydrogels Aqueous solutions Hydrophilic pastes

W/O, water-in-oil; O/W, oil-in-water; W/S, water-in-silicone.

Furthermore, it is important to take into account the skin type during vehicle/base selection for facial application. Facial skin and sensitive areas are critical, especially when facing prolonged topical treatment. Dry skin needs some occlusion to increase hydration, while oily skin needs the opposite. For sensitive or reactive skin, it is important to select non-irritant excipients, such as non-ionic emulsifiers, and a more inert composition, such as cream gels or glycoside emulsions. Table 4 suggests some vehicles that can be chosen, especially for facial skin.

Table 4. Vehicle selection according to the facial-skin type.

Dry Skin	Oily Skin	Combination Skin	Sensitive Skin
W/O cream	O/W cream (<30% F.C.)	O/W cream (<30% F.C.)	O/W cream (>50% F.C.)
O/W cream (>50% F.C.)	W/S cream	W/S cream	Oils
	Emulgel	Glycoside cream	Glycoside cream
	Hydrogel		Emulgel

W/O, water-in-oil; O/W, oil-in-water; W/S, water-in-silicone; F.C., fat content.

Ultimately, the purpose of a topical vehicle/base is to carry and deliver a drug, contribute to its stability, retain the substance at the site of action, and facilitate its skin permeation. However, regarding skin disorders, the vehicle can play a role that is complementary to that of the drug [50] and contribute to the therapy by modulating the skin's water content [51–53], improving the lipid–skin barrier [54,55], or regenerating skin cells [56]. Van Zuuren et al. conducted a systematic review of five randomized clinical trials to assess the effects of moisturizers on eczema and found that the moisturizing effect produced better results when added to the drug than a placebo vehicle or no moisturizer [57]. The use of enriched topical vehicles with non-drug substances to improve the skin barrier can improve dermatitis and decrease the use of corticosteroids [58]. Hydrophilic bases and cleansing lotions showed a better tolerance to benzoyl peroxide formulations by reducing skin irritation [59,60]. The positive effect of the vehicle/base on skin-disorder treatment still needs to be further explored.

In addition to their skin condition, the needs of the patient must also be accounted for when prescribing the treatment regimen. When patients present with impairments in motoric function (e.g., rheumatoid arthritis), the ability to open closure systems, squeeze tubes, rub formulations onto the skin, or reach less accessible areas can be impaired. In these cases, fluid vehicles are preferred, and the package should be easy to handle. The elderly is also a special population presenting a variable degree of frailty. In cases of blindness, packages should present braille inscriptions, whereas if a mild degree of cognitive impairment is present, the instructions for use should be easy to understand, and the packaging should be simple [61].

3.1.2. Patient Preferences for Topical Medicines

Several studies underlined that patient preferences need to be considered when prescribing topical treatments to maximize adherence and improve clinical outcomes [12,62–67]. The topical application procedure includes four steps: (a) removal from a container (pick-up), (b) the primary sensation upon the first contact with the skin, (c) the secondary sensation during spreading on the skin, and (d) the final impression, through skin residue. Each patient applies semisolid/liquid formulations to the skin with a slightly different motion and their mechanical and sensory features are closely looked at by patients during topical application [68]. The mechanical properties of different topical anti-psoriatic medicines have been shown to vary substantially, demonstrating that topical vehicles can be perceived in very different ways during their application on the skin [14]. Vehicles also differ in their hydrophilic/lipophilic character, as mentioned before, which results in differences between the sensations they create in the skin. Vehicle excipients can also influence skin moisturization and tolerability [31]. All these differences can influence patient satisfaction and justify, at least partially, their preferences.

A limited number of studies have addressed patient preferences regarding topical products. Patient preferences can vary according to the skin disease and the location of the affected area [69]. For example, the preferences of acne patients (n = 19) were found to be markedly different from those of patients suffering from atopic dermatitis (n = 18) [69]. Regarding lesion location, patients might avoid using ointments in locations where their clothes might come into contact with the medicated area to avoid staining their clothes. A preference for more fluid forms for hairy regions, such as the scalp, is also common. Furthermore, in one study, age group, ethnicity, and gender were also shown to influence preferences for particular vehicles/bases (n = 404) [70]. The patients younger than 40 years preferred lotions, while patients aged over 40 preferred creams. An analysis based on gender showed that females preferred creams, while males preferred lotions and ointments. A strong preference for ointments was found in black-skinned patients, while for white-skinned patients, cream was the preferred form. Few vehicles/bases were included in the survey, and the reasons behind these preferences were not studied. Since it was established that skin condition and anatomic location influence vehicle preference, the results obtained without controlling these variables have limited value.

Fisher et al. studied the influence of ethnicity on vehicle preference for the scalp and found that compared with Caucasian patients (n = 100), African American patients (n = 100) mostly prefer ointments for treating scalp conditions over other topical preparations. A general assumption is that ointment will prevent hair shaft frizzing and drying [71].

Concerning vehicle-type preferences, acne patients were shown to tend to prefer washes, creams, and lotions [62,72]. A conjoint analysis conducted to determine patient preferences for topical antibiotic treatments for acne found that the patients preferred gel formulations to lotions (n = 67) [73]. Interestingly, this analysis revealed that the patients' experiences using the medications had a substantial effect on their reported preferences. While hydrogels were not popular choices before treatment, they became the preferred dosage form by far after ending the treatment. A new tretinoin lotion formulated with a polymeric emulsion technology for the uniform delivery of micronized tretinoin and moisturizing excipients was associated with fewer irritant effects and a greater preference compared with a tretinoin cream [62]. The preferred attributes reported for acne medications included: *easy to dispense/dispense the right amount, non-drying, product goes on/spreads smoothly, no residue,* and *creamy* [69].

Atopic dermatitis patients were shown to prefer creams [69]. When comparing different leave-on emollients, the patients valued *hydrating activity* (67%), and *greasiness* (51%), but not color or scent (n = 250) [74]. Atopic dermatitis patients considered the following condition-specific features relevant [69]: *is not noticeable to others/conceals area, good consistency, cooling, no residue,* and *soothing effect.* Attributes such as *easy to apply* (32%), *easy absorption* (6.8%), and *cooling effect* (6.8%) were also noted in a study involving both patients and caregivers (n = 103) [75]. Topical treatments were consistently described as being *greasy* and/or *messy,* inconvenient to carry or travel with, and time-consuming to apply. The burden described by both adolescents and caregivers in association with frequent topical-treatment administration was higher than for adults, highlighting the influence of demographics on patient preferences. Faster *dermal absorption* and the opportunity to test samples were mentioned by adolescents (n = 15) as preferences regarding treatment-specific attributes [76].

Systematic reviews summarize the findings of all the relevant individual studies and thus provide a higher level of evidence. A systematic review that addressed atopic dermatitis patients and caregivers found that the main preference factors for topical medicines were *odorless treatments, low visibility,* and *sparing use,* with little impact on daily life [77]. However, these preferences were supported by low-certainty evidence when compared with concerns about adverse effects. Fear of side effects, such as steroid phobia, can result in non-adherence to medication; this is a major issue to be addressed in the patient-centric design process by carefully selecting the drug and designing the vehicle to minimize the most troublesome adverse skin effects [78].

Patients with **rosacea** were reported to be neutral regarding their current treatments [79,80] but frequently reported concerns, such as efficacy and side effects, were not associated with treatment satisfaction (n = 216) [80]. Concerns about topical treatments rather than preferences regarding topical attributes were evaluated in these studies and, thus, specific preferences were not established. *Application residue* and, less frequently, *smell* or *texture* were rated as formulation-dependent concerns by a minority of the patients. More tolerable topical treatments that do not elicit burning, itch, and dryness were identified as unmet needs. Foams with azelaic acid have been studied as therapeutic alternatives to hydrogels, with azelaic acid or metronidazole showing good tolerability and efficacy [79,80].

Satisfaction with topical treatment and vehicle preference has been more extensively studied for **psoriasis**, probably because is a chronic disease with high prevalence and a low treatment-adherence rate [81]. Psoriasis patients (n = 17) have shown preferences for creams, ointments, and foams (particularly for the scalp) [69]. A small study on 20 patients showed that topical suspensions were preferred to ointments [82], which was consistent with other findings demonstrating a low level of satisfaction with treatment with *messy ointments* [83]. One of the attributes that were significantly highly rated for the suspension was comfort under clothing. In other studies, possible solutions suggested by patients with psoriasis to increase their satisfaction with topical treatments were *less greasy, sticky*, and *smelly formulations* [8,67]. The use of corticosteroid solutions by psoriasis patients has been proposed as a good alternative for patients who dislike greasy preparations, although these solutions are sometimes associated with burning or stinging. When spray-on solutions are overly expensive for patients, a possible alternative is to place a generic corticosteroid solution in an inexpensive spray bottle. When alcohol-based solutions cause excessive stinging, an oily vehicle can be prescribed for spray-on application [84]. Solution- and foam-based corticosteroid vehicles were also preferred to ointments, gels, and creams in a small study (n = 20) [83]. Adam et al. performed a retrospective study and analyzed the impact of changing drug bases for psoriasis from ointment or gel to aerosol foam, and they found a successful transition in 85% of the patients, with improved treatment adherence and better quality of life [85]. Foam bases were also preferred by plaque-psoriasis patients as easy-to-use topical-drug options [86–89]. Emerging vehicles/bases for psoriasis treatment are continuously investigated. New hydrophilic vehicles obtained with PAD technology protect drugs against hydrolysis, ensuring the stability of the calcipotriene/betamethasone combination while being more patient-friendly than current formulations for psoriasis treatment [90].

The three most highly valued attributes of topical products noted by psoriasis patients were as follows: *allow dressing shortly after application, good moisturizing properties*, and *use only once daily*. These were followed by *good absorption, does not leave stains, does not cause itching or burn*, and *does not run-off* [91]. These findings were consistent with those of another study, which highlighted *ease of application*, the *time needed for application*, the *cost of replacing stained clothes and bed linen, absorption*, and *messiness* as important characteristics for patient use [83]. A systematic review (n = 12) on psoriasis patients' preferences regarding topical treatments found that overall, the patients preferred medicines that are *easy to apply, less messy*, and *have a pleasant scent* [67]. This review also emphasized that there is no single topical-drug product that suits everyone, as well as the importance of shared decision making.

The attributes that were reported simultaneously by patients with plaque psoriasis, atopic dermatitis, and acne were absorbed/disappears/dries quickly, available in various formulations, does not bleach or stain skin/hair/clothing, is not greasy/oily, is not sticky/tacky, is long-lasting/long-acting/stays on/lasts through sweating or hand washing, is fragrance- or odor-free, is easy to apply/simple to use, can use all the time, and moisturizing [69]. However, the ranking of these attributes in terms of importance was not reported.

For **seborrheic dermatitis**, little information is available, A ketoconazole-foam formulation for the treatment of seborrheic dermatitis was included in a more integrated analysis aiming to demonstrate that foams are preferable to other topical vehicles (n = 3398). The proportion of dermatological patients who preferred foam over other vehicles used in the past was greater than 60% when compared to cream, 70% compared to gel, and 60% compared to ointment [92].

The results obtained from the studies assessing vehicle preference are, however, limited by the numbers of vehicles compared, which are usually low, and the small sample sizes. Many studies on patient preferences regarding topical vehicles compared only two vehicles [62,82] or relied on patient perspectives/beliefs rather than experiences of using the vehicle [70]. The identification of dosage form also needs to be properly described. For instance, a gel can refer to a hydrogel or an oleogel, which have very different properties.

From the point of view of drug-product design, studying the topical attributes deemed most relevant by patients is meaningful and provides a rational basis for drug-product design. More studies, with larger sample sizes, addressing other skin conditions, and of good methodological quality are needed [93]. Systematic reviews for each skin condition would be highly useful. Based on a review of current studies on preferences regarding topical treatments Gutknecht et al. recommended that preferences have to be recorded in such a way that they are representative of the affected patients. Questions should be also asked comprehensibly and openly, and the options described should be realistic [93].

For pigmentary disorders, information on patient preferences is scarce. Combi-kits with sunscreen day cream and night cream were found to be very convenient, helping users to remember to apply the medication [94]. New drug-delivery systems for vitiligo treatment were proposed based on phospholipid-based carrier systems, which are thought to improve skin penetration and increase drug localization while putatively improving adherence because of their moisturizing effect, favorable rheological properties, and reduced side effects [95]. Lecithin organogels are among the phospholipid-based approaches studied for vitiligo treatment.

Preferences cannot be predicted by a single variable, such as demographics; hence, more clinical studies are needed to better understand the preferences of patients suffering from skin disorders [12]. From the industrial point of view, commercializing individualized products is not feasible. A product that meets every patient's expectations is also practically impossible to achieve, since preferences often vary between individuals [96]. Patient interviews can be performed before defining the treatment regimen. Giving patients the option of participating in their choice of medication could prove critical to treatment adherence and, ultimately, clinical efficacy. From the point of view of healthcare practice, one possible way to meet patients' preferences for topical vehicles is to allow them to try samples before establishing the treatment regimen. Pharmaceutical compounding also plays a key role in obtaining individualized medicines that are not available in the market [97]. The process of patient-centric compounding design was previously proposed [97], supported by close interactions between the patient, clinician, and pharmacist.

3.2. Target Product Profile (TPP)

The definition of the drug-product profile should take into account the needs and preferences of a given patient population and then translate this information into a profile that is as universal as possible. The drug product is considered the presentation of the topical treatment to the end user (patient/caregiver/health care provider) and includes the vehicle/base, formulation composition, dose, dosing frequency, primary, secondary, and tertiary packaging, dosing devices, and instructions for use. The triad of disease needs + patient needs + patient preferences is the cornerstone of the PCDPD process. Considerations regarding the packaging of topical products and TPP for selected skin disorders are addressed below.

3.2.1. Packaging

The packages conventionally used for semisolid topical products are mainly tubes. Packages or applicators that ease the application by avoiding the use of the hands (sometimes called "no-mess applicators") were recently introduced to the market. The avoidance of the use of hands during rub-in decreases the time spent on washing hands and the putative discomfort of the residue on the hands. Other devices that are used to help to define the amount to be applied in lesions are also available [98].

Recent technological advances, such as 3-D printing, offer an unlimited number of possibilities regarding package design. Instructions for use and for defining the correct amount to be used (e.g., the size of a pea, a finger-tip unit) can also be included within the package, which contributes to the education of patients and improves adherence [61].

3.2.2. Target Product Profile for Selected Skin Disorders

Skin disorders were grouped according to the symptomatology and type of lesion, and a generic TPP was proposed for each illustrative disorder. All of the disorders had a general inflammatory character associated with some skin lesions and symptoms that differentiated them.

In general, the vehicles/bases used should be non-irritant and easy to spread to avoid friction. Many skin conditions, such as eczematous disorders, occur with inflammation, exhibiting erythema and edema.

Eczema is characterized by inflammatory lesions of diverse etiology but with similar characteristics: erythema, vesicles, and desquamation. Different phases can be distinguished in eczema, and so the vehicles/bases should be selected accordingly: (a) in acute phase with erythema, vesicles, exudation, drying vehicles with absorbing capacity, such as suspensions, are preferred; (b) in subacute phase with peeling, excoriation, crusts, and, often, secondary infection, the vehicles should have non-occlusive characteristics, such as those of pastes (e.g., calamine lotion or zinc paste); (c) in the chronic phases of dry lesions, such as lichenification (thickening, darkening, skin folding), the vehicles should have a more occlusive and emollient capacity, such as that of ointments (Figure 2) [99].

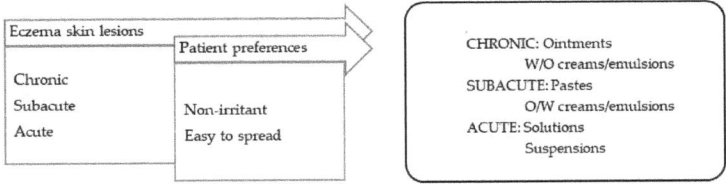

Figure 2. TPP for formulations for eczema-lesion treatment and most suitable vehicles/bases.

1. Scaly and xerotic disorders.

    Formulations for disorders with scaliness and dry skin should be, in general, occlusive, lubricating, and emollient (Figure 3). The skin conditions in this category include psoriasis, ichthyosis, keratosis pillaris, and xerosis.

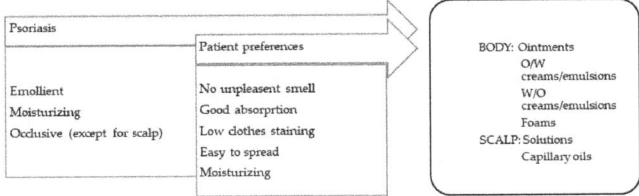

Figure 3. TPP for formulations for psoriasis treatment and most suitable vehicles/bases.

Psoriasis is a chronic erythematous–squamous disease with a high psychosocial impact. Lesions, or psoriatic plaques, present erythema, infiltration, and flaking. Plaque psoriasis, the most common form of the disease, can affect extensive areas of the skin, scalp, and nails. Itching and local pain are symptoms that are frequently reported by patients. Other forms of psoriasis are known, such as flexural psoriasis (on areas of sensitive skin), guttate psoriasis (after streptococcal infections), pustular psoriasis (featuring the presence of pustules, which are generally palmoplantar), erythrodermic psoriasis (a severe and generalized form of erythema), and arthropathic psoriasis (associated with inflammation of the joints, particularly the hands and feet) [99].

2. Long-term inflammatory disorders.

Rosacea is essentially a form of facial inflammatory dermatitis characterized by erythema and, in a more advanced stage, by papulopustular lesions [99]. The vehicles/bases for rosacea treatment should have low fat contents and be non-irritant (Figure 4).

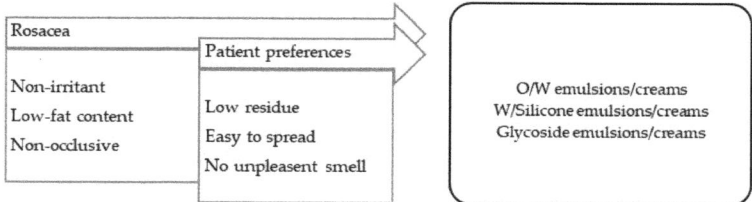

Figure 4. TPP for formulations for rosacea treatment and most suitable vehicles/bases.

3. Seborrheic disorders.

In general, the vehicles/bases used should have low fat contents and not leave skin residue. Seborrheic conditions occur in high-sebaceous-gland-density locations, such as the face, trunk, or scalp, and include seborrheic dermatitis and acne.

Seborrheic dermatitis is a form of chronic inflammatory dermatitis located in areas with an excess of sebum and a high prevalence of *Malassezia furfur* [99]. For applications on the body, O/W creams or emulsions low in fat should be used. For the scalp, O/W emulsions are less appealing, since they require clothing to be protected; instead surfactant-based shampoos should be used for washing and treatment, as well as capillary oils with silicones, which are slightly oily and confer emollience, and aqueous solutions for a drying effect (Figure 5).

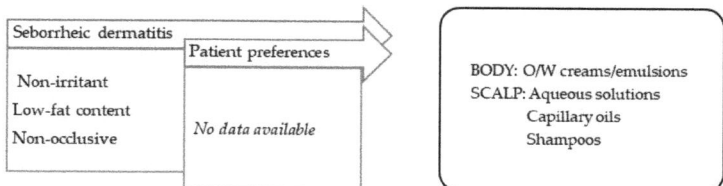

Figure 5. TPP for formulations for treatment of seborrheic dermatitis and most suitable vehicles/bases.

Acne is an inflammation of the sebaceous glands with bacterial colonization (*Cutibacterium acnes*). Its lesions differ in severity and evolve, and include hyperkeratosis and comedones (non-inflammatory), papules and erythema (inflammatory), pustules and cysts (pustular), nodules, and scars (cicatricial) [99]. It should be noted that the vehicles for this pathology must contain reduced fat contents, and therapeutic practice is slightly complex because it often resorts to the use of drugs (Figure 6).

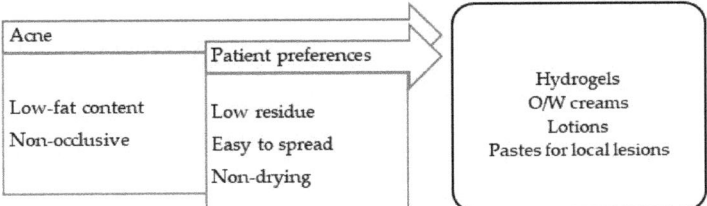

Figure 6. TPP for formulations for acne treatment and most suitable vehicles/bases.

4. Pruritic disorders.

Pruritus is a common symptom that is widely spread in many diseases, not only of cutaneous origin, but also of systemic origin (neurologic, psychiatric, endocrine, hematologic, and others). Pruritus skin lesions present additional symptoms, which may include inflammation (erythema, edema), or dry and scaly skin—both of which may present with excoriations caused by scratching and lichenification, if chronic [99]. The vehicles and bases for these conditions should be adapted to the prevalent symptoms.

Skin conditions such as atopic dermatitis and urticaria are illustrative of pruritic dermatosis.

Atopic dermatitis is a chronic inflammatory dermatitis associated with intense pruritus [99]. In the acute phase, and if there is edema, the vehicle must be siccative (such as aqueous solutions), and when the exudation ceases, the vehicle can be changed to emulsions with a different fat contents, according to the occlusive effect required. Atopic dermatitis requires maintenance, in which the hydration of the skin is essential; numerous emulsified vehicles and oils can be enriched with moisturizing substances (Figure 7).

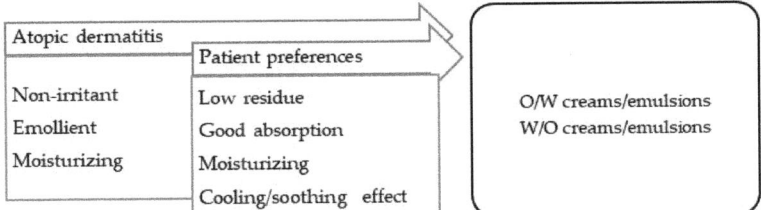

Figure 7. TPP for formulations for treatment of atopic dermatitis and most suitable vehicles/bases.

5. Pigmentation disorders.

Hyperpigmentation (dark macules) results from an increase in melanin production or in the proliferation of melanocytes, originating in epidermal or dermal melanin deposition. The absence of local melanocytes leads to vitiligo, an hypopigmentary skin (white macules) disorder, possibly autoimmune in origin. In addition to a certain inflammatory grade, both lesions are characterized by apparently normal skin with no other symptoms, although they differ in terms of their extension [99]. A variety of vehicles/bases can be applied to ensure: (a) the vehiculation of several types of drug, (b) a non-irritation effect to counterbalance some sensitizing substances, and (c) adaptation to the location and extension of lesions. The most commonly used vehicles/bases are emulsions, creams, and stick bars for easy use (Figure 8).

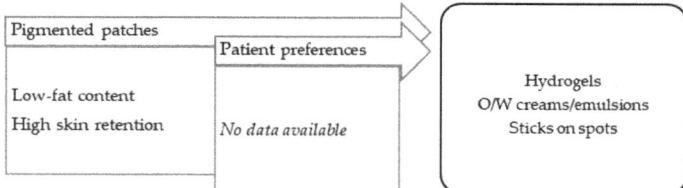

Figure 8. TPP for formulations for treatment of pigmentation disorders and most suitable vehicles/bases.

The treatment of dermatoses with mixed symptomatology must target the most troublesome symptoms at the point of treatment prescription, in association with the patient's specific skin condition and comorbidities. In all cases, the patient's needs should be accounted for when prescribing the treatment regimen. These include visual, motor, and cognitive impairments, as well as poor hand sensitivity and the need for help in applying the treatment.

4. Conclusions

Topical medicines have been associated with poor adherence despite being considered the mainstay of dermatological treatments.

Patient-centric drug-product pharmaceutical design can be a useful tool to improve adherence in dermatology by taking into consideration both the disease and the patient's needs and preferences to improve the acceptability of the drug product. The target profile of the drug product, based on the lesions' characteristics and location, the symptomatology of the underlying skin disease, and the patient's preferences, supports the selection of the most appropriate dosage form and formulation composition. The systematization of target product profiles provided herein can help members of the pharmaceutical industry to offer topical drug products with more universal profiles. Furthermore, it also of utmost importance to clinicians to support the selection of the most suitable topical medicine, as well as the prescription of customized compounding formulations. After optimized formulations are obtained, they should be characterized in terms of the features that are relevant from the patient's perspective to confirm their suitability with the TPP, or the need for reformulation. Increases in patient satisfaction with topical treatments should also be verified in comparison with standard treatments in a sample population. Patient-centric design, however, should not be regarded as a single intervention, but rather as a strategy that complements other interventions aimed at improving medication adherence.

The main purpose of vehicles is to ensure drugs' stability and their delivery, in therapeutic doses, to the sites of action. After establishing the most suitable vehicle/base, the final decision should be centered on the patient's preferences, since it is certain that a drug product will not be effective if it is not used. Medicine rejection may be countered by tailoring vehicles to individualized patient preferences. Many formulations are available to help clinicians to prescribe customized treatments. Clinicians can also rely on the technical expertise of pharmacists. Allowing patients to try samples of different vehicles before establishing the treatment regimen can be also very helpful, especially when the identification of patient preferences is troublesome.

Insights regarding the development of new vehicles with better organoleptic features, as well as new studies on patient preferences and on the therapeutic effects of topical vehicles on clinical outcomes, need to be continuously analyzed and translated in the update of the TPPs for the most common skin disorders.

Author Contributions: Conceptualization, I.F.A.; writing—original draft preparation, I.F.A. and R.O.; writing—review and editing, I.F.A. and R.O.; supervision, I.F.A. All authors have read and agreed to the published version of the manuscript.

Funding: This research received no external funding.

Institutional Review Board Statement: Not applicable.

Informed Consent Statement: Not applicable.

Data Availability Statement: No new data were created or analyzed in this study. Data sharing is not applicable to this article.

Acknowledgments: The authors would like to acknowledge the support of FCT—Fundação para a Ciência e a Tecnologia, I.P., within projects UIDP/04378/2020 and UIDB/04378/2020 of the Research Unit on Applied Molecular Biosciences—UCIBIO—and project LA/P/0140/2020 of the Associate Laboratory Institute for Health and Bioeconomy—i4HB.

Conflicts of Interest: The authors declare no conflict of interest.

References

1. Ana Teixeira, M.T.; Almeida, V.; Almeida, I.F. Adherence to Topical Treatment in Psoriasis. In *Adherence to Medical Plans for Active and Healthy Ageing*; Costa, E., Giardini, A., Monaco, A., Eds.; Nova Science Publishers, Incorporated: New York, NY, USA, 2017.
2. Augustin, M.; Holland, B.; Dartsch, D.; Langenbruch, A.; Radtke, M.A. Adherence in the treatment of psoriasis: A systematic review. *Dermatology* **2011**, *222*, 363–374. [CrossRef]
3. Miyachi, Y.; Hayashi, N.; Furukawa, F.; Akamatsu, H.; Matsunaga, K.; Watanabe, S.; Kawashima, M. Acne management in Japan: Study of patient adherence. *Dermatology* **2011**, *223*, 174–181. [CrossRef]
4. Snyder, A.; Farhangian, M.; Feldman, S.R. A review of patient adherence to topical therapies for treatment of atopic dermatitis. *Cutis* **2015**, *96*, 397–401.
5. Teixeira, A.; Oliveira, C.; Teixeira, M.; Rita Gaio, A.; Lobo, J.M.S.; de Almeida, I.F.M.; Almeida, V. Development and Validation of a Novel Questionnaire for Adherence with Topical Treatments in Psoriasis (QATOP). *Am. J. Clin. Dermatol.* **2017**, *18*, 571–581. [CrossRef]
6. Tveit, K.S.; Duvetorp, A.; Østergaard, M.; Skov, L.; Danielsen, K.; Iversen, L.; Seifert, O. Treatment use and satisfaction among patients with psoriasis and psoriatic arthritis: Results from the NORdic PAtient survey of Psoriasis and Psoriatic arthritis (NORPAPP). *J. Eur. Acad. Dermatol. Venereol.* **2019**, *33*, 340–354. [CrossRef]
7. Schaarschmidt, M.L.; Umar, N.; Schmieder, A.; Terris, D.D.; Goebeler, M.; Goerdt, S.; Peitsch, W.K. Patient preferences for psoriasis treatments: Impact of treatment experience. *J. Eur. Acad. Dermatol. Venereol.* **2013**, *27*, 187–198. [CrossRef]
8. Fouéré, S.; Adjadj, L.; Pawin, H. How patients experience psoriasis: Results from a European survey. *J. Eur. Acad. Dermatol. Venereol.* **2005**, *19* (Suppl. S3), 2–6. [CrossRef]
9. Brown, K.K.; Rehmus, W.E.; Kimball, A.B. Determining the relative importance of patient motivations for nonadherence to topical corticosteroid therapy in psoriasis. *J. Am. Acad. Dermatol.* **2006**, *55*, 607–613. [CrossRef]
10. Teixeira, A.; Teixeira, M.; Almeida, V.; Gaio, R.; Torres, T.; Magina, S.; Cunha, C.; Sousa Lobo, J.M.; Almeida, I.F. Does the Vehicle Matter? Real-World Evidence on Adherence to Topical Treatment in Psoriasis. *Pharmaceutics* **2021**, *13*, 1539. [CrossRef]
11. Puig, L.; Carrascosa, J.M.; Belinchón, I.; Fernández-Redondo, V.; Carretero, G.; Ruiz-Carrascosa, J.C.; Careaga, J.M.; de la Cueva, P.; Gárate, M.T.; Ribera, M. Adherence and Patient Satisfaction With Topical Treatment in Psoriasis, and the Use, and Organoleptic Properties of Such Treatments: A Delphi Study With an Expert Panel and Members of the Psoriasis Group of the Spanish Academy of Dermatology and Venereology. *Actas Dermo-Sifiliográficas* **2013**, *104*, 488–496. [CrossRef]
12. Iversen, L.; Jakobsen, H.B. Patient Preferences for Topical Psoriasis Treatments are Diverse and Difficult to Predict. *Dermatol. Ther.* **2016**, *6*, 273–285. [CrossRef] [PubMed]
13. Council of Europe. *European Pharmacopoeia, 10th Edition 2020*; Directorate for the Quality of Medicines and HealthCare of the Council of Europe (EDQM): Strasbourg, France, 2019.
14. Teixeira, A.; Vasconcelos, V.; Teixeira, M.; Almeida, V.; Azevedo, R.; Torres, T.; Sousa Lobo, J.M.; Costa, P.C.; Almeida, I.F. Mechanical Properties of Topical Anti-Psoriatic Medicines: Implications for Patient Satisfaction with Treatment. *AAPS PharmSciTech* **2019**, *20*, 36. [CrossRef] [PubMed]
15. *Encyclopedia of Pharmaceutical Technology*, 3rd ed.; Swarbrick, J., Ed.; CRC Press: Boca Raton, FL, USA, 2007.
16. Taylor, K.M.G.; Aulton, M.E. *Aulton's Pharmaceutics: The Design and Manufacture of Medicines*, 6th ed.; Taylor, K.M.G., Aulton, M.E., Eds.; Elsevier: Amsterdam, The Netherlands, 2021.
17. Lukic, M.; Pantelic, I.; Savic, S. An Overview of Novel Surfactants for Formulation of Cosmetics with Certain Emphasis on Acidic Active Substances. *Tenside Surfactants Deterg.* **2016**, *53*, 7–19. [CrossRef]
18. Pal, A.; Mondal, M.H.; Adhikari, A.; Bhattarai, A.; Saha, B. Scientific information about sugar-based emulsifiers: A comprehensive review. *RSC Adv.* **2021**, *11*, 33004–33016. [CrossRef]
19. Ajazuddin; Alexander, A.; Khichariya, A.; Gupta, S.; Patel, R.J.; Giri, T.K.; Tripathi, D.K. Recent expansions in an emergent novel drug delivery technology: Emulgel. *J. Control. Release* **2013**, *171*, 122–132. [CrossRef]
20. Somasundaran, P.; Mehta, S.C.; Purohit, P. Silicone emulsions. *Adv. Colloid Interface Sci.* **2006**, *128–130*, 103–109. [CrossRef]
21. Mancuso, A.; Tarsitano, M.; Udongo, B.P.; Cristiano, M.C.; Torella, D.; Paolino, D.; Fresta, M. A comparison between silicone-free and silicone-based emulsions: Technological features and in vivo evaluation. *Int. J. Cosmet. Sci.* **2022**, *44*, 514–529. [CrossRef]

22. Ohsedo, Y. N-Alkylhydantoins as New Organogelators and Their Ability to Create Thixotropic Mixed Molecular Organogels. *Gels* **2022**, *8*, 638. [CrossRef]
23. Ambreen, Z.; Faran, S.A.; Daniel, A.; Khalid, S.H.; Khan, I.U.; Asif, M.; Rehman, A.; Mehmood, H.Q.; Asghar, S. Physicochemical, rheological and antifungal evaluation of miconazole nitrate organogels for topical delivery. *Pak. J. Pharm. Sci.* **2022**, *35*, 1215–1221.
24. Jun Yang, S.; Yoon, K.S. Preparation and Evaluation of Pluronic Lecithin Organogels in Cosmetics. *J. Cosmet. Sci.* **2021**, *72*, 325–346.
25. Kircik, L.H. Vehicles Always Matter. *J. Drugs Dermatol.* **2019**, *18*, s99. [PubMed]
26. Hoc, D.; Haznar-Garbacz, D. Foams as unique drug delivery systems. *Eur. J. Pharm. Biopharm.* **2021**, *167*, 73–82. [CrossRef] [PubMed]
27. Daniels, R.; Knie, U. Galenics of dermal products–vehicles, properties and drug release. *J. Dtsch. Dermatol. Ges.* **2007**, *5*, 367–383. [CrossRef] [PubMed]
28. Weiss, S.C. Conventional topical delivery systems. *Dermatol. Ther.* **2011**, *24*, 471–476. [CrossRef]
29. Rosen, J.; Landriscina, A.; Friedman, A.J. Principles and approaches for optimizing therapy with unique topical vehicles. *J. Drugs Dermatol.* **2014**, *13*, 1431–1435.
30. Mayba, J.N.; Gooderham, M.J. A Guide to Topical Vehicle Formulations. *J. Cutan. Med. Surg.* **2018**, *22*, 207–212. [CrossRef]
31. Barnes, T.M.; Mijaljica, D.; Townley, J.P.; Spada, F.; Harrison, I.P. Vehicles for Drug Delivery and Cosmetic Moisturizers: Review and Comparison. *Pharmaceutics* **2021**, *13*, 2012. [CrossRef]
32. EMA. Reflection Paper on the Use of Extrapolation in the Development of Medicines for Paediatrics (EMA/189724/2018). Available online: https://www.ema.europa.eu/en/documents/scientific-guideline/adopted-reflection-paper-use-extrapolation-development-medicines-paediatrics-revision-1_en.pdf (accessed on 20 February 2023).
33. EMA. Guideline on Pharmaceutical Development of Medicines for Paediatric Use (EMA/CHMP/QWP/805880/2012 Rev.2). Available online: https://www.ema.europa.eu/en/documents/scientific-guideline/guideline-pharmaceutical-development-medicines-paediatric-use_en.pdf (accessed on 20 February 2023).
34. EMA. Reflection paper on the pharmaceutical development of medicines for use in the older population (EMA/CHMP/QWP/292439/2017). Available online: https://www.ema.europa.eu/en/documents/scientific-guideline/reflection-paper-pharmaceutical-development-medicines-use-older-population-first-version_en.pdf (accessed on 20 February 2023).
35. FDA. Patient-Focused Drug Development: Methods to Identify What Is Important to Patients. Available online: https://www.fda.gov/media/131230/download (accessed on 20 February 2023).
36. Perfetto, E.M.; Burke, L.; Oehrlein, E.M.; Epstein, R.S. Patient-Focused Drug Development: A New Direction for Collaboration. *Med. Care* **2015**, *53*, 9–17. [CrossRef]
37. Chalasani, M.; Vaidya, P.; Mullin, T. Enhancing the incorporation of the patient's voice in drug development and evaluation. *Res. Involv. Engagem.* **2018**, *4*, 10. [CrossRef]
38. Zvonareva, O.; Cravet, C.; Richards, D.P. Practices of patient engagement in drug development: A systematic scoping review. *Res. Involv. Engagem.* **2022**, *8*, 29. [CrossRef]
39. ICH. Proposed ICH guideline work to advance patient focused drug development. Available online: https://www.ema.europa.eu/en/documents/scientific-guideline/ich-reflection-paper-proposed-ich-guideline-work-advance-patient-focused-drug-development_en.pdf (accessed on 20 February 2023).
40. Stegemann, S.; Ternik, R.L.; Onder, G.; Khan, M.A.; van Riet-Nales, D.A. Defining Patient Centric Pharmaceutical Drug Product Design. *AAPS J.* **2016**, *18*, 1047–1055. [CrossRef] [PubMed]
41. Timpe, C.; Stegemann, S.; Barrett, A.; Mujumdar, S. Challenges and opportunities to include patient-centric product design in industrial medicines development to improve therapeutic goals. *Br. J. Clin. Pharmacol.* **2020**, *86*, 2020–2027. [CrossRef] [PubMed]
42. Algorri, M.; Cauchon, N.S.; Christian, T.; O'Connell, C.; Vaidya, P. Patient-Centric Product Development: A Summary of Select Regulatory CMC and Device Considerations. *J. Pharm. Sci.* **2023**, *112*, 922–936. [CrossRef] [PubMed]
43. Ogbonna, J.D.N.; Cunha, E.; Attama, A.A.; Ofokansi, K.C.; Ferreira, H.; Pinto, S.; Gomes, J.; Marx, Í.M.G.; Peres, A.M.; Lobo, J.M.S.; et al. Overcoming Challenges in Pediatric Formulation with a Patient-Centric Design Approach: A Proof-of-Concept Study on the Design of an Oral Solution of a Bitter Drug. *Pharmaceuticals* **2022**, *15*, 1331. [CrossRef] [PubMed]
44. Shariff, Z.; Kirby, D.; Missaghi, S.; Rajabi-Siahboomi, A.; Maidment, I. Patient-Centric Medicine Design: Key Characteristics of Oral Solid Dosage Forms that Improve Adherence and Acceptance in Older People. *Pharmaceutics* **2020**, *12*, 905. [CrossRef]
45. Drumond, N. Future Perspectives for Patient-Centric Pharmaceutical Drug Product Design with Regard to Solid Oral Dosage Forms. *J. Pharm. Innov.* **2020**, *15*, 318–324. [CrossRef]
46. Oliveira, R.S.; da Silva, D.F.; Mota, S.; Garrido, J.; Garrido, E.M.; Lobo, J.M.S.; Almeida, I.F. Design of an Emulgel for Psoriasis Focused on Patient Preferences. *Appl. Sci.* **2022**, *12*, 3260. [CrossRef]
47. Cook, N.S.; Cave, J.; Holtorf, A.P. Patient Preference Studies During Early Drug Development: Aligning Stakeholders to Ensure Development Plans Meet Patient Needs. *Front. Med.* **2019**, *6*, 82. [CrossRef]
48. Stegemann, S.; Sheehan, L.; Rossi, A.; Barrett, A.; Paudel, A.; Crean, A.; Ruiz, F.; Bresciani, M.; Liu, F.; Shariff, Z.; et al. Rational and practical considerations to guide a target product profile for patient-centric drug product development with measurable patient outcomes—A proposed roadmap. *Eur. J. Pharm. Biopharm.* **2022**, *177*, 81–88. [CrossRef]
49. Surber, C.; Smith, E.W. The mystical effects of dermatological vehicles. *Dermatology* **2005**, *210*, 157–168. [CrossRef]
50. Danby, S.G.; Draelos, Z.D.; Gold, L.F.S.; Cha, A.; Vlahos, B.; Aikman, L.; Sanders, P.; Wu-Linhares, D.; Cork, M.J. Vehicles for atopic dermatitis therapies: More than just a placebo. *J. Dermatol. Treat.* **2022**, *33*, 685–698. [CrossRef]

51. Crowther, J.M.; Sieg, A.; Blenkiron, P.; Marcott, C.; Matts, P.J.; Kaczvinsky, J.R.; Rawlings, A.V. Measuring the effects of topical moisturizers on changes in stratum corneum thickness, water gradients and hydration in vivo. *Br. J. Dermatol.* **2008**, *159*, 567–577. [CrossRef]
52. Spada, F.; Barnes, T.M.; Greive, K.A. Skin hydration is significantly increased by a cream formulated to mimic the skin's own natural moisturizing systems. *Clin. Cosmet. Investig. Dermatol.* **2018**, *11*, 491–497. [CrossRef] [PubMed]
53. Danby, S.G.; Andrew, P.V.; Taylor, R.N.; Kay, L.J.; Chittock, J.; Pinnock, A.; Ulhaq, I.; Fasth, A.; Carlander, K.; Holm, T.; et al. Different types of emollient cream exhibit diverse physiological effects on the skin barrier in adults with atopic dermatitis. *Clin Exp. Dermatol.* **2022**, *47*, 1154–1164. [CrossRef] [PubMed]
54. Lodén, M. Effect of moisturizers on epidermal barrier function. *Clin. Dermatol.* **2012**, *30*, 286–296. [CrossRef] [PubMed]
55. Draelos, Z.D. New treatments for restoring impaired epidermal barrier permeability: Skin barrier repair creams. *Clin. Dermatol.* **2012**, *30*, 345–348. [CrossRef] [PubMed]
56. Murasawa, Y.; Furuta, K.; Noda, Y.; Nakamura, H.; Fujii, S.; Isogai, Z. Ointment vehicles regulate the wound-healing process by modifying the hyaluronan-rich matrix. *Wound Repair Regen.* **2018**, *26*, 437–445. [CrossRef] [PubMed]
57. van Zuuren, E.J.; Fedorowicz, Z.; Christensen, R.; Lavrijsen, A.; Arents, B.W.M. Emollients and moisturisers for eczema. *Cochrane Database Syst. Rev.* **2017**, *2*, Cd012119. [CrossRef]
58. Spigariolo, C.B.; Ferrucci, S.M. Efficacy and tolerability of a repairing moisturizing cream containing amino-inositole and urea 10% in adults with chronic eczematous dermatitis of the hands. *Ital. J. Dermatol. Venerol.* **2023**, *158*, 42–48. [CrossRef]
59. Fakhouri, T.; Yentzer, B.A.; Feldman, S.R. Advancement in benzoyl peroxide-based acne treatment: Methods to increase both efficacy and tolerability. *J. Drugs Dermatol.* **2009**, *8*, 657–661.
60. Hoffman, L.K.; Bhatia, N.; Zeichner, J.; Kircik, L.H. Topical Vehicle Formulations in the Treatment of Acne. *J. Drugs Dermatol.* **2018**, *17*, s6–s10. [PubMed]
61. Menditto, E.; Orlando, V.; De Rosa, G.; Minghetti, P.; Musazzi, U.M.; Cahir, C.; Kurczewska-Michalak, M.; Kardas, P.; Costa, E.; Sousa Lobo, J.M.; et al. Patient Centric Pharmaceutical Drug Product Design-The Impact on Medication Adherence. *Pharmaceutics* **2020**, *12*, 44. [CrossRef] [PubMed]
62. Draelos, Z.; Tanghetti, E.; Guenin, E. Vehicle Formulation Impacts Tolerability and Patient Preference: Comparison of Tretinoin Branded Lotion and Generic Cream. *J. Drugs Dermatol.* **2022**, *21*, 875–880. [CrossRef]
63. Tan, X.; Feldman, S.R.; Chang, J.; Balkrishnan, R. Topical drug delivery systems in dermatology: A review of patient adherence issues. *Expert Opin. Drug Deliv.* **2012**, *9*, 1263–1271. [CrossRef]
64. Patel, N.U.; D'Ambra, V.; Feldman, S.R. Increasing Adherence with Topical Agents for Atopic Dermatitis. *Am. J. Clin. Dermatol.* **2017**, *18*, 323–332. [CrossRef]
65. Umar, N.; Yamamoto, S.; Loerbroks, A.; Terris, D. Elicitation and use of patients' preferences in the treatment of psoriasis: A systematic review. *Acta Derm. Venereol.* **2012**, *92*, 341–346. [CrossRef]
66. de Wijs, L.E.M.; van Egmond, S.; Devillers, A.C.A.; Nijsten, T.; Hijnen, D.; Lugtenberg, M. Needs and preferences of patients regarding atopic dermatitis care in the era of new therapeutic options: A qualitative study. *Arch. Dermatol. Res.* **2023**, *315*, 75–83. [CrossRef] [PubMed]
67. Svendsen, M.T.; Feldman, S.R.; Tiedemann, S.N.; Sørensen, A.S.S.; Rivas, C.M.R.; Andersen, K.E. Psoriasis patient preferences for topical drugs: A systematic review. *J. Dermatol. Treat.* **2021**, *32*, 478–483. [CrossRef]
68. Park, E.-K.; Song, K.-W. Rheological evaluation of petroleum jelly as a base material in ointment and cream formulations: Steady shear flow behavior. *Arch. Pharmacal Res.* **2010**, *33*, 141–150. [CrossRef]
69. Eastman, W.J.; Malahias, S.; Delconte, J.; DiBenedetti, D. Assessing attributes of topical vehicles for the treatment of acne, atopic dermatitis, and plaque psoriasis. *Cutis* **2014**, *94*, 46–53.
70. Figenshau, K.; Kimmis, B.D.; Reicherter, P. Variations in preference for topical vehicles among demographic groups. *Cutis* **2020**, *106*, 40–43. [CrossRef] [PubMed]
71. Fisher, E.J.; Adams, B.B. African American and Caucasian patients' vehicle preference for the scalp. *J. Am. Acad. Dermatol.* **2008**, *58*, S46–S47. [CrossRef] [PubMed]
72. Kircik, L.H.; Green, L.; Guenin, E.; Khalid, W.; Alexander, B. Dermal sensitization, safety, tolerability, and patient preference of tazarotene 0.045% lotion from five clinical trials. *J. Dermatolog. Treat.* **2022**, *33*, 2241–2249. [CrossRef] [PubMed]
73. Kellett, N.; West, F.; Finlay, A.Y. Conjoint analysis: A novel, rigorous tool for determining patient preferences for topical antibiotic treatment for acne. A randomised controlled trial. *Br. J. Dermatol.* **2006**, *154*, 524–532. [CrossRef] [PubMed]
74. Kunkiel, K.; Natkańska, N.; Nędzi, M.; Zawadzka-Krajewska, A.; Feleszko, W. Patients' preferences of leave-on emollients: A survey on patients with atopic dermatitis. *J. Dermatol. Treat.* **2022**, *33*, 1143–1145. [CrossRef]
75. Ervin, C.; Crawford, R.; Evans, E.; Feldman, S.R.; Zeichner, J.; Zielinski, M.A.; Cappelleri, J.C.; DiBonaventura, M.; Takiya, L.; Myers, D.E. Patient and caregiver preferences on treatment attributes for atopic dermatitis. *J. Dermatol. Treat.* **2022**, *33*, 2225–2233. [CrossRef] [PubMed]
76. Kosse, R.C.; Bouvy, M.L.; Daanen, M.; de Vries, T.W.; Koster, E.S. Adolescents' Perspectives on Atopic Dermatitis Treatment-Experiences, Preferences, and Beliefs. *JAMA Dermatol.* **2018**, *154*, 824–827. [CrossRef]
77. Maleki-Yazdi, K.A.; Heen, A.F.; Zhao, I.X.; Guyatt, G.H.; Suzumura, E.A.; Makhdami, N.; Chen, L.; Winders, T.; Wheeler, K.E.; Wang, J.; et al. Values and Preferences of Patients and Caregivers Regarding Treatment of Atopic Dermatitis (Eczema): A Systematic Review. *JAMA Dermatol.* **2023**, *159*, 320–330. [CrossRef]

78. Contento, M.; Cline, A.; Russo, M. Steroid Phobia: A Review of Prevalence, Risk Factors, and Interventions. *Am. J. Clin. Dermatol.* **2021**, *22*, 837–851. [CrossRef]
79. Williamson, T.; Cameron, J.; McLeod, K.; Turner, B.; Quillen, A.; LaRose, A. Patient Concerns and Treatment Satisfaction in Patients Treated with Azelaic Acid Foam for Rosacea. *SKIN J. Cutan. Med.* **2018**, *2*, S36. [CrossRef]
80. Williamson, T.; Cheng, W.Y.; McCormick, N.; Vekeman, F. Patient Preferences and Therapeutic Satisfaction with Topical Agents for Rosacea: A Survey-Based Study. *Am. Health Drug Benefits* **2018**, *11*, 97–106. [PubMed]
81. Damiani, G.; Bragazzi, N.L.; Karimkhani Aksut, C.; Wu, D.; Alicandro, G.; McGonagle, D.; Guo, C.; Dellavalle, R.; Grada, A.; Wong, P.; et al. The Global, Regional, and National Burden of Psoriasis: Results and Insights From the Global Burden of Disease 2019 Study. *Front. Med.* **2021**, *8*, 743180. [CrossRef] [PubMed]
82. Sandoval, L.; Huang, K.; Harrison, J.; Clark, A.; Feldman, S. Calcipotriene 0.005%-Betamethasone Dipropionate 0.064% Ointment Versus Topical Suspension in the Treatment of Plaque Psoriasis: A Randomized Pilot Study of Patient Preference. *Cutis* **2014**, *94*, 304–309. [PubMed]
83. Housman, T.S.; Mellen, B.G.; Rapp, S.R.; Fleischer, A.B., Jr.; Feldman, S.R. Patients with psoriasis prefer solution and foam vehicles: A quantitative assessment of vehicle preference. *Cutis* **2002**, *70*, 327–332. [PubMed]
84. Hill, D.; Farhangian, M.E.; Feldman, S.R. Increasing adherence to topical therapy in psoriasis through use of solution medication. *Dermatol. Online J.* **2016**, *22*, 16. [CrossRef]
85. Adam, D.N.; Abdulla, S.J.; Fleming, P.; Gooderham, M.J.; Ashkenas, J.; McCracken, C.B. Transition of Topical Therapy Formulation in Psoriasis: Insights from a Canadian Practice Reflective. *Skin Therapy Lett.* **2022**, *27*, 6–11.
86. Chung, M.; Yeroushalmi, S.; Hakimi, M.; Bartholomew, E.; Liao, W.; Bhutani, T. A critical review of halobetasol propionate foam (0.05%) as a treatment option for adolescent plaque psoriasis. *Expert Rev. Clin. Immunol.* **2022**, *18*, 997–1003. [CrossRef]
87. Bhatia, N.; Stein Gold, L.; Kircik, L.H.; Schreiber, R. Two Multicenter, Randomized, Double-Blind, Parallel Group Comparison Studies of a Novel Foam Formulation of Halobetasol Propionate, 0.05% vs Its Vehicle in Adult Subjects With Plaque Psoriasis. *J Drugs Dermatol.* **2019**, *18*, 790–796.
88. Aschoff, R.; Bewley, A.; Dattola, A.; De Simone, C.; Lahfa, M.; Llamas-Velasco, M.; Martorell, A.; Pavlovic, M.; Sticherling, M. Beyond-Mild Psoriasis: A Consensus Statement on Calcipotriol and Betamethasone Dipropionate Foam for the Topical Treatment of Adult Patients. *Dermatol. Ther.* **2021**, *11*, 1791–1804. [CrossRef]
89. Dattola, A.; Silvestri, M.; Bennardo, L.; Passante, M.; Rizzuto, F.; Dastoli, S.; Patruno, C.; Bianchi, L.; Nisticò, S.P. A novel vehicle for the treatment of psoriasis. *Dermatol. Ther.* **2020**, *33*, e13185. [CrossRef]
90. Pinter, A.; Green, L.J.; Selmer, J.; Praestegaard, M.; Gold, L.S.; Augustin, M. A pooled analysis of randomized, controlled, phase 3 trials investigating the efficacy and safety of a novel, fixed dose calcipotriene and betamethasone dipropionate cream for the topical treatment of plaque psoriasis. *J. Eur. Acad. Dermatol. Venereol.* **2022**, *36*, 228–236. [CrossRef] [PubMed]
91. Vasconcelos, V.; Teixeira, A.; Almeida, V.; Teixeira, M.; Ramos, S.; Torres, T.; Sousa Lobo, J.M.; Almeida, I.F. Patient preferences for attributes of topical anti-psoriatic medicines. *J. Dermatol. Treat.* **2019**, *30*, 659–663. [CrossRef] [PubMed]
92. Weiss, S.; Wyres, M.; Brundage, T. A novel foam vehicle is consistently preferred by patients for dermatologic conditions. *J. Am. Acad. Dermatol.* **2011**, *64*, AB50. [CrossRef]
93. Gutknecht, M.; Schaarschmidt, M.L.; Herrlein, O.; Augustin, M. A systematic review on methods used to evaluate patient preferences in psoriasis treatments. *J. Eur. Acad. Dermatol. Venereol.* **2016**, *30*, 1454–1464. [CrossRef] [PubMed]
94. Nair, P.A.; Vora, R.V.; Jivani, N.B.; Gandhi, S.S. A study of clinical profile and quality of life in patients with scabies. *Int. J. Res. Dermatol.* **2021**, *7*, 508–512. [CrossRef]
95. Garg, B.J.; Saraswat, A.; Bhatia, A.; Katare, O.P. Topical treatment in vitiligo and the potential uses of new drug delivery systems. *Indian J. Dermatol. Venereol. Leprol.* **2010**, *76*, 231–238. [CrossRef]
96. Felix, K.; Unrue, E.; Inyang, M.; Cardwell, L.A.; Oussedik, E.; Richardson, I.; Feldman, S.R. Patients preferences for different corticosteroid vehicles are highly variable. *J. Dermatol. Treat.* **2020**, *31*, 147–151. [CrossRef]
97. Carvalho, M.; Almeida, I.F. The Role of Pharmaceutical Compounding in Promoting Medication Adherence. *Pharmaceuticals* **2022**, *15*, 1091. [CrossRef]
98. Savary, J.; Ortonne, J.P.; Aractingi, S. The right dose in the right place: An overview of current prescription, instruction and application modalities for topical psoriasis treatments. *J. Eur. Acad. Dermatol. Venereol.* **2005**, *19* (Suppl. S3), 14–17. [CrossRef]
99. Buxton, P.K.; Morris-Jones, R. *ABC of Dermatology*, 5th ed.; Paul, K., Buxton, R.M.-J., Eds.; BMJ Books: London, UK, 2013.

Disclaimer/Publisher's Note: The statements, opinions and data contained in all publications are solely those of the individual author(s) and contributor(s) and not of MDPI and/or the editor(s). MDPI and/or the editor(s) disclaim responsibility for any injury to people or property resulting from any ideas, methods, instructions or products referred to in the content.

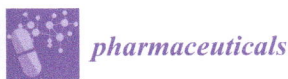

Review

Exploring the Application of Micellar Drug Delivery Systems in Cancer Nanomedicine

Qi Wang [1], Keerthi Atluri [2], Amit K. Tiwari [3,4] and R. Jayachandra Babu [1,*]

1. Department of Drug Discovery and Development, Auburn University, Auburn, AL 36849, USA
2. Product Development Department, Alcami Corporation, Morrisville, NC 27560, USA
3. Department of Pharmacology and Experimental Therapeutics, University of Toledo, Toledo, OH 43614, USA
4. Department of Cell and Cancer Biology, University of Toledo, Toledo, OH 43614, USA
* Correspondence: ramapjb@auburn.edu

Abstract: Various formulations of polymeric micelles, tiny spherical structures made of polymeric materials, are currently being investigated in preclinical and clinical settings for their potential as nanomedicines. They target specific tissues and prolong circulation in the body, making them promising cancer treatment options. This review focuses on the different types of polymeric materials available to synthesize micelles, as well as the different ways that micelles can be tailored to be responsive to different stimuli. The selection of stimuli-sensitive polymers used in micelle preparation is based on the specific conditions found in the tumor microenvironment. Additionally, clinical trends in using micelles to treat cancer are presented, including what happens to micelles after they are administered. Finally, various cancer drug delivery applications involving micelles are discussed along with their regulatory aspects and future outlooks. As part of this discussion, we will examine current research and development in this field. The challenges and barriers they may have to overcome before they can be widely adopted in clinics will also be discussed.

Keywords: micelle; polymer; drug delivery; stimuli sensitive; regulatory; clinical trials

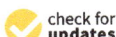

Citation: Wang, Q.; Atluri, K.; Tiwari, A.K.; Babu, R.J. Exploring the Application of Micellar Drug Delivery Systems in Cancer Nanomedicine. *Pharmaceuticals* **2023**, *16*, 433. https://doi.org/10.3390/ph16030433

Academic Editors: Silviya Petrova Zustiak and Era Jain

Received: 17 February 2023
Revised: 7 March 2023
Accepted: 8 March 2023
Published: 12 March 2023

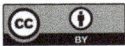

Copyright: © 2023 by the authors. Licensee MDPI, Basel, Switzerland. This article is an open access article distributed under the terms and conditions of the Creative Commons Attribution (CC BY) license (https://creativecommons.org/licenses/by/4.0/).

1. Introduction

Cancer continues to be one of the leading causes of death throughout the world, despite extensive research and advances in treatment. With nanotechnology, materials can be manipulated and engineered at the nanometer scale, revolutionizing cancer treatment. To better understand how nanotechnology can be applied to the diagnosis and how to deliver chemotherapy drugs directly to cancer cells for targeted drug delivery systems is currently the subject of intense study. Drug transport, imaging, immune system development, diagnostics, and therapy all benefit from the use of nanomaterials. Several nanomaterials, such as liposomes and polymeric micelles used for the treatment of cancer, have been approved by regulatory authorities in several countries, including the United States and Europe, and a few other nanomedicines are currently under clinical investigation. Hypoxia, acidosis, and vascular anomalies are some of the features that the tumor microenvironment (TME) differs from normal tissues [1,2].

Low pH, high glutathione (GSH) concentrations, excess production of reactive oxygen species (ROS), and severe hypoxia are some of the typical features of TME. Tumor development, metastasis, and medication resistance may result from tumors with these features because they create a conducive internal environment for tumor cells to survive. These features could be used to develop targeted nanomedicine delivery systems that selectively release drugs only in tumor tissues with minimal systemic drug exposures. Stimuli responsive nanoparticles can release drugs only in response to certain stimuli, prolonging blood circulation and enhancing cancer cell absorption while also improving biosafety. They can also maintain stability under physiological conditions. As a result, there is great potential that the development of TME-responsive smart nanomedicine may improve the efficiency of existing cancer treatments [3,4].

1.1. Targeting TME with a Low pH

Although the extracellular pH of healthy tissue is carefully controlled at around 7.4, it is frequently dysregulated in pathological conditions such as ischemia, inflammation, and neoplasia. Due to tumor cell anaerobic glycolysis and lactic acid generation, the TME is generally acidic. Tumors prefer anaerobic glycolysis even when exposed to oxygen, a phenomenon known as the Warburg effect [5]. Numerous investigations have demonstrated that the unregulated energy metabolism, inadequate perfusion, and accumulation of lactic acid (Warburg effect) cause the extracellular space of tumor tissue to be weakly acidic, with a pH range from 6.5 to 6.8 [6–8]. Recent studies have shown the development of pH responsive nanomedicines due to the high acidity in the tumor extracellular environment being a characteristic pathological hallmark of solid tumor tissues in comparison to the neutral environment of normal tissues. Therefore, acidity permeates the TME, and delivery devices targeting low extracellular pH would permit very selective delivery of cargo to the tumors in vivo [9–11].

1.2. Targeting TME with High Level of GSH

GSH is a thiol compound made of cysteine, glutamate, and glycine. It is essential for the body to have a normal concentration of GSH because it has antioxidant and detoxifying properties [6]. To keep the cellular redox state in check, GSH is an essential component as one of the most prevalent reductive cellular metabolites. GSH mediates the formation and breakdown of disulfide bonds, making it an important player in the regulation of protein folding. The reported GSH content in tumor cells is significantly greater than that in normal cells. About 2–10 mM of GSH is present intracellularly, which is a considerable increase over the 2–20 M levels found in the extracellular matrix and blood. Additionally, compared to normal tissues, tumor tissues had a GSH concentration that was ten times higher [3,12,13]. As oxidized glutathione (GSSG) is catabolized in the cytosol into GSH by GSH reductases and nicotinamide adenine dinucleotide phosphate (NADP), the cytosol contains 1000 times more GSH than the surrounding environment or plasma. For this reason, disulfide bonds have been included in nanomedicine to promote selective drug release in the tumor cytosol via GSH as a particular marker [6,14,15].

1.3. Targeting Hypoxia TME

Hypoxia is a defining feature of solid tumors and is intimately associated with invasion, metastasis, and medication resistance. Blood arteries in solid tumors are unable to adequately distribute oxygen and nutrients to all areas due to their uneven structure, which causes tumor cells to become hypoxic temporarily or permanently. From the tumor surface to the center, the oxygen partial pressure gradually drops. The oxygen partial pressure in some locations can be as low as 0–2.5 mmHg, which creates a hypoxic environment around the tumor compared to the normal tissue's 30–40 mmHg oxygen partial pressure [3,6,16]. The oxygen partial pressure in normal tissues is around 30 mmHg, whereas it steadily drops from the outside to the inside of tumor tissues and reaches a low level (5 mmHg) in some areas; and in some solid tumors, it may even be close to 0 mmHg. Hypoxia in the TME can upregulate hypoxia-inducible factors (HIFs), a protein dimerization made up of the HIF-(oxygen-sensitive subunit) and HIF-(constitutively expressed subunit) subunits that can promote tumor growth and metastasis. This hypoxic adaptation influences activities like cell energy metabolism, endocytic receptor internalization, transmembrane receptor recirculation, and transportation by altering the general biochemical environment around cells [3,17,18]. Hypoxia is becoming the main focus of both diagnosis and treatment because of the obvious differences between tumor tissue and normal tissue. In order to treat and image tumors, hypoxia can therefore be exploited as an endogenous stimulation. Quinone, nitroaromatic, and azobenzene derivatives are the principal functional groups that react to hypoxia and have been widely used as hypoxia-responsive nanomedicine or nanoprobes [6,19–22]. Hypoxia sensitive polymers have shown potential in developing trigger-release nanomedicine responses to specific TME conditions.

1.4. Targeting TME with High Level of ROS

The concentration of ROS, which is 2–5 times greater in tumor tissues than in normal tissues, has been reported. The production of ROS, particularly hydrogen peroxide (H_2O_2), is essential for several physiological activities [23,24]. Through processes involving the mitochondrial respiratory chain and nicotinamide adenine dinucleotide phosphate oxidase, the majority of tumor cells create more ROS than normal cells. Based on the high amounts of ROS in tumor tissues, many ROS-responsive polymers have been investigated. These include unsaturated lipids, sulfur, selenium, tellurium, and other ROS-sensitive groups. High ROS level has been used as a stimulus to trigger drug release from nanomedicine in TME [25,26].

1.5. Targeting Specific Enzymes in TME

Some enzymes are overexpressed in tumor tissues compared to regular tissues. Matrix metalloproteinases (MMPs), hyaluronidase, glucosidase, and esterase are all examples of enzymes that are oversecreted in the TME. Drugs can be released in the TME from nanomedicines by having them modified with enzyme substrates [3,27,28]. MMPs, which are overexpressed in the extracellular environment of many malignancies, are an attractive target for drug release triggers [29].

1.6. The Enhanced Permeability and Retention (EPR) Effect and Its Application in Nanomedicine Delivery

To be effective, nanomedicines need to do more than simply circulate throughout the body. Thus, the preferential accumulation of nanomedicines in solid tumors is important for the advancement of anticancer therapy. The EPR effect increases the retention of the macromolecules and mediates the prominent accumulation of drug carriers in tumors. With the systemic injection, long-circulating PEGylated nanoparticles have a better chance of targeting tumors due to the increased EPR effect. Circulating nanomedicines can preferentially concentrate in tumors because the apertures prevalent throughout the tumor vasculature (>400 nm) are considerably greater than those of endothelial fenestrae in the liver [30–32]. Tumors have a varied blood supply and permeability, which may induce an inhomogeneity in the delivery of nanomedicines across the tumor sites. The EPR effect is the primary mechanism through which nanoparticles accumulate in tumor tissue. Nanoparticles have more difficulty moving through the vasculature of any given tissue, whereas tiny molecules can do so with relative ease. Because tumors and healthy tissues have distinct vascular networks, malignancies are a major source of the EPR effect [33]. Therefore, the carriers should have a prolonged blood half-life and successful extravasation and deep penetration from the blood compartment into tumor tissues, as well as have the ability to exploit the EPR effect for tumor targeting and uniformly distribute adequate dosages of drugs [34,35].

1.7. Micelles as Nanomedicine Delivery Systems

The nanomedicine approach to delivering hydrophobic drugs is becoming a common and effective strategy for overcoming the challenges associated with drug delivery. In order to achieve the desired therapeutic response, an adequate quantity of the active drug must arrive at the site of action, and the effective concentration of the drug must be kept at the target location for a predetermined amount of time. However, this process is hampered for the vast majority of drugs due to several obstacles. These include rapid degradation of drugs in an in vivo environment, inadequate pharmacokinetics (PK), a lack of selectivity for the tissues that are being targeted, and the possibility of systemic toxicity [34]. In order to encapsulate drugs, nanoparticulate medicines such as polymer-based micelles have been utilized. Nanomedicines have the potential to accomplish both sustained circulation and accumulation at the target site [36].

To form polymeric micelles, biocompatible synthetic polymers or natural macromolecules can be used. The core-forming segments are primarily responsible for determining important aspects of the polymeric micelle, such as shape, stability, drug-loading capacity, and drug-release profile [37,38]. When compared to conventional drug delivery systems, the nanosize of the micelles makes it possible for the drug to extravasate via the leaky vasculature more effectively. The hydrophilic polymeric coating will make it possible for them to avoid being detected by the reticuloendothelial system while they are in circulation. Because of the hydrophilic shell of the micelle, nanoparticles are able to maintain their steric stability and experience less non-specific absorption by the reticuloendothelial system (RES). This results in a longer period of time spent circulating throughout the body. In order for micelles to be successfully delivered, they need to maintain a steady circulation in the blood compartment while avoiding undesired interactions with blood components and the RES. Micelles should also selectively extravasate at the sick (tumor) location, where the target cells can pick them up and release them intracellularly. Micelles should also extravasate at the diseased site. Micelles can be administered directly into the bloodstream, which allows for rapid and uniform distribution throughout the body. This route is often used for cancer treatments, as it allows for targeted delivery of chemotherapy drugs to tumor sites. The other routes of administration such as oral, transmucosal or topical administration are utilized to deliver micellar formulation for various localized non-cancer diseases.

Nanomedicine with a macromolecular or particulate nature can aggregate in the tumor tissues and remain in the TME in order to prolong its retention time at the target location since the arterial walls are damaged and leaky, and the lymphatic drainage is poor. Over the course of the last few decades, various types of micelles have been explored for their potential use in the administration of chemotherapy drugs in cancer therapy [39–42]. Though various types of stimuli responsive micelles have been reported in the literature for various therapeutic uses, the materials that are used in the construction of micelles in recent years are not well documented, which is the focus of this review. Furthermore, this review provides recent updates on the clinical trials and procedures related to regulatory submissions for micellar nanocarrier systems.

2. Characteristic Features of Micelles

Because of the mechanical and physical properties that they possess, certain polymers and surfactants have the ability to self-assemble into specific systems. The fact that it puts itself together can help the structure be more stable. The concentration at which the polymers or surfactants prefer to assemble themselves in ordered micellar structures is referred to as the Critical Micelle Concentration (CMC). Since the surface tension of a solution is affected by the concentration of the polymer in the solution, it is possible to utilize surface tension to calculate CMC. The fluorometric method, the approach based on surface tension, the method based on light scattering, the method based on electric conductivity, the method based on osmotic pressure, the method based on the surface plasmon resonance, and the method based on electric conductivity are some of the more common methods used to determine CMCs. Micelles are formed through the self-assembly of amphiphilic polymers at the CMC. The Krafft point, also known as critical micelle temperature (CMT), is the minimum temperature at which the detergent will form micelles. At its CMT, the solubility of a surfactant is equal to its critical micelle concentration, indicating that the surfactant can form micelles. For detergents, insolubility causes precipitation at temperatures below CMT at or above the detergent's CMC. Micelles are produced when block copolymers, random block copolymers, and grafted polymers self-assemble into their desired structures. Transmission electron microscopy, atomic force microscopy, small-angle neutron scattering, small-angle X-ray scattering, dynamic light scattering, and electron paramagnetic resonance spectroscopy are some of the methods that are used to characterize the micelles [43–48].

Polymeric micelles are self-assembled in aqueous environments from amphiphilic polymers, which are the building blocks of polymeric micelles, as shown in Figure 1. The construction of these amphiphilic polymers involves the use of a variety of polymeric building components. The blocks are able to be customized depending on the need for an optimal balance of hydrophobic and lipophilic groups, size, drug loading capability, micellization ability, and stability in the systemic circulation. When the concentration reaches CMC or even higher, the amphiphilic polymers will self-assemble into micelles in the shape of spheres. The brush-like structure of the head, which is hydrophilic, combines to form the shell, while the hydrophobic tail aggregates to form the inner core of the structure. Through the use of hydrophobic interactions, hydrophobic drugs can be contained inside this core. The hydrophilic units that are present in the micelle's shell will engage in interactions with the water molecules that are in its immediate environment. The micelles are highly stable in the liquid state in the aqueous solution [43,49,50]. The size and shape of micelles can be analyzed by scanning electron microscopy and transmission electron microscopy.

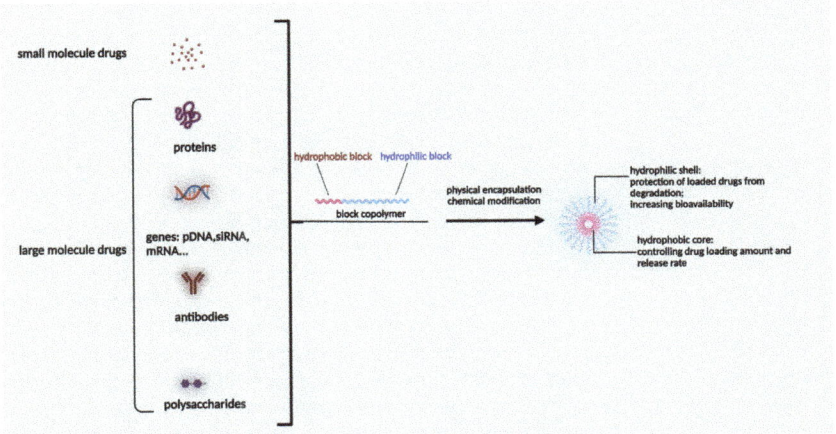

Figure 1. Structure of polymeric micelles for loading small and large molecule drugs. Created with BioRender.com.

The drug loading is affected by its hydrophobic interaction with the micellar core, as well as polar interactions and hydrogen bonding to some extent [51]. The drug loading efficiency can also be affected by the hydrophobic block chain length, the substituted groups, and the block copolymer aggregates [52]. The micellar structures in the physiological environment should be stable and long circulating to enable their uptake by the tumor tissue and should not cause any side effects during their fate in the body.

The physical stability of micelles is dependent on the CMC, which is determined by the hydrophilic and hydrophobic nature of the polymer, and polymers with long hydrophobic chains show lower stability. The physical state of the micelle core, amount of solvent, size of the hydrophobic block, and hydrophobic/hydrophilic balance of the polymer determine the physical stability of the micelles. The physical stability of polymeric micelles can be higher for materials with low CMC values. Increased intra-micellar interactions and covalent cross-linking of the micelle core can also increase physical stability [53]. The drug loading efficiency and physical stability were increased by attaching fatty acids to the core of polyethylene oxide-poly(aspartic acid) (PEO-P(Asp)) micelles, modifying the core with structures capable of forming intra-micellar structures and electrostatic interactions, and covalent cross-linking [52,54].

3. Polymers Used for Micelle Formation

The assembly of the block copolymer, the arrangement of the polymers, the stability of micelles, and their biodistribution are all determined by the segments of the block copolymer. When choosing polymers, on the other hand, it is important to take into account the structure of the micelle complex as well as the inherent safety of these polymers. These polymers make it possible for micelles to dissolve and be expelled from the body, hence preventing any adverse long-term effects [41]. The covalent binding of drugs to polymers that dissolve in water can extend their half-life in the bloodstream and reduce their toxicity to healthy cells and tissue. Polymers have been modified by including polyethylene glycol (PEG) to prevent opsonization and lengthen their circulation time, incorporating targeting ligands, and employing pH-sensitive or hypothermic polymer conjugates [55,56].

PEG is the most popular and most effective stealth polymer in the field of polymer-based drug delivery is PEG. Twenty years have passed since the introduction of the first PEGylated products for sale. Hypersensitivity, unexpected changes in pharmacokinetic behavior, toxic side products, an antagonism arising from the easy degradation of the polymer, and the resulting possible accumulation in the body may all need consideration. PEG is very soluble in organic solvents, making it simple to modify its end groups. PEG is an excellent polymer for use in biological systems, since it is soluble in water and has a low intrinsic toxicity. The hydrophilicity of PEG improves the solubility of hydrophobic medicines or carriers in water. It improves the physical and thermal stability of pharmaceuticals and eliminates or greatly decreases drug aggregation in vivo and in storage [57,58]. Polysaccharides are a wide variety of polymeric substances with natural origins, known as polysaccharides. Polysaccharides are found naturally, are renewable, pose no health risks, and break down quickly. They are created through the glycosidic bonding of monosaccharides. The architecture of polysaccharides can be either linear or branching, depending on the type of monosaccharide unit. Polysaccharides have a variety of reactive groups, such as hydroxyl, amino, and carboxylic acid groups, which further suggests the potential for chemical alteration. These functional groups can be used to modify polysaccharides with small molecules, polymers, and crosslinkers, and the resulting modified polysaccharides have proven to be useful building blocks in the development of novel biomaterials for use in a wide range of biomedical settings, including as drug delivery carriers, cell-encapsulating biomaterials, and tissue engineering scaffolds. Further increasing diversity, polysaccharide molecular weight can range from hundreds to thousands of Daltons. The majority of polysaccharides are susceptible to enzymatic breakdown as a result of their natural existence in the body. Polysaccharides can be recycled for use as storage, structural support, or even cell signaling by breaking them down into their monomer or oligomer building parts through enzyme catalysis [59–64]. Regarding Poly[N-(2-hydroxypropyl) methacrylamide], pHPMA, research into pHPMA's potential as a polymeric micelle building block has focused on both its use as a hydrophilic shell component and its use as a hydrophobic core derivative. As a potential building block of polymeric micelles with a hydrophilic, shell-forming property, pHPMA is a promising contender. In comparison to PEG, pHPMA is advantageous due to its multifunctionality, which permits the conjugation of numerous therapeutic or targeting molecules to a single polymer chain without compromising biocompatibility or non-immunogenicity [65–68]. Regarding Poly(amino acids), because of their many useful properties, including biodegradability, biocompatibility, and the availability of side functional groups, poly(amino acid) and its derivatives are commonly used to form polymeric micelles. These materials have several applications due to their many desirable properties, including biodegradability, biocompatibility, and a high number of side functional groups. With the right design of hydrophobic segments and the right amount of side functional groups, these polymeric micelles often exhibit a high drug loading capacity for both hydrophobic and hydrophilic agents. Due to the adaptability of their chemical structures and the availability of functional groups on polymer, micelles of amphiphilic poly(amino acid) copolymers can load a wide variety of potential pharmaceuticals through non-covalent contact. Engineering of the polymeric structure also allows for a high drug loading capacity in these micelles. Special strategies, such as crosslinking and layer-by-layer coating, may thereby further stabilize the drug-loaded micelles in terms of physical loading [69–71]. Regarding polyethers, developments in polyether-based amphiphilic nanocarriers have made it possible to easily distribute active components while avoiding the toxicity, unwanted side effects, and hypersensitivity reactions associated with conventional surfactants. Delivering active components at high dilutions in the bloodstream is now possible thanks to the low CMCs of these nanocarriers. PEG often conjugates with these polyethers. The PEG-based amphiphilic nanocarriers show optimal biocompatibility over cellular and systemic levels. They may have drawbacks, including degradation under stress, accumulation in the body above an uncertain excretion limit, and interaction with the immune system. Since PEG has very uninteresting end group functionality, there is not much room for alteration at the polyether backbone to modify [34,72]. Regarding polyesters (such as poly(L, D-lactide), PLA), PLA has the mechanical and physical qualities that may be designed to fit a wide variety of uses, and PLA is also biodegradable via hydrolysis and enzymatic activity, and it has a low immunogenicity characteristic. The Food and Drug Administration (FDA) has authorized various formulations incorporating PLA, further demonstrating its suitability for rapid clinical translation. These biomaterials can be made into a wide variety of useful products, including sutures, scaffolds, cell carriers, medication delivery systems, and more. Numerous studies, both laboratory and human, have been conducted on PLA. Liposomes, polymeric nanoparticles, dendrimers, and micelles are only a few of the nanoparticle drug carriers that can be loaded with PLA to encapsulate hydrophobic anti-tumor medicines and protect the body from their systemic toxicity. It is an ever-evolving discipline that sees modest improvements in the clinical translation of these technologies from preclinical experimental settings [73,74]. A summary of the polymers commonly used for polymeric micelles is listed in Tables 1 and 2.

Table 1. Features of hydrophilic polymers commonly used for polymeric micelles.

Polymer	Structure	Advantages	Disadvantages	Ref
PEG		Clinically approved Stealth behavior Prolonged blood circulation Diminished RES uptake Enhanced permeability and retention effect	Unexpected changes in PK behavior Non-biodegradable	[57,58]
Polysaccharides		Non-toxic Biodegradable Stealth behavior Facilitating mucoadhesion Enhanced targeting of specific tissues Enhanced a reduction in the inflammatory response Easy for modification	Its degradation (oxidation) characteristics at high temperatures (above their melting point), which are often required in industrial processes Toxicity due to impurities	[59–63]
pHPMA		Non-toxic Non-immunogenic Biocompatible Pendant groups readily engineered	Only a few soluble drug conjugates have entered clinical trials Complicated synthesis The unsatisfactory characteristics of the conjugate molecules The tendency for such conjugates to perform differently in preclinical animal models than in the human body	[65–68,75]
Poly(acrylic acid)		pH sensitive, mucoadhesive Biodegradable Biocompatible	Poor mechanical properties, its structures need to be modified for use	[69–71,76]

Table 1. Cont.

Polymer	Structure	Advantages	Disadvantages	Ref
Poly(glutamic acid)		pH sensitive Biodegradable Biocompatible Easy for chemical modification	α- poly(glutamic acid) synthetically produced has a lower molecular mass which limits its application High cost of production	[71,77]
Polyvinyl alcohol		Widely used for cross-linking synthesis Biocompatible Non-immunogenic Non-toxic	Under wet conditions, its properties are diminished because of the plasticizing action of water molecules	[78–80]
Poly(N-vinyl-2-pyrrolidone)		Containing cationic groups for modification	Non-biodegradable Hygroscopic	[81–83]
Poly(N-isopropyl acrylamide) (PNIAAm)		Thermo sensitive controlling payload release	In vivo studies are still pending for most copolymers, grafted polymers, and biopolymer-conjugates investigated up to today due to high cost and ethical restrictions for in vivo analysis to test their viability	[84,85]
Poly(ethylene imine)		Facilitating to escape from endosome and payload release in cytoplasm Facilitating cellular uptake	Positively charged with toxicity Difficult to release negatively charged payloads due to strong electro attraction	[86]

Table 2. Features of hydrophobic polymers commonly used for polymeric micelles.

Polymer	Structure	Advantage	Disadvantage	Ref
Poly(histidine) (PHIS)		hydrophilic at acidic pH condition; hydrophobic at pH around 7.4, pH sensitive Biocompatible Biodegradable Facilitating to escape from endosome and payload release in cytoplasm	Poly(histidine) is too sensitive to environmental pH, which could affect the stability of the core The chain length also affects the anticancer efficacy and the pH responsive drug release rate	[87,88]
Polyethers (i.e., poly(propylene oxide; block copolymers such as Pluronics)	Pluronics:	Widely used, commercially available Non-expensive Pluronics are thermoresponsive.	Low affinity with drug molecules	[34,72]
Polyesters (i.e., poly(lactide), poly(lactide-co-glycolide), poly(ε-caprolactone), poly(β-amino ester)), poly(glycolic acid), poly(lactide-co-caprolactone))	Poly(lactide) (PLA): Poly(lactide-co-glycolide) (PLGA): Poly(ε-caprolactone) (PCL): Poly(glycolic acid) (PGA): Poly(lactide-co-caprolactone) (PLCA):	Biodegradable and biocompatible. These are the most used polymers for drug delivery. They show excellent control on the drug release rates. Poly(β-amino ester) is pH sensitive, providing stimuli-responsive drug release, and is used for gene carriers and increased cell uptake due to positive charges. Poly(glycolic acid) is thermoplastic, enabling a stimuli response.	High hydrophobicity and subsequently entrapment by macrophages through the opsonization process, long-term degradation time, and low loading for hydrophilic drugs. PLA induces the production of lactic acid due to polymer degradation, which leads to the formation of an acidic microenvironment. PLA shows initial burst release with significant drug loss and drug-related toxicity. PCL has a slow degradation time. Poly(β-amino ester): cationic charges may be toxic to cells. Poly(glycolic acid) has a fast degradation time with fast drug release.	[34,73,89–93]

4. Micelles in Tumor Targeted Drug Release

Polymeric micelles are a novel type of drug delivery system that offers a variety of advantages. These advantages include fewer adverse effects of systematic toxicity, more selective targeting to specific tissues due to stimuli-sensitive polymeric materials, storage stability, and resistance toward dilution. In addition, the nanoscale sizes of polymeric micelles are distributed in an extremely confined manner. The vast majority of polymeric micelles containing hydrophobic small molecules were designed with the intention of delivering hydrophobic anticancer drugs, the administration of which normally necessitates the injection of surfactants as well as organic solvents. Micelles, because of their core-shell structure, have the ability to shield pharmaceuticals against oxidation in both in vitro and in vivo settings. It is also feasible to produce polymeric micelles by using the appropriate pharmacological chemicals [34].

Anticancer drugs need frequent dosing during the course of treatment to keep an effective concentration of the drug in the tumor sites. The severity of chronic toxicities and even the development of acquired drug resistance can both be a consequence of this. Therefore, polymeric micelles are highly advantageous for stabilizing the drugs in aqueous conditions, shielding the agents from the outside environment within their core, maintaining stable blood circulation, and specifically accumulating in solid tumors where they can release the loaded drugs in a controlled manner. This is because they can shield the agents from the outside environment within their core. Moreover, they are advantageous for maintaining stable blood circulation. Drugs can be physically incorporated into the core of micelles by one of the two methods: (i) by the interaction with the hydrophobic core-forming segment of the polymer, or (ii) they can be conjugated to the polymer backbone using labile bonds, which can be cleaved under specific conditions to recover the active drug [36,43,94].

To achieve targeted drug release, the micelles system has been modified to make it responsive to stimuli within the tumors. The nanoparticles and micelles are programmed to deteriorate or disassemble in response to the stimuli that are present at the target site or that are applied externally in order to free the payload that is inside. External stimuli include light, temperature, and localized magnetic fields, whereas TME-specific ligands include pH, upregulated enzymes, and a hypoxic environment. Due to the fact that they have shifted their metabolism away from that of normal cells, tumor cells create lactic acid as a result of their adaptation to anaerobic glycolysis [95,96]. A number of enzymes, including matrix metalloproteinases, have been found to have their activity levels increased near the tumor site. Because of the weakened blood arteries, the solid tumor's core has a poor oxygen supply. This is because oxygen cannot get to the core. As a result, various markers of hypoxia have been found to be increased in solid tumors. The easiest way to make polymeric micelles sensitive to stimuli is to introduce linkers that are sensitive to pH, enzymes, or hypoxia between the hydrophobic core and the hydrophilic corona. This makes it so that when a stimuli-trigger is applied, the linker breaks down, causing the micelles to disassemble and release the drug inside [29,34,43,94]. The stimuli-sensitive polymers used for micelle formation are shown in Table 3.

Table 3. Stimuli polymeric micelles for drug delivery.

Stimuli	Polymeric Carrier	Payload	Release Mechanism	Application	Ref
pH	Poly(L-histidine)-b-poly(ethylene glycol)/poly(L-lactic acid)-b-poly(ethylene glycol-folate	Doxorubicin	Protonation of PHIS	PHIS destabilizes micelles and triggers doxorubicin release	[97]
	Poly(ethylene glycol-block-poly[(1,4-butanediol)-diacrylate-β-5-amino-1-pentanol]/2,3-dimethylmaleic anhydride-polyethyleneimine-b-poly[(1,4-butanediol)-diacrylate-β-5-amino-1-pentanol]	Paclitaxel	Protonation of poly[(1,4-butanediol)-diacrylate-β-5-amino-1-pentanol]	2,3-dimethylmaleic anhydride enhances micelles internalization; poly[(1,4-butanediol)-diacrylate-β-5-amino-1-pentanol] dissociates micelles and triggers paclitaxel release	[98]
	Methyl poly(ethylene glycol)ether-b-poly (β-amino esters)-b-poly lactic acid	Doxorubicin	Protonation of poly(β-amino esters)	Poly(β-amino esters decreases hydrophobicity of micelles at acidic condition and triggers doxorubicin release	[99]
	Poly(ethylene glycol)-poly(L-histidine)-poly(L-lactide)	Doxorubicin	Protonation of PHIS	PHIS swells and relocates to the surface of the micelles to trigger doxorubicin release	[100]
	Methoxy-poly (ethylene glycol)-b-poly (ε-caprolactone)-b-poly (diethylaminoethyl methacrylate)	Curcumin	Protonation of poly (diethylaminoethyl methacrylate)	Poly (diethylaminoethyl methacrylate) switch from hydrophobic to hydrophilic to change micelles structure and triggers release Curcumin	[101]
	Poly(2-(diisopropylamino)ethyl methacrylate-co-2-(2′,3′,5′-triiodobenzoyl)ethyl methacrylate)	Dextran/Doxorubicin	Protonation of poly(2-(diisopropylamino)	Poly(2-(diisopropylamino) switch from a hydrophobic to a hydrophilic state under acidic conditions upon protonation, which deceases the stability of micelles and triggers drug release	[102]
	Methyl ether poly(ethylene glycol)-poly (β-amino ester)	Camptothecin	Protonation of poly(β-amino ester)	Poly(β-amino ester facilitates a pH-dependant micellization/demicellization transition and triggers camptothecin	[103]
	Poly (ethylene glycol) methyl ether-b-(poly lactic acid-co-poly(β-amino esters))	Doxorubicin	Protonation of poly(β-amino ester)	Poly(β-amino ester) destabilizes micelles and triggers doxorubicin release	[104]
	Methoxy poly (ethylene oxide)-b-poly (aspartate-hydrazide)	Doxorubicin/SN-38	Hydrolisis of Hydrazone bond	Se-Se bond exerting redox responsiveness and Hydrazone bond hydrolyzing decrease micelles stability and trigger Doxorubicin/SN-38 release	[105]
	Hyaluronic acid-S-S-Podophyllotoxin	Podophyllotoxin	Cleavage of acid-sensitive ester bonds	Ester bonds and disulfide bonds cleave to decrease micelle stability and podophyllotoxin releases from micelles	[106]

Table 3. Cont.

Stimuli	Polymeric Carrier	Payload	Release Mechanism	Application	Ref
ROS	Hydrazide functionalized methoxy poly(ethylene glycol)-block-poly(ε-caprolactone)	LCA	Electrorepulsion between LCA and the copolymer	Loss of ionic interaction between LCA and micelles triggers LCA release	[107]
	Chitosan coated hyaluronic acid-oleic acid	Doxorubicin/siPD-L1	Protonation of the amino group of COS	Decomposition of copolymer shell, the swelling of COS, and disulfide bond cleavage trigger drug release	[108]
	Methoxypolyethylene glycols-b-poly (6-O-methacryloyl-d-galactopyranose)-disulfide bond-doxorubicin	Doxorubicin	Destability of hydrazone bonds	The destability of hydrazone bonds decrease micelles stability; the break of disulfide bonds causes decreased hydrophobicity in the micellar inner cores and dissociates the conjugates to release doxorubicin	[109]
	Polyethylene glycol-p(2-aminoethyl methacrylate hydrochloride-camptothecin conjugated hydroxyethyl methacrylate-oxalyl chloride	β-Lapachone/camptothecin	Breaking the H_2O_2-cleavable linkage from camptothecin	The removal of camptothecin enhances the disassembly of the micelles and drug release	[110]
	Poly(β-thioether ester)-poly (ethylene glycol)-lipoic acid	Doxorubicin	Thioether group and disulfide bond cleavage	The cleavage of disulfide bonds and β-thiopropionate linkers decrease in core crosslinking density and trigger doxorubicin release	[111]
	Methoxy poly(ethylene glycol)-thioketal-poly(ε-caprolactone)	Doxorubicin	Thioketal bond cleavage	π-π interactions increase drug loading; thioketal bond cleavage increases doxorubicin release	[112]
	Poly(l-methionine-block-l-lysine)-PLGLAG-methoxy poly(ethylene glycol)	Doxorubicin	MMP-sensitive linkers (PLGLAG) cleavage	Poly-l-lysine chains assist the cellular penetration by electrostatic interactions; thioether converts to a sulfoxide moiety to cause a phase transitions and micelle structure break to release Doxorubicin	[113]
	CD147-Carboxymethyl chitosan-phenylboronic acid pinacol ester	Doxorubicin/CD147	Oxidation of phenylboronic acid pinacol ester	The micelles exert CD147 targeting effect; ROS depolymerizes micelles and triggers doxorubicin release	[114]
	Poly(ethylene glycol)-poly[aspartamidoethyl (p-boronobenzyl)diethylammonium bromide]	miR-34a mimic/volasertib (BI6727)	Boronic acid reaction	Boronic acid produces tertiary amines and p-quinone methide to enhance micelle degradation and release drugs	[115]
	Poly(propylene sulfide)-poly(N-isopropylacrylamide)	Doxorubicin	Hydrophobic (thioether)-to-hydrophilic (sulfoxide, sulfone) transition of thioether	Poly(propylene sulfide) decreases micelles stability and triggers doxorubicin release	[116]

Table 3. *Cont.*

Stimuli	Polymeric Carrier	Payload	Release Mechanism	Application	Ref
	Methyl ether poly(ethylene glycol)-poly(ester-thioether)	Doxorubicin	Oxidation of thioether	Enhance drug loading content via the π-π interaction	[117]
	Poly(ethylene glycol)-poly(N6-carbobenzyloxy-l-lysine)-poly(β-benzyl-l-aspartate)	Doxorubicin	Thioketal bond cleavage	The primary-amine-rich pLys block would provide interlace sites for the ROS cleavable cross-linker and then increases doxorubicin release	[118]
	Imidazole groups conjugate polyethylene glycol-conjugated triphenylphosphonium	Doxorubicin	TK bonds cleavage	Imidazole groups protonation and TK bonds cleavage release doxorubicin	[119]
Hypoxia	Poly(ethylene glycol)-*block*-poly(methacrylic acid-*co*-2-nitroimidazole methacrylate)	Doxorubicin	2-nitroimidazole converting to hydrophilic 2-aminoimidazole	2-nitroimidazole groups enhances expansion and self-disassembly of micelles, then triggers doxorubicin release	[120]
	Polyethyleneimine-C6-2-nitroimidazole	siRNA	2-nitroimidazole converting to hydrophilic 2-aminoimidazole	2-nitroimidazole elicits a loose structure to facilitate the siRNA dissociation in the cytoplasm	[121]
	Poly(ethylene glycol-poly(ε-(4-nitro)benzyloxycarbonyl-l-lysine)	Doxorubicin	Degradation of poly(ε-(4-nitro)benzyloxycarbonyl-l-lysine)	Self-immolation of poly(ε-(4-nitrobenzyloxycarbonyl-l-lysine) derivative triggers doxorubicin release	[122]
	Poly(ethylene glycol)-azobenzene-polyethyleneimine-DOPE	siRNA/ Doxorubicin	Cleavage of azobenzene	Cleavage of azobenzene triggers PEG shedding and leads to drug release	[123]
	Methoxy poly(ethylene glycol)-azobenzene-4,4-diamino-poly(d,l-lactide)	Docetaxel	Reductive cleavage of azobenzene	Reductive cleavage leads to structural change of self-assembled micelles and triggers docetaxel release	[124]
	Folic acid-poly(ethylene glycol)-2-nitroimidazole	Sorafenib	Hydrophobic-to-hydrophilic transition of nitro of nitroimidazole	Cohesion of the hydrophobic core of the micelles is weakened; hydrophobic inner core weakens the binding force of the hydrophobic drug, which is more prone to drug leakage and promotes sorafenib release	[125]
	Alendronate-poly(ethylene glycol)-azobenzene-poly-l-lysine	Doxorubicin	Reductive cleavage of azobenzene	Azobenzene cleavage for micelle disassembly triggers doxorubicin release	[126]
	Glucose-poly(ethylene glycol)-azobenzene-IR808-S-S-Paclitaxel	Paclitaxel	Reductive cleavage of azobenzene	Glucose modification promotes cellular uptake; azobenzene cleavage triggers IR808-S-S-PTX release; disulfide bond cleavage triggers paclitaxel release	[127]

Table 3. Cont.

Stimuli	Polymeric Carrier	Payload	Release Mechanism	Application	Ref
Enzyme	Polyethylene glycol-block-poly(acrylic acid)	Doxorubicin	Amidase cleavaging the covalent linked doxorubicin from the micelles	Amidase causes the breakage of amide bond between doxorubicin molecules and polymers, and then triggers disassembly of the micelles to facilitate the doxorubicin release	[128]
	Monomethyl poly(ethylene glycol)-ss-camptothecin/phenylboronic acid-poly(ethylene glycol)-4,4′-(diazene-1,2-diyl)benzoyl-poly(ε-caprolactone)	Camptothecin	Azoreductase	Azoreductase and NADPH facilitates the azobenzene bonds cleavage and GSH facilitate disulfide bond cleavage, which trigger camptothecin release	[129]
	Poly(ethylene glycol)-peptide-polyethyleneimine-1,2-dioleoyl-sn-glycero-3-phosphoethanolamine	Paclitaxel/siRNA	Metalloproteinase 2 cleavage	Polyethyleneimine increases cellular uptake and delivers siRNA and facilitates endosome escape; MMP2 decreases micelles stability and release drugs	[130]
	Methoxypolyethylene glycol amine-glutathione-palmitic acid	Dexamethasone	Glutathione reductase	Glutathione reductase breaks micelles structure and triggers dexamethasone release	[131]
	Poly(ethylene glycol)-b-poly(l-tyrosine)	JQ1	Proteinase K	π–π stacking for efficient and stable encapsulation of JQ1; PTyr degradation by proteinase K triggers JQ1 release	[132]
	D-α-tocopherol polyethylene glycol 3350 succinate-Gly-Pro-Leu-Gly-Val-Arg-doxorubicin/FA-Asp-Glu-Val-Asp-doxorubicin	Doxorubicin	Matrix metalloproteinase (MMP-9); caspase-3	MMP-9 increases micelles endocytosis; caspase-3 increases doxorubicin release	[133]
Thermo	Monomethoxy poly(ethylene glycol)-deoxycholic acid	Estradiol	Lower critical solution temperature (LCST) transition of the micelles facilitating dehydration of the PEG shell	Thermosensitive micelles with a rigid core minimizes the initial burst release of estradiol encapsulated by coating the shell at a temperature above its LCST through the thermal transition	[134]
	Poly(t-butyl acrylate-co-acrylic acid)-b-poly(N-isopropylacrylamide)/chitosan-g-poly(N-isopropylacrylamide)	Doxorubicin	Poly(N-isopropylacrylamide) exerting temperature responsiveness	The pH-sensitive poly(t-butyl acrylate-co-acrylic acid) encapsulates doxorubicin by electrostatic interactions; and the poly(N-isopropylacrylamide) plays the role of aqueous solubilization and responses to temperature changes, and triggers doxorubicin release	[135]
	Poly(N-isopropylacrylamide-b-butylmethacrylat	Adriamycin	Poly(N-isopropylacrylamide) phase transistion	Poly(N-isopropylacrylamide) reverses micelle structure to trigger Adriamycin release	[136]

Table 3. *Cont.*

Stimuli	Polymeric Carrier	Payload	Release Mechanism	Application	Ref
Magnetic	P-(N,N-isopropylacrylamide-co-N-hydroxymethylacrylamide)-b-caprolactone	Doxorubicin	Poly(N-isopropylacrylamide) phase transisition	Poly(N-isopropylacrylamide) reverses micelle structure to trigger doxorubicin release	[137]
	RGD-poly[(N-isopropylacrylamide-r-acrylamide)-b-L-lactic acid]/oleic acid-SPIONs	Paclitaxel	Magnetic hyperthermia	Hydrophobic PLA segments incorporates SPIONs and paclitaxel, RGD serves as a targeting moiety, and SPIONs concentrate paclitaxel to targeted sites	[138]
	Poly(phenyl isocyanide)s	Doxorubicin/Fe_3O_4 nanoparticles	Magnetic hyperthermia	The loading of magnetic Fe_3O_4 nanoparticles contributes to the hyperthermia performance; effective drug release due to the morphology change of thermoresponsive poly(phenyl isocyanide)s	[139]

4.1. pH Sensitive Micelles

To specifically target TME with specific acidity, polymeric micelles derived from pH-sensitive block copolymers have been developed. The physical or chemical properties of segments from these micelles are sensitive to moderate shifts in pH values. Particle shrinkage or disruption can be induced by the segment, leading to rapid release kinetics from the micelles at tumor sites. These pH sensitive micelles can use slight pH changes to modify the micelles' biodistribution and their interactions with tissues and cells. These characteristics allow encapsulated drugs to circumvent issues, including nonspecific toxicity, insufficient tumor selectivity, and the emergence of multidrug resistance in tumor cells [140,141]. If the pH of the surrounding environment changes, protons will be absorbed by the block copolymer if it contains weak acidic groups or released if it has weak basic groups. The extracellular pH of healthy tissues and blood is 7.4, whereas it is between 6.0 and 6.5 in malignant tissues. Researchers have used the endosomal and lysosomal pH disparity between healthy and cancerous tissues as a trigger for the release of chemotherapy drugs. The pH-sensitive micelles can be twisted to help release drugs under moderately acidic circumstances outside or inside the tumor cells, which improves therapeutic efficacy and reduces unwanted effects because of the presence of an ionic block or an acid-labile link [142,143].

A few research reports have recently been published based on pH-sensitive micelles' applications. Zeng et al. prepared mixed micelles from curcumin-hyaluronic acid conjugate (HC) and D-α-tocopherol acid polyethylene glycolsuccinate as carriers and dasatinib as the core. The mixed micelles were designed for co-delivery of curcumin and dasatinib for increased solubility and stability of the drugs and to increase the circulation time of micelles for an EPR effect. The system also utilized active targeting via the use of hyaluronic acid to the CD44 protein in tumor cells. The pH-sensitive ester bonds in the HC conjugate activated the micelles and release drugs in the tumor micro-acid environment. The co-delivery of curcumin and dasatinib from hyaluronic acid-based micelles effectively targeted CD4 overexpressed HepG2 cells and produced a synergistic effect. The micelles showed significant inhibition of tumor growth and reduced toxic side effects in a mouse solid tumor model of liver cancer [144]. A novel pH-sensitive drug delivery system for daunorubicin was created using poly (oligo (ethylene glycol) methyl ether methacrylate and 2-aminoethyl methacrylate hydrochloride (AMA) and 4-azibo benzyl methacrylate and 2-aminoethyl methacrylate hydrochloride. The micelles were with a particle size of 132 nm and showed 13 and 73% drug release at pH 5.0 and 7.4, respectively. The cytotoxicity against HeLa cells suggested its potential for enhanced cancer therapy. The pH-sensitive and charge-conversion micelles exhibited potential for use in cancer therapy [145]. The combination of Paclitaxel, Etoposide, and Rapamycin targets different pathways to kill cancer cells, but their low water solubility limits their clinical use. To overcome this, pH-sensitive polymeric micelles made of methyl PEG-pH-PCL polymer were developed to improve solubility and delivery to cancer cells. The pH-sensitive polymeric micelles display varying drug release behaviors based on the differential pH of tumors and healthy tissues. As the pH decreases, as in tumors, the release rate of each drug increases, resulting in improved drug levels in tumor cells. The micelles showed improved bioavailability of drugs compared to respective solutions. These drug-loaded monomethoxy PEG-pH-PCL micelles were therefore considered a beneficial option for gastric cancer treatment [146]. Lin et al. reported a pH sensitive micelle system based on O-(2-aminoethyl)-O'-methylpoly(ethylene glycol) 5000, 1-(3-aminopropyl) imidazole, and cinnamate onto polysuccinimide. The hydrophobic anticancer drug paclitaxel was successfully encapsulated within the polymeric micelles. Before being cross-linked in a low-pH environment, the drug-loaded micelles released the drug in a single burst due to the micelle-unimer transition of the polymer in the buffer solution. They demonstrated that at pH 7.4, the core cross-linked micelles released a relatively small amount of the drug, while the uncross-linked micelles released a significant amount of drug over time. This suggests that the drug circulation time can be increased, and premature drug release can be prevented by cross-linking the core of the micelles. At pH 7.4, the uncross-linked molecular state from the micelles did not provide enough protection for the paclitaxel in the core. As a result, even in physiological fluids at pH 7.4, the drugs could gradually be released from the un-cross-linked carriers before reaching the targeted cells. Drugs released too soon from uncross-linked micelle carriers in bodily fluid suggested the significance of developing micelles with cross-linked molecular states as drug carriers [147]. Song et al. developed a pH/reduction-responsive micelle for the simultaneous delivery of siPD-L1 and doxorubicin to increase the effectiveness of chemotherapy in treating cancer. The reduction-sensitive and CD44-targeting amphiphilic micelles (Hyluorpnic acid-ss-oleic acid, HAssOA) were created by joining oleic acid (OA) and hyluoronic acid (HA) with cystine. Then, doxorubicin-loaded micelles (D@HAssOA) were created by nanoprecipitating doxorubicin into the hydrophobic core of micelles. Electrostatic contact was used to coat positively charged cationic chitosan oligosaccharides (COS) on the surface of D@HAssOA in order to effectively deliver siPD-L1, as shown in Figure 2. Next, DOX and siPD-L1 co-delivering micelles (R/C/D@HAssOA) were created by electrostatic interaction loading siPD-L1. In weak acid and reduction (pH 5.0 + 10 mM GSH), doxorubicin and siPD-L1 release dramatically increased [108]. An amphiphilic triblock pH-sensitive poly(β-amino ester)-g-poly(ethylene glycol) methyl ether-cholesterol (PAE-g-MPEG-Chol) was reported to show an excellent drug release profile under different pH conditions. Doxorubicin was encapsulated into the polymeric micelles with a high drug-loading concentration. The in vitro doxorubicin release from the micelles was distinctly enhanced, with the pH decreasing from 7.4 to 6.0. Micelles exhibited excellent pH sensitivity. The release of doxorubicin was slow at a pH of 7.4. The cumulative release for the doxorubicin/polymer system was roughly 33% after 24 h, indicating that most of the drug remained in the micellar core. The doxorubicin release rate was significantly increased at pH 6.0. The drug-loaded devices showed regulated release dependent on pH change and with 35% of the drug released after 3 h and approximately 95% released after 24 h. The greater protonation of amino groups in PAE moieties under lower pH conditions may account for the loosened micelle structure. In addition, the increasing charge density on the micelle surface increased electrostatic repulsion between PAE units, which resulted in the disorganized micelle [148].

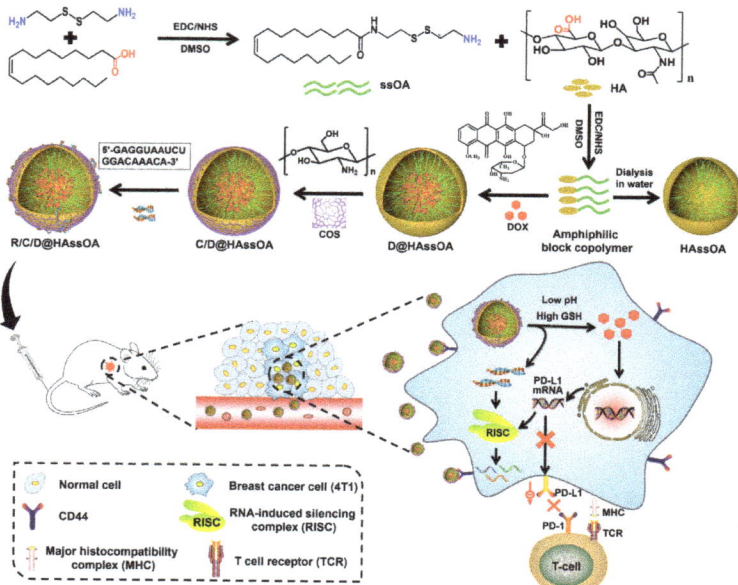

Figure 2. Schematic illustration of pH/redox dual-sensitive R/C/D@HAssOA synthesis and controlled release. Reprinted with permission from ref. [108]. Copyright © 2022 Elsevier B.V.

4.2. ROS Sensitive Micelles

The high level of ROS in cancer cells makes them more susceptible to damage from external ROS than normal cells that can maintain redox balance. Thus, increasing ROS production to levels greater than the hazardous threshold within cancer cells has emerged as a viable way to eliminate tumors. TME characteristics include hypoxia, moderate acidity, and elevated levels of H_2O_2. The presence of hypoxia in the TME facilitates tumor metastasis and increases the resistance of tumors to ROS-based cancer therapies. It has been shown that tumor oxygenation, which could significantly increase oxygen concentrations in hypoxic tumors, can help combat tumor hypoxia and make hypoxic tumors more susceptible to ROS-generated cancer therapy by exploiting the excessive buildup of ROS, particularly disease tissues [149–151]. In small doses, ROS, a chemical species derived from oxygen, can alter cell signaling pathways and stimulate cell growth. Increasing ROS concentration results in "oxidative stress", since antioxidants (such as catalase or superoxide dismutase) are no longer effective in neutralizing ROS. As a result, ROS-sensitive micelles have been developed to target cancer cells specifically [25,152].

A few ROS sensitive micelles have been reported recently. For example, a dual-responsive micelle for the delivery of doxorubicin and a cyclopalladated anti-cancer agent was reported. In this micelle, the drugs were combined within the micelle's hydrophobic core, and the micelle were decorated with an outer hydrophilic layer of PEG and β-cyclodextrin conjugate. The micelle was destabilized in response to high levels of ROS found in cancer cells or in an acidic environment, leading to the release of the drugs. The study demonstrated that the anti-cancer effects of co-delivery micelles were improved compared to free drugs in vitro [153]. Liang et al. reported the development of a ROS-responsive micelle for the co-delivery of dexamethasone and hypericin for photodynamic therapy of cancer. The micelles delivered dexamethasone to inhibit migration, invasion, and angiogenesis of vein endothelial cells, promoting the delivery of oxygen and drug-loaded micelles to the tumor site. Within the tumors, endogenous ROS partially cleaved the outer shell of the micelle to release the drugs, and an external light source was used to excite hypericin and produce ROS, leading to effective cell apoptosis. The upregulated ROS further cleaved the micelles, achieving a self-circulating burst release of hypericin and dexamethasone. This ROS-responsive platform can be used as a feasible strategy to combat cancers [154]. Sulfur-based polypeptides can show ROS-responsive structural changes, thereby providing ROS triggered release from the micellar systems. For example, a new selenium-based polypeptide with higher sensitivity to ROS-response has been developed so that they even respond to much lower levels of ROS in terms of triggered drug release. The micelles were prepared from Se-Benzyl-l-Selenocysteine N-Carboxyanhydride and methyl PEG-NH_2. The amphiphilic copolymer was loaded with doxorubicin. These micelles selectively released their payload in tumor cells with ROS [155]. PEG biodegradable polymeric micelles with PLA, PCL, and PLGA hydrophobic blocks have been widely used as drug carriers due to their excellent biocompatibility and biodegradability [26,117,156–158]. Recently, a ROS-sensitive methyl poly(ethylene glycol)-poly(ester-thioether) micelles were developed and showed enhanced cellular uptake and anticancer efficacy, as shown in Figure 3. The ROS-sensitivity of the self-assembled micelles was investigated in the presence of different ROS reagents. Once the concentration of H_2O_2 was increased to 500 mM, the size of micelles was about 70 nm for 2 h and more than 500 nm for 4 h. It revealed that the micelles were more sensitive to high H_2O_2 concentrations. A similar size variation behavior of the micelles was observed in the other two ROS reagents of Fenton's reagent and NaClO. From the size variation results, it could be concluded that the micelles were more sensitive to the ROS reagent. The methyl poly(ethylene glycol)-poly(ester-thioether) micelles showed the most efficient anticancer activity compared to methyl poly(ethylene glycol)-poly(thioketal-ester) and methyl poly(ethylene glycol)-poly(thioketal-ester-thioether) micelles [117].

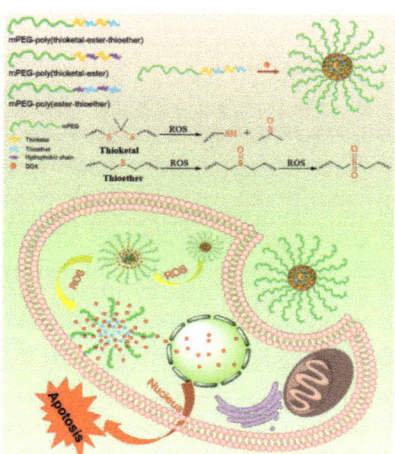

Figure 3. The illustration of ROS-responsive nanoparticles to induce cell apoptosis. Reprinted with permission from ref. [117]. Copyright © 2019 Elsevier B.V.

4.3. Hypoxia Sensitive Micelles

Because hypoxic cells have distinct microenvironments, a decrease in oxygen partial pressure permits tumor-specific drug delivery. Oxygen-sensitive sensors reveal that TMEs contain much less oxygen than healthy tissues. Research shows that chronic low oxygen levels alter tumor biology [94,159]. De novo angiogenesis is the process by which tumor cells generate new blood vessels in response to the inadequate blood supply. However, due to vascular hyperpermeability and accelerated permeation, these newly created blood arteries are leaky due to their discontinuous endothelium and the blockage of lymphatic drainage. Increased interstitial fluid pressure results from hypoxia-induced vascular leakage and aberrant lymphatic drainage in the tumor [160,161]. A viable technique to overcome the rising resistance to accomplish deep penetration in tumors is to progressively increase the driving force. Nitroimidazoles, nitrobenzyl alcohols, and azo linkers are representative types of hypoxia-responsive groups [16,162,163]. As a result, the hydrophobicity and surface charge of the nano-carriers undergo dramatic alterations when subjected to hypoxic circumstances. Effective drug delivery systems result from a change in hydrophilicity in response to hypoxia [162].

Hypoxia sensitive micelles have shown great potentials in cancer therapy. For example, hypoxia-sensitive polymeric micelles were constructed by using a hydrophilic angelica polysaccharide, which is linked to ferrocene (using azobenzene linker), and then the side chain was covalently modified with arachidonic acid. The polymer micelles were engineered to be hypoxia-responsive and achieve selective enhancement of ferroptosis in solid tumors. In these micelles, when curcumin was incorporated, the micelles can respond to hypoxia to release drugs, and that hypoxia can enhance cell uptake and improve the proliferation inhibitory activity of HepG2 cells. This novel micellar platform has potential for the development of ferroptosis and delivery of anti-cancer drugs [164]. Mixed micelles made of folic acid and 2-(2-nitroimidazole) ethylamine conjugated poly (2-hydroxyethyl methacrylate-co-dimethylaminoethyl methacrylate-co-styrene) polymers that contain both paclitaxel and quantum dots were developed. These micelles have good drug encapsulation, storage stability, and sustained drug release properties, and exhibit enhanced cytotoxicity in MCF-7 cells and improved cellular uptake, especially under hypoxic conditions. The system also has excellent tumor targeting and hypoxia-responsive properties, and can be used for real-time in vivo imaging [165]. Recently, researchers developed hypoxia-responsive polymer micelles based on methoxyl poly(ethylene glycol)-co-poly(aspartate-nitroimidazole). The micelles were loaded with dicoumarol and sorafenib. Under low oxygen conditions, micelles cause the depletion of NADPH and inactivate quinone oxidoreductase 1, leading to the repression of hypoxia-inducible factor-1 alpha (HIF-1α). The degradation of HIF-1α increases the vulnerability of cancer cells to sorafenib-induced apoptosis, leading to increased cytotoxicity and the activation of caspase 3 and cytochrome C. The results of this study suggest that the hypoxia-responsive polymer micelles could provide a new approach for addressing hypoxia-induced drug resistance in chemotherapy [166]. Nanocarriers with positively charged surfaces have been proven in several studies to penetrate tumors more effectively. In order to overcome this problem, a hypoxia-sensitive micelle was designed, which may increase its positive surface charge in response to hypoxia gradients and therefore accomplish deep penetration in tumors. PCL served as the nanocarrier's core, and PEG and 4-nitrobenzyl chloroformate (NBCF)-modified polylysine (PLL) formed the outer shell. During blood circulation, the NBCF-modified PLL was protected by the PEG, which provided it the capacity to block its quick removal by the immune system. Once the nanocarrier arrived at the tumor site, the hypoxic microenvironment prompted partial NBCF breakdown, which recovered the amine groups of PLL, resulting in a significant shift in the surface to be positively charged, allowing for tumor penetration. As the nanocarrier entered the core of the tumor, the decrease in oxygen content led to the further degradation of the NBCF-modified PLL, resulting in an increased positive surface charge which further promoted the deep penetration. The subsequent in vitro and in vivo investigations validated that RM/doxorubicin had a superior penetration ability and increased inhibitory efficacy on tumor tissues, which suggested its prospective applicability in cancer therapy [162]. In a recent study, a GLUT1 targeting and tumor micro-environment responsive polyprodrug-based micelle was developed, as shown in Figure 4. Amphiphilic polyprodrug conjugate glucose-PEG-aminoazobenzene-IR808-S-S-paclitaxel was constructed by using the prodrug IR808-S-S-paclitaxel as the hydrophobic block and then modifying the glycosylated PEG as the hydrophilic shell via a hypoxia sensitive linker p-aminoazobenzene. The micelles self-assembled when dissolved in water. Under the GSH reductive TME, the prodrug IR808-S-S-paclitaxel burst into paclitaxel and IR808, which then targeted tubulin and mitochondria, respectively. The micelle could be specifically transported by the GLUT1 of tumor cells and efficiently delivered paclitaxel and IR808 to the tubulin and mitochondria under the TME, ultimately leading to cell apoptosis through destroying mitochondria and depleting ATP production [127].

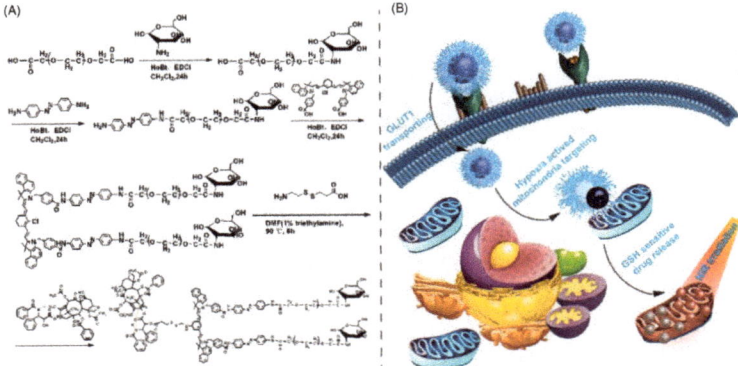

Figure 4. (**A**) The synthetic process of Glu-PEG-Azo-IR808-S-S-PTX conjugate; (**B**) its action mechanism after self-assembled into micelle. Abbreviations: Glu: glucose; Azo: azobenzene; PTX: Paclitaxel. Reprinted with permission from ref. [127]. Copyright 2021, published by Informa UK Limited, trading as Taylor & Francis Group.

4.4. Enzyme Sensitive Micelles

The ability to selectively release their active cargo at the targeting site makes enzymatically degradable polymeric micelles promising drug delivery devices. Clearance of the delivery system is facilitated by enzymatic breakdown of the polymeric nanocarriers [167]. To transport an enzyme-sensitive substrate, these nanocarriers use the selectivity and specificity of enzymes found in cancer cells. Almost all enzyme-sensitive DDSs require extrinsic enzymes. Matrix metalloproteinases (MMPs) are the extracellular enzyme most usually employed for controlled drug discharge. Angiogenesis, invasion, metastasis, and migration are the four hallmarks of cancer, and it has been shown that MMPs play a vital role in the degradation of cell adhesion molecules. Overexpressed MMPs in the extracellular environment of many malignancies make them a promising target for drug release triggers in cancer treatment [29,94,168,169].

Han et al. constructed a polypeptide-based micellar system that is responsive to the enzyme MMP-2 for tumor immune microenvironment reprogramming. The micelles encapsulated an aryl hydrocarbon receptor inhibitor in its hydrophobic core and anti-CD28 is loaded through an MMP-sensitive peptide segment. The micelles are passively delivered to the tumor tissues and ensure the controlled release of both drugs in response to the enriched MMP-2 expression in the TME. The results of in vivo and in vitro studies show that the Dual-SHRP system performed well as a breast cancer immunotherapy, increasing the percentage of CD8+ T cells and decreasing the ratio of immunosuppressive lymphocytes within the tumor [170]. A glucose transporter-mediated and MMP2-triggered mitochondrion-targeting conjugate [glucose-PEG–peptide–triphenylphosponium–polyamidoamine-paclitaxel] composed of a polyamidoamine (PAMAM) dendrimer and enzymatic detachable glucose-PEG was constructed for mitochondrial delivery of paclitaxel, as shown in Figure 5. This conjugate was shown to target mitochondria via the glucose transporter and to be activated by MMP2. The conjugate's sphere-shaped particles, sensitivity to MMP2, and sensitivity to GSH all play a role in the release of paclitaxel. The core of the conjugate was a PAMAM dendrimer polymer, which was co-modified with mitochondria-targeting molecular triphenylphosphine via an amido bond and model drug paclitaxel via a disulfide bond; the paclitaxel was then conjugated with the long circulating PEG layer via the MMP2-sensitive peptide. As a result, the increased EPR effect allowed the conjugates to effectively accumulate in tumor tissue. After the system binds to GLUT1 on tumor cells, the MMP2-sensitive peptide linker was disrupted, and the PEG layer separated from PAMAM. The triphenylphosphine then directed the conjugate to the mitochondria, where paclitaxel was promptly released through a reductive process into the cytoplasm and mitochondria. Overcoming tumor cell multidrug resistance required a high enough intracellular concentration of paclitaxel to block the efflux action of P-glycoprotein (P-gp) while directly acting on the mitochondria to cut off the energy source of P-gp [171].

4.5. Thermo Sensitive Micelles

The temperature has been identified as one of the triggers for cancer drug delivery applications. Thermosensitive synthetic polymers include PNIPAM, poly(N-vinylcaprolactam (PNVCL), poly(N-vinylisobutyramide), poly(N-vinyl-n-butyramide), poly(2-isopropyl-2-oxazoline, and poly[2-(2-ethoxy)ethoxyethoxyethyl vinyl ether]. PNIPAM, as one of the most common thermo-responsive polymers, has a LCST in an aqueous solution at 32 °C. Once the LCST has been reached, the polymer will become water soluble. Above the LCST, however, it loses its solubility in water due to a decrease in the strength of the hydrogen bonds that hold the polymer and the water together and an increase in the importance of the hydrophobic interaction [94]. In an aqueous media, pNIPAAm can undergo a phase change that can be reversed due to temperature changes [172–174].

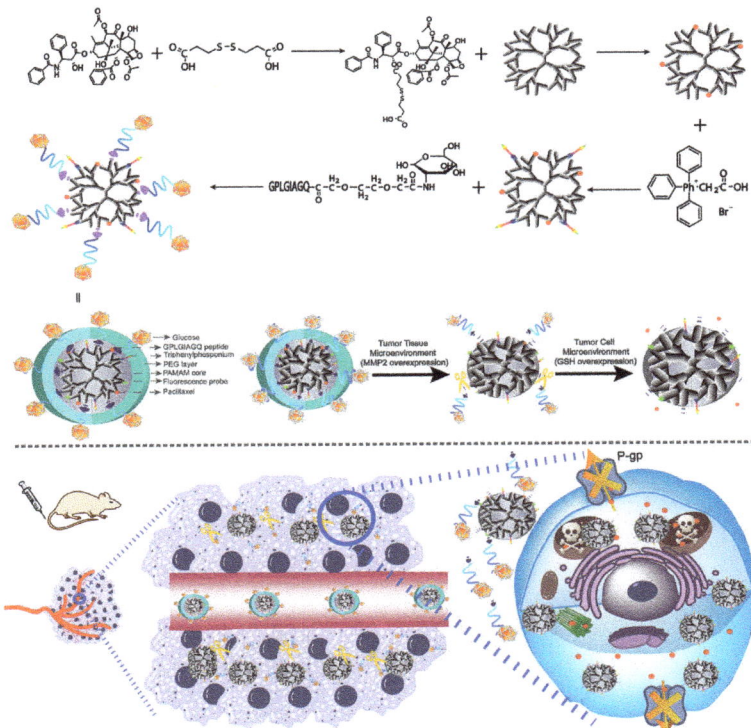

Figure 5. Schematic illustration of the synthesis route of the glucose-PEG–peptide–triphenylphosponium–PAMAM–PTX conjugate and its action mechanism of overcoming multidrug resistance. Abbreviation: PTX: paclitaxel. Reprinted with permission from ref. [171]. Copyright © 2018 American Chemical Society.

Here are some recent applications of thermosensitive micelles. A thermosensitive co-polymer hydrogel system made from gelatin and Pluronic® F127 was developed. This system is capable of a sustained release of a nitric oxide donor and an antibody-blocking immune checkpoint cytotoxic T-lymphocyte-associated protein-4. The unique gel formation and degradation properties of the hydrogel allow for drug retention at the tumor site and triggering release by the TME, and the formation of in situ micelles with the size enables lymphatic uptake. This platform thus represents a technology highly amenable to clinical translation to enable nitric oxide's immune-modulatory functions to improve the therapeutic index of immune checkpoint blockade therapy [175]. Yu et al. fabricated sodium alginate-graft-poly(N-isopropylacrylamide) (SA-g-PNIPAM) biocompatible thermo-sensitive micelles by electrostatic interactions between divalent cationic metal ions and anionic SA-g-PNIPAM. The influence of temperature on the release of 5-Fluorouracil (5-FU) from SA-g-PNIPAM complex micelles was examined at below and above the LCST. At 37 °C, the drug release of the 5-FU was obviously higher than that released at 25 °C. The temperature at 25 °C was lower than the cloud-point temperature of polymeric micelles. The molecular chains of PNIPAM were stretched due to the solvation of water. It was difficult for drugs encapsulated in micelles to come out. However, when the temperature reached 37 °C, the PNIPAM chains became hydrophobic, which led to the partial dissociation of polymer micelles and accelerated the drug release. 5-FU acquired energy as the temperature increased, and, as a result, the inter-molecular forces between 5-FU and polymer micelles weakened. Based on these mechanisms, the drug release of 5-FU at 37 °C was higher than that released at 25 °C. This behavior demonstrated that the release rate of 5-FU was controlled by changing external conditions [176,177].

Han et al. reported deoxycholic acid-conjugated monomethoxy polyethylene glycol (mPEG-DC) forming thermosensitive micelles with rigid cores. The mPEG-DC thermosensitive micelles were employed to deliver estradiol to the target site of action. After 16 days, there was no noticeable increase in the estradiol release from the thermosensitive mPEG-DC micelles. The LCST behavior of the aqueous polymer solution coated the estradiol-enclosed micelles with monomethoxy polyethylene glycol shells, explaining why there was no initial burst. The LCST of the aqueous mPEG-DC solution was determined to be between 30 and 35 °C and was found to be concentration independent over the range of 0.1 to 10.0 wt.%. The DC core of the mPEG-DC micelles remained, as evidenced by the fact that it continued to exist as a collapsed peak at LCST. Furthermore, unlike with free estradiol, the release of estradiol from the micelle was diffusion-controlled rather than an explosive release at the outset. The micelle exhibited thermoreversible behavior [134].

Another heavily studied thermo-sensitive polymer is Pluronic F127, due to its exceptional thermal response and its role in regulating drug release. Pluronic F127 is made of poly(ethylene oxide), poly(propylene oxide), and poly(ethylene oxide). However, Pluronic F127's potential applications as drug delivery systems are hampered by its unacceptably high CMC and low LCST. The modification of hydrophobic polyester blocks on Pluronic F127 is a potential solution to this issue because it improves the copolymer's biocompatibility and biodegradability while also increasing its stability and LCST. The decreasing temperature has been reported to be effective in forming a temperature-triggered "on-off" nanocarrier in F127 [178–180].

Guo et al. fabricated Pluronic F127-PLA (FP) copolymer decorated with folic acid ligands-based thermo-sensitive micelles with an active targeting capacity, as shown in Figure 6. These amphiphilic copolymer-formed micelles in an aqueous solution can be taken up by FR-overexpressed tumor cells via receptor-mediated endocytosis and then rapidly released inside the cells under modest hyperthermia (40 °C). The critical solution temperature of FP100 micelles (containing a PLA segment with a polymerization degree of 100) was 39.2 °C and were suitable for use at or near body temperature. While the anticancer drug doxorubicin was released slowly from FP100 micelles at room temperature (37 °C), its concentration was rapidly increased by the shrinkage of thermo-sensitive segments at an enhanced temperature (40 °C). FP100 micelles exhibited excellent thermo sensitivity with a suitable LCST value of 39.2 °C. Under low hyperthermia (40 °C), the encapsulated anticancer drug in these micelles was rapidly released while it remained stable at 37 °C [178].

4.6. Magnetic Sensitive Micelles

Nanoparticles of magnesium oxide (MgO), magnetite (Fe_3O_4), and maghemite (Fe_3O_3) are widely employed to create magnetic sensitivity. It is because of their extraordinary super paramagnetism and diminutive size that they are commonly referred to as superparamagnetic iron oxide nanoparticles. In the presence of a magnetic field, they become attracted to it, but this attraction quickly dissipates once the field is no longer there. Studies have found that controlled drug release is accomplished through two distinct mechanisms: magnetic field-induced hyperthermia and magnetic field-guided drug targeting. Hyperthermia-based magnetically induced drug release systems have been investigated throughout the past few decades [94,168,181,182].

Lin et al. reported a dual targeting method for the anti-neoplastic medicine paclitaxel using magnetic particles and an RGD peptide to achieve more cell cytotoxicity with a reduced drug dose. The amphiphilic polymer poly[(N-isopropylacrylamide-r-acrylamide)-b-L-lactic acid] (PNAL) was used as micelle-forming materials to solve the problems of water-insolubility of oleic acid-stabilized superparamagnetic iron oxide nanoparticles (SPIONs) and low incorporation efficiency of hydrophobic paclitaxel with SPION nanocarriers. The magnetic particles were then concentrated on the target cells by the influence of an external magnetic field generated by magnets. Hydrophilic PNA interacts with the aqueous environment, while hydrophobic segments form aggregates inside the micelles, where carboxylic acid stabilized-SPIONs and hydrophobic medicines can be included. PNAL-SPIONs are modified with a targeting moiety, a peptide called GGGGRGD that contains an RGD sequence and has a short linker linked to it by homo-crosslinking. The physical targeting and biochemical targeting of the micelles had a synergistic effect [138].

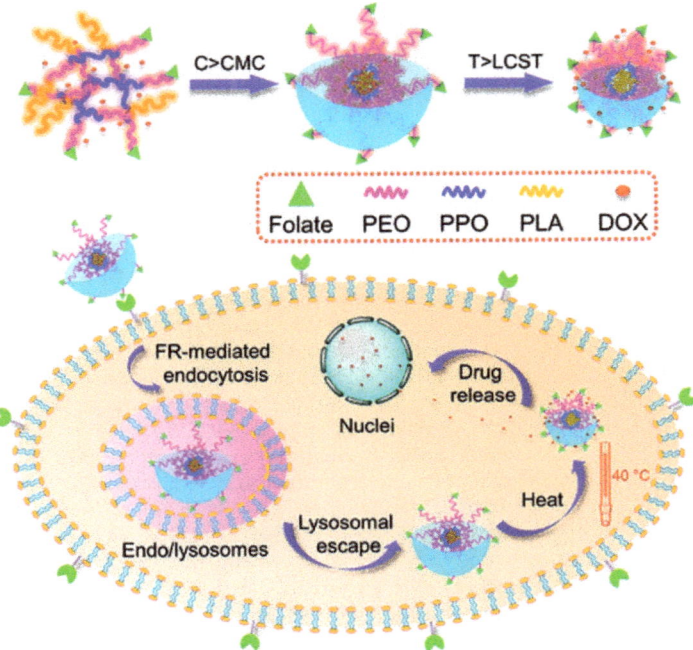

Figure 6. Schematic Representation of Thermosensitive Nanocarrier Working as a Targeted Drug Delivery System with Controlled Drug Release. Reprinted with permission from ref. [178]. Copyright © 2014 American Chemical Society.

Micelles based on copolymers of PCL and PEG bearing folate on the PEG distal ends, denoted as folate–PEG–PCL, were developed by Yang et al. and were used to encapsulate the anticancer drug doxorubicin and superparamagnetic iron oxide (SPIO), as shown in Figure 7. Micelles with sizes of fewer than 100 nm contained both SPIO nanoparticles and the anticancer medication doxorubicin. The micelles were superparamagnetic at ambient temperature but became ferrimagnetic at 10 K. In vitro studies showed that these polymeric micelles could serve as an efficient dual targeting nanoplatform for the delivery of anticancer medicines. Micelles functionalized with folate were recognized and taken up by tumor cells that overexpressed folate receptors; an external magnetic field improved the efficiency with which the SPIO-loaded and folate-functionalized micelles were transported into the tumor cells. The micelles showed excellent efficacy and potentials to deliver drugs and SPIO [183].

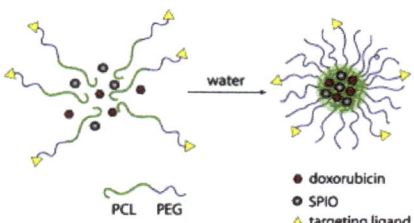

Figure 7. Schematic illustration of metal ions induced complex micelles for drug encapsulation. Reprinted with permission from ref. [183]. Copyright © 2018 Elsevier B.V.

5. Fate of Micelles Post Administration

The fate of nanoparticles is decided by their physicochemical properties such as size, surface charge, and hydrophobicity. For example, follicle associated epithelia mediated transcellular uptake of smaller nanomaterial is higher compared to larger ones [42,184–186]. Cellular entry of nanoparticles through the endocytotic route include clathrin- and caveola-mediated endocytosis, pinocytosis, potocytosis, and patocytosis [187]. Contrarily, larger particles are opsonized and removed by the reticuloendothelial system (RES) related macrophagial phagocytosis. Considering the opsonization phenomenon, the nanoparticles are engineered such that the surfaces are coated with hydrophilic material, including surfactants such as polysorbate 80, hydrophilic polymers such as poloxamers, PEGs, PEO, poloxamine, etc. [188]. Surface charge and strategic functionalization can result in a transcellular transport of nanodrugs. For example, positive surface charge of the nanodrug can complex with the anionic moieties (sulfate sialic acid, sugars) of mucin resulting in enhanced transcellular transport across mucus and internalization by epithelial cells [184]. In addition, paracellular transport is enhanced in nanodrugs composed of bioadhesive polymers. The delivery of nanodrugs can be made targeted by modifying the surfaces of nanodrugs with antibodies, proteins etc. [189]. Targeted action can improve therapeutic potential and decrease toxicity. Nanotechnology-based drug delivery systems are administered either via injection, orally, or by a transdermal route [190–192]. Currently, the ongoing nanoparticle studies also include the pulmonary route of delivery through inhalations. In the majority of these cases, inhaled particles other than nanoparticles have limited duration of action as they undergo pulmonary clearance, including mucociliary and macrophage clearance [190–192]. Nanoparticles, in contrast, have long residence times as they avoid mucociliary and macrophage clearance and, thereby, enhance the therapeutic action of encapsulated active moieties [193].

Micellar nanoparticles have been proven to demonstrate a therapeutic potential for pharmaceutical drug delivery and are considered a potential alternative to liposomes. The concept of micelles has been undertaken due to their ability to solubilize the API and enhance blood circulation time, resulting in targeted delivery and enhanced therapeutic efficacy. However, the circulation time of micelles in the blood depends on biodistribution, metabolism, and clearance, which depends, in turn, on the physicochemical properties of micelles such as the size and shape, core properties, surface modifications, and surface charge as well as targeting ligand functionalization [194]. Due to the minimal surface area, micelles of ~3–5 nm size are not cleared by macrophages and thus are excreted by the kidney. Small particles easily cross tight endothelial junctions and reach extravascular extracellular space (EES) and target organs, and thus exhibit wide distributions [194,195]. However, large-size (≥10 nm) particles are easily cleared through the liver and spleen. Small-sized polymeric micelles take advantage of the EPR effect and passively diffuse through the endothelial lining, and due to poor lymphatic drainage, they remain at the site of inflammation site and thus show targeted site-specific action [196]. Despite the stability, the leaky nature of ω-methoxy poly (ethylene glycol)-b-(N-(2-benzoyloxypropyl) methacrylamide) polymer used for curcumin delivery with more than a 70% release in plasma at 37 °C has negated the advantage of the EPR effect [197]. The same effect of curcumin leakage was also shown in other forms of delivery liposomes (180 nm) and intralipid nanoparticles (280 nm) [198].

Thus, the physicochemical properties and the effect of drug and polymeric/lipidic material and their interaction must be considered while aiming for an optimal formulation. In addition, and as discussed earlier, the size, shape, and surface charge are important for micellar biodistribution and clearance. Even though positively charged micelles are readily taken up by the RES compared to neutral and negatively charged micelles, the rate of cellular uptake and blood circulation time were found to be low in negatively charged micelles [194]. For instance, the pharmacokinetic activity of Tyr-PEG/PDLLA (neutral) and Tyr-Glu-PEG/PDLLA (anionic) micelles in mice showed that although both exhibited similar blood clearance kinetics, anionic micelles demonstrated approximately a 10 times lower biodistribution in the liver and the spleen compared to neutral micelles, due to synergic steric and electrostatic repulsion [198,199]. In addition, the composition of the core also determines the fate (biodistribution, clearance) of micelles. A study was performed to evaluate the clearance of paclitaxel-loaded pluronic P105 micelles and mixed micelles composed of similar copolymer with the addition of hydrophobic lamella [200]. The mixed micelles with additional hydrophobic lamella exhibited a significant decrease in clearance compared to just paclitaxel-loaded pluronic P105 micelles, and this can be due to the increased stability of micelles against liver uptake due to increased hydrophobic interactions in the core of micelles [200].

Following IV, administration micelles were proven to show better tissue distribution and clearance, resulting in better clinical outcomes compared to free drugs. For instance, micellar nanoparticles administered vial liquid eye drops, resulting in reduced elimination of drugs from the precorneal area compared to free drugs, and thereby increasing the therapeutic duration of action. Self-micellizing solid dispersion of tranilast using an amphiphilic block copolymer of 2-methacryloyloxyethyl phosphorylcholine (MPC) unit and a n-butyl methacrylate (BMA) unit ([poly(MPC-co-BMA)]) rapidly formed micelles of 100–150 nm diameter and showed a significant improvement in dissolution behavior [201]. Furthermore, a 50-fold enhancement of oral bioavailability and accelerate absorption of tranilast was observed in rats. In another study, the accumulation of polymeric micelles of a size of 65 nm into a subcutaneous BxPC3 tumor was observed and compared to a liposomal doxorubicin (Doxil) carrier with a size of 108 nm [201]. The results indicate that the permeability of smaller micelles into deeper tumor tissue (the region distant from blood vasculature) was higher compared to the larger liposomes, with micellar formulation showing significantly stronger anti-tumor activity than the liposome with the aid of TGF-b inhibitor [201].

6. Clinical Trials on Micellar Drug Delivery Systems

Many clinical studies on micellar drug delivery are in progress that aim to enhance the pharmacokinetic (PK) profiles and reduce toxicity effects in cancer therapy. The results from these studies suggest that micelles improve the pharmacokinetics and pharmacodynamics of anti-cancer drugs [202]. One such novel formulation is Genexol®-PM, which is a paclitaxel formulation encapsulated in polymeric micelles (PEG-PLA).

Paclitaxel on its own has low water solubility, and therefore Taxol, a solution in Cremophor EL/ethanol, was developed. However, Cremophor has been associated with several side effects, such as hypersensitivity, nephrotoxicity, neurotoxicity, neuropathy, and neutropenia [203–205]. Hence, micellar formulations with no Cremophor have been developed. A Genexol®-PM 30 mg injection is used in chemotherapy to treat various cancers, including breast cancer and ovarian cancer. It has been approved for use in Bulgaria, Hungary, and South Korea, and is being evaluated in Phase II trials in the US. The same drug is marketed under the name Cynviloq™ in other countries. Compared to Taxol®, Genexol®-PM has a high drug solubilizing capacity of about 25%, higher maximum tolerated doses, and median lethal dose, and it demonstrates linear PK behavior. Additionally, it has been shown to have higher tumor accumulation, decreased myelosuppression, and effective

P-gp inhibition. Several other micellar formulations are in different stages of stage clinical trials for the treatment of various cancers (Table 4). These trials are aimed at exploring the potential of micellar drug delivery in cancer treatment. All the information of the clinical trials in Table 4 was from https://clinicaltrials.gov (accessed on 31 January 2023).

Table 4. The clinical trials of polymeric micelles.

Clinical Trial/Drug	Polymeric Carrier	Condition	Status	Phase	Participants	Clinical Trials ID
Pm-Pac/Paclitaxel	PEG-PLA	Non-Small Cell Lung Cancer	Unknown	Phase 3	454	NCT02667743
Genexol-PM/Paclitaxel	PEG-PLA	Taxane-Pretreated Recurrent Breast Cancer	Unknown	Phase 4	90	NCT00912639
	PEG-PLA	Advanced Non-Small Cell Lung Cancer	Completed	Phase 2	276	NCT01023347
	PEG-PLA	Advanced Ovarian Cancer	Unknown	Phase1/2	74	NCT00886717
	PEG-PLA	Advanced Urothelial Cancer Previously Treated with Gemcitabine and Platinum	Completed	Phase 2	37	NCT01426126
	PEG-PLA	Advanced Pancreatic Cancer	Completed	Phase 2	43	NCT00111904
	PEG-PLA	Advanced Hepatocelluar Carcinoma after Failure of Sorafenib	Terminated	Phase 2	5	NCT03008512
	PEG-PLA	Advanced Non-small-cell Lung Cancer	Completed	Phase 2	45	NCT01770795
	PEG-PLA	Gynecologic Cancer (Adult Solid Tumor)	Unknown	Phase 1	18	NCT02739529
	PEG-PLA	Pancreatic Cancer	Completed	Phase 1	18	NCT00882973
	PEG-PLA	Metastatic or Locally Recurrent Breast Cancer	Completed	N/A	111	NCT02064829
NANOXEL-M/Docetaxel	PEG-PLA	Esophageal Squamous Cell Carcinoma	Unknown	Phase 2	38	NCT03585673
	PEG-PLA	Recurrent or Metastatic Head and Neck Squamous Cell Carcinoma	Unknown	Phase 2	31	NCT02639858
NC-6004/Cisplatin	PEG-Poly (glutamic acid)	Recurrent and/or Metastatic Squamous Cell Carcinoma of the Head and Neck	Terminated	Phase 1	4	NCT02817113
	PEG-Poly (glutamic acid)	Locally Advanced or Metastatic Pancreatic Cancer	Completed	Phase 3	310	NCT02043288
NK105/Paclitaxel	PEG-Polyaspartate	Metastatic or Recurrent Breast Cancer	Completed	Phase 3	436	NCT01644890
NC-4016/Oxaliplatin	PEG-Poly (glutamic acid)	Advanced Solid Tumors or Lymphoma	Completed	Phase 1	34	NCT03168035
NC 6300/Epirubicin	PEG-Polyaspartate	Advanced Solid Tumors or Advanced, Metastatic, or Unresectable Soft Tissue Sarcoma	Unknown	Phase1b/2	150	NCT03168061
NK012/SN-38	PEG-Poly (glutamic acid)	Advanced Solid Tumors Followed by a Dose Expansion Phase in Patients with Metastatic Colorectal Cancer	Completed	Phase 1	35	NCT01238939
	PEG-Poly (glutamic acid)	Sensitive Relapsed and Refractory Relapsed Small-Cell Lung Cancer	Completed	Phase 2	72	NCT00951613
	PEG-Poly (glutamic acid)	Locally Advanced Non-Resectable and Metastatic Breast Cancer Patients with Triple Negative Phenotype	Completed	Phase 2	61	NCT00951054
	PEG-Poly (glutamic acid)	Refractory Solid Tumors	Completed	Phase 1	39	NCT00542958
	PEG-Poly (glutamic acid)	Advanced Solid Tumors Followed by a Dose Expansion Phase in Patients with Triple Negative Metastatic Breast Cancer	Completed	Phase 1	4	NCT01238952

Table 4. The clinical trials of polymeric micelles.

Clinical Trial/Drug	Polymeric Carrier	Condition	Status	Phase	Participants	Clinical Trials ID
BIND-014/Docetaxel	PEG-PLA	Metastatic Castration-Resistant Prostate Cancer	Completed	Phase 2	42	NCT01812746
	PEG-PLA	Non-Small Cell Lung Cancer	Completed	Phase 2	64	NCT01792479
	PEG-PLA	Advanced or Metastatic Cancer	Completed	Phase 1	58	NCT01300533
	PEG-PLA	KRAS Mutation Positive or Squamous Cell Non-Small Cell Lung Cancer	Completed	Phase 2	69	NCT02283320
	PEG-PLA	Urothelial Carcinoma, Cholangiocarcinoma, Cervical Cancer and Squamous Cell Carcinoma of the Head and Neck	Terminated	Phase 2	73	NCT02479178
Paclitaxel Micelles	Micelles (polymer unknown)	Advanced Solid Tumor	Not yet recruiting	Phase 1	98	NCT04778839
Docetaxel Polymeric Micelles	Micelles (polymer unknown)	Advanced Malignant Solid Tumors	Not yet recruiting	Phase 2	110	NCT05254665
Cisplatin Micelles (HA132)	Micelles (polymer unknown)	Advanced Malignant Solid Tumors	Not yet recruiting	Phase 1/2	126	NCT05478785
PLZ4-coated paclitaxel micelles (PPM)	PEG-Cholic acid	Non-myoinvasive Bladder Cancer	Recruiting	Phase 1	29	NCT05519241

Abbreviation: PEG-PLA: poly(ethylene glycol)-poly(lactide).

6.1. Paclitaxel Micellar Formulations

Paclitaxel is a taxane class drug with potential anti-cancer properties, as it blocks the breakdown of free tubulin microtubules. Taxol® is a form of Paclitaxel that uses a mixture of polyoxyethylene castor oil and dehydrated alcohol, but the required doses often result in acute allergic reactions due to the non-ionic surfactant [206,207]. Genexol-PM, made by Samyang Co. in Seoul, is a less toxic version of Paclitaxel, formulated as a 25-nm diameter micellar complex of PEG and PLA. It was produced by dissolving the block copolymer and drug in acetonitrile, evaporating the solvent, and then dissolving the resulting gel in preheated water to form paclitaxel-filled micelles [208]. Genexol-PM is approved for the treatment of breast, lung, and ovarian cancers, and is undergoing clinical evaluation for use in other cancers (Table 4). Clinical studies of Genexol-PM in pancreatic and urothelial cancers showed that the drug was well tolerated and showed good antitumor activity [209].

The NK105 drug delivery system (Nippon Kayaku Co., Tokyo, Japan.) is a polymeric micelle na-noparticle that encapsulates paclitaxel. It has a diameter of about 85 nm and is comprised of an amphiphilic copolymer made up of a hydrophilic block of PEG and a hydrophobic block of polyaspartate modified with 4-phenyl-1-butanol. The copolymer is designed to create a microenvironment within the micelle core that enables high drug loading and retention, with the goal of producing a drug carrier that retains the drug after intravenous administration. This first-generation technology results in a prolonged half-life of the drug (more than 10 h) compared to Taxol (30 min), and the second-generation nano-formulations in clinical development include drugs that are covalently conjugated or chelated to the core-forming block of the micelles [210,211]. It was developed as a safer alternative to traditional paclitaxel formulations, which are solubilized in ethanol or poly-oxyethylene castor oil and can cause serious hypersensitivity reactions and anaphylactic shock. In vivo studies in mice showed that the Cmax and AUC were increased 3- and 25-fold, respectively, with NK105 compared to free paclitaxel [210]. A Phase II clinical study with NK105 showed a 15-fold higher AUC than conventional paclitaxel. The efficacy of NK105 has been attributed to its EPR, a unique phenomenon in solid tumor tissue, and previous clinical studies have shown its potential—with a good response rate in advanced gastric cancer, and with a partial response or stable disease in solid tumors and breast cancer [212,213]. In a Phase III trial, NK105 (a nanoparticle drug delivery formulation of paclitaxel) was compared to paclitaxel for the treatment of metastatic or recurrent breast cancer. Both treatments were given to patients in a 28-day cycle, with NK105 given at 65 mg/m^2 and paclitaxel at 80 mg/m^2. The primary endpoint was progression-free survival, but the results showed that both treatments had similar efficacy with a median progression-free survival of 8.4 and 8.5 months for NK105 and paclitaxel, respectively. The safety profile of the two treatments was similar, but the incidence of peripheral sensory neuropathy was lower in patients receiving NK105. The patient-reported outcomes for peripheral sensory neuropathy were significantly better in the NK105 group [214]. The Phase III studies on NK105 resulted in a failure to meet endpoints. Nippon Kayaku Co. stated that the study's main objective, which was progression-free survival, failed to meet its predetermined statistical standards. However, the drug NK105 was well-tolerated compared to paclitaxel. Currently the paclitaxel micellar formulations, Cynvilog (polymer-based) Paclical polymer-based), are approved in South Korea and Russia, respectively [211].

Nanoxel-PM is a docetaxel-loaded PEG2000-PDLLA1765 micellar formulation with 25 nm sized particles (Samyang company, Seoul, Korea). The formulation was created by dissolving docetaxel and copolymer in ethanol, evaporating the solvent, and then dispersing the matrix in water. D-mannitol was added as a cryoprotectant. The bioequivalence of Nanoxel-PM to Taxotere® was determined to be within 100% ± 20% which were performed on based on mice, rats, and beagle dogs. Clinical trials for Nanoxel-PM have been registered but no results have been published [215,216].

Paccal Vet is a new form of PTX combined with a surfactant-based derivative of retinoic acid for treatment of mast cell tumors in dogs. In a study of 29 dogs, 59% showed complete or partial responses with a median progression-free survival of 247 days. A Phase III study showed Paccal Vet to be clinically safe and effective with better response rates than lomustine, and fewer adverse effects. Paccal Vet has been granted MUMS status and approved by the FDA for use in certain types of dog cancer but can only be used for the approved indications [209].

Triolimus (Co-D Therapeutics) is a polymeric micelle drug delivery system that contains a combination of three drugs: paclitaxel, rapamycin (mTOR inhibitor), and tanespimycin (Hsp90 inhibitor). It is a 30–40 nm diameter PEG-b-PLA micelle formulation. Triolimus has received orphan drug designation for angiosarcoma and is in late-stage preclinical evaluation for the treatment of breast cancer, non-small cell lung cancer, and angiosarcoma. The use of a polymeric nanomedicine delivering multiple drugs is close to entering the market through clinical trials [217,218].

6.2. SN38 (Irinotecan Metabolite (NK012) Micelles

NK012 is a polymeric micelle formulation of SN-38, the active metabolite of irinotecan [219]. NK012 releases its active ingredient via hydrolysis and does not require metabolic conversion by enzymes. This makes it a promising agent for clinical use, as its ability to suppress tumor growth and its antitumor effects in various cell types, including human tumors, are stronger than those of the active metabolite. In addition, NK012 accumulates in high concentrations in tumors and has been shown to result in less severe diarrhea compared to the active metabolite in preclinical studies [220]. A clinical study evaluated the efficacy and safety of NK012 in Japanese patients with unresectable metastatic colorectal cancer through a multicenter open-label Phase II trial. The study consisted of 58 patients divided into two groups, with group A as the primary efficacy population. The primary endpoint was the response rate, which was 3.8% in group A, with median progression-free survival and overall survival of 3.30 months and 15.03 months, respectively. The most common adverse drug reaction was neutropenia, while the incidence of grade three diarrhea was low or zero. No treatment-related deaths were reported. The study concluded that the response rate of NK012 monotherapy was similar to that of irinotecan monotherapy reported in a Phase III trial, but the initial dose of 28 mg/m^2 may be too high for colorectal cancer patients who have previously been treated with oxaliplatin-based chemotherapy [221]. NK012 is a polymeric micelle formulation of SN-38, the active metabolite of irinotecan [200].

6.3. Anthracycline Class Drugs—Micellar Formulations

The NK911 is a micellar formulation of doxorubicin that is composed of a copolymer of PEG and polyaspartic acid developed in Japan. Doxorubicin is partially attached to the side chains of aspartic acid to increase its hydrophobicity, resulting in a hydrophobic core within the micelle. This allows for the encapsulation of free doxorubicin, making the loaded drug responsible for its antitumor activity [222]. The NK911 micelles have a small size of around 40 nm and have been shown to accumulate in solid tumors in mice, leading to a Phase I clinical trial with 23 patients with metastatic or recurrent solid tumors. The trial aimed to study the pharmacokinetic profile of the nanotherapeutic through the maximum tolerated dose and toxicity, with administration starting at 6 mg/m^2 doxorubicin equivalent every 3 weeks. The NK911 micelles showed an increased plasma half-life and plasma concentrations of the drug compared to free doxorubicin but had lower stability in plasma compared to liposomal doxorubicin. The most common side effect was neutropenia, but the treatment was generally well tolerated and had a good safety profile [223]. A Phase II clinical trial was proposed with a recommended dose of 50 mg/m^2 every 3 weeks, but it is unclear if it proceeded.

Sp1049C, developed by Supratek Pharma Inc. in Canada, is a 30 nm diameter mi-cellar formulation that contains doxorubicin (8.2%) loaded into a blend of two Pluronic block copolymers (Pluronic F127 and Pluronic L61 with a ratio of 1:8). Pluronic F127 serves to stabilize the micelles while Pluronic L61 enhances the effectiveness of the treatment by inhibiting P-gp efflux transporter [224]. In a Phase I clinical trial, this formulation was evaluated in 26 patients with advanced solid tumors. The trial administered doses ranging from 5 to 90 mg/m^2 every 3 weeks for at least six cycles. The pharmacokinetics showed linearity and a longer half-life than conventional doxorubicin. The maximum tolerated dose was 70 mg/m^2, and side effects included myelosuppression, alopecia, stomatitis, and transient lethargy. No patients showed a complete or partial response, but 30.8% had stable disease for a median time of 17.5 weeks [225]. A Phase II trial showed notable single-agent activity and an acceptable safety profile in 21 patients with advanced adenocarcinoma of the esophagus and gastroesophageal junction. The objective response rate was 47%, median overall survival was 10 months, and median progression-free survival was 6.6 months. The predominant toxicity was neutropenia [226]. A Phase III trial for gastrointestinal cancer was conducted but no results have been published.

NC-6300/K-912 is a pro-drug conjugate made by linking the chemotherapy drug epirubicin to PEG-poly(α,β-aspartic acid) through an acid-sensitive hydrazone bond. This results in a micellar formulation with a particle size of 40–80 nm and selectively accumulates in tumor tissue due to the EPR effect and the release of the drug in acidic tumor environments. In a Phase I clinical trial, 19 patients with advanced or recurrent solid tumors were given doses of NC-6300/K-912 to determine safety, recommended dosage, tolerability, and pharmacokinetics. The maximum tolerated dose was found to be 170 mg/m^2 and 1 patient out of 19 had a partial response, with an objective response rate of 5%. The trial showed that NC-6300/K-912 was well tolerated, with lower toxicity compared to conventional epirubicin [227,228].

6.4. NC-4016/Oxaliplatin Micelles

NC-4016 is a PEG-b-poly (L-glutamic acid) copolymer-based micelle of size 40 nm developed to deliver oxaliplatin for advanced solid tumor treatment to decrease drug-related toxicity. Oxaliplatin is incorporated into the micelles in its active metabolite form dichloro (1,2-diamino cyclohexane) platinum(II) (DACHPt) [229]. In vivo studies in a mouse model demonstrated that the antitumor effects of NC-4016 are comparable to oxaliplatin. Other animal studies have also demonstrated higher efficacy in tumor models, including human pancreatic, murine colon carcinoma, and melanoma [230]. Compared to oxaliplatin alone, oxaliplatin loaded micelles showed enhanced stability in physiological conditions, with extended blood circulation time and with more than a 1000-fold increase in plasma drug concentration from 0 to 72 h.

6.5. NC-6004/Cisplatin Micelles

NC-6004 (NanoplatinTM) is a PEG-b-poly (l-glutamic acid) based polymeric micelle formulation for cisplatin delivery with a micelle size ~28 nm [231]. NC-6004 is composed of micelles of size ~30 nm. NC-6004 is made by reacting the sodium salt of PEG-P(Glu) and Cisplatin in water to create Cisplatin-incorporating micelles. Cisplatin is released from NC-6004 in the presence of chloride ions through an exchange reaction between the carboxylic groups in P(Glu) and chloride ions. A micelle-based formulation was developed to alter the bio-distribution and PK profile, thereby increasing the tumor accumulation and efficacy [232].

A Phase I clinical trial of NC-6004 for advanced solid tumors was conducted in the UK, with doses ranging from 10 to 120 mg/m^2. The maximum tolerated dose (MTD) was determined to be 120 mg/m^2 due to renal impairment and hypersensitivity reactions. The recommended dose for Phase II was 90 mg/m^2. There was no complete or partial response in patients, with 41.2% of patients having stable disease. The median progression-free survival was 49 days, and 82.4% of patients died or had tumor progression. A Phase I clinical trial of NC-6004 in combination with gemcitabine for advanced solid tumors was conducted in Japan. The most common side effects were decreases in neutrophil and white blood cell count. The MTD was determined to be 90 mg/m^2, and the recommended dose for Phase II was 60 mg/m^2 [233]. In addition, another Phase I/II study was performed in Taiwan and Singapore on 19 patients who had pancreatic cancer and were treated with a combination therapy of NC-6004 and gemcitabine. This study also recommends a Phase II dose for the combination therapy to be 90 mg/m^2, and the results indicated good activity and tolerability [234]. A combination Therapy With NC-6004 and Gemcitabine in advanced solid tumors or non-small cell lung, biliary, and bladder Cancer (NanoCarrier Co., Ltd., Chiba, Japan) was submitted for clinical trials with a dose escalation, but no results were reported [235].

6.6. BIND-014/Docetaxel Micelles

BIND-0 Docetaxel is a taxoid that is derived from the European yew and is more potent than paclitaxel as a microtubule depolymerization inhibitor. It is used in the treatment of various cancers, including breast, lung, ovarian, and gastric cancers. However, the clinical formulation of docetaxel, Taxotere, can cause adverse effects, such as hypersensitivity reactions, hemolysis, and peripheral neuropathy [236]. BIND-014 is a nanoparticle composed of PEG-PLA, decorated with a prostate-specific membrane antigen inhibitor and encapsulating docetaxel [237]. A Phase I study of BIND-014 showed it was well-tolerated with predictable and manageable toxicity [238]. A Phase II study of BIND-014 in combination with prednisone in patients with metastatic prostate cancer showed an overall response rate of 32% and a median progression-free survival of 9.9 months [239]. Another Phase II study of BIND-014 as second-line therapy in patients with Stage III/IV non-small cell lung cancer showed a disease control rate of 63% in patients with KRAS mutations [240]. However, BIND-014 was not effective in later trials against cervical and head-and-neck cancers, leading the company to discontinue its development in 2016 [241].

7. Regulatory Submissions

A schematic showing the regulatory process of a nanoparticle (including micellar nanoparticles) based drug delivery system is shown in Figure 8. Several clinical trials are in progress to investigate the safety and efficacy of micelles, but their scalability remains an issue to transfer basic research to clinical practice to commercialization. In addition, a lack of detailed understanding of the PK/pharmacodynamics (PD) aspects, clearance rate, and in vivo degradation profiles of the materials and micelles needs extensive research. Thus far, most of the IVIVC profiles are only confined to lethal dose (LD50), inhibitory concentration (IC50), and maximum tolerated dose (MTD). However, to obtain a complete toxicity profile, an inclusion of acute and sub-acute models, such as genotoxicity and gene expression pattern determination, must be considered. Additionally, due to the toxicity resulting from the size and altered physicochemical properties, due to the type of polymers used in the micelle construction, a separate registration requirement might be needed for micelles [242–244].

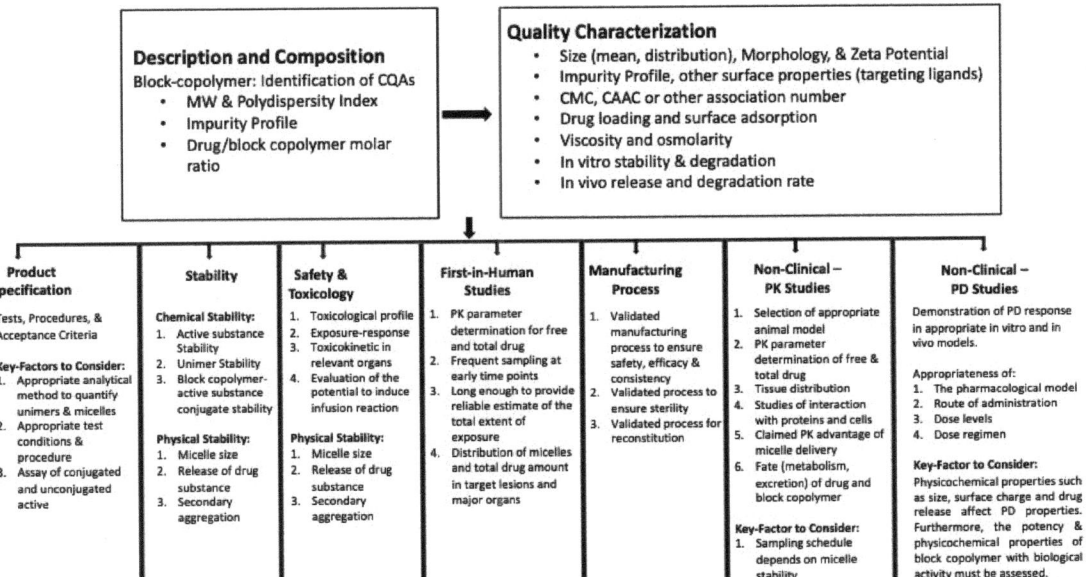

Figure 8. Schematic of regulatory process of a nanoparticle (including micellar nanoparticles) based drug delivery system. Abbreviations: CQA: critical quality arrtribute; MW: molecular weight; CMC: Critical Micelle Concentration; CAAC: Critical Assembly/Aggregate Concentration; PK: pharmacokinetics; PD: pharmacodynamics.

ICH Pharmaceutical Development Q8(R2) guideline encompasses the regulation of the pharmaceutical development of any novel formulation. Similar to other regulated products, such as a drug, device, or biologic, the Food and Drug Administration (FDA) is the regulatory authority for the approval of nanomedicines in humans in the USA [244]. However, the nanoscale size of micelles requires rigorous characterization and testing to determine the safety and efficacy profiles in humans. Extensive assessment and characterization of micelles is addressed in an EMA reflection paper published in 2013 [244,245]. The paper describes various aspects of product development, including its characterization, specifications, stability, non-clinical pharmacokinetic and pharmacodynamic aspects, and first-in-human studies. Furthermore, the paper also discusses the physicochemical characterization of actives and polymers and their chemical stability with an impurity profile. Physical characterization includes CMC, micelle size, and surface charge, micelle shape and morphology, micellar stability in plasma, and drug release in biorelevant conditions. To summarize, the key highlights of the reflection paper include micelle characterization as a representative of product specifications for its physicochemical stability, pharmacokinetics and pharmacokinetics, and toxicology studies. To exemplify, considering the stability of micelles and the fate (site and release) of the micelles and drug, PK and PD studies should be designed accordingly [244,245].

Due to the absence of compendial methods for the integrity of micelles and their release rate, in-house methods must be set up and validated accordingly to ensure repeatability and reproducibility. Methods should be developed such that the method should be able to predict the release both in the circulation and the targeted site of action to mimic the physiological environment of micelle. In addition, the method should be sensitive enough to verify batch-to-batch variability. In vitro–in vivo correlation (IVIVC) for micelles is not always straightforward, as the predictivity of in vitro tests is a critical issue. Only a few research articles have tried to address IVIVC by establishing a correlation between in vitro drug release and drug pharmacokinetics. For example, Zhang et al. established IVIVC for PEG-PCL micelles, where they found that 70% of micelles were intact in an in vitro experiment versus the 60% that were found to be in bloodstream in vivo after 72 h [246,247].

In addition, Liu et al. demonstrated the stability profiles of micelles in the bloodstream in vivo correlated with in vitro stability by employing AF4 coupled with fluorescence and DLS, which was able to study interactions between micelles and different plasma proteins. However, this concept cannot be generalized, as evident from the work published by Bagheri et al. using similar techniques to determine the fate of curcumin-loaded polymeric micelles. Although the data indicated an agreement between micelle circulation time and in vitro data in plasma using AF4, curcumin clearance was faster in vivo than in vitro, which was then attributed to curcumin/blood cell interaction [247]. These results suggest that the selected polymers, drugs, and their interaction with the blood and plasma components in vivo can have a significant impact on the method predictivity. Owing to these issues, it is recommended to set up a method considering the physicochemical interaction of the drug product in vivo, and the method should always be drug and formulation specific.

In summary, stability, extensive physicochemical characterization, and the development and validation of specific methods constitute the main barriers to micellar clinical development. Thus, it is recommended to address these concerns in order to reduce the gap between preliminary research and the progression toward commercialization.

8. Conclusions and Future Outlooks

Polymeric micelles have gained attention as a promising nanocarrier for drug delivery because of their advantageous properties. The biocompatibility and low toxicity of micelles improve their circulation in the body, and they can solubilize hydrophobic drugs, making them more effective for treating various diseases.

In this review, different aspects of micelle development and application were discussed, including the selection of polymers, the responsive release of drugs, the fate of micelle administration in the body, regulatory considerations, and clinical trials.

The micellar formulations for cancer treatment are very promising. One of the key advantages of micelles is their ability to target specific cancer cells and improve the intratumor concentrations with increased potency of anti-cancer drugs. Micelles can be designed to target cancer cells by using specific targeting moieties, such as antibodies or peptides, which can enhance the selectivity and specificity of drug delivery.

In addition, micelles have the potential to overcome cancer drug resistance, which is a major challenge in the treatment of many cancers. The drugs loaded within the protective micelle structure are protected or shielded from efflux pumps and other mechanisms responsible for developing drug resistance. Micelles also offer combination drug therapies by serving as a co-delivery vehicle. The stimuli-responsive polymers can also release drugs in response to specific triggers, such as changes in pH or temperature, which could improve the accuracy and effectiveness of drug delivery to cancer cells.

Micelles have shown considerable success at the clinical level. Several micelles have been approved by FDA and become commercially available. The clinical translation of micelles has seen major progress in recent years. For example, Genexol®-PM and NANOXEL-M are examples of commercially available micelles mentioned in this review. However, a few obstacles still exist in micelle application. Despite their versatility, micelles still face challenges, such as delivering low payloads to target sites and ensuring clinical safety. However, researchers are actively working to overcome these challenges by designing copolymers for micelles and studying their behavior in vivo. By further developing novel copolymers used for micelles and investigating micelle in vivo kinetics, these obstacles may be overcome, and more effective therapies for a wide range of diseases may be developed.

Author Contributions: Q.W.; writing—original draft, writing—review and editing, figure drawing; K.A.; writing—original draft, writing—review and editing; A.K.T.; visualization, writing—review and editing; R.J.B.; visualization, supervision, writing—original draft, writing—review and editing. All authors have read and agreed to the published version of the manuscript.

Funding: This work received no external funding.

Institutional Review Board Statement: Not applicable.

Informed Consent Statement: Not applicable.

Data Availability Statement: Data sharing not applicable.

Acknowledgments: The authors acknowledge the funding support from Auburn University Presidential Graduate Research Fellowship (to Q.W.). The authors would like to thank the funding agency, the Department of Defense Breast Cancer Research Program Level 2 award (1W81XWH-21-1-0053) (to A.K.T.). The views expressed in this article are the opinions of the authors and may not reflect the official policy or position of the Department of the Army, Department of Defense, or the United States Government.

Conflicts of Interest: The authors declare no conflict of interest.

References

1. Huai, Y.; Hossen, M.N.; Wilhelm, S.; Bhattacharya, R.; Mukherjee, P. Nanoparticle Interactions with the Tumor Microenvironment. *Bioconjug. Chem.* **2019**, *30*, 2247–2263. [CrossRef] [PubMed]
2. Domingues, C.; Santos, A.; Alvarez-Lorenzo, C.; Concheiro, A.; Jarak, I.; Veiga, F.; Barbosa, I.; Dourado, M.; Figueiras, A. Where Is Nano Today and Where Is It Headed? A Review of Nanomedicine and the Dilemma of Nanotoxicology. *ACS Nano* **2022**, *16*, 9994–10041. [CrossRef] [PubMed]
3. Zhou, W.; Jia, Y.; Liu, Y.; Chen, Y.; Zhao, P. Tumor Microenvironment-Based Stimuli-Responsive Nanoparticles for Controlled Release of Drugs in Cancer Therapy. *Pharmaceutics* **2022**, *14*, 2346. [CrossRef]
4. Mbugua, S.N. Targeting Tumor Microenvironment by Metal Peroxide Nanoparticles in Cancer Therapy. *Bioinorg. Chem. Appl.* **2022**, *2022*, 5041399. [CrossRef] [PubMed]
5. Fan, T.; Sun, G.; Sun, X.; Zhao, L.; Zhong, R.; Peng, Y. Tumor Energy Metabolism and Potential of 3-Bromopyruvate as an Inhibitor of Aerobic Glycolysis: Implications in Tumor Treatment. *Cancers* **2019**, *11*, 317. [CrossRef]
6. Peng, S.; Xiao, F.; Chen, M.; Gao, H. Tumor-Microenvironment-Responsive Nanomedicine for Enhanced Cancer Immunotherapy. *Adv. Sci.* **2022**, *9*, e2103836. [CrossRef]
7. Dharmaratne, N.U.; Kaplan, A.R.; Glazer, P.M. Targeting the Hypoxic and Acidic Tumor Microenvironment with pH-Sensitive Peptides. *Cells* **2021**, *10*, 541. [CrossRef]
8. Qiu, N.; Du, X.; Ji, J.; Zhai, G. A review of stimuli-responsive polymeric micelles for tumor-targeted delivery of curcumin. *Drug Dev. Ind. Pharm.* **2021**, *47*, 839–856. [CrossRef]
9. Du, J.-Z.; Sun, T.-M.; Song, W.-J.; Wu, J.; Wang, J. A tumor-acidity-activated charge-conversional nanogel as an intelligent vehicle for promoted tumoral-cell uptake and drug delivery. *Angew. Chem. Int. Ed. Engl.* **2010**, *49*, 3621–3626. [CrossRef] [PubMed]
10. Du, J.-Z.; Mao, C.-Q.; Yuan, Y.-Y.; Yang, X.-Z.; Wang, J. Tumor extracellular acidity-activated nanoparticles as drug delivery systems for enhanced cancer therapy. *Biotechnol. Adv.* **2014**, *32*, 789–803. [CrossRef]
11. Miao, P.; Sheng, S.; Sun, X.; Liu, J.; Huang, G. Lactate dehydrogenase a in cancer: A promising target for diagnosis and therapy. *IUBMB Life* **2013**, *65*, 904–910. [CrossRef]
12. Cheng, R.; Feng, F.; Meng, F.; Deng, C.; Feijen, J.; Zhong, Z. Glutathione-responsive nano-vehicles as a promising platform for targeted intracellular drug and gene delivery. *J. Control. Release Off. J. Control. Release Soc.* **2011**, *152*, 2–12. [CrossRef]
13. Kurtoglu, Y.E.; Navath, R.S.; Wang, B.; Kannan, S.; Romero, R.; Kannan, R.M. Poly(amidoamine) dendrimer–drug conjugates with disulfide linkages for intracellular drug delivery. *Biomaterials* **2009**, *30*, 2112–2121. [CrossRef]
14. Peng, S.; Men, Y.; Xie, R.; Tian, Y.; Yang, W. Biodegradable phosphorylcholine-based zwitterionic polymer nanogels with smart charge-conversion ability for efficient inhibition of tumor cells. *J. Colloid Interface Sci.* **2019**, *539*, 19–29. [CrossRef] [PubMed]
15. Men, Y.; Peng, S.; Yang, P.; Jiang, Q.; Zhang, Y.; Shen, B.; Dong, P.; Pang, Z.; Yang, W. Biodegradable Zwitterionic Nanogels with Long Circulation for Antitumor Drug Delivery. *ACS Appl. Mater. Interfaces* **2018**, *10*, 23509–23521. [CrossRef] [PubMed]
16. Thambi, T.; Deepagan, V.G.; Yoon, H.Y.; Han, H.S.; Kim, S.H.; Son, S.; Jo, D.G.; Ahn, C.H.; Suh, Y.D.; Kim, K.; et al. Hypoxia-responsive polymeric nanoparticles for tumor-targeted drug delivery. *Biomaterials* **2014**, *35*, 1735–1743. [CrossRef]
17. Okuda, K.; Okabe, Y.; Kadonosono, T.; Ueno, T.; Youssif, B.G.; Kizaka-Kondoh, S.; Nagasawa, H. 2-Nitroimidazole-tricarbocyanine conjugate as a near-infrared fluorescent probe for In Vivo imaging of tumor hypoxia. *Bioconjug. Chem.* **2012**, *23*, 324–329. [CrossRef]
18. Moyer, M.W. Targeting hypoxia brings breath of fresh air to cancer therapy. *Nat. Med.* **2012**, *18*, 636–637. [CrossRef]
19. Wilson, W.R.; Hay, M.P. Targeting hypoxia in cancer therapy. *Nat. Rev. Cancer* **2011**, *11*, 393–410. [CrossRef] [PubMed]
20. Frezza, C.; Zheng, L.; Tennant, D.A.; Papkovsky, D.B.; Hedley, B.A.; Kalna, G.; Watson, D.G.; Gottlieb, E. Metabolic profiling of hypoxic cells revealed a catabolic signature required for cell survival. *PLoS ONE* **2011**, *6*, e24411. [CrossRef]

21. Mosesson, Y.; Mills, G.B.; Yarden, Y. Derailed endocytosis: An emerging feature of cancer. *Nat. Rev. Cancer* **2008**, *8*, 835–850. [CrossRef] [PubMed]
22. Wang, Y.; Roche, O.; Yan, M.S.; Finak, G.; Evans, A.J.; Metcalf, J.L.; Hast, B.E.; Hanna, S.C.; Wondergem, B.; Furge, K.A.; et al. Regulation of endocytosis via the oxygen-sensing pathway. *Nat. Med.* **2009**, *15*, 319–324. [CrossRef] [PubMed]
23. Srinivas, U.S.; Tan, B.W.Q.; Vellayappan, B.A.; Jeyasekharan, A.D. ROS and the DNA damage response in cancer. *Redox Biol.* **2019**, *25*, 101084. [CrossRef]
24. Peng, X.; Gandhi, V. ROS-activated anticancer prodrugs: A new strategy for tumor-specific damage. *Ther. Deliv.* **2012**, *3*, 823–833. [CrossRef]
25. Bai, J.; Jia, X.; Zhen, W.; Cheng, W.; Jiang, X. A Facile Ion-Doping Strategy to Regulate Tumor Microenvironments for Enhanced Multimodal Tumor Theranostics. *J. Am. Chem. Soc.* **2018**, *140*, 106–109. [CrossRef] [PubMed]
26. Shim, M.S.; Xia, Y. A Reactive Oxygen Species (ROS)-Responsive Polymer for Safe, Efficient, and Targeted Gene Delivery in Cancer Cells. *Angew. Chem. Int. Ed.* **2013**, *52*, 6926–6929. [CrossRef] [PubMed]
27. Qiu, N.; Gao, J.; Liu, Q.; Wang, J.; Shen, Y. Enzyme-Responsive Charge-Reversal Polymer-Mediated Effective Gene Therapy for Intraperitoneal Tumors. *Biomacromolecules* **2018**, *19*, 2308–2319. [CrossRef] [PubMed]
28. Li, Y.; Gao, J.; Zhang, C.; Cao, Z.; Cheng, D.; Liu, J.; Shuai, X. Stimuli-Responsive Polymeric Nanocarriers for Efficient Gene Delivery. *Top. Curr. Chem.* **2017**, *375*, 27. [CrossRef] [PubMed]
29. Liu, D.; Yang, F.; Xiong, F.; Gu, N. The Smart Drug Delivery System and Its Clinical Potential. *Theranostics* **2016**, *6*, 1306–1323. [CrossRef]
30. Matsumura, Y.; Maeda, H. A new concept for macromolecular therapeutics in cancer chemotherapy: Mechanism of tumoritropic accumulation of proteins and the antitumor agent smancs. *Cancer Res.* **1986**, *46*, 6387–6392.
31. Suk, J.S.; Xu, Q.; Kim, N.; Hanes, J.; Ensign, L.M. PEGylation as a strategy for improving nanoparticle-based drug and gene delivery. *Adv. Drug Deliv. Rev.* **2016**, *99*, 28–51. [CrossRef]
32. Hobbs, S.K.; Monsky, W.L.; Yuan, F.; Roberts, W.G.; Griffith, L.; Torchilin, V.P.; Jain, R.K. Regulation of transport pathways in tumor vessels: Role of tumor type and microenvironment. *Proc. Natl. Acad. Sci. USA* **1998**, *95*, 4607–4612. [CrossRef]
33. Wolfram, J.; Zhu, M.; Yang, Y.; Shen, J.; Gentile, E.; Paolino, D.; Fresta, M.; Nie, G.; Chen, C.; Shen, H.; et al. Safety of Nanoparticles in Medicine. *Curr. Drug Targets* **2015**, *16*, 1671–1681. [CrossRef] [PubMed]
34. Cabral, H.; Miyata, K.; Osada, K.; Kataoka, K. Block Copolymer Micelles in Nanomedicine Applications. *Chem. Rev.* **2018**, *118*, 6844–6892. [CrossRef] [PubMed]
35. Tang, L.; Yang, X.; Yin, Q.; Cai, K.; Wang, H.; Chaudhury, I.; Yao, C.; Zhou, Q.; Kwon, M.; Hartman, J.A.; et al. Investigating the optimal size of anticancer nanomedicine. *Proc. Natl. Acad. Sci. USA* **2014**, *111*, 15344–15349. [CrossRef]
36. Ghosh, B.; Biswas, S. Polymeric micelles in cancer therapy: State of the art. *J. Control. Release* **2021**, *332*, 127–147. [CrossRef] [PubMed]
37. Marzbali, M.Y.; Khosroushahi, A.Y. Polymeric micelles as mighty nanocarriers for cancer gene therapy: A review. *Cancer Chemother. Pharmacol.* **2017**, *79*, 637–649. [CrossRef] [PubMed]
38. Morshed, R.A.; Cheng, Y.; Auffinger, B.; Wegscheid, M.L.; Lesniak, M.S. The potential of polymeric micelles in the context of glioblastoma therapy. *Front. Pharmacol.* **2013**, *4*, 157. [CrossRef] [PubMed]
39. Kabanov, A.; Batrakova, E.; Alakhov, V.Y. Pluronic block copolymers as novel polymer therapeutics for drug and gene delivery. *J. Control. Release Off. J. Control. Release Soc.* **2002**, *82*, 189–212. [CrossRef] [PubMed]
40. Peer, D.; Karp, J.M.; Hong, S.; Farokhzad, O.C.; Margalit, R.; Langer, R. Nanocarriers as an emerging platform for cancer therapy. *Nat. Nanotechnol.* **2007**, *2*, 751–760. [CrossRef]
41. Kataoka, K.; Harada, A.; Nagasaki, Y. Block copolymer micelles for drug delivery: Design, characterization and biological significance. *Adv. Drug Deliv. Rev.* **2001**, *47*, 113–131. [CrossRef]
42. Petros, R.A.; DeSimone, J.M. Strategies in the design of nanoparticles for therapeutic applications. *Nat. Rev. Drug Discov.* **2010**, *9*, 615–627. [CrossRef] [PubMed]
43. Perumal, S.-A.; Atchudan, R.; Lee, W. A Review of Polymeric Micelles and Their Applications. *Polymers* **2022**, *14*, 2510. [CrossRef]
44. Topel, Ö.; Çakır, B.A.; Budama, L.; Hoda, N. Determination of critical micelle concentration of polybutadiene-block-poly(ethyleneoxide) diblock copolymer by fluorescence spectroscopy and dynamic light scattering. *J. Mol. Liq.* **2013**, *177*, 40–43. [CrossRef]
45. Amos, D.A.; Markels, J.H.; Lynn, S.; Radke, C.J. Osmotic Pressure and Interparticle Interactions in Ionic Micellar Surfactant Solutions. *J. Phys. Chem. B* **1998**, *102*, 2739–2753. [CrossRef]
46. Pérez-Rodríguez, M.; Prieto, G.; Rega, C.; Varela, L.M.; Sarmiento, F.; Mosquera, V. A Comparative Study of the Determination of the Critical Micelle Concentration by Conductivity and Dielectric Constant Measurements. *Langmuir* **1998**, *14*, 4422–4426. [CrossRef]
47. Scholz, N.; Behnke, T.; Resch-Genger, U. Determination of the Critical Micelle Concentration of Neutral and Ionic Surfactants with Fluorometry, Conductometry, and Surface Tension—A Method Comparison. *J. Fluoresc.* **2018**, *28*, 465–476. [CrossRef]
48. Heakal, F.E.-T.; Elkholy, A.E. Gemini surfactants as corrosion inhibitors for carbon steel. *J. Mol. Liq.* **2017**, *230*, 395–407. [CrossRef]
49. Li, X.; Zhang, Y.; Fan, Y.; Zhou, Y.; Wang, X.; Fan, C.; Liu, Y.; Zhang, Q. Preparation and evaluation of novel mixed micelles as nanocarriers for intravenous delivery of propofol. *Nanoscale Res. Lett.* **2011**, *6*, 275. [CrossRef]

50. Bae, Y.; Nishiyama, N.; Fukushima, S.; Koyama, H.; Yasuhiro, M.; Kataoka, K. Preparation and Biological Characterization of Polymeric Micelle Drug Carriers with Intracellular pH-Triggered Drug Release Property: Tumor Permeability, Controlled Subcellular Drug Distribution, and Enhanced In Vivo Antitumor Efficacy. *Bioconjug. Chem.* **2005**, *16*, 122–130. [CrossRef]
51. Nagarajan, R.; Barry, M.; Ruckenstein, E. Unusual selectivity in solubilization by block copolymer micelles. *Langmuir* **1986**, *2*, 210–215. [CrossRef]
52. Xiong, X.-B.; Falamarzian, A.; Garg, S.M.; Lavasanifar, A. Engineering of amphiphilic block copolymers for polymeric micellar drug and gene delivery. *J. Control. Release* **2011**, *155*, 248–261. [CrossRef]
53. Lu, Y.; Zhang, E.; Yang, J.; Cao, Z. Strategies to improve micelle stability for drug delivery. *Nano Res.* **2018**, *11*, 4985–4998. [CrossRef]
54. Lavasanifar, A.; Samuel, J.; Sattari, S.; Kwon, G.S. Block copolymer micelles for the encapsulation and delivery of amphotericin B. *Pharm. Res.* **2002**, *19*, 418–422. [CrossRef]
55. Markman, J.L.; Rekechenetskiy, A.; Holler, E.; Ljubimova, J.Y. Nanomedicine therapeutic approaches to overcome cancer drug resistance. *Adv. Drug Deliv. Rev.* **2013**, *65*, 1866–1879. [CrossRef] [PubMed]
56. Minko, T. Soluble polymer conjugates for drug delivery. *Drug Discov. Today Technol.* **2005**, *2*, 15–20. [CrossRef]
57. Knop, K.; Hoogenboom, R.; Fischer, D.; Schubert, U.S. Poly(ethylene glycol) in Drug Delivery: Pros and Cons as Well as Potential Alternatives. *Angew. Chem. Int. Ed.* **2010**, *49*, 6288–6308. [CrossRef] [PubMed]
58. Zhang, F.; Liu, M.; Wan, H. Discussion about several potential drawbacks of PEGylated therapeutic proteins. *Biol. Pharm. Bull.* **2014**, *37*, 335–339. [CrossRef]
59. Zhang, N.; Wardwell, P.R.; Bader, R.A. Polysaccharide-based micelles for drug delivery. *Pharmaceutics* **2013**, *5*, 329–352. [CrossRef]
60. Thanou, M.; Verhoef, J.C.; Junginger, H.E. Chitosan and its derivatives as intestinal absorption enhancers. *Adv. Drug Deliv. Rev.* **2001**, *50* (Suppl. 1), S91–S101. [CrossRef] [PubMed]
61. Patra, J.K.; Das, G.; Fraceto, L.F.; Campos, E.V.R.; Rodriguez-Torres, M.D.P.; Acosta-Torres, L.S.; Diaz-Torres, L.A.; Grillo, R.; Swamy, M.K.; Sharma, S.; et al. Nano based drug delivery systems: Recent developments and future prospects. *J. Nanobiotechnol.* **2018**, *16*, 71. [CrossRef] [PubMed]
62. Pertici, G. 1—Introduction to bioresorbable polymers for biomedical applications. In *Bioresorbable Polymers for Biomedical Applications*; Perale, G., Hilborn, J., Eds.; Woodhead Publishing: Amsterdam, The Netherlands, 2017; pp. 3–29. [CrossRef]
63. Poole-Warren, L.A.; Patton, A.J. 1—Introduction to biomedical polymers and biocompatibility. In *Woodhead Publishing Series in Biomaterials*; Poole-Warren, L., Martens, P., Green, R., Eds.; Woodhead Publishing: Amsterdam, The Netherlands, 2016; pp. 3–31. [CrossRef]
64. Wen, Y.; Oh, J.K. Recent Strategies to Develop Polysaccharide-Based Nanomaterials for Biomedical Applications. *Macromol. Rapid Commun.* **2014**, *35*, 1819–1832. [CrossRef] [PubMed]
65. Luo, K.; Yang, J.; Kopečková, P.; Kopeček, J. Biodegradable Multiblock Poly[N-(2-hydroxypropyl)methacrylamide] via Reversible Addition-Fragmentation Chain Transfer Polymerization and Click Chemistry. *Macromolecules* **2011**, *44*, 2481–2488. [CrossRef] [PubMed]
66. Alfurhood, J.A.; Sun, H.; Kabb, C.P.; Tucker, B.S.; Matthews, J.H.; Luesch, H.; Sumerlin, B.S. Poly(N-(2-Hydroxypropyl) Methacrylamide)-Valproic Acid Conjugates as Block Copolymer Nanocarriers. *Polym. Chem.* **2017**, *8*, 4983–4987. [CrossRef]
67. Kopecek, J.; Kopecková, P.; Minko, T.; Lu, Z. HPMA copolymer-anticancer drug conjugates: Design, activity, and mechanism of action. *Eur. J. Pharm. Biopharm. Off. J. Arb. Fur Pharm. Verfahr. e.V.* **2000**, *50*, 61–81. [CrossRef]
68. Tucker, B.S.; Sumerlin, B.S. Poly(N-(2-hydroxypropyl) methacrylamide)-based nanotherapeutics. *Polym. Chem.* **2014**, *5*, 1566–1572. [CrossRef]
69. Soni, V.; Pandey, V.; Tiwari, R.; Asati, S.; Tekade, R.K. Chapter 13—Design and Evaluation of Ophthalmic Delivery Formulations. In *Advances in Pharmaceutical Product Development and Research*; Tekade, R.K., Ed.; Academic Press: Cambridge, MA, USA, 2019; pp. 473–538. [CrossRef]
70. Liu, H.; Chen, H.; Cao, F.; Peng, D.; Chen, W.; Zhang, C. Amphiphilic Block Copolymer Poly (Acrylic Acid)-B-Polycaprolactone as a Novel pH-sensitive Nanocarrier for Anti-Cancer Drugs Delivery: In-Vitro and In-Vivo Evaluation. *Polymers* **2019**, *11*, 820. [CrossRef]
71. Xu, H.; Yao, Q.; Cai, C.; Gou, J.; Zhang, Y.; Zhong, H.; Tang, X. Amphiphilic poly(amino acid) based micelles applied to drug delivery: The In Vitro and In Vivo challenges and the corresponding potential strategies. *J. Control. Release Off. J. Control. Release Soc.* **2015**, *199*, 84–97. [CrossRef] [PubMed]
72. Chen, Z.; FitzGerald, P.A.; Kobayashi, Y.; Ueno, K.; Watanabe, M.; Warr, G.G.; Atkin, R. Micelle Structure of Novel Diblock Polyethers in Water and Two Protic Ionic Liquids (EAN and PAN). *Macromolecules* **2015**, *48*, 1843–1851. [CrossRef]
73. Urbánek, T.; Jäger, E.; Jäger, A.; Hrubý, M. Selectively Biodegradable Polyesters: Nature-Inspired Construction Materials for Future Biomedical Applications. *Polymers* **2019**, *11*, 1061. [CrossRef]
74. Tyler, B.; Gullotti, D.; Mangraviti, A.; Utsuki, T.; Brem, H. Polylactic acid (PLA) controlled delivery carriers for biomedical applications. *Adv. Drug Deliv. Rev.* **2016**, *107*, 163–175. [CrossRef] [PubMed]
75. Ulbrich, K.; Holá, K.; Šubr, V.; Bakandritsos, A.; Tuček, J.; Zbořil, R. Targeted Drug Delivery with Polymers and Magnetic Nanoparticles: Covalent and Noncovalent Approaches, Release Control, and Clinical Studies. *Chem. Rev.* **2016**, *116*, 5338–5431. [CrossRef]

76. Dehbari, N.; Tavakoli, J.; Khatrao, S.S.; Tang, Y. In Situ polymerized hyperbranched polymer reinforced poly (acrylic acid) hydrogels. *Mater. Chem. Front.* **2017**, *1*, 1995–2004. [CrossRef]
77. Balogun-Agbaje, O.A.; Odeniyi, O.A.; Odeniyi, M.A. Drug delivery applications of poly-γ-glutamic acid. *Futur. J. Pharm. Sci.* **2021**, *7*, 125. [CrossRef]
78. Delbecq, F.; Kawakami, K. Self-assembly study and formation of hydrophobized PVA dense and stable nanoparticles loaded with cholesterol or a steroid-type drug. *J. Colloid Interface Sci.* **2014**, *428*, 57–62. [CrossRef] [PubMed]
79. Deng, W.; Chen, J.; Kulkarni, A.; Thompson, D.H. Poly(ethylene glycol)-poly(vinyl alcohol)-adamantanate: Synthesis and stimuli-responsive micelle properties. *Soft Matter* **2012**, *8*, 5843–5846. [CrossRef]
80. Gaaz, T.S.; Sulong, A.B.; Akhtar, M.N.; Kadhum, A.A.H.; Mohamad, A.B.; Al-Amiery, A.A. Properties and Applications of Polyvinyl Alcohol, Halloysite Nanotubes and Their Nanocomposites. *Molecules* **2015**, *20*, 22833–22847. [CrossRef]
81. Torchilin, V.P.; Trubetskoy, V.S. Which polymers can make nanoparticulate drug carriers long-circulating? *Adv. Drug Deliv. Rev.* **1995**, *16*, 141–155. [CrossRef]
82. Takeuchi, H.; Kojima, H.; Yamamoto, H.; Kawashima, Y. Evaluation of circulation profiles of liposomes coated with hydrophilic polymers having different molecular weights in rats. *J. Control. Release Off. J. Control. Release Soc.* **2001**, *75*, 83–91. [CrossRef]
83. Kuang, C.; Yusa, S.; Sato, T. Micellization and Phase Separation in Aqueous Solutions of Thermosensitive Block Copolymer Poly(N-isopropylacrylamide)-b-poly(N-vinyl-2-pyrrolidone) upon Heating. *Macromolecules* **2019**, *52*, 4812–4819. [CrossRef]
84. Wei, H.; Cheng, S.-X.; Zhang, X.-Z.; Zhuo, R.-X. Thermo-sensitive polymeric micelles based on poly(N-isopropylacrylamide) as drug carriers. *Prog. Polym. Sci.* **2009**, *34*, 893–910. [CrossRef]
85. Lanzalaco, S.; Armelin, E. Poly(N-isopropylacrylamide) and Copolymers: A Review on Recent Progresses in Biomedical Applications. *Gels* **2017**, *3*, 36. [CrossRef] [PubMed]
86. Lv, J.; Yang, J.; Hao, X.; Ren, X.; Feng, Y.; Zhang, W. Biodegradable PEI modified complex micelles as gene carriers with tunable gene transfection efficiency for ECs. *J. Mater. Chem. B* **2016**, *4*, 997–1008. [CrossRef] [PubMed]
87. Xie, L.; Liu, R.; Chen, X.; He, M.; Zhang, Y.; Chen, S. Micelles Based on Lysine, Histidine, or Arginine: Designing Structures for Enhanced Drug Delivery. *Front. Bioeng. Biotechnol.* **2021**, *9*, 744657. [CrossRef] [PubMed]
88. Abdelaziz, H.M.; Abdelmoneem, M.A.; Abdelsalam, K.; Freag, M.S.; Elkhodairy, K.A.; Elzoghby, A.O. *Chapter 9—Poly(Amino Acid) Nanoparticles as a Promising Tool for Anticancer Therapeutics*; Kesharwani, P., Paknikar, K., Gajbhiye, V., Eds.; Academic Press: Cambridge, MA, USA, 2019; pp. 167–204. [CrossRef]
89. Ghasemi, R.; Abdollahi, M.; Emamgholi Zadeh, E.; Khodabakhshi, K.; Badeli, A.; Bagheri, H.; Hosseinkhani, S. mPEG-PLA and PLA-PEG-PLA nanoparticles as new carriers for delivery of recombinant human Growth Hormone (rhGH). *Sci. Rep.* **2018**, *8*, 9854. [CrossRef]
90. Nair, N.R.; Sekhar, V.C.; Nampoothiri, K.M.; Pandey, A. 32—Biodegradation of Biopolymers. In *Production, Isolation and Purification of Industrial Products*; Pandey, A., Negi, S., Singh-Nee Nigam, P., Soccol, C.R., Eds.; Elsevier: Amsterdam, The Netherlands, 2017; pp. 739–755. [CrossRef]
91. De Oliveira, J.; Vandenberghe, L.P.S.; Zawadzki, S.F.; Rodrigues, C.; de Carvalho, J.C.; Soccol, C.R. 28—Production and Application of Polylactides. In *Production, Isolation and Purification of Industrial Products*; Pandey, A., Negi, S., Singh-Nee Nigam, P., Soccol, C.R., Eds.; Elsevier: Amsterdam, The Netherlands, 2017; pp. 633–653. [CrossRef]
92. Elmowafy, E.M.; Tiboni, M.; Soliman, M.E. Biocompatibility, biodegradation and biomedical applications of poly(lactic acid)/poly(lactic-co-glycolic acid) micro and nanoparticles. *J. Pharm. Investig.* **2019**, *49*, 347–380. [CrossRef]
93. Lu, X.; Yang, X.; Meng, Y.; Li, S. Temperature and pH dually-responsive poly(β-amino ester) nanoparticles for drug delivery. *Chin. J. Polym. Sci.* **2017**, *35*, 534–546. [CrossRef]
94. Hari, S.K.; Gauba, A.; Shrivastava, N.; Tripathi, R.M.; Jain, S.K.; Pandey, A.K. Polymeric micelles and cancer therapy: An ingenious multimodal tumor-targeted drug delivery system. *Drug Deliv. Transl. Res.* **2022**, *13*, 135–163. [CrossRef]
95. Biswas, S.; Kumari, P.; Lakhani, P.M.; Ghosh, B. Recent advances in polymeric micelles for anti-cancer drug delivery. *Eur. J. Pharm. Sci. Off. J. Eur. Fed. Pharm. Sci.* **2016**, *83*, 184–202. [CrossRef]
96. Dai, Y.; Chen, X.; Zhang, X. Recent advances in stimuli-responsive polymeric micelles via click chemistry. *Polym. Chem.* **2019**, *10*, 34–44. [CrossRef]
97. Kim, D.; Lee, E.S.; Park, K.; Kwon, I.C.; Bae, Y.H. Doxorubicin Loaded pH-sensitive Micelle: Antitumoral Efficacy against Ovarian A2780/DOXR Tumor. *Pharm. Res.* **2008**, *25*, 2074–2082. [CrossRef] [PubMed]
98. Tang, S.; Meng, Q.; Sun, H.; Su, J.; Yin, Q.; Zhang, Z.; Yu, H.; Chen, L.; Gu, W.; Li, Y. Dual pH-sensitive micelles with charge-switch for controlling cellular uptake and drug release to treat metastatic breast cancer. *Biomaterials* **2017**, *114*, 44–53. [CrossRef]
99. Yang, C.; Xue, Z.; Liu, Y.; Xiao, J.; Chen, J.; Zhang, L.; Guo, J.; Lin, W. Delivery of anticancer drug using pH-sensitive micelles from triblock copolymer MPEG-b-PBAE-b-PLA. *Mater. Sci. Eng. C* **2018**, *84*, 254–262. [CrossRef] [PubMed]
100. Liu, R.; Li, D.; He, B.; Xu, X.; Sheng, M.; Lai, Y.; Wang, G.; Gu, Z. Anti-tumor drug delivery of pH-sensitive poly(ethylene glycol)-poly(L-histidine-)-poly(L-lactide) nanoparticles. *J. Control. Release* **2011**, *152*, 49–56. [CrossRef] [PubMed]
101. Li, Y.; Leng, M.; Cai, M.; Huang, L.; Chen, Y.; Luo, X. pH responsive micelles based on copolymers mPEG-PCL-PDEA: The relationship between composition and properties. *Colloids Surf. B Biointerfaces* **2017**, *154*, 397–407. [CrossRef]
102. Liu, P.; Huang, P.; Kang, E.-T. pH-Sensitive Dextran-Based Micelles from Copper-Free Click Reaction for Antitumor Drug Delivery. *Langmuir* **2021**, *37*, 12990–12999. [CrossRef]

103. Min, K.H.; Kim, J.-H.; Bae, S.M.; Shin, H.; Kim, M.S.; Park, S.; Lee, H.; Park, R.-W.; Kim, I.-S.; Kim, K.; et al. Tumoral acidic pH-responsive MPEG-poly(β-amino ester) polymeric micelles for cancer targeting therapy. *J. Control. Release* 2010, *144*, 259–266. [CrossRef]
104. Zhang, C.Y.; Yang, Y.Q.; Huang, T.X.; Zhao, B.; Guo, X.D.; Wang, J.F.; Zhang, L.J. Self-assembled pH-responsive MPEG-b-(PLA-co-PAE) block copolymer micelles for anticancer drug delivery. *Biomaterials* 2012, *33*, 6273–6283. [CrossRef]
105. Gebrie, H.T.; Addisu, K.D.; Darge, H.F.; Birhan, Y.S.; Thankachan, D.; Tsai, H.-C.; Wu, S.-Y. pH/redox-responsive core cross-linked based prodrug micelle for enhancing micellar stability and controlling delivery of chemo drugs: An effective combination drug delivery platform for cancer therapy. *Biomater. Adv.* 2022, *139*, 213015. [CrossRef]
106. Li, M.; Zhao, Y.; Sun, J.; Chen, H.; Liu, Z.; Lin, K.; Ma, P.; Zhang, W.; Zhen, Y.; Zhang, S.; et al. pH/reduction dual-responsive hyaluronic acid-podophyllotoxin prodrug micelles for tumor targeted delivery. *Carbohydr. Polym.* 2022, *288*, 119402. [CrossRef]
107. Isik, G.; Kiziltay, A.; Hasirci, N.; Tezcaner, A. Lithocholic acid conjugated mPEG-b-PCL micelles for pH responsive delivery to breast cancer cells. *Int. J. Pharm.* 2022, *621*, 121779. [CrossRef]
108. Song, P.; Lu, Z.; Jiang, T.; Han, W.; Chen, X.; Zhao, X. Chitosan coated pH/redox-responsive hyaluronic acid micelles for enhanced tumor targeted co-delivery of doxorubicin and siPD-L1. *Int. J. Biol. Macromol.* 2022, *222*, 1078–1091. [CrossRef]
109. Wang, L.; Tian, B.; Zhang, J.; Li, K.; Liang, Y.; Sun, Y.; Ding, Y.; Han, J. Coordinated pH/redox dual-sensitive and hepatoma-targeted multifunctional polymeric micelle system for stimuli-triggered doxorubicin release: Synthesis, characterization and In Vitro evaluation. *Int. J. Pharm.* 2016, *501*, 221–235. [CrossRef] [PubMed]
110. Dai, L.; Li, X.; Duan, X.; Li, M.; Niu, P.; Xu, H.; Cai, K.; Yang, H. A pH/ROS Cascade-Responsive Charge-Reversal Nanosystem with Self-Amplified Drug Release for Synergistic Oxidation-Chemotherapy. *Adv. Sci.* 2019, *6*, 1801807. [CrossRef] [PubMed]
111. Hu, Y.; Deng, M.; Yang, H.; Chen, L.; Xiao, C.; Zhuang, X.; Chen, X. Multi-responsive core-crosslinked poly (thioether ester) micelles for smart drug delivery. *Polymer* 2017, *110*, 235–241. [CrossRef]
112. Sun, C.; Liang, Y.; Hao, N.; Xu, L.; Cheng, F.; Su, T.; Cao, J.; Gao, W.; Pu, Y.; He, B. A ROS-responsive polymeric micelle with a π-conjugated thioketal moiety for enhanced drug loading and efficient drug delivery. *Org. Biomol. Chem.* 2017, *15*, 9176–9185. [CrossRef]
113. Yoo, J.; Rejinold, N.S.; Lee, D.; Jon, S.; Kim, Y.-C. Protease-activatable cell-penetrating peptide possessing ROS-triggered phase transition for enhanced cancer therapy. *J. Control. Release* 2017, *264*, 89–101. [CrossRef] [PubMed]
114. Qu, C.; Li, J.; Zhou, Y.; Yang, S.; Chen, W.; Li, F.; You, B.; Liu, Y.; Zhang, X. Targeted Delivery of Doxorubicin via CD147-Mediated ROS/pH Dual-Sensitive Nanomicelles for the Efficient Therapy of Hepatocellular Carcinoma. *AAPS J.* 2018, *20*, 34. [CrossRef]
115. Xin, X.; Lin, F.; Wang, Q.; Yin, L.; Mahato, R.I. ROS-Responsive Polymeric Micelles for Triggered Simultaneous Delivery of PLK1 Inhibitor/miR-34a and Effective Synergistic Therapy in Pancreatic Cancer. *ACS Appl. Mater. Interfaces* 2019, *11*, 14647–14659. [CrossRef]
116. Tang, M.; Hu, P.; Zheng, Q.; Tirelli, N.; Yang, X.; Wang, Z.; Wang, Y.; Tang, Q.; He, Y. Polymeric micelles with dual thermal and reactive oxygen species (ROS)-responsiveness for inflammatory cancer cell delivery. *J. Nanobiotechnol.* 2017, *15*, 39. [CrossRef]
117. Xu, L.; Zhao, M.; Gao, W.; Yang, Y.; Zhang, J.; Pu, Y.; He, B. Polymeric nanoparticles responsive to intracellular ROS for anticancer drug delivery. *Colloids Surf. B Biointerfaces* 2019, *181*, 252–260. [CrossRef]
118. Zhang, Y.; Guo, Q.; An, S.; Lu, Y.; Li, J.; He, X.; Liu, L.; Zhang, Y.; Sun, T.; Jiang, C. ROS-Switchable Polymeric Nanoplatform with Stimuli-Responsive Release for Active Targeted Drug Delivery to Breast Cancer. *ACS Appl. Mater. Interfaces* 2017, *9*, 12227–12240. [CrossRef]
119. Xu, H.; Yang, M.; Du, Y.; Gao, T.; Liu, Y.; Xiong, L.; Peng, N. Self-assembly of micelles with pH/ROS dual-responsiveness and mitochondrial targeting for potential anti-tumor applications. *New J. Chem.* 2022, *46*, 21235–21244. [CrossRef]
120. Deng, Y.; Yuan, H.; Yuan, W. Hypoxia-responsive micelles self-assembled from amphiphilic block copolymers for the controlled release of anticancer drugs. *J. Mater. Chem. B* 2019, *7*, 286–295. [CrossRef]
121. Kang, L.; Fan, B.; Sun, P.; Huang, W.; Jin, M.; Wang, Q.; Gao, Z. An effective tumor-targeting strategy utilizing hypoxia-sensitive siRNA delivery system for improved anti-tumor outcome. *Acta Biomater.* 2016, *44*, 341–354. [CrossRef]
122. Thambi, T.; Son, S.; Lee, D.S.; Park, J.H. Poly(ethylene glycol)-b-poly(lysine) copolymer bearing nitroaromatics for hypoxia-sensitive drug delivery. *Acta Biomater.* 2016, *29*, 261–270. [CrossRef]
123. Filipczak, N.; Joshi, U.; Attia, S.A.; Berger Fridman, I.; Cohen, S.; Konry, T.; Torchilin, V. Hypoxia-sensitive drug delivery to tumors. *J. Control. Release* 2022, *341*, 431–442. [CrossRef]
124. Lu, M.; Huang, X.; Cai, X.; Sun, J.; Liu, X.; Weng, L.; Zhu, L.; Luo, Q.; Chen, Z. Hypoxia-Responsive Stereocomplex Polymeric Micelles with Improved Drug Loading Inhibit Breast Cancer Metastasis in an Orthotopic Murine Model. *ACS Appl. Mater. Interfaces* 2022, *14*, 20551–20565. [CrossRef] [PubMed]
125. Meng, T.; Li, Y.; Tian, Y.; Ma, M.; Shi, K.; Shang, X.; Yuan, H.; Hu, F. A Hypoxia-Sensitive Drug Delivery System Constructed by Nitroimidazole and its Application in the Treatment of Hepatocellular Carcinoma. *AAPS PharmSciTech* 2022, *23*, 167. [CrossRef]
126. Long, M.; Liu, X.; Huang, X.; Lu, M.; Wu, X.; Weng, L.; Chen, Q.; Wang, X.; Zhu, L.; Chen, Z. Alendronate-functionalized hypoxia-responsive polymeric micelles for targeted therapy of bone metastatic prostate cancer. *J. Control. Release* 2021, *334*, 303–317. [CrossRef] [PubMed]
127. Ma, P.; Wei, G.; Chen, J.; Jing, Z.; Wang, X.; Wang, Z. GLUT1 targeting and hypoxia-activating polymer-drug conjugate-based micelle for tumor chemo-thermal therapy. *Drug Deliv.* 2021, *28*, 2256–2267. [CrossRef] [PubMed]

128. Zhang, M.; Zhang, S.; Zhang, K.; Zhu, Z.; Miao, Y.; Qiu, Y.; Zhang, P.; Zhao, X. Self-assembly of polymer-doxorubicin conjugates to form polyprodrug micelles for pH/enzyme dual-responsive drug delivery. *Colloids Surf. A Physicochem. Eng. Asp.* **2021**, *622*, 126669. [CrossRef]
129. Zhang, L.; Wang, Y.; Zhang, X.; Wei, X.; Xiong, X.; Zhou, S. Enzyme and Redox Dual-Triggered Intracellular Release from Actively Targeted Polymeric Micelles. *ACS Appl. Mater. Interfaces* **2017**, *9*, 3388–3399. [CrossRef] [PubMed]
130. Zhu, L.; Perche, F.; Wang, T.; Torchilin, V.P. Matrix metalloproteinase 2-sensitive multifunctional polymeric micelles for tumor-specific co-delivery of siRNA and hydrophobic drugs. *Biomaterials* **2014**, *35*, 4213–4222. [CrossRef] [PubMed]
131. Lima, A.C.; Reis, R.L.; Ferreira, H.; Neves, N.M. Glutathione Reductase-Sensitive Polymeric Micelles for Controlled Drug Delivery on Arthritic Diseases. *ACS Biomater. Sci. Eng.* **2021**, *7*, 3229–3241. [CrossRef] [PubMed]
132. Zhang, Z.; Zhang, Q.; Xie, J.; Zhong, Z.; Deng, C. Enzyme-responsive micellar JQ1 induces enhanced BET protein inhibition and immunotherapy of malignant tumors. *Biomater. Sci.* **2021**, *9*, 6915–6926. [CrossRef]
133. Wan, D.; Zhu, Q.; Zhang, J.; Chen, X.; Li, F.; Liu, Y.; Pan, J. Intracellular and extracellular enzymatic responsive micelle for intelligent therapy of cancer. *Nano Res.* **2022**, *16*, 2851–2858. [CrossRef]
134. Han, J.O.; Lee, H.J.; Jeong, B. Thermosensitive core-rigid micelles of monomethoxy poly(ethylene glycol)-deoxy cholic acid. *Biomater. Res.* **2022**, *26*, 16. [CrossRef]
135. Li, G.; Guo, L.; Meng, Y.; Zhang, T. Self-assembled nanoparticles from thermo-sensitive polyion complex micelles for controlled drug release. *Chem. Eng. J.* **2011**, *174*, 199–205. [CrossRef]
136. Chung, J.E.; Yokoyama, M.; Yamato, M.; Aoyagi, T.; Sakurai, Y.; Okano, T. Thermo-responsive drug delivery from polymeric micelles constructed using block copolymers of poly (N-isopropylacrylamide) and poly (butylmethacrylate). *J. Control. Release* **1999**, *62*, 115–127. [CrossRef]
137. Wang, X.; Li, S.; Wan, Z.; Quan, Z.; Tan, Q. Investigation of thermo-sensitive amphiphilic micelles as drug carriers for chemotherapy in cholangiocarcinoma In Vitro and In Vivo. *Int. J. Pharm.* **2014**, *463*, 81–88. [CrossRef]
138. Lin, M.M.; Kang, Y.J.; Sohn, Y.; Kim, D.K. Dual targeting strategy of magnetic nanoparticle-loaded and RGD peptide-activated stimuli-sensitive polymeric micelles for delivery of paclitaxel. *J. Nanoparticle Res.* **2015**, *17*, 248. [CrossRef]
139. Wang, Q.; Xiao, J.; Su, Y.; Huang, J.; Li, J.; Qiu, L.; Zhan, M.; He, X.; Yuan, W.; Li, Y. Fabrication of thermoresponsive magnetic micelles from amphiphilic poly(phenyl isocyanide) and Fe_3O_4 nanoparticles for controlled drug release and synergistic thermochemotherapy. *Polym. Chem.* **2021**, *12*, 2132–2140. [CrossRef]
140. Lei, B.; Sun, M.; Chen, M.; Xu, S.; Liu, H. pH and Temperature Double-Switch Hybrid Micelles for Controllable Drug Release. *Langmuir* **2021**, *37*, 14628–14637. [CrossRef] [PubMed]
141. Cheng, C.-C.; Sun, Y.T.; Lee, A.W.; Huang, S.Y.; Fan, W.L.; Chiao, Y.H.; Tsai, H.C.; Lai, J.Y. Self-Assembled Supramolecular Micelles with pH-Responsive Properties for More Effective Cancer Chemotherapy. *ACS Biomater. Sci. Eng.* **2020**, *6*, 4096–4105. [CrossRef] [PubMed]
142. Sethuraman, V.; Janakiraman, K.; Krishnaswami, V.; Kandasamy, R. Recent Progress in Stimuli-Responsive Intelligent Nano Scale Drug Delivery Systems: A Special Focus Towards pH-Sensitive Systems. *Curr. Drug Targets* **2021**, *22*, 947–966. [CrossRef]
143. Suarato, G.; Li, W.; Meng, Y. Role of pH-responsiveness in the design of chitosan-based cancer nanotherapeutics: A review. *Biointerphases* **2016**, *11*, 04B201. [CrossRef]
144. Zeng, X.; Zhang, Y.; Xu, X.; Chen, Z.; Ma, L.; Wang, Y.; Guo, X.; Li, J.; Wang, X. Construction of pH-sensitive targeted micelle system co-delivery with curcumin and dasatinib and evaluation of anti-liver cancer. *Drug Deliv.* **2022**, *29*, 792–806. [CrossRef]
145. Lei, J.; Song, Y.; Li, D.; Lei, M.; Tan, R.; Liu, Y.; Zheng, H. pH-sensitive and charge-reversal Daunorubicin-conjugated polymeric micelles for enhanced cancer therapy. *J. Appl. Polym. Sci.* **2022**, *139*, 51535. [CrossRef]
146. Jo, M.J.; Shin, H.J.; Yoon, M.S.; Kim, S.Y.; Jin, C.E.; Park, C.-W.; Kim, J.-S.; Shin, D.H. Evaluation of pH-Sensitive Polymeric Micelles Using Citraconic Amide Bonds for the Co-Delivery of Paclitaxel, Etoposide, and Rapamycin. *Pharmaceutics* **2023**, *15*, 154. [CrossRef]
147. Lin, W.; Kim, D. pH-Sensitive Micelles with Cross-Linked Cores Formed from Polyaspartamide Derivatives for Drug Delivery. *Langmuir* **2011**, *27*, 12090–12097. [CrossRef] [PubMed]
148. Zhang, C.Y.; Xiong, D.; Sun, Y.; Zhao, B.; Lin, W.J.; Zhang, L.J. Self-assembled micelles based on pH-sensitive PAE-g-MPEG-cholesterol block copolymer for anticancer drug delivery. *Int. J. Nanomed.* **2014**, *9*, 4923–4933. [CrossRef] [PubMed]
149. Ruan, C.; Su, K.; Zhao, D.; Lu, A.; Zhong, C. Nanomaterials for Tumor Hypoxia Relief to Improve the Efficacy of ROS-Generated Cancer Therapy. *Front. Chem.* **2021**, *9*, 649158. [CrossRef] [PubMed]
150. Horie, M.; Tabei, Y. Role of oxidative stress in nanoparticles toxicity. *Free Radic. Res.* **2021**, *55*, 331–342. [CrossRef]
151. Zuberek, M.; Grzelak, A. Nanoparticles-Caused Oxidative Imbalance. *Adv. Exp. Med. Biol.* **2018**, *1048*, 85–98. [CrossRef]
152. Chen, H.; He, W.; Guo, Z. An H_2O_2-responsive nanocarrier for dual-release of platinum anticancer drugs and O_2: Controlled release and enhanced cytotoxicity against cisplatin resistant cancer cells. *Chem. Commun.* **2014**, *50*, 9714–9717. [CrossRef] [PubMed]
153. Lu, X.; Du, G.; Zhang, Z.; Gong, G.; Cai, W.; Wu, L.; Zhao, G. Fabrication of Redox- and pH-Sensitive Self-Assembled Nano-Micelles with Pegylated β-Cyclodextrin for Codelivery of Doxorubicin and Cyclopalladated Ferrocene. *Eur. J. Inorg. Chem.* **2022**, *2022*, e202101061. [CrossRef]
154. Liang, R.; Wong, K.H.; Yang, Y.; Duan, Y.; Chen, M. ROS-responsive dexamethasone micelles normalize the tumor microenvironment enhancing hypericin in cancer photodynamic therapy. *Biomater. Sci.* **2022**, *10*, 1018–1025. [CrossRef]

155. Ge, C.; Zhu, J.; Wu, G.; Ye, H.; Lu, H.; Yin, L. ROS-Responsive Selenopolypeptide Micelles: Preparation, Characterization, and Controlled Drug Release. *Biomacromolecules* **2022**, *23*, 2647–2654. [CrossRef]
156. Goyal, K.; Konar, A.; Kumar, B.S.H.; Koul, V. Lactoferrin-conjugated pH and redox-sensitive polymersomes based on PEG-S-S-PLA-PCL-OH boost delivery of bacosides to the brain. *Nanoscale* **2018**, *10*, 17781–17798. [CrossRef] [PubMed]
157. Li, P.; Song, H.; Zhang, H.; Yang, P.; Zhang, C.; Huang, P.; Kong, D.; Wang, W. Engineering biodegradable guanidyl-decorated PEG-PCL nanoparticles as robust exogenous activators of DCs and antigen cross-presentation. *Nanoscale* **2017**, *9*, 13413–13418. [CrossRef]
158. Liang, Y.; Deng, X.; Zhang, L.; Peng, X.; Gao, W.; Cao, J.; Gu, Z.; He, B. Terminal modification of polymeric micelles with π-conjugated moieties for efficient anticancer drug delivery. *Biomaterials* **2015**, *71*, 1–10. [CrossRef] [PubMed]
159. Rao, N.V.; Ko, H.; Lee, J.; Park, J.H. Recent Progress and Advances in Stimuli-Responsive Polymers for Cancer Therapy. *Front. Bioeng. Biotechnol.* **2018**, *6*, 110. [CrossRef]
160. Jing, X.; Yang, F.; Shao, C.; Wei, K.; Xie, M.; Shen, H.; Shu, Y. Role of hypoxia in cancer therapy by regulating the tumor microenvironment. *Mol. Cancer* **2019**, *18*, 157. [CrossRef] [PubMed]
161. Roma-Rodrigues, C.; Mendes, R.; Baptista, P.; Fernandes, A.R. Targeting Tumor Microenvironment for Cancer Therapy. *Int. J. Mol. Sci.* **2019**, *20*, 840. [CrossRef] [PubMed]
162. Zhen, J.; Tian, S.; Liu, Q.; Zheng, C.; Zhang, Z.; Ding, Y.; An, Y.; Liu, Y.; Shi, L. Nanocarriers responsive to a hypoxia gradient facilitate enhanced tumor penetration and improved anti-tumor efficacy. *Biomater. Sci.* **2019**, *7*, 2986–2995. [CrossRef]
163. Li, Y.; Sun, Y.; Li, J.; Su, Q.; Yuan, W.; Dai, Y.; Han, C.; Wang, Q.; Feng, W.; Li, F. Ultrasensitive Near-Infrared Fluorescence-Enhanced Probe for In Vivo Nitroreductase Imaging. *J. Am. Chem. Soc.* **2015**, *137*, 6407–6416. [CrossRef]
164. Liu, X.; Wu, Z.; Guo, C.; Guo, H.; Su, Y.; Chen, Q.; Sun, C.; Liu, Q.; Chen, D.; Mu, H. Hypoxia responsive nano-drug delivery system based on angelica polysaccharide for liver cancer therapy. *Drug Deliv.* **2022**, *29*, 138–148. [CrossRef]
165. Xu, Y.; Chen, P.; Tang, L.; Zhang, X.; Shi, F.; Ning, X.; Bi, J.; Qu, Y.; Liu, H. Hypoxia responsive and tumor-targeted mixed micelles for enhanced cancer therapy and real-time imaging. *Colloids Surf. B Biointerfaces* **2022**, *215*, 112526. [CrossRef]
166. Wang, Z.; Mu, X.; Yang, Q.; Luo, J.; Zhao, Y. Hypoxia-responsive nanocarriers for chemotherapy sensitization via dual-mode inhibition of hypoxia-inducible factor-1 alpha. *J. Colloid Interface Sci.* **2022**, *628*, 106–115. [CrossRef]
167. Slor, G.; Olea, A.R.; Pujals, S.; Tigrine, A.; De La Rosa, V.R.; Hoogenboom, R.; Albertazzi, L.; Amir, R.J. Judging Enzyme-Responsive Micelles by Their Covers: Direct Comparison of Dendritic Amphiphiles with Different Hydrophilic Blocks. *Biomacromolecules* **2021**, *22*, 1197–1210. [CrossRef] [PubMed]
168. Na, K.; Sethuraman, V.T.; Bae, Y.H. Stimuli-sensitive polymeric micelles as anticancer drug carriers. *Anticancer Agents Med. Chem.* **2006**, *6*, 525–535. [CrossRef]
169. Reddy, B.P.K.; Yadav, H.K.S.; Nagesha, D.K.; Raizaday, A.; Karim, A. Polymeric Micelles as Novel Carriers for Poorly Soluble Drugs—A Review. *J. Nanosci. Nanotechnol.* **2015**, *15*, 4009–4018. [CrossRef]
170. Han, Z.; Gong, C.; Li, J.; Guo, H.; Chen, X.; Jin, Y.; Gao, S.; Tai, Z. Immunologically modified enzyme-responsive micelles regulate the tumor microenvironment for cancer immunotherapy. *Mater. Today Bio* **2022**, *13*, 100170. [CrossRef]
171. Ma, P.; Chen, J.; Bi, X.; Li, Z.; Gao, X.; Li, H.; Zhu, H.; Huang, Y.; Qi, J.; Zhang, Y. Overcoming Multidrug Resistance through the GLUT1-Mediated and Enzyme-Triggered Mitochondrial Targeting Conjugate with Redox-Sensitive Paclitaxel Release. *ACS Appl. Mater. Interfaces* **2018**, *10*, 12351–12363. [CrossRef] [PubMed]
172. Luo, L.-J.; Lai, J.-Y. Amination degree of gelatin is critical for establishing structure-property-function relationships of biodegradable thermogels as intracameral drug delivery systems. *Mater. Sci. Eng. C Mater. Biol. Appl.* **2019**, *98*, 897–909. [CrossRef] [PubMed]
173. Nakayama, M.; Chung, J.E.; Miyazaki, T.; Yokoyama, M.; Sakai, K.; Okano, T. Thermal modulation of intracellular drug distribution using thermoresponsive polymeric micelles. *React. Funct. Polym.* **2007**, *67*, 1398–1407. [CrossRef]
174. Qi, M.; Li, G.; Yu, N.; Meng, Y.; Liu, X. Synthesis of thermo-sensitive polyelectrolyte complex nanoparticles from CS-g-PNIPAM and SA-g-PNIPAM for controlled drug release. *Macromol. Res.* **2014**, *22*, 1004–1011. [CrossRef]
175. Kim, J.; Francis, D.M.; Sestito, L.F.; Archer, P.A.; Manspeaker, M.P.; O'Melia, M.J.; Thomas, S.N. Thermosensitive hydrogel releasing nitric oxide donor and anti-CTLA-4 micelles for anti-tumor immunotherapy. *Nat. Commun.* **2022**, *13*, 1479. [CrossRef] [PubMed]
176. Yu, N.; Li, G.; Gao, Y.; Jiang, H.; Tao, Q. Thermo-sensitive complex micelles from sodium alginate-graft-poly(N-isopropylacrylamide) for drug release. *Int. J. Biol. Macromol.* **2016**, *86*, 296–301. [CrossRef]
177. Li, M.; Meng, Y.; Guo, L.; Zhang, T.; Liu, J. Formation of thermo-sensitive polyelectrolyte complex micelles from two biocompatible graft copolymers for drug delivery. *J. Biomed. Mater. Res. A* **2014**, *102*, 2163–2172. [CrossRef]
178. Guo, X.; Li, D.; Yang, G.; Shi, C.; Tang, Z.; Wang, J.; Zhou, S. Thermo-triggered Drug Release from Actively Targeting Polymer Micelles. *ACS Appl. Mater. Interfaces* **2014**, *6*, 8549–8559. [CrossRef] [PubMed]
179. Lee, S.H.; Choi, S.H.; Kim, S.H.; Park, T.G. Thermally sensitive cationic polymer nanocapsules for specific cytosolic delivery and efficient gene silencing of siRNA: Swelling induced physical disruption of endosome by cold shock. *J. Control. Release Off. J. Control. Release Soc.* **2008**, *125*, 25–32. [CrossRef] [PubMed]
180. Chen, S.; Li, Y.; Guo, C.; Wang, J.; Ma, J.; Liang, X.; Yang, L.-R.; Liu, H.-Z. Temperature-responsive magnetite/PEO-PPO-PEO block copolymer nanoparticles for controlled drug targeting delivery. *Langmuir* **2007**, *23*, 12669–12676. [CrossRef]

181. Gupta, A.K.; Naregalkar, R.R.; Vaidya, V.D.; Gupta, M. Recent advances on surface engineering of magnetic iron oxide nanoparticles and their biomedical applications. *Nanomedicine* **2007**, *2*, 23–39. [CrossRef]
182. Wang, Y.; Kohane, D.S. External triggering and triggered targeting strategies for drug delivery. *Nat. Rev. Mater.* **2017**, *2*, 17020. [CrossRef]
183. Yang, X.; Chen, Y.; Yuan, R.; Chen, G.; Blanco, E.; Gao, J.; Shuai, X. Folate-encoded and Fe_3O_4-loaded polymeric micelles for dual targeting of cancer cells. *Polymer* **2008**, *49*, 3477–3485. [CrossRef]
184. Francis, M.F.; Cristea, M.; Winnik, F.M. Exploiting the vitamin B12 pathway to enhance oral drug delivery via polymeric micelles. *Biomacromolecules* **2005**, *6*, 2462–2467. [CrossRef]
185. Jain, A.; Jain, S.K. In Vitro and cell uptake studies for targeting of ligand anchored nanoparticles for colon tumors. *Eur. J. Pharm. Sci.* **2008**, *35*, 404–416. [CrossRef]
186. Roger, E.; Lagarce, F.; Garcion, E.; Benoit, J.-P. Biopharmaceutical parameters to consider in order to alter the fate of nanocarriers after oral delivery. *Nanomedicine* **2010**, *5*, 287–306. [CrossRef]
187. Vega-Villa, K.R.; Takemoto, J.K.; Yáñez, J.A.; Remsberg, C.M.; Forrest, M.L.; Davies, N.M. Clinical toxicities of nanocarrier systems. *Adv. Drug Deliv. Rev.* **2008**, *60*, 929–938. [CrossRef]
188. Rieux, A.; Fievez, V.; Garinot, M.; Schneider, Y.-J.; Préat, V. Nanoparticles as potential oral delivery systems of proteins and vaccines: A mechanistic approach. *J. Control. Release Off. J. Control. Release Soc.* **2006**, *116*, 1–27. [CrossRef]
189. Onoue, S.; Yamada, S.; Chan, H.-K. Nanodrugs: Pharmacokinetics and safety. *Int. J. Nanomed.* **2014**, *9*, 1025–1037. [CrossRef] [PubMed]
190. Wang, K.; Shen, R.; Meng, T.; Hu, F.; Yuan, H. Nano-Drug Delivery Systems Based on Different Targeting Mechanisms in the Targeted Therapy of Colorectal Cancer. *Molecules* **2022**, *27*, 2981. [CrossRef]
191. Kesharwani, P.; Gupta, U. *Nanotechnology-Based Targeted Drug Delivery Systems for Brain Tumors*; Academic Press: Cambridge, MA, USA, 2018.
192. Baranyai, Z.; Baranyai, Z.; Soria-Carrera, H.; Alleva, M.; Millán-Placer, A.C.; Lucía, A.; Martín-Rapún, R.; Aínsa, J.A.; de la Fuente, J.M. Nanotechnology-Based Targeted Drug Delivery: An Emerging Tool to Overcome Tuberculosis. *Adv. Ther.* **2021**, *4*, 2000113. [CrossRef]
193. Kirch, J.; Guenther, M.; Doshi, N.; Schaefer, U.F.; Schneider, M.; Mitragotri, S.; Lehr, C.M. Mucociliary clearance of micro- and nanoparticles is independent of size, shape and charge—An Ex Vivo and In Silico approach. *J. Control. Release Off. J. Control. Release Soc.* **2012**, *159*, 128–134. [CrossRef]
194. Alexis, F.; Pridgen, E.; Molnar, L.K.; Farokhzad, O.C. Factors Affecting the Clearance and Biodistribution of Polymeric Nanoparticles. *Mol. Pharm.* **2008**, *5*, 505–515. [CrossRef] [PubMed]
195. Perin, F.; Motta, A.; Maniglio, D. Amphiphilic copolymers in biomedical applications: Synthesis routes and property control. *Mater. Sci. Eng. C* **2021**, *123*, 111952. [CrossRef] [PubMed]
196. Vonarbourg, A.; Passirani, C.; Saulnier, P.; Benoit, J.-P. Parameters influencing the stealthiness of colloidal drug delivery systems. *Biomaterials* **2006**, *27*, 4356–4373. [CrossRef] [PubMed]
197. Naksuriya, O.; Shi, Y.; van Nostrum, C.F.; Anuchapreeda, S.; Hennink, W.E.; Okonogi, S. HPMA-based polymeric micelles for curcumin solubilization and inhibition of cancer cell growth. *Eur. J. Pharm. Biopharm. Off. J. Arb. Fur Pharm. Verfahr. e.V* **2015**, *94*, 501–512. [CrossRef] [PubMed]
198. Duan, X.; Li, Y. Physicochemical characteristics of nanoparticles affect circulation, biodistribution, cellular internalization, and trafficking. *Small* **2013**, *9*, 1521–1532. [CrossRef]
199. Yamamoto, Y.; Nagasaki, Y.; Kato, Y.; Sugiyama, Y.; Kataoka, K. Long-circulating poly(ethylene glycol)-poly(D,L-lactide) block copolymer micelles with modulated surface charge. *J. Control. Release Off. J. Control. Release Soc.* **2001**, *77*, 27–38. [CrossRef] [PubMed]
200. Wang, Y.; Li, Y.; Zhang, L.; Fang, X. Pharmacokinetics and biodistribution of paclitaxel-loaded pluronic P105 polymeric micelles. *Arch. Pharm. Res.* **2008**, *31*, 530–538. [CrossRef]
201. Onoue, S.; Kojo, Y.; Suzuki, H.; Yuminoki, K.; Kou, K.; Kawabata, Y.; Yamauchi, Y.; Hashimoto, N.; Yamada, S. Development of novel solid dispersion of tranilast using amphiphilic block copolymer for improved oral bioavailability. *Int. J. Pharm.* **2013**, *452*, 220–226. [CrossRef] [PubMed]
202. Hwang, D.; Ramsey, J.D.; Kabanov, A. Polymeric micelles for the delivery of poorly soluble drugs: From nanoformulation to clinical approval. *Adv. Drug Deliv. Rev.* **2020**, *156*, 80–118. [CrossRef]
203. Lu, Y.; Park, K. Polymeric micelles and alternative nanonized delivery vehicles for poorly soluble drugs. *Int. J. Pharm.* **2013**, *453*, 198–214. [CrossRef]
204. Cabral, H.; Kataoka, K. Progress of drug-loaded polymeric micelles into clinical studies. *J. Control. Release Off. J. Control. Release Soc.* **2014**, *190*, 465–476. [CrossRef]
205. Gong, J.; Chen, M.; Zheng, Y.; Wang, S.; Wang, Y. Polymeric micelles drug delivery system in oncology. *J. Control. Release Off. J. Control. Release Soc.* **2012**, *159*, 312–323. [CrossRef] [PubMed]
206. Yang, C.-P.H.; Horwitz, S.B. Taxol($^{®}$): The First Microtubule Stabilizing Agent. *Int. J. Mol. Sci.* **2017**, *18*, 1733. [CrossRef]
207. Kim, S.C.; Kim, D.W.; Shim, Y.H.; Bang, J.S.; Oh, H.S.; Wan Kim, S.; Seo, M.H. In Vivo evaluation of polymeric micellar paclitaxel formulation: Toxicity and efficacy. *J. Control. Release Off. J. Control. Release Soc.* **2001**, *72*, 191–202. [CrossRef] [PubMed]

208. Fan, Z.; Chen, C.; Pang, X.; Yu, Z.; Qi, Y.; Chen, X.; Liang, H.; Fang, X.; Sha, X. Adding vitamin E-TPGS to the formulation of Genexol-PM: Specially mixed micelles improve drug-loading ability and cytotoxicity against multidrug-resistant tumors significantly. *PLoS ONE* **2015**, *10*, e0120129. [CrossRef]
209. Zheng, X.; Xie, J.; Zhang, X.; Sun, W.; Zhao, H.; Li, Y.; Wang, C. An overview of polymeric nanomicelles in clinical trials and on the market. *Chin. Chem. Lett.* **2021**, *32*, 243–257. [CrossRef]
210. Hamaguchi, T.; Matsumura, Y.; Suzuki, M.; Shimizu, K.; Goda, R.; Nakamura, I.; Nakatomi, I.; Yokoyama, M.; Kataoka, K.; Kakizoe, T. NK105, a paclitaxel-incorporating micellar nanoparticle formulation, can extend In Vivo antitumour activity and reduce the neurotoxicity of paclitaxel. *Br. J. Cancer* **2005**, *92*, 1240–1246. [CrossRef] [PubMed]
211. Sofias, A.M.; Dunne, M.; Storm, G.; Allen, C. The battle of 'nano' paclitaxel. *Adv. Drug Deliv. Rev.* **2017**, *122*, 20–30. [CrossRef] [PubMed]
212. Mukai, H.; Kato, K.; Esaki, T.; Ohsumi, S.; Hozomi, Y.; Matsubara, N.; Hamaguchi, T.; Matsumura, Y.; Goda, R.; Hirai, T.; et al. Phase I study of NK105, a nanomicellar paclitaxel formulation, administered on a weekly schedule in patients with solid tumors. *Invest New Drugs* **2016**, *34*, 750–759. [CrossRef] [PubMed]
213. Kato, K.; Chin, K.; Yoshikawa, T.; Yamaguchi, K.; Tsuji, Y.; Esaki, T.; Sakai, K.; Kimura, M.; Hamaguchi, T.; Shimada, Y. Phase II study of NK105, a paclitaxel-incorporating micellar nanoparticle, for previously treated advanced or recurrent gastric cancer. *Invest New Drugs* **2012**, *30*, 1621–1627. [CrossRef]
214. Fujiwara, Y.; Mukai, H.; Saeki, T.; Ro, J.; Lin, Y.C.; Nagai, S.E.; Lee, K.S.; Watanabe, J.; Ohtani, S.; Kim, S.B.; et al. A multi-national, randomised, open-label, parallel, phase III non-inferiority study comparing NK105 and paclitaxel in metastatic or recurrent breast cancer patients. *Br. J. Cancer* **2019**, *120*, 475–480. [CrossRef]
215. Lee, S.-W.; Yun, M.H.; Jeong, S.W.; In, C.H.; Kim, J.Y.; Seo, M.H.; Pai, C.M.; Kim, S.O. Development of docetaxel-loaded intravenous formulation, Nanoxel-PM™ using polymer-based delivery system. *J. Control. Release* **2011**, *155*, 262–271. [CrossRef] [PubMed]
216. Bernabeu, E.; Cagel, M.; Lagomarsino, E.; Moretton, M.; Chiappetta, D.A. Paclitaxel: What has been done and the challenges remain ahead. *Int. J. Pharm.* **2017**, *526*, 474–495. [CrossRef]
217. Triolimus, C.-D. Therapeutics. Available online: https://co-drx.com/pipeline/triolimus/2023 (accessed on 17 February 2023).
218. Hasenstein, J.R.; Shin, H.-C.; Kasmerchak, K.; Buehler, D.; Kwon, G.S.; Kozak, K.R. Antitumor Activity of Triolimus: A Novel Multidrug-Loaded Micelle Containing Paclitaxel, Rapamycin, and 17-AAGMolecular Multitargeting with Triolimus. *Mol. Cancer Ther.* **2012**, *11*, 2233–2242. [CrossRef]
219. Kubiak, T. Polymeric capsules and micelles as promising carriers of anticancer drugs. *Polym. Med.* **2022**, *52*, 35–48. [CrossRef] [PubMed]
220. Si, J.; Zhao, X.; Gao, S.; Huang, D.; Sui, M. Advances in delivery of Irinotecan (CPT-11) active metabolite 7-ethyl-10-hydroxycamptothecin. *Int. J. Pharm.* **2019**, *568*, 118499. [CrossRef] [PubMed]
221. Hamaguchi, T.; Tsuji, A.; Yamaguchi, K.; Takeda, K.; Uetake, H.; Esaki, T.; Amagai, K.; Sakai, D.; Baba, H.; Kimura, M.; et al. A phase II study of NK012, a polymeric micelle formulation of SN-38, in unresectable, metastatic or recurrent colorectal cancer patients. *Cancer Chemother. Pharmacol.* **2018**, *82*, 1021–1029. [CrossRef] [PubMed]
222. Nakanishi, T.; Fukushima, S.; Okamoto, K.; Suzuki, M.; Matsumura, Y.; Yokoyama, M.; Okano, T.; Sakurai, Y.; Kataoka, K. Development of the polymer micelle carrier system for doxorubicin. *J. Control. Release Off. J. Control. Release Soc.* **2001**, *74*, 295–302. [CrossRef]
223. Matsumura, Y.; Hamaguchi, T.; Ura, T.; Muro, K.; Yamada, Y.; Shimada, Y.; Shirao, K.; Okusaka, T.; Ueno, H.; Ikeda, M.; et al. Phase I clinical trial and pharmacokinetic evaluation of NK911, a micelle-encapsulated doxorubicin. *Br. J. Cancer* **2004**, *91*, 1775–1781. [CrossRef]
224. Kabanov, A.; Batrakova, E.; Alakhov, V.Y. Pluronic® block copolymers for overcoming drug resistance in cancer. *Adv. Drug Deliv. Rev.* **2002**, *54*, 759–779. [CrossRef]
225. Danson, S.; Ferry, D.; Alakhov, V.; Margison, J.; Kerr, D.; Jowle, D.; Brampton, M.; Halbert, G.; Ranson, M. Phase I dose escalation and pharmacokinetic study of pluronic polymer-bound doxorubicin (SP1049C) in patients with advanced cancer. *Br. J. Cancer* **2004**, *90*, 2085–2091. [CrossRef] [PubMed]
226. Valle, J.W.; Armstrong, A.; Newman, C.; Alakhov, V.; Pietrzynski, G.; Brewer, J.; Campbell, S.; Corrie, P.; Rowinsky, E.K.; Ranson, M. A phase 2 study of SP1049C, doxorubicin in P-glycoprotein-targeting pluronics, in patients with advanced adenocarcinoma of the esophagus and gastroesophageal junction. *Invest New Drugs.* **2011**, *29*, 1029–1037. [CrossRef] [PubMed]
227. Takahashi, A.; Yamamoto, Y.; Yasunaga, M.; Koga, Y.; Kuroda, J.; Takigahira, M.; Harada, M.; Saito, H.; Hayashi, T.; Kato, Y.; et al. NC-6300, an epirubicin-incorporating micelle, extends the antitumor effect and reduces the cardiotoxicity of epirubicin. *Cancer Sci.* **2013**, *104*, 920–925. [CrossRef]
228. Mukai, H.; Kogawa, T.; Matsubara, N.; Naito, Y.; Sasaki, M.; Hosono, A. A first-in-human Phase 1 study of epirubicin-conjugated polymer micelles (K-912/NC-6300) in patients with advanced or recurrent solid tumors. *Invest New Drugs* **2017**, *35*, 307–314. [CrossRef]
229. Ueno, T.; Ueno, T.; Endo, K.; Hori, K.; Ozaki, N.; Tsuji, A.; Kondo, S.; Wakisaka, N.; Murono, S.; Kataoka, K.; et al. Assessment of antitumor activity and acute peripheral neuropathy of 1, 2-diaminocyclohexane platinum (II)-incorporating micelles (NC-4016). *Int. J. Nanomed.* **2014**, *9*, 3005. [CrossRef] [PubMed]

230. Wang, K.; Liu, L.; Zhang, T.; Zhu, Y.L.; Qiu, F.; Wu, X.G.; Wang, X.L.; Hu, F.Q.; Huang, J. Oxaliplatin-incorporated micelles eliminate both cancer stem-like and bulk cell populations in colorectal cancer. *Int. J. Nanomed.* **2011**, *6*, 3207.
231. Osada, A. NC-6004, a novel cisplatin nanoparticle, in combination with pembrolizumab for head and neck cancer. *Integr. Clin. Med.* **2019**, *3*. [CrossRef]
232. Uchino, H.; Matsumura, Y.; Negishi, T.; Koizumi, F.; Hayashi, T.; Honda, T.; Nishiyama, N.; Kataoka, K.; Naito, S.; Kakizoe, T. Cisplatin-incorporating polymeric micelles (NC-6004) can reduce nephrotoxicity and neurotoxicity of cisplatin in rats. *Br. J. Cancer* **2005**, *93*, 678–687. [CrossRef]
233. Plummer, R.; Wilson, R.H.; Calvert, H.; Boddy, A.V.; Griffin, M.; Sludden, J.; Tilby, M.J.; Eatock, M.; Pearson, D.G.; Ottley, C.J.; et al. A Phase I clinical study of cisplatin-incorporated polymeric micelles (NC-6004) in patients with solid tumours. *Br. J. Cancer* **2011**, *104*, 593–598. [CrossRef] [PubMed]
234. Volovat, S.R.; Ciuleanu, T.E.; Koralewski, P.; Olson, J.E.G.; Croitoru, A.; Koynov, K.; Stabile, S.; Cerea, G.; Osada, A.; Bobe, I.; et al. A multicenter, single-arm, basket design, phase II study of NC-6004 plus gemcitabine in patients with advanced unresectable lung, biliary tract, or bladder cancer. *Oncotarget* **2020**, *11*, 3105. [CrossRef]
235. NCT02240238. Available online: https://beta.clinicaltrials.gov/study/NCT02240238 (accessed on 31 January 2023).
236. van Oosterom, A.T.; Schriivers, D. Docetaxel (Taxotere®), a review of preclinical and clinical experience. Part II: Clinical experience. *Anticancer Drugs* **1995**, *6*, 356–368. [CrossRef]
237. Zhao, P.; Astruc, D. Docetaxel nanotechnology in anticancer therapy. *ChemMedChem* **2012**, *7*, 952–972. [CrossRef]
238. Von Hoff, D.D.; Mita, M.M.; Ramanathan, R.K.; Weiss, G.J.; Mita, A.C.; LoRusso, P.M.; Burris, H.A.; Hart, L.L., 3rd; Low, S.C.; Parsons, D.M.; et al. Phase I study of PSMA-targeted docetaxel-containing nanoparticle BIND-014 in patients with advanced solid tumors. *Clin. Cancer Res.* **2016**, *22*, 3157–3163. [CrossRef]
239. Autio, K.A.; Dreicer, R.; Anderson, J.; Garcia, J.A.; Alva, A.; Hart, L.L.; Milowsky, M.I.; Posadas, E.M.; Ryan, C.J.; Graf, R.P.; et al. Safety and efficacy of BIND-014, a docetaxel nanoparticle targeting prostate-specific membrane antigen for patients with metastatic castration-resistant prostate cancer: A phase 2 clinical trial. *JAMA Oncol.* **2018**, *4*, 1344–1351. [CrossRef]
240. Natale, R.; Socinski, M.A.; Hart, L.L.; Lipatov, O.N.; Spigel, D.R.; Gershenhorn, B.; Weiss, G.J.; Kazmi, S.; Karaseva, N.A.; Gladkov, O.A.; et al. 41 Clinical activity of BIND-014 (docetaxel nanoparticles for injectable suspension) as second-line therapy in patients (pts) with Stage III/IV non-small cell lung cancer. *Eur. J. Cancer* **2014**, *50*, 19. [CrossRef]
241. Ledford, H. Bankruptcy filing worries developers of nanoparticle cancer drugs. *Nature* **2016**, *533*, 304–305. [CrossRef] [PubMed]
242. Li, P.; Kumar, A.; Ma, J.; Kuang, Y.; Luo, L.; Sun, X. Density gradient ultracentrifugation for colloidal nanostructures separation and investigation. *Sci. Bull.* **2018**, *63*, 645–662. [CrossRef] [PubMed]
243. Choi, Y.H.; Han, H.-K. Nanomedicines: Current status and future perspectives in aspect of drug delivery and pharmacokinetics. *J. Pharm. Investig.* **2018**, *48*, 43–60. [CrossRef] [PubMed]
244. Ghezzi, M.; Pescina, S.; Padula, C.; Santi, P.; Del Favero, E.; Cantù, L.; Nicoli, S. Polymeric micelles in drug delivery: An insight of the techniques for their characterization and assessment in biorelevant conditions. *J. Control. Release* **2021**, *332*, 312–336. [CrossRef] [PubMed]
245. Committee for Medicinal Products for Human Use; European Medicine Agency Joint MHLW/EMA Reflection Paper on the Development of Block Copolymer Micelle Medicinal Products. 2013. Available online: https://www.ema.europa.eu/en/documents/scientific-guideline/draft-joint-ministry-health-labour-welfare/european-medicines-agency-reflection-paper-development-block-copolymer-micelle-medicinal-products_en.pdf (accessed on 17 February 2023).
246. Zhang, H.; Li, H.; Cao, Z.; Du, J.; Yan, L.; Wang, J. Investigation of the In Vivo integrity of polymeric micelles via large Stokes shift fluorophore-based FRET. *J. Control. Release* **2020**, *324*, 47–54. [CrossRef] [PubMed]
247. Liu, J.; Zeng, F.; Allen, C. Influence of serum protein on polycarbonate-based copolymer micelles as a delivery system for a hydrophobic anti-cancer agent. *J. Control. Release* **2005**, *103*, 481–497. [CrossRef]

Disclaimer/Publisher's Note: The statements, opinions and data contained in all publications are solely those of the individual author(s) and contributor(s) and not of MDPI and/or the editor(s). MDPI and/or the editor(s) disclaim responsibility for any injury to people or property resulting from any ideas, methods, instructions or products referred to in the content.

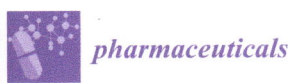

Review

Commercially Available Enteric Empty Hard Capsules, Production Technology and Application

Aleš Franc, David Vetchý and Nicole Fülöpová *

Department of Pharmaceutical Technology, Faculty of Pharmacy, Masaryk University, 612 42 Brno, Czech Republic
* Correspondence: 507073@muni.cz; Tel.: +420-(5)-4156-2868

Abstract: Currently, there is a growing need to prepare small batches of enteric capsules for individual therapy or clinical evaluation since many acidic-sensitive substances should be protected from the stomach's acidic environment, including probiotics or fecal material, in the fecal microbiota transplantation (FMT) process. A suitable method seems to be the encapsulation of drugs or lyophilized alternatively frozen biological suspensions in commercial hard enteric capsules prepared by so-called Enteric Capsule Drug Delivery Technology (ECDDT). Manufacturers supply these types of capsules, made from pH-soluble polymers, in products such as AR Caps®, EnTRinsic™, and Vcaps® Enteric, or capsules made of gelling polymers that release their content as the gel erodes over time when passing through the digestive tract. These include DRcaps®, EMBO CAPS® AP, BioVXR®, or ACGcaps™ HD. Although not all capsules in all formulations meet pharmaceutical requirements for delayed-release dosage forms in disintegration and dissolution tests, they usually find practical application. This literature review presents their composition and properties. Since ECDDT is a new technology, this article is based on a limited number of references.

Keywords: hard capsules; commercial capsules; enteric administration; acid resistance; encapsulation; ECDDT technology

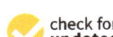

Citation: Franc, A.; Vetchý, D.; Fülöpová, N. Commercially Available Enteric Empty Hard Capsules, Production Technology and Application. *Pharmaceuticals* **2022**, *15*, 1398. https://doi.org/10.3390/ph15111398

Academic Editors: Silviya Petrova Zustiak and Era Jain

Received: 27 October 2022
Accepted: 11 November 2022
Published: 13 November 2022

Publisher's Note: MDPI stays neutral with regard to jurisdictional claims in published maps and institutional affiliations.

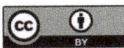

Copyright: © 2022 by the authors. Licensee MDPI, Basel, Switzerland. This article is an open access article distributed under the terms and conditions of the Creative Commons Attribution (CC BY) license (https://creativecommons.org/licenses/by/4.0/).

1. Introduction

In 1982, only 17.5% of newly licensed products were presented as hard gelatin capsules. By 1996, the percentage had already reached 34% [1]. In 2001, capsules accounted for approximately 20% of all prescriptions dispensed [2]. Thus, technically, is it possible to produce an oral solid dosage form containing a drug with limited stability, poor compressibility, or inappropriate organoleptic properties. Most patients also prefer capsules due to their easy swallowing and inert taste [3]. The drug is encapsulated here as a mixture of different excipients to the hard capsule, consisting of a lower part (body) into which the mixture is filled and closed with an upper part of the capsule (cap). Laboratory machines (manual capsule filling machines) [4,5] or semi-automatic alternatively automatic devices (capsule filling machines) [1,3,6] are usually used for encapsulation in pharmacies or research fields. Materials used for manufacturing both capsule parts are often dried glycerogelatin or, more recently, cellulose derivates, mostly hydroxypropyl methylcellulose (HPMC) or other derivatives, and different hydrophilic polymers. At the same time, natural polymers created without using genetically modified organisms (GMOs) and preservatives are being sought [3,7]. There is also a growing demand for new materials in terms of functionality, enabling the dosage form to be delayed, prolonged, or pulsed release [8,9]. In addition, with the development of the administration of locally acting drugs (e.g., for the treatment of Crohn's disease or colorectal cancer) or probiotics, polymers have been used to protect the dosage forms and their contents as they pass through the gastrointestinal tract (GIT) to its distal parts [10,11]. Recently, there has been an effort to produce enteric capsules in laboratory conditions for small groups of patients, especially in clinical or preclinical trials. These capsules could also be used in fecal microbiota transplantation (FMT), where the damaged intestinal microbiome of the patient is replaced with modified, frozen, or lyophilized stool from a suitable donor (or with lyophilized bacterial cultures from stool). FMT would otherwise have to be performed with nasojejunal tubes or enemas [12–14]. As transplants are prepared directly in hospital wards, there is a need to ensure that the process is reproducible, individualized, and feasible without special equipment [13,15]. Coating hard capsules with encapsulated content using enteric polymers is the most common way to achieve acid resistance of pharmaceutical drug form. In clinical practice, it is impossible to use industrial equipment (coaters), but simply immersing the capsules in the polymer dispersion (immersion method) was offered, which often yielded not satisfactory results [16]. In the last 10 years, several manufacturers have focused on producing empty enteric capsules without requiring subsequent coating for simplification and reproducibility of the process [17]. Therefore, Enteric Capsule Drug Delivery Technology (ECDDT) was created, where pharmaceutically approved enteric polymers are incorporated into the capsule shell to provide acid resistance without another coating. This review article describes several commercially available hard capsules prepared by the ECDDT method and their properties [18].

2. Enterosolvency of Solid Dosage Forms

Legislation provides synonyms such as delayed-release, gastro-resistant, or enteric-coated for oral enteric dosage forms that resist the acidic environment in the stomach, and then dissolve in the unified simulated environment of the small intestine [19].

Average fasting stomach pH values range from 1.5 to 1.9, but due to inter- and intra-individual variability in the human population, they could be less than 1.0 or even 5.0–6.0. Therefore, after a meal, values could shift from 3.0 to 7.0. The small intestine consists of the duodenum, the jejunum, and the ileum. The duodenum pH values range from 6.0 to 6.5, the jejunum around 6.8, and the ileum up to 7.4 [20,21]. Pharmacopoeial and industry guidelines for enteric capsules require two specific tests to verify acid resistance of drug form, namely disintegration and dissolution. The common principle is to expose the capsule to an acidic and then neutral environment.

For disintegration, the capsules must not show signs of disintegration or crack in simulated gastric juice (SGF) with pH 1.2, within 60 to 120 min (according to requirements of different pharmacopeias), usually without the use of 'disks'. Subsequently, capsules must disintegrate in simulated intestinal juice (SIF), with pH 6.8, usually with 'disks', within 60 min to meet the pharmacopeia limits [22]. Disks are used when specified to prevent floating capsules in the disintegration medium [19]. For the dissolution test, the capsules could release a maximum of 10% content in SGF within 120 min under defined conditions and subsequently a minimum of 80% in pH 4.5–7.5 buffer, usually within 120 min [19,23]. There are also several slightly different conditions and limits across pharmacopeias, presented in Table 1 [22,24–26].

Table 1. Conditions and limits in three different pharmacopeias (European, Unites States, Japanese) [19,22–26].

Pharmacopoeia/Abbreviation	European Pharmacopoeia/Ph. Eur.		United States Pharmacopoeia/USP		Japanese Pharmacopoeia/JP	
	A. Disintegration test					
Conditions [1]	1.	2.	1.	2.	1.	2.
Time (min)	120	60	60	MON	120	60
Disks	No	Yes	MON	MON	No	Yes
Limits (units)	0/6	6/6	0/6	MON	0/6	6/6

Table 1. Cont.

Pharmacopoeia/Abbreviation	European Pharmacopoeia/Ph. Eur.		United States Pharmacopoeia/USP		Japanese Pharmacopoeia/JP	
	B. Dissolution test					
Conditions [1]	1.	2.	1.	2.	1.	2.
Time (min)	120	45/MON	120	45/MON	120	MON
Limits (%)	≤10	Q + 5	≤10	Q + 5	≤10	Q_{MON} + 5
Pharmacopoeia procedure [2]	Method A Continual two-step dissolution Method B Separated two-step dissolution		Method A Continual two-step dissolution Method B Separated two-step dissolution		If not specified, proceed with both stages of the test separately	

[1] Experimental conditions in disintegration and dissolution tests (first (1.) in pH 1.2; second (2.) in pH 6.8); [2] Two methods for proceeding with the dissolution test (A—Placed first in acid stage, then add the required amount of buffer to an acid solution; B—First placed in acid stage, then replaced to buffer stage); MON—Specified in individual pharmacopeial monographs; Q—the dissolution end time (total dissolution time) given by the general lower limit (amount of released API 75.0% if not specified in the individual pharmacopeial monograph); Q_{MON}—Amount of released API specified in the monograph.

3. Enteric Polymers

For enteric coating or the ECDDT formation of pharmaceutical dosage form, pharmaceutical technology offers so-called pH-dependent and gel-forming polymers, or a combination thereof.

3.1. pH-Dependent Enteric Polymers

Due to their acidic nature, these polymers prevent the drug's dissolution in the stomach's acidic environment, but allows its release in the neutral environment of the small intestine [27]. Acidic poly-(meth)-acrylate copolymers or cellulose and vinyl derivatives are commonly used in phthalates, acetates, trimellitates, succinates, or acetate succinates form. They usually dissolve at pH 5–7 [28] (see Table 2). In the case of ECDDT formation, these polymers are combined with HPMC, with more favorable properties than gelatin for this application, forming the body shell and capsule cap [29].

Table 2. Overview of the most common pH-dependent enteric polymers [28,30–32].

Commercial Name/Abbreviation [1]	Chemical Name	Solubility at pH Values [2]
Eudragit® FS	A copolymer of methyl acrylate, methyl methacrylate, and methacrylic acid in a ratio of 7:3:1	7.0
Eudragit® S	A copolymer of methacrylic acid and methyl methacrylate in a ratio of 1:2	7.0
Eudragit® L	A copolymer of methacrylic acid and methyl methacrylate in a ratio of 1:1	6.0
Eudragit® FL	A mixture of a copolymer of ethyl methacrylate and methyl methacrylate with a copolymer of methacrylic acid and ethyl methacrylate in a ratio of 1:1	5.5
CAS	Cellulose acetate succinate	5.8–6.2
CAP	Cellulose acetate phthalate	5.5–6.2
CAT	Cellulose trimellitate	5.2–5.5
HPMCAS	Hydroxypropyl methylcellulose acetate succinate	5.5–6.8
HPMCP	Hydroxypropyl methylcellulose phthalate	5.0–5.5
PVAP	Polyvinyl acetate phthalate	5.0–5.5

[1] Abbreviation of enteric polymers are used in a whole article according to this table; [2] This is the value at which the polymer dissolves; this could vary for some substances depending on the ratio of substituents, with literature values often differing slightly.

3.2. Gel-Forming Polymers for Enteric Coating

These polymers form a gel layer on the surface of the dosage form when passing through the GIT. The gel layer prevents active pharmaceutical ingredient (API) release from the dosage form in the proximal parts of the GIT (especially in the stomach area). The hydrogel layer is subsequently degraded by two mechanisms, either by spontaneous erosion or by the action of enzymes. Natural substances as polysaccharides (agar, alginates, amylopectin, amylose, arabic gum, arabinogalactan, carrageenan, curdlan, cyclodextrin, dextran esters, dextran's, gellan gum, glucuronate, guar gum, chitosan, inulin, modified starches, pectin, pullulan, xanthan, xylan, respectively); proteins (collagen, hyaluronic acid); proteoglycans (chondroitin sulfate) [11,28,32–34], and others, could be incorporated into the capsule shell in ECDDT technology. Another possibility is to use HPMC [35] or its mixture with natural substances in the ECDDT process [29].

4. Related Excipients Used in the Formulation of the Capsule Shell

Film-forming substances from several cellulose derivatives, (meth)-acrylate copolymers, and gelatin create fragile films, therefore, contain plasticizers, most often from several alcoholic sugars, polyols, and their esters or selected polyethers or acylglycerols [36]. In addition, acidic enteric polymers need alkaline substances to dissolve in water, such as ammonia or hydroxides, carbonates, and phosphates of some alkaline metals and earth, which are added to dispersions [37,38]. Gelling substances, like polysaccharides, can be gelled with monovalent or divalent cations of selected alkaline metals and earth [39]. For the easier dispersion of the individual components and the wettability of the finished capsules, the dispersions can also contain several water-soluble and insoluble surfactants [40]. All these components together form homogeneous liquid dispersions, and after drying, solid dispersions in the form of a capsule shell are obtained. The detailed mechanism of action of these substances at the molecular level is described in the literature [7]. The substance groups mentioned above are qualitatively presented in concrete solutions in the overview of inventions in the summary of inventions (see Table A1).

5. Brief Description of the Production and Filling of Hard Capsules

In 1846, pharmacist J. C. Lehuby patented two-piece empty hard gelatin capsules, made by dipping metal pins into glycerogelatin. In 1877, another pharmacist, F. A. Hubel, standardized the pins and produced two-part capsules consisting of a body and cap with a size range labeled as 00, 0, 1, 2, 3, 4, and 5 (from the largest size 00 to the smallest size 5) [1]. This labeling of capsules is still used today (see Table 3). In 1931, the company Parke, Davis & Co. (Detroit, MI, USA; now part of Pfizer Corporation, New York, NY, USA) patented the first hard capsule machine [40]. The principle was to prepare a glycerogelatin, with the possible addition of pigment and preservative, and heat it to the required temperature (usually between 45 and 55 °C) [3,7]. A rotating oval pin is then dipped into the prepared, heated solution to ensure uniformity of the application of glycerogelatin. Subsequently, the glycerogel deposition is dried, pulled off from the pin, and trimmed or eventually branded. The capsule bodies and caps are produced separately [3,41]. Later, polymers such as HPMC (the required temperature for hydrogel is approximately 70 °C), pH-dependent, and gel-forming polymers began to be used in the capsule manufacturing process [42,43]. If it is convenient to form an inner and outer shell by coating, immersion could be repeated in different polymer dispersions (double immersion technology). This procedure is preferably used to prepare the outer enteric coating [17]. Until 1968, the capsules had straight, smooth walls, while later conical shapes and various grooves were designed (e.g., Snap-fit (Lock-caps), Eta-lock, Coni-snap, Coni-snap supro capsules) to facilitate the closure of the body with the cap (see Figure 1) [3,40]. Manual and semi-automatic devices could be used for encapsulation in laboratory conditions. API, or its mixture with a suitable filler, is here filled into the capsule bodies and enclosed with a cap [44]. In the industry, automatic devices are used with two leading technologies for filling capsules. The first is tamping (the capsule filling is pressed into the capsule's body and closed with the cap) [45]. The second technology is damping or dosator (the capsule filling is pressed into a roller, inserted into the capsule's body, and enclosed by a cap) [46]. Although the detailed capsule production process is not part of this review article, it is already well-known and described in the available literature [47].

Table 3. Sizes, volumes, weights, dimensions of capsule parts (body, cap), and the whole capsule [48–50].

Size	000	00EL	00	0EL	0	1EL	1	2EL	2	3	4	5
Body length (mm)	22.2	22.2	20.2	20.2	18.4	17.7	16.6	16.7	15.3	13.6	12.2	9.3
Cap length (mm)	12.9	12.9	11.7	11.7	10.7	10.5	9.8	9.7	8.9	8.1	7.2	6.2
Capsule length (mm)	26.1	25.3	23.3	23.1	21.7	20.4	19.4	19.3	18.0	15.9	14.3	11.1
Weight (mg) [1]	163	130	118	107	96	81	76	66	61	48	38	28
Volume (mL)	1.37	1.02	0.91	0.78	0.68	0.54	0.50	0.41	0.37	0.30	0.25	0.13

[1] Some manufacturers list the same weight of gelatin and HPMC capsules.

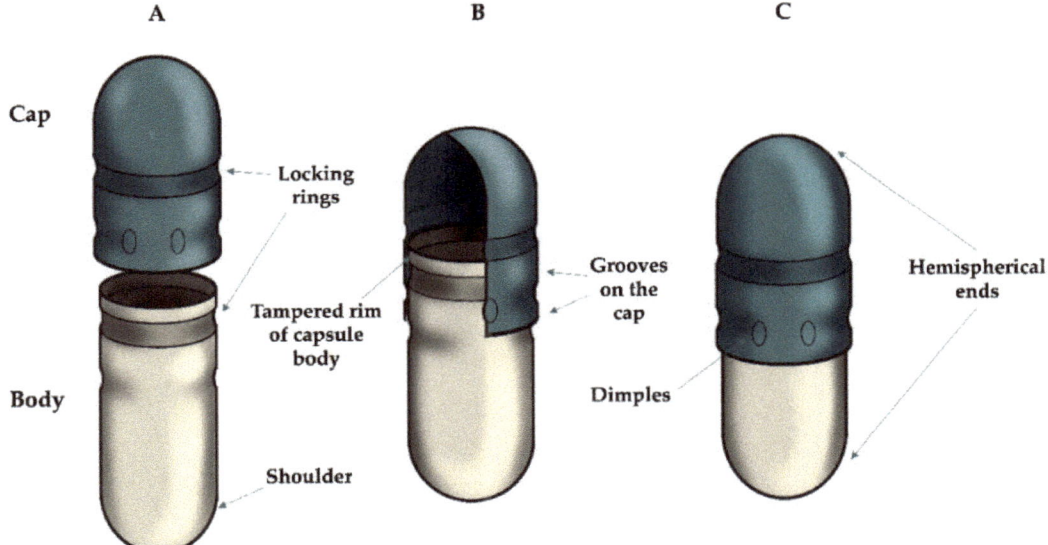

Figure 1. Structure of the common type of enteric hard capsule prepared with ECDDT (Snap-fit type): (A) open position with two capsule parts (cap, body); (B) pre-closed position; (C) closed position of hard capsule.

6. Patent Research of Empty Enteric Capsules

A patent search was conducted from the Google Patents and EspaceNet patent databases using the keywords "enteric", "acid resistant", "delayed release", "hollow", "empty", "shell", "hard", and "capsule" in various combinations. In addition, the cited patents from each application and related documents offered by the databases were searched. Documents describing the encapsulation of specific drugs by the in situ method were excluded from the final determination. The cited documents do not distinguish between an "application" and a granted "patent", which allows for maintaining the "priority" necessary to track the development of knowledge and preserve the intent of the review article. The technology description indicates whether it is a single-shell capsule (indicated as Capsule in the table), a double-shell capsule (indicated as Inner and Outer shell), or an Outer shell only. The individual excipients are taken from the patent 'claims' in the order listed. Functional groups of excipients, such as film-forming agents, pH-dependent polymers, and gelling agents, are separated by the conjunction "and". Commas separate individual groups. These functional groups are not directly mentioned in this research but are implied by the preceding text.

It should be noted that the final composition of the capsules does not necessarily contain all the declared substances, but their use and their combination protect the stated inventiveness. However, these are usually inventions companies own for mass production; not all are commercially available. Instead, they preserve compositions and technologies from the use by other manufacturers, which is currently the primary role of patent protection [51]. Fifty-one relevant patents from 1942 to 2022 were selected and sorted diachronically, in Appendix A. Although these technologies have been around since the 1940s, the funnel graph below shows the increase in patent applications in the last decade. The growing demand for encapsulation of acid-labile and biological materials is evident (see Figure 2). The funnel plot also correlates with the incidence of clinical trials, especially in the last 10 years (see Section 8, clinical trials performed with enteric capsules).

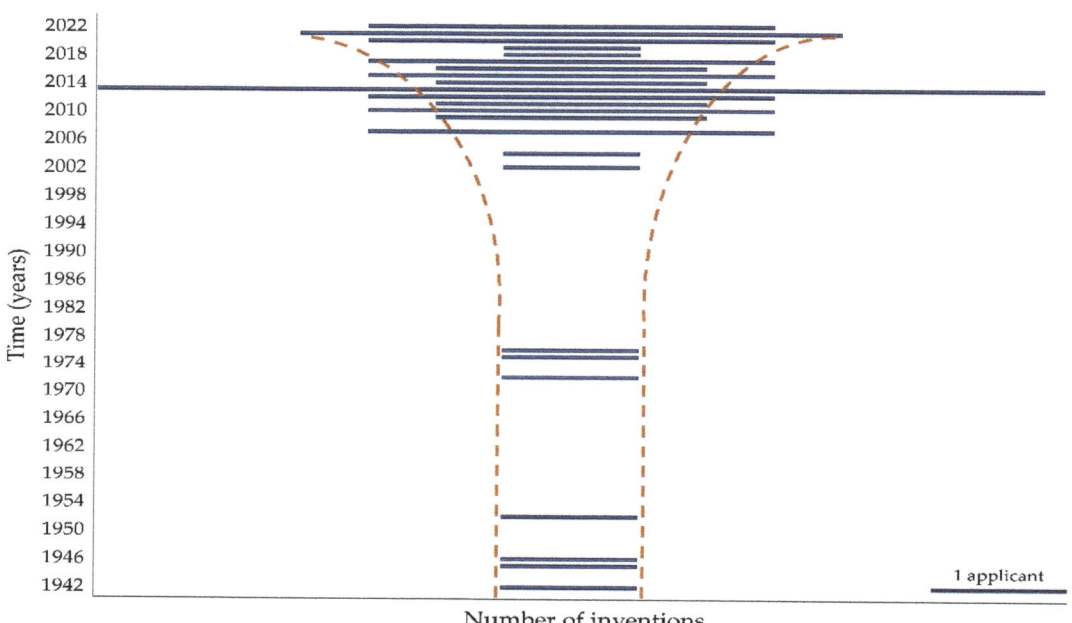

Figure 2. The funnel plot. Approximate growth of patent applications in time.

7. Commercially Hard Capsules Prepared by ECDDT

The capsule shell contains the pH-dependent or gel-forming polymers mentioned above. If the capsules are administered in the FMT process, patients could be premedicated with a proton pump inhibitor, changing the pH in the stomach to 5. However, it could lead to the dissolution of pH-dependent enteric polymers already in the proximal parts of the GIT. Therefore, using capsules made of gel-forming polymers may be preferable here. On the other hand, using pH-dependent polymers avoids premedication [52].

7.1. ECDDT Prepared from pH-Dependent Polymers

The first possibility of ECDDT is to manufacture capsule shells from pH-dependent polymers based on acidic cellulose derivatives, for now in phthalates, and acetate succinates forms or from their combinations with HPMC. Based on this principle, the pharmaceutical company CapsCanada (Windsor, ON, Canada) introduced AR Caps® and Capsugel® (Lonza Company, Greenwood, SC, USA) and launched two capsules under the trade name EnTRinsic™ and Vcaps® Enteric.

7.1.1. AR Caps® Capsules

The capsules were introduced in 2013 and have been on the market since 2015 [29]. They are made from HPMC and HPMCP in a ratio of 4:6 [53]. Due to a low moisture content of 4–10% in the capsule shell, the manufacturer recommends them for hygroscopic and hydrolyzing drugs. In addition, capsules are stable over a wide range of air humidity and are not subject to cross-linking [54]. The product information claims that AR Caps® capsules are stable for 60 min in the SGF. Their disintegration begins in the SIF, and capsules are completely released in the duodenum within 60 min [54,55]. Nevertheless, a related study by Al-Tabakha M. et al. shows that AR Caps® capsules filled with paracetamol do not meet the USP requirements for disintegration and dissolution for the delayed-release dosage form. Capsules disintegrate earlier than 60 min in SGF and release more than 15.7% of their content during the 120 min in SGF, and only 46.8% in 45 min in the continuous dissolution test. The study also finds no significant difference in the protection of hygroscopic material (concretely polyvinylpyrrolidone) compared to conventional HPMC capsules [29]. However, AR Caps® capsules were used in a study by Marcial G.E et al. to encapsulate lyophilized bacteria *Lactobacillus johnsonii N6.2* investigated as a potential substance for preventing the development of diabetes, where they provide suitable results for administering biological material to the GIT [56]. Capsules are available in sizes ranging from 000 to 5 [55].

7.1.2. EnTRinsic™ Capsules

The company Capsugel® launched the product in 2015, claiming it was the first capsules prepared by ECDDT with complete enteric protection [57]. The capsule shell is made of pure CAP with a pin dipping process using commercially available machines without any other additive, with 2–7% water content. The thickness of the capsule shell achieves acid resistance. The capsules should dissolve at a pH above 5.5 due to the polymer used for their production [58,59]. According to the manufacturer, capsules fully comply with Ph. Eur., USP, and JP requirements [60]. In a related study, Benameur H. et al. concluded that EnTRinsic™ capsules with esomeprazole meet USP disintegration and dissolution specifications for delayed-release drug form and are bioequivalent to gastro-resistant Nexium® capsules produced by AstraZeneca Plc (Cambridge, UK) [18,61]. In addition, a clinical study by Sager M. et al. investigated the amount of caffeine released from EnTRinsic™ capsules using saliva detection and magnetic resonance imaging (MRI) in vivo after a meal. Results from 14 out of 16 subjects demonstrated the ability to protect the capsule content in the gastric environment because of their disintegration only in the small intestine [62]. Furthermore, capsules were successfully used in the clinical evaluation of lyophilizate-containing bacteria of the human microbiome [63]. Sizes 0 and 3 are commercially available, other sizes could be supplied to order [60].

7.1.3. Vcaps® Enteric Capsules

The capsules were launched in 2015 [64]. They consist of HPMC and HPMCAS, contain less than 6.0% water, and are not subject to cross-linking [65]. The manufacturer, Capsugel®, declares that the capsules have been evaluated in vitro and in vivo with various substances, such as paracetamol, dimethyl fumarate, budesonide, or bisacodyl compliantly with USP, Ph. Eur., and JP requirements for delayed release [66]. In addition, Varga A. et al. demonstrated that capsules could be used to encapsulate frozen or lyophilized FMT with results comparable to administration by nasogastric or nasojejunal tubes [52]. Monschke M. et al. also used Vcaps® Enteric capsules to encapsulate amorphous drug dispersions to prevent their disruption in the acidic stomach area, resulting in the delayed release of dosage form during passage in the small intestine [67]. Vcaps® Enteric capsules were also applied for encapsulation of sprayed-dried pectin microparticles with peptides (Lanreotide acetate; Octreotide acetate) with satisfactory results in dissolution testing (total dissolution time of peptides from the capsule after 120 min in the intestinal area) [68]. The manufacturer usually supplies size 0 as standard, with other sizes available to order [69].

7.2. ECDDT Prepared from Gel-Forming Polymers

The second principle of ECDDT is producing a capsule shell from a mixture of gel-forming polymers such as pectin or gellan gum, often in combination with HPMC or another formative agent. Various companies worldwide are using this technology to produce their enteric capsule products. For example, company Capsugel® (Lonza Company, Colmar, France) introduced capsules DRcaps™; Suhueng Capsule (Seoul, South Korea) produced EMBO CAPS® AP; BioCaps® (El Monte, CA, USA) launched BioVXR; and the company ACG (Mumbai, India) manufactured capsules under the trade name ACGcaps™ HD.

7.2.1. DRcaps™ Capsules

In 2011, Capsugel® launched DRcaps™ capsules consisting of HPMC and gellan gum (a heteropolysaccharide of glucose, rhamnose, and glucuronic acid containing acidic functional groups, allowing pH-dependent dissolution [70]) in the ratio of 95:5 [71]. The water content in their structure is 4–7% allows, according to the manufacturer's encapsulation of hygroscopic drugs [72]. While conventional hard gelatin capsules disintegrate approximately 5 min after administration in SGF [73], DRcaps™ starts to disintegrate 45 min later in the dissolution test. Besides, according to an in vivo scintigraphy test made by the producer, complete disintegration occurs in the small intestine after 20 min [74]. According to Al-Tabakha M. et al., DRcaps™ capsules with paracetamol do not meet the USP requirements for disintegration and dissolution tests because they disintegrated in SGF within 60 min. In the dissolution test, capsules released 19.6% of API in SGF after 120 min, and subsequently, in SIF, only 34.2% within 45 min [29]. A similar result was reached by Grimm M. et al., with even a third less capsule content released in SIF [75]. DRcaps™ capsules were also used in a study by Youngster I. et al. as a prospective dosage form in FMT. DRcaps™ capsules were filled with fecal material with trypan blue as a dye and deep frozen. The capsules began to release dye after 115 min at pH $\geq$ 3 [76]. A longer time was achieved by inserting capsule size 0 into capsule size 00 (so-called Cap-in-Cap system). The total disintegration time in SGF ranged from 148 $\pm$ 42 to 168 $\pm$ 38 min depending on the capsule's contents. MRI then confirmed the gastric passage at fasting and API release in the small intestine [75]. In a study by Marzorati M. et al., DRcaps™ capsules containing encapsulated bacterial strain *Bifidobacterium longum* or acid-labile enzymes were used. During an in vitro dissolution test, the capsules showed satisfactory results in capsule content protection when they stayed intact in the stomach area and disintegrated entirely at the beginning of the simulated small intestine. Additionally, DRcaps™ capsules preserved bacterial viability in the capsule even after long-term storage [77]. Classic HPMC capsules and DRcaps™ were compared by the Cap-in-Cap method in different combinations. Only doubled DRcaps™ capsules showed pharmacopeial acid resistance [78]. However, significant protection of the hygroscopic drug was not demonstrated after comparison with conventional HPMC capsules [29]. The commercially available sizes of DRcaps™ capsules are from 000 to 4 [79].

7.2.2. EMBO CAPS® AP Capsules

The capsules appeared on the market in 2018. They consist of HPMC and pectin, with 5–7% water content [80]. According to the manufacturer, they release 12.0% after 120 min in SGF and more than 90.0% of the unspecified API after 30 min in SIF [81]. However, Grimm M. et al. discovered that capsules in the dissolution test released over 20.0% of paracetamol as their content during 120 min in SGF and subsequently more than 90.0% in 45 min in SIF [75]. These results do not comply with the limit requirements of the USP, so they cannot be considered enteric. The producer declares their use for encapsulating probiotics and hygroscopic materials [56] and it is already used for encapsulating bacterial lyophilizates and plant extracts in market products [82]. They are available in the size range of 00EL–4 [83].

7.2.3. BioVXR® Capsules

BioVXR capsules were patented in 2016. A producer, the company BioCaps®, does not fully disclose the composition of its product, except for HPMC [75]. However, the associated patent mentions using polymers such as pectin, propylene glycol, alginate, or xanthan gum and gelling agents such as gellan gum or carrageenan [84]. According to the producer, BioVXR® capsules are fully acid-resistant, with no more than 6.95% of the capsule content leaked in 120 min in SGF during the dissolution test, then in SIF within 45 min 89.1% of unspecified API [85]. A mixture of HPMC, gellan gum, and pectin roughly corresponds to this dissolution profile according to the patent composition [84]. Yet, results from the dissolution test provided by Grimm M. et al. showed a drug release of 48.5% from BioVXR® capsules at 120 min in SGF, and subsequently in SIF less than 80.0% after 45 min, which does not meet the requirements of the delayed-release drug form [75]. Capsules are available in sizes 00, 0, and 1 [86].

7.2.4. ACGcaps™ HD Capsules

The capsules, consisting of HPMC, with other components not specified, were introduced in 2019 as a part of the company's HPMC capsule line [87,88]. According to the manufacturer, the capsules disintegrate by a dual mechanism, i.e., also depending on the transit time through the GIT [89], and could be used for encapsulation hygroscopic drug due to their low moisture of capsule shell and resistance to cross-linking [90]. In addition, the product information states solubility at pH > 5.5 [91]. A study by Ashish V. et al. examined ACGcaps™ HD capsules with lyophilized or oil-based content of *Lactobacillus casei* for 120 min in SGF, and then for 360 min in SIF at an electromagnetic stirrer. Viability detected by in vitro cultivation of the collected samples after tests showed no significant release of capsule content in SGF, while 70.0–90.0% was released in SIF [87]. However, this is not a pharmacopoeial method for examining delayed-release drug forms. Nevertheless, these capsules are more suitable for lyophilized bacteria *Lactobacillus fermentum* compared to conventional gelatin capsules [35]. The ACG company offers capsules in sizes from 000 to 5 [89,90].

The individual commercially manufactured enteric capsules, their manufacturer, quality composition and the pharmacopoeial assumptions mentioned in the text above are summarized in Table 4.

Table 4. Overview of commercially produced capsules using ECDDT.

Product Name	Manufacturer/Country of Origin	Composition of Capsule	Pharmacopoeial Acid Resistance
A. Capsules prepared from pH-dependent polymers			
AR Caps®	CapsCanada/Canada	HPMC, HMPCP	No [29]
EnTRinsic™	Capsugel®/USA	CAP	Ph. Eur., USP, JP [60]
VCaps® Enteric	Capsugel®/USA	HPMC, HPMCAS	Ph. Eur., USP, JP [66]
B. Capsules prepared from gel-forming polymers			
DRcaps™	Capsugel®/France	HPMC, gellan gum	No [29]
EMBO CAPS® AP	Suhueng Capsule/Republic of Korea	HPMC, pectin	No [75]
BioVXR®	BioCaps®/USA	HPMC, gellan gum/pectin [1]	No [75]
AGCcaps™ HD	ACG/India	HPMC [2]	Not specified

[1] Derived composition based on an associated patent [84]; [2] other components are not listed.

8. Clinical Studies Performed with Enteric Capsules

A search for clinical studies was conducted from Google Scholar, ScienceDirect, and Scopus using the keywords "enteric", "acid resistant", "delayed release", "capsule product name", "capsule", "clinical", "individual treatment", "trial", "study", and in various combinations. A list of clinical studies is presented in correlation with a funnel plot to show the success of introducing this enteric dosage form in recent years (Table 5; Figure 2). According to a recent clinical systematic reviews and meta-analyses, a series of studies with enteric capsules have been conducted [13,92]; however, it is not always possible to identify the specific enteric capsule type and its manufacturer. Table 5 summarizes those clinical trials for which this information (capsule type, manufacturer) has been published.

Table 5. Overview of clinical studies with enteric capsules arranged in chronological order.

Clinical Study	Type of Capsule	Specification of Dosage Form	Single Dose/A Total Dose of Capsules	Capsule Content	Clinical Indication	Patient Population	Clinical Success Rate
Walker, E.G., et al., 2022 [93]	DRcaps™	-	2/2	Bitter extract of *Humulus lupulus*	Regulating Energy Intake (EI)	19	EI ↓ 17.54%
Reid I. et al., 2022 [94]	Vcaps® Enteric	One capsule with 20 mg of API	1; 2; 3/NA	Zoledronic acid (ZA); ZA as microparticles	Safety in bone resorption	5	Positive after one week
Zain N. et al., 2022 [95]	DRcaps™	-	5/5	Lyophilized bacteria in FMT	rCDI [1]	7	86%
Varga A. et al., 2021 [52]	Vcaps® Enteric	-	5–11/NA	Various parts of fecal suspension	rCDI	28	82.14%
Reigadas E. et al., 2020 [96]	DRcaps™	Cap-in-Cap system	4–5/NA	Lyophilized bacteria in FMT	rCDI	32	87.5%
Leong K. S. W. et al., 2019 [97]	DRcaps™	Cap-in-Cap system [2]	14/28	Frozen bacteria in FMT	Obesity/insulin resistance in adolescent	80	NA
Jiang Z., et al., 2018 [98]	AR CAPS®	-	NA/27	Lyophilized bacteria in FMT	rCDI	31	84%
Chehri M. et al., 2018 [99]	DRcaps™	Cap-in-Cap system	25 (daily)/75	Frozen bacteria in FMT	rCDI	9	88.9%
Halkjær S. et al., 2018 [100]	DRcaps™		25 (daily)/ 12 days	Frozen fecal in FMT	Irritable Bowel Syndrome (IBS)	52	36.4
Staley C. et al., 2017 [101]	DRcaps™	Cap-in-Cap system	2–4/NA	Lyophilized bacteria in FMT	rCDI	49	88%
Khana S. et al., 2016 [102]	DRcaps™	-	15/30 1–12/NA	Various numbers of bacteria	rCDI	15 15	80% 86.7%
Hirsch B. et al., 2015 [103]	DRcaps™	Cap-in-Cap system + gelatin capsule [3]	6–22/NA	Frozen bacteria in FMT	rCDI	19	89%
Youngster I. et al., 2014 [76]	DRcaps™	Cap-in-Cap system	NA/30	Frozen bacteria in FMT	rCDI	20	90%
Jones M. et al., 2012 [104]	DRcaps™	-	2 (daily)/126	Lyophilized bacteria *Lactobacillus reuteri* NCIMB 30242	Hypercholesterolemia	131	LDL-C [4] ↓ 11.64%
Jones M. et al., 2012 [105]	DRcaps™	-	2 (daily)/126	Lyophilized bacteria *Lactobacillus reuteri*	Clinical safety of *Lactobacillus reuteri*	131	Positive; Not quantified

[1] System of two capsules encapsulated into each other; [2] recurrent clostridium difficile infections; [3] system of two capsules encapsulated into each other + gelatin capsule as a third cover layer; [4] low-density lipoprotein-cholesterol. NA—not applicable.

In clinical or preclinical trials, for documentation and a better understanding of the capsule behavior after its administration to the GIT, non-invasive imaging techniques are used. Techniques such as MRI [75], single-photon emission computed tomography (SPECT) [106] and X-ray imaging could track movement through the tract [107]. Of additional imaging techniques, computed tomography (CT) allows 3D imaging of soft tissue structures. In combination with positron emission tomography (PET), CT could investigate the in vivo behavior of capsules in the GIT [108] (see Figure 3).

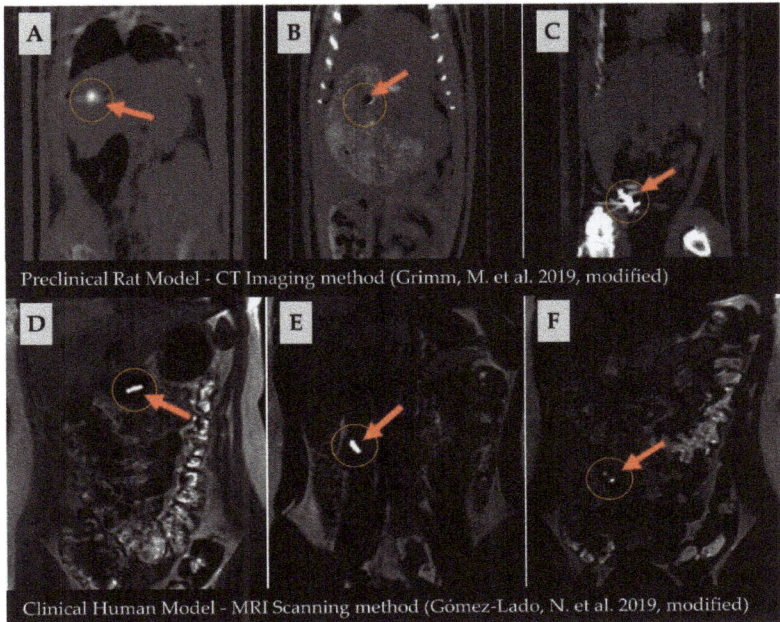

Figure 3. Documentation of the behavior of the enteric capsule after administration into the organism with two methods (MRI; CT) [75,108]; preclinical study performed on multiple rat models (differences in transit time could occur): (**A**)—capsule in the stomach after administration, (**B**)—disintegrated capsule in the stomach after 540 min, (**C**)—disintegrated capsule in caecum after 180 min; clinical study performed on one human model: (**D**)—capsule in the stomach after 5 min, (**E**)—capsule in ileum after 150 min, (**F**)—disintegrated capsule in ileum after 210 min. Reprinted from Eur. J. Pharm. Sci., 129. Grimm, M.; Ball, K.; Scholz, E.; Schneider, F.; Sivert, A.; Benameur, H.; Kromrey, M.L.; Kühn, J.P.; Weitschies, W. Characterization of the Gastrointestinal Transit and Disintegration Behavior of Floating and Sinking Acid-Resistant Capsules Using a Novel MRI Labeling Technique, 163–172, Copyright (2019), with permission from Elsevier.

9. Conclusions

Over the last decade, capsules prepared by ECDDT have started to appear on the worldwide market. Their shells are formed by synthetic and semi-synthetic pH-dependent polymers, which prevent dissolution in the acidic stomach environment or swelling natural or semi-synthetic polymers, which gel-forming properties extend the disintegration of drug form into the small intestine area. Although their commercial availability allows industrial manufacturing and preparation of drugs under laboratory conditions in pharmacies, pharmacopoeial limits for acid resistance may only sometimes be achieved with their use. Nevertheless, all capsules from the manufacturers mentioned above could help protect the encapsulated material from the acidic stomach environment. In addition, preventing release in the gastric environment can be enhanced by repeatedly encapsulating the drug capsules in a larger capsule (Cap-in-Cap). At the same time, the limits of pharmacopeia are not always guaranteed in pH 6.8 conditions. Another complication is the encapsulation of frozen FMT, which thaws during GIT passage. Due to the neutral environment, the capsule shell melts in the stomach, causing damage to the FMT.

Furthermore, specifically, when preparing a filling made of FMT, ethical problems arise on the part of patients. Currently, there are several trends to overcome the previous complications. One possibility is the application of an internal insoluble layer, which would prevent the capsule from dissolving from the inside, but which would disintegrate due to the impact of intestinal motility. Another developing option is manufacturing capsules directly in hospital pharmacies using 3D printing, allowing, for instance, a more precise adjustment of the release according to the thickness of the capsule wall. Finally, the cultivation of bacterial repopulation consortia is beginning to be considered in practice. It would solve the ethical aspect of FMT encapsulation by replacing it with selective cultures grown ex vivo.

Author Contributions: A.F. and N.F. wrote the review with the help of D.V.; D.V. reviewed the text; A.F. and N.F. prepared the review structure; D.V. managed funding acquisition. All authors have read and agreed to the published version of the manuscript.

Funding: This work was supported by Masaryk University (project MUNI/IGA/0942/2021).

Institutional Review Board Statement: Not applicable.

Informed Consent Statement: Not applicable.

Data Availability Statement: Not applicable.

Acknowledgments: Special appreciation is expressed to Matúš Lazor for capsule graphic design.

Conflicts of Interest: The authors declare no conflict of interest.

Appendix A

Table A1. Summary of inventions of enteric capsules between 1942 and 2022.

Publication [1]	Applicant	Priority	Composition [2] (Capsule; INNER SHELL of the Capsule; Outer Shell of the Capsule)/Technology
CN115068436	Jiangsu Zodiac Pharmaceutical Co., Ltd.	2022-06-23	Inner shell (HPMC, and carrageenan, gellan gum, agar, and potassium ions); Outer shell (HPMCP, and Tween® 80)
CN112546016	Zhejiang Wanli University	2022-04-22	Capsule (HPMCP, agar, potassium chloride, and Tween® 80 in ammonium)
CN114376982	Guangdong Pharmacology University	2022-01-18	Inner shell (chitosan); Outer shell (Eudragit® L 100, and HPMC)
EP3881834	Jiangsu Lefan Capsule Co., Ltd.	2021-09-22	Capsule (pullulan, carrageenan, glycerol, and SLS)
CN215875588	Zhejiang Xinchang Kangping Capsule Co., Ltd.	2021-08-30	Capsule (gelated alginate)/Provided with a special positioning lock ring
CN112569204	Hubei Humanwell Pharmaceutical Excipients Co., Ltd.	2021-03-30	Inner shell (HPMS, HPMC, and pullulan, guar gum, carrageenan, xanthan gum, agar, and emulsifier); Outer shell (HPMCP)
CN109846852	Chongqing Hengsheng Pharmaceutical Capsule Co., Ltd.	2021-02-26	Capsule (HPMC, potassium chloride, calcium acetate/carbonate/citrate, sodium alginate)
WO2022112422	Capsugel®, France/Belgium	2020-11-25	Inner shell (gelatin, starch, PVA, and HPMC); Outer shell (HPMCAS, HPMCP, CAP)
CN111467318	Hubei Humanwell Pharmaceutical Excipients Co., Ltd.	2020-07-31	Inner shell (tragacanth, gellan gum, carrageenan, konjac gum, xanthan gum, guar gum, agar, and calcium ions, and emulsifier, and coated with chitin, and sodium carbonate)
KR102272658	Suheung Capsule	2020-05-26	Capsule (gelatin, and methoxylamide pectin, and buffer, and emulsifier)
TW201912150	Qualicaps®	2019-04-01	Capsule (HPMC, MC, HPC, and Eudragit® L, Eudragit® NE, Eudragit® NM, Eudragit® FS 30D and HPMCP, HPMCAS, CAP, and PVA, and plasticizer, and surfactant)
CN109528689	Jiangsu Zodiac Pharmaceutical Co., Ltd.	2018-12-24	Inner shell (carrageenan, sesbania gum, maltitol, potassium chloride, PVAP); Outer shell (PVAP, and surfactant)
WO2019020134	Novamed	2017-07-24	Capsule (HPMC, CMC, gelatin, and gellan gum, guar gum, tragacanth, agar, alginate)

Table A1. Cont.

Publication [1]	Applicant	Priority	Composition [2] (Capsule; INNER SHELL of the Capsule; Outer Shell of the Capsule)/Technology
CN106902093	Huaqiao University	2017-01-24	Capsule (alginate, and gellan gum, xanthan gum, carragheen, konjac glucomannan, locust bean gum, guar gum, arabic gum, and potassium ions, and HPMC, HPC, CMC, HPS)
CN106924211	Qingdao Blue Valley Pharmaceutical	2017-01-18	Inner shell (HPMC, and carrageenan); Outer shell (low acyl gellan gum, and calcium chloride, acetic acid, calcium lactate)
US2021220285	Capsugel®, Belgium	2016-07-22	Capsule (HPMCAS, HPMCP, CAP, PVAP, and HPMC, and ammonia, ethanolamine)
KR102335455	Shinetsu Chemical Co., Ltd.	2016-07-12	Capsule (HPMCAS, ammonia)
US9452141	Dah Feng Capsule Co., Ltd.	2015-05-01	Outer shell (gellan gum, pectin, pullulan, HPMC, and potassium chloride)
CN104434870	Shaoxing Kangke Capsule Co., Ltd.	2015-03-25	Capsule (gelatin, and SLS, and sodium alginate)
TWI587880	Dah Feng Capsule Co., Ltd.	2015-03-24	Outer shell (gelatin/ poly triglucose, PVA, modified starch, HPMC, and gellan gum, carrageenan, and monovalent/ divalent salt)
CN104288120	Shaoxing Kangke Capsule Co., Ltd.	2014-10-16	Capsule (HPMC, and pectin, and SLS, Tween® 80, and glycerol, PEG, and sodium alginate, agar, carrageenan)
CN103919752	Lou Zhi	2014-05-07	Capsule (HPMCP, and PEG, glycerol, castor oil)
CN103520134	Songlin Liu	2013-10-29	Capsule (HPMCP, and PPG, glycerol, castor oil)
CN103394093	Chongqing Hengsheng Medicinal Capsules	2013-08-11	Capsule (HPMC, and carrageenan, and potassium chloride)
CN103394092	Chongqing Hengsheng Medicinal Capsules	2013-08-11	Capsule (HPMC, and gellan gum, and calcium chloride)
CN103417511	Chongqing Hengsheng Medicinal Capsules	2013-08-11	Capsule (HPMC, and carrageenan, and calcium chloride)
CN103432096	Chongqing Hengsheng Medicinal Capsules	2013-08-11	Capsule (HPMC, and carrageenan and potassium citrate)
CN103330695	Shaoxing Kangke Capsule Co., Ltd.	2013-06-05	Capsule (HPMC, and SLS, Tween® 80, glycerol, PEG, and sodium alginate, agar, carrageenan)
US10172803	Capsugel®, Belgium	2013-03-07	Capsule (HPMC, and calcium stearate, magnesium stearate, carnauba wax, and guar gum, pectin, carrageenan, xanthan gum, locust bean gum, alginate, alginic acid, tamarind gum, glucomannan, agar, curdlan, gellan gum, collagen)
TWI554290	Samsung Fine Chemicals	2012-06-05	Capsule (HPMC, HPMCP, and ammonia, sodium hydroxide, and potassium hydroxide)
JP2018058870	Capsugel®, Belgium	2012-05-02	Capsule (Eudragit® L 100, Eudragit® S 100, Eudragit® RS 100, CAP, CAT, HPMCAS, HPMCP, HPMC, HEC, EC, HPC, CMC, MC, and sorbitan monoesters, sorbitan POE esters, glycerol, PEG, castor oil, SLS, TEC, triacetin); Other similar compounds are also listed.
US2015080479	Son Jin Ryul, Park Eun Hee	2012-03-26	Capsule (HPMCP, and HPMC, and calcium hydroxide, and ammonia, sodium hydroxide, and potassium hydroxide, and TEC, triacetin, PEG, PPG, and surfactants)
EP3566698	Capsugel®, Belgium	2011-11-09	Capsule (CAP, CAT, HPMCAS, CMEC, PVAP, and monovalent/divalent carbonates and hydroxides)
KR20120100305	Samsung Fine Chemicals	2011-03-03	Capsule (HPMCP, and HPMC, and calcium hydroxide, and sodium hydroxide, potassium hydroxide, and hydrogenated corn syrup, TEC, triacetin, PEG, PPG)

Table A1. Cont.

Publication [1]	Applicant	Priority	Composition [2] (Capsule; INNER SHELL of the Capsule; Outer Shell of the Capsule)/Technology
EP3354335	Capsugel®, Belgium	2010-10-26	Capsule (CAP, and HPMC, HPC, EC, MC, CMEC, HPMCAS, HPMCP, and sorbitan monoesters and POE esters, glycerol, PEG, glycol, ricin oleate, SLS, TEC, triacetin, and POE-POP-POE triblock polymers); Other similar compounds are also listed.
US9603933	Son Jin Ryul, Baek Hyon Ho	2010-10-21	Capsule (HPMCP, and HPMC, and ammonia, sodium hydroxide, potassium hydroxide, calcium hydroxide, and SLS, sugar ester)
US8710105	Son Jin Ryul, Baek Hyon Ho	2010-06-11	Capsule (HPMCP, HPMCAS, HPMC, MC, carrageenan, agar, sodium alginate, gellan gum, pectin, sodium hydroxide, ammonia, potassium hydroxide, calcium hydroxide)
US8852631	Capsugel®, Belgium	2009-09-24	Capsule (gellan gum, and HPMC)
WO2011030952	Samsung Fine Chemicals	2009-09-11	Capsule (gellan gum, and HPMCP, and HPMCAS, and HPMC, MC, and neutralizing agent)
CN101433526	Shanghai Huiyuan Plant Capsule Co., Ltd.	2007-11-13	Outlet shell (HPS, carrageenan, and calcium chloride, sodium carbonate, and CA)
WO2009062356	Shanghai Huiyuan Vegetal Capsule Co., Ltd.	2007-11-13	Capsule (PVAP acrylic resin, acetyl pullulan, CAP, 1, 2, 4-benzene tricarboxylic acid acetate, HPMCP, HPMC 1,2,4-benzenetricarboxylate, CAS, succinic acid, acetic acid, HPMC, and monovalent and divalent hydroxides and carbonates, and acetylated gellan gum, carrageenan, agar, pectin, sodium alginate, xanthan gum, scutellaria, paulownia gum, locust bean gum, red algae gum, tamarind gum, tara gum, sclerotium glucan, alginate, carbomers)
US2010113620	Aston University	2007-03-29	Capsule (HPMC, and alginate, and gellan gum, sodium, and potassium ions, and PEG)
US6752953	Yung Shin Pharmaceutical Co.	2004-06-22	Capsule (cellulose nitrate, CTA, CAP, MC, EC, HPC, HPMC, HPMCP, and Eudragit® L, Eudragit® S, Eudragit® E, Eudragit® RL, Eudragit® RS, and glycerin, PPG, PEG, DEP, DBP, DBS, TEC, acetyl TEC, acetyl TBC, triacyl glycerol, castor oil); Other similar compounds are also listed.
WO2004012701	Ajit Singh, Meena Parashuraman	2002-08-02	Capsule (gelatin, and methacrylic acid copolymer, CAP, HPMCP, PVAP, and ammonia, sodium carbonate, sodium bicarbonate, sodium hydroxide, and TEC, DBP, DEP, benzyl phenyl formate, sorbitol, PEG)
US4138013	Parke, Davis & Co.	1976-08-27	Capsule (HPMC, and CAP, gelatin, the copolymer of methacrylic acid, and methacrylic acid ester)
GB1529901	Parke, Davis & Co.	1975-04-17	Capsule (gelatin and CAP, HPMCP, the copolymer of methacrylic acid with methacrylic acid ester)
DE2336807	Parke, Davis & Co.	1972-07-20	Capsule (gelatin, and HPMCP with softener)
GB743014	Kodak Ltd.	1952-05-01	Capsule (ethyl ether CP, CAP, both prepared in situ)
GB638284	Parke, Davis & Co.	1946-03-25	Capsule (gelatin, and glycerol, and in situ prepared CAP, and sodium carbonate)
GB610538	Gelatin Products Corp.	1945-11-05	Capsule (gelatin, and glycerol, in situ prepared CAP, and sodium carbonate)
US2390088	Gelatin Products Corp.	1942-09-24	Capsule (gelatin, and glycerol, CAP, and sodium carbonate)

[1] Each patent has a unique patent number that allows it to be found in the patent database; [2] abbreviations of the compositions of capsules used in summary without previous explanation are alphabetically ordered in brackets (CA—cellulose acetate; CP—cellulose phthalate; CMC—carboxymethyl cellulose; CMEC—carboxymethyl ethyl cellulose; DBP—dibutyl phthalate; DBS—dibutyl sebacate; DEP—diethyl phthalate; HEC—hydroxyethylcellulose; HEP—hydroxyethyl starch; HPS—hydroxypropyl starch; MC—methylcellulose; PEG—polyethylene glycol; POE—polyoxymethylene; POP—polyoxypropylene; PPG—propylene glycol; SLS—sodium lauryl sulfate; TBC—tributyl citrate; TEC—triethyl citrate).

References

1. Stegemann, S.; Tian, W.; Morgen, M.; Brown, S. Hard Capsules in Modern Drug Delivery. In *Pharmaceutical Formulation: The Science and Technology of Dosage Forms*, 1st ed.; Tovey, G.D., Ed.; Royal Society of Chemistry: London, UK, 2018. [CrossRef]
2. Overgaard, A.B.A.; Møller-Sonnergaard, J.; Christrup, L.L.; Højsted, J.; Hansen, R. Patients' Evaluation of Shape, Size and Colour of Solid Dosage Forms. *Pharm. World Sci.* **2001**, *23*, 185–188. [CrossRef] [PubMed]
3. Augsburger, L.L. Pharmaceutical Dosage Forms. In *Pharmaceutical Dosage Forms*; Augsburger, L.L., Hoag, S.W., Eds.; CRC Press: Boca Raton, FL, USA; London, UK, 2017. [CrossRef]
4. Franc, A.; Kubová, K.; Elbl, J.; Muselík, J.; Vetchý, D.; Šaloun, J.; Opatřilová, R. Diazepam Filled Hard Capsules Intended for Detoxification of Patients Addicted to Benzodiazepines and Z-Drugs. *Eur. J. Hosp. Pharm.* **2019**, *26*, 10–15. [CrossRef] [PubMed]
5. Hannula, A.M.; Marvola, M.; Kopra, T. Release of Ibuprofen from Hard Gelatin Capsule Formulations: Effect of Various Additives and Filling Method. *Acta Pharm.* **1989**, *98*.
6. Nair, R.; Vemuri, M.; Agrawala, P.; Kim, S. Investigation of Various Factors Affecting Encapsulation on the In-Cap Automatic Capsule-Filling Machine. *AAPS PharmSciTech* **2004**, *5*, 46–53. Available online: https://link.springer.com/content/pdf/10.1208/pt050457.pdf (accessed on 19 September 2022). [CrossRef]
7. Gullapalli, R.P.; Mazzitelli, C.L. Gelatin and Non-Gelatin Capsule Dosage Forms. *J. Pharm. Sci.* **2017**, *106*, 1453–1465. [CrossRef] [PubMed]
8. Sabadková, D.; Franc, A.; Muselík, J.; Neumann, D.; Vetchý, D. Pulsatile Drug Delivery Systems. *Chem. Listy* **2015**, *109*, 353–359. Available online: http://www.chemicke-listy.cz/ojs3/index.php/chemicke-listy/article/view/369 (accessed on 19 September 2022).
9. Sivert, A.; Wald, R.; Craig, C.; Benameur, H. Strategies for Modified Release Oral Formulation Development. In *Oral Drug Delivery for Modified Release Formulations*; Wiley: Hoboken, NJ, USA, 2022; pp. 235–252. Available online: https://onlinelibrary.wiley.com/doi/abs/10.1002/9781119772729.ch13 (accessed on 10 October 2022).
10. Bhutiani, N.; Schucht, J.E.; Miller, K.R.; McClave, S.A. Technical Aspects of Fecal Microbial Transplantation (FMT). *Curr. Gastroenterol. Rep.* **2018**, *20*, 30. [CrossRef]
11. Dvořáčková, K.; Franc, A.; Kejdušová, M. Drug Delivery to the Large Intesine. *Chem. Listy* **2013**, *107*, 522–529. Available online: http://chemicke-listy.cz/ojs3/index.php/chemicke-listy/article/view/6455 (accessed on 29 September 2022).
12. Kaito, S.; Toya, T.; Yoshifuji, K.; Kurosawa, S.; Inamoto, K.; Takeshita, K.; Suda, W.; Kakihana, K.; Honda, K.; Hattori, M.; et al. Fecal Microbiota Transplantation with Frozen Capsules for a Patient with Refractory Acute Gut Graft-versus-Host Disease. *Blood Adv.* **2018**, *2*, 3097–3101. [CrossRef]
13. Ramai, D.; Zakhia, K.; Fields, P.J.; Ofosu, A.; Patel, G.; Shahnazarian, V.; Lai, J.K.; Dhaliwal, A.; Reddy, M.; Chang, S. Fecal Microbiota Transplantation (FMT) with Colonoscopy Is Superior to Enema and Nasogastric Tube While Comparable to Capsule for the Treatment of Recurrent Clostridioides Difficile Infection: A Systematic Review and Meta-Analysis. *Dig. Dis. Sci.* **2021**, *66*, 369–380. [CrossRef]
14. Zheng, L.; Ji, Y.-Y.; Wen, X.-L.; Duan, S.-L. Fecal Microbiota Transplantation in the Metabolic Diseases: Current Status and Perspectives. *World J. Gastroenterol.* **2022**, *28*, 2546–2560. [CrossRef] [PubMed]
15. Huyghebaert, N.; Vermeire, A.; Remon, J.P. Alternative Method for Enteric Coating of HPMC Capsules Resulting in Ready-to-Use Enteric-Coated Capsules. *Eur. J. Pharm. Sci.* **2004**, *21*, 617–623. [CrossRef] [PubMed]
16. Fülöpová, N.; Pavloková, S.; DeBono, I.; Vetchý, D.; Franc, A. Development and Comparison of Various Coated Hard Capsules Suitable for Enteric Administration to Small Patient Cohorts. *Pharmaceutics* **2022**, *14*, 1577. [CrossRef] [PubMed]
17. Barbosa, J.A.C.; Al-Kauraishi, M.M.; Smith, A.M.; Conway, B.R.; Merchant, H.A. Achieving Gastroresistance without Coating: Formulation of Capsule Shells from Enteric Polymers. *Eur. J. Pharm. Biopharm.* **2019**, *144*, 174–179. [CrossRef] [PubMed]
18. Benameur, H. Enteric Capsule Drug Delivery Technology–Achieving Protection without Coating. *Drug Dev. Deliv.* **2015**, *15*, 34–37. Available online: https://drug-dev.com/capsule-technology-enteric-capsule-drug-delivery-technology-achieving-protection-without-coating/ (accessed on 15 September 2022).
19. Ph. Eur. MMXVII. *European Pharmacopoeia*, 9th ed.; European Pharmacopoeia Commission: Strasbourg, France, 2017.
20. Dvořáčková, K.; Rabišková, M.; Muselík, J.; Gajdziok, J.; Bajerová, M. Coated Hard Capsules as the PH-Dependent Drug Transport Systems to Ileo-Colonic Compartment. *Drug Dev. Ind. Pharm.* **2011**, *37*, 1131–1140. [CrossRef]
21. Vraníková, B.; Franc, A.; Gajdziok, J.; Vetchý, D. Biorelevant dissolution media simulating digestive tract conditions. *Chem. Listy* **2016**, *110*, 126–132. Available online: http://www.chemicke-listy.cz/ojs3/index.php/chemicke-listy/article/view/233/233 (accessed on 12 October 2022).
22. Donauer, N.; Lobenberg, R. A Mini Review of Scientific and Pharmacopeial Requirements for the Disintegration Test. *Int. J. Pharm.* **2007**, *345*, 2–8. [CrossRef]
23. *United States Pharmacopeia*, 43rd ed.; United States Pharmacopeia Convention Committee of Revision: Rockville, MD, USA, 2021.
24. *The Japanese Pharmacopeia*, 17th ed.; Society of Japanese Pharmacopoeia: Tokyo, Japan, 2016.
25. Katona, M.T.; Kakuk, M.; Szabó, R.; Tonka-Nagy, P.; Takács-Novák, K.; Borbás, E. Towards a Better Understanding of the Post-Gastric Behavior of Enteric-Coated Formulations. *Pharm. Res.* **2022**, *39*, 201–211. [CrossRef]
26. Al-Gousous, J.; Langguth, P. European versus United States Pharmacopeia Disintegration Testing Methods for Enteric-Coated Soft Gelatin Capsules. *Dissolution Technol.* **2015**, *22*, 6–8. [CrossRef]

27. Mašková, E.; Kubová, K.; Vetchý, D. Use of (Meth) Acrylate Copolymers in Controlled Release Matrix Tablet Technology. *Chem. Listy* **2015**, *109*, 14–20. Available online: http://www.chemicke-listy.cz/ojs3/index.php/chemicke-listy/article/view/408 (accessed on 15 October 2022).
28. Maderuelo, C.; Lanao, J.M.; Zarzuelo, A. Enteric Coating of Oral Solid Dosage Forms as a Tool to Improve Drug Bioavailability. *Eur. J. Pharm. Sci.* **2019**, *138*, 105019. [CrossRef] [PubMed]
29. Al-Tabakha, M.M.; Arida, A.I.; Fahelelbom, K.M.S.; Sadek, B.; Abu Jarad, R.A. Performances of New Generation of Delayed Release Capsules. *J. Young Pharm.* **2014**, *7*, 36–44. [CrossRef]
30. Liu, F.; McConnell, E.; Pygall, S. *Update on Polymers for Oral Drug Delivery*, 1st ed.; Smithers Rapra Technology: Shawburry, UK, 2011.
31. Edgar, K.J. Cellulose Esters in Drug Delivery. *Cellulose* **2006**, *14*, 49–64. [CrossRef]
32. Barbosa, J. Going Natural: Using Polymers from Nature for Gastroresistant Applications. *Br. J. Pharm.* **2017**, *2*, 14–30. [CrossRef]
33. Sinha, V.R.; Kumria, R. Polysaccharides in Colon-Specific Drug Delivery. *Int. J. Pharm.* **2001**, *224*, 19–38. [CrossRef]
34. Layek, B.; Mandal, S. Natural Polysaccharides for Controlled Delivery of Oral Therapeutics: A Recent Update. *Carbohydr. Polym.* **2020**, *230*, 115617. [CrossRef]
35. Rodríguez, M.T.S.; Urbano, H.C.; Muñoz de los Ríos, D.; Lara-Villoslada, F.; Martínez, M.A.R.; Hernández, M.E.M. Evaluation of Viability of Lactobacillus fermentum CECT 5716 in Gelatin and Gastroresistant Capsules. *J. Pharm. Pharmacol.* **2016**, *4*, 413–418. [CrossRef]
36. Saringat, H.B.; Alfadol, K.I.; Khan, G.M. The Influence of Different Plasticizers on Some Physical and Mechanical Properties of Hydroxypropyl Methylcellulose Free Films. *Pak. J. Pharm. Sci.* **2005**, *18*, 25–38.
37. De Oliveira, H.P.; Albuquerque, J.J.F.; Nogueiras, C.; Rieumont, J. Physical Chemistry Behavior of Enteric Polymer in Drug Release Systems. *Int. J. Pharm.* **2009**, *366*, 185–189. [CrossRef]
38. Dudhat, K.R. The Overview of Oral Solid Dosage Forms and Different Excipients Used for Solid Dosage Formulation. *Glob. Acad. J. Pharm. Drug Res.* **2022**, *4*, 66–72. [CrossRef]
39. Coviello, T.; Matricardi, P.; Marianecci, C.; Alhaique, F. Polysaccharide Hydrogels for Modified Release Formulations. *J. Control. Release* **2007**, *119*, 5–24. [CrossRef] [PubMed]
40. Podczeck, F.; Jones Brian, E. *Pharmaceutical Capsules*; Jones, B.E., Podczeck, F., Eds.; Pharmaceutical Press: London, UK, 2004.
41. Murachanian, D. Two-piece hard capsules for pharmaceutical formulation. *J. GXP Compliance* **2010**, *14*, 31–42.
42. Zhang, L.; Wang, Y.; Liu, H.; Yu, L.; Liu, X.; Chen, L.; Zhang, N. Developing Hydroxypropyl Methylcellulose/Hydroxypropyl Starch Blends for Use as Capsule Materials. *Carbohydr. Polym.* **2013**, *98*, 73–79. [CrossRef]
43. Al-Tabakha, M.M. HPMC Capsules: Current Status and Future Prospects. *J. Pharm. Pharmaceut. Sci.* **2010**, *13*, 428–442. Available online: https://journals.library.ualberta.ca/jpps/index.php/JPPS/article/view/8870/7398 (accessed on 20 August 2022). [CrossRef]
44. Hard Gelatin Capsules: Formulation and Manufacturing Considerations. Available online: https://www.pharmappsroach.com/hard-gelatin-capsules-formulation-and-manufacturing-considerations (accessed on 19 September 2022).
45. Podczeck, F. The Development of an Instrumented Tamp-Filling Capsule Machine I. *Eur. J. Pharm. Sci.* **2000**, *10*, 267–274. [CrossRef]
46. Kruisz, J.; Faulhammer, E.; Rehrl, J.; Scheibelhofer, O.; Witschnigg, A.; Khinast, J.G. Residence Time Distribution of a Continuously-Operated Capsule Filling Machine: Development of a Measurement Technique and Comparison of Three Volume-Reducing Inserts. *Int. J. Pharm.* **2018**, *550*, 180–189. [CrossRef]
47. Deodhar, C.P. *Soft and Empty Hard Gelatine Capsule Technology*; Nirali Prakashan: Bombai, India, 2019.
48. Capsule Sizes. Available online: https://www.saintytec.com/softgel-sizes (accessed on 20 September 2022).
49. Sizes_HPMC Capsule. Available online: https://www.saintytec.com/hpmc-capsule (accessed on 20 September 2022).
50. Capsule Sizes. Available online: https://www.medisca.com/Files/ReferenceCharts/Capsule%20Size%20Reference%20Chart%20-%20MUS%20&%20MCA.pdf (accessed on 20 September 2022).
51. Cohen, W.M.; Goto, A.; Nagata, A.; Nelson, R.R.; Walsh, J.P. R&D Spillovers, Patents and the Incentives to Innovate in Japan and the United States. *Res. Policy* **2002**, *31*, 1349–1367.
52. Varga, A.; Kocsis, K.; Sipos, D.; Kása, P.; Vigvári, S.; Pál, S.; Dembrovszky, F.; Farkas, K.; Péterfi, Z. How to Apply FMT More Effectively, Conveniently and Flexible–A Comparison of FMT Methods. *Front. Cell. Infect. Microbiol.* **2021**, *11*, 657320. [CrossRef]
53. AR CAPS® Enteric Capsules. Available online: https://www.cphi-online.com/ar-caps-enteric-capsules-prod476709.html (accessed on 15 July 2022).
54. Gastric acid Resistant Capsules_ARCAPS®. CapsCanada. Available online: https://capscanada.com/products/acid-resistant-capsules (accessed on 15 July 2022).
55. Technical Data Sheet AR Caps Acid Resistant Capsules. Available online: https://www.gocaps.com/wp-content/uploads/2021/04/AR-Caps-Technical-Data-SheetPR00373576.pdf (accessed on 15 July 2022).
56. Marcial, G.E.; Ford, A.L.; Haller, M.J.; Gezan, S.A.; Harrison, N.A.; Cai, D.; Meyer, J.L.; Perry, D.J.; Atkinson, M.A.; Wasserfall, C.H.; et al. Lactobacillus Johnsonii N6.2 Modulates the Host Immune Responses: A Double-Blind, Randomized Trial in Healthy Adults. *Front. Immunol.* **2017**, *8*, 655. [CrossRef]
57. Capsugel_EnTRinsic Drug Delivery Technology Platform. Available online: https://www.capsugel.com/news/capsugel-launches-breakthrough-entrinsic-drug-delivery-technology-platform (accessed on 6 June 2022).

58. EnTRinsic Drug Delivery Technology. Available online: https://pharma.lonza.co.jp/-/media/Lonza/knowledge/Small-Molecules/Tech%20Briefs/Lonza_tech-brief_Targeted-enTRinsic_ODP.pdf (accessed on 10 June 2022).
59. Rowe, R.C.; Sheskey, P.J.; Weller, P.J. *Handbook of Pharmaceutical Excipients*; The Pharmaceutical Press: London, UK, 2003.
60. Capsugel. New Intrinsically Enteric Capsule Technology for Pharmaceutical Drug Development. 2017. Available online: https://www.youtube.com/watch?v=yKAb_oKMuTY (accessed on 9 September 2022).
61. Lee, H.W.; Kang, W.Y.; Jung, W.; Gwon, M.-R.; Cho, K.; Yoon, Y.-R.; Seong, S.J. Pharmacokinetics and Pharmacodynamics of YYD601, a Dual Delayed-Release Formulation of Esomeprazole, Following Single and Multiple Doses in Healthy Adult Volunteers Under Fasting and Fed Conditions. *Drug Des. Devel. Ther.* **2022**, *16*, 619–634. [CrossRef] [PubMed]
62. Sager, M.; Grimm, M.; Aude, P.; Schick, P.; Merdivan, S.; Hasan, M.; Kromrey, M.-L.; Sivert, A.; Benameur, H.; Koziolek, M.; et al. In Vivo Characterization of EnTRinsic™ Drug Delivery Technology Capsule after Intake in Fed State: A Cross-Validation Approach Using Salivary Tracer Technique in Comparison to MRI. *J. Control. Release* **2019**, *313*, 24–32. [CrossRef] [PubMed]
63. Benameur, H. EnTRinsic™ Drug Delivery Technology for Live Biotherapeutics (Microbiomes). Recent Achievements and Further Challenges in Drug Delivery Research. In Proceedings of the 12th France-Japan Drug Delivery Systems Symposium, Abbaye des Vaux de Cernay, France, 9–12 October 2016. Available online: https://www.umr-cnrs8612.universite-paris-saclay.fr/docs/pdf/Prog-Symposium-Japon-2016.pdf#page=19 (accessed on 15 September 2022).
64. Jančálková, M. Capsule Coating for Faecal Transplant Transport. Master's Thesis, Masaryk University, Brno, Czech Republic, 2021.
65. Vcaps® Enteric Capsules_Capsugel®. Available online: https://www.capsugel.com/biopharmaceutical-products/vcaps-enteric-capsules (accessed on 19 September 2022).
66. Capsugel_Vcaps® Enteric. Available online: http://alfresco-static-files.s3.amazonaws.com/alfresco_images/pharma/2018/10/11/0592de88-9026-4c61-b660-f5fd790b7cea/PharmTech_Europe_July2018.pdf#page=38 (accessed on 10 September 2022).
67. Monschke, M.; Kayser, K.; Wagner, K.G. Influence of Particle Size and Drug Load on Amorphous Solid Dispersions Containing PH-Dependent Soluble Polymers and the Weak Base Ketoconazole. *AAPS PharmSciTech* **2021**, *22*, 44. [CrossRef] [PubMed]
68. Li, T.; Wan, B.; Jog, R.; Costa, A.; Burgess, D.J. Pectin Microparticles for Peptide Delivery: Optimization of Spray Drying Processing. *Int. J. Pharm.* **2022**, *613*, 121384. [CrossRef]
69. Vcaps Enteric. Available online: https://cpsl-web.s3.amazonaws.com/kc/Vcaps-Enteric_Oct-2017.pdf?mtime=20171017051951 (accessed on 10 September 2022).
70. Barbosa, J.A.C.; Abdelsadig, M.S.E.; Conway, B.R.; Merchant, H.A. Using Zeta Potential to Study the Ionisation Behaviour of Polymers Employed in Modified-Release Dosage Forms and Estimating Their PKa. *Int. J. Pharm. X* **2019**, *1*, 100024. [CrossRef] [PubMed]
71. Certificate of analysis: Empty DRcaps™ capsules. In *Capsugel*; Lonza Company: Colmar, France, 2020.
72. DRcaps_Capsules. Available online: https://s3.amazonaws.com/cpsl-web/kc/library/c1a-32029_DRCaps-A4_FIN.PDF (accessed on 10 September 2022).
73. Tuleu, C.; Khela, M.K.; Evans, D.F.; Jones, B.E.; Nagata, S.; Basit, A.W. A Scintigraphic Investigation of the Disintegration Behaviour of Capsules in Fasting Subjects: A Comparison of Hypromellose Capsules Containing Carrageenan as a Gelling Agent and Standard Gelatin Capsules. *Eur. J. Pharm. Sci.* **2007**, *30*, 251–255. [CrossRef]
74. Amo, R. DRcaps Capsules Achieve Delayed Release Properties for Nutritional Ingredients in Human Clinical Study. Capsugel. 2021. Available online: https://www.pharmaexcipients.com/wp-content/uploads/2021/01/DRcaps%C2%AE-Capsules-Achieve-Delayed-Release-Properties-for-Nutritional-Ingredients-in-Human-Clinical-Study.pdf (accessed on 10 September 2022).
75. Grimm, M.; Ball, K.; Scholz, E.; Schneider, F.; Sivert, A.; Benameur, H.; Kromrey, M.L.; Kühn, J.P.; Weitschies, W. Characterization of the Gastrointestinal Transit and Disintegration Behavior of Floating and Sinking Acid-Resistant Capsules Using a Novel MRI Labeling Technique. *Eur. J. Pharm. Sci.* **2019**, *129*, 163–172. [CrossRef]
76. Youngster, I.; Russell, G.H.; Pindar, C.; Ziv-Baran, T.; Sauk, J.; Hohmann, E.L. Oral, Capsulized, Frozen Fecal Microbiota Transplantation for Relapsing Clostridium Difficile Infection. *JAMA* **2014**, *312*, 1772–1778. [CrossRef]
77. Marzorati, M.; Possemiers, S.; Verhelst, A.; Cadé, D.; Madit, N.; Van de Wiele, T. A Novel Hypromellose Capsule, with Acid Resistance Properties, Permits the Targeted Delivery of Acid-Sensitive Products to the Intestine. *LWT-Food Sci. Technol.* **2015**, *60*, 544–551. [CrossRef]
78. Rump, A.; Weiss, F.N.; Schulz, L.; Kromrey, M.L.; Scheuch, E.; Tzvetkov, M.V.; White, T.; Durkee, S.; Judge, K.W.; Jannin, V.; et al. The Effect of Capsule-in-Capsule Combinations on in Vivo Disintegration in Human Volunteers: A Combined Imaging and Salivary Tracer Study. *Pharmaceutics* **2021**, *13*, 2002. [CrossRef]
79. Empty Capsules. Available online: https://www.purecapsules.co.uk/index.php/product/index/mid/76 (accessed on 14 August 2022).
80. Embocaps®. Available online: https://www.embocaps.com/sub/capsule-advantage-design.php (accessed on 12 August 2022).
81. EMBO CAPS AP_Brochure. Available online: https://www.embocaps.com/sub/brochure/products-ap.pdf (accessed on 15 August 2022).
82. Probiotics Swanson®. Available online: https://www.swansonvitamins.com/ncat1/Health+Concerns/ncat2/Digestive+System/ncat3/Probiotics/q (accessed on 13 August 2022).
83. Embo caps®_Suheung Capsule Co. Available online: https://www.cphi-online.com/embo-caps-prod047905.html (accessed on 19 July 2022).
84. Chang, R.J.; Wu, C.J.; Lin, Y.H. Acid Resistant Capsule Shell Composition, Acid Resistant Capsule Shell and Its Preparing Process. U.S. Patent No. 9,452,141 B1, 27 September 2016.

85. BioVXR Acid Resistant Capsules. Available online: https://www.dfc.com.tw/archive/product/item/files/BioVXR%20brochure%202022.pdf (accessed on 16 August 2022).
86. Acid Resistant Vegetable Capsules Bio-VXR. Available online: https://biocaps.net/portfolio/acid-resistant-vegetable-capsules (accessed on 19 August 2022).
87. Sangve, A.V.; Bansode, S.S.; Menon, M.D. Evaluation of Side selective release of Probiotics from an HPMC Delayed release capsule. Disso India-Chandigarh. In Proceedings of the 7th International Annual Symposium, Chandigarh, India, 12–13 September 2019. Available online: https://spds.in/wp-content/uploads/2020/07/Disso-India-Chandhigarh-scientifica-abstract-book-2019-dt-30-8-19.pdf (accessed on 5 October 2022).
88. ACG_Formulation: Flexibility with New Era HPMC Capsules. Available online: https://ondrugdelivery.com/wp-content/uploads/2020/07/109_Jul_2020_ACG.pdf (accessed on 10 September 2022).
89. ACG Capsule Brochure. Available online: https://issuu.com/acggroup/docs/capsule_20range_20brochure-web_20us (accessed on 10 September 2022).
90. ACGcapsTM_ ACG. Available online: https://www.acg-world.com/archives/capsules/hpmc-capsules/acgcapstm-hr (accessed on 12 September 2022).
91. ACGCAPS_HD_Capsules. Available online: https://www.justdial.com/jdmart/Mumbai/ACGCAPS-HD-Capsules/pid-2020831557/022P427056 (accessed on 12 September 2022).
92. Cold, F.; Baunwall, S.M.D.; Dahlerup, J.F.; Petersen, A.M.; Hvas, C.L.; Hansen, L.H. Systematic Review with Meta-Analysis: Encapsulated Faecal Microbiota Transplantation–Evidence for Clinical Efficacy. Therap. Adv. Gastroenterol. 2021, 14, 175628482110410. [CrossRef] [PubMed]
93. Walker, E.G.; Lo, K.R.; Pahl, M.C.; Shin, H.S.; Lang, C.; Wohlers, M.W.; Poppitt, S.D.; Sutton, K.H.; Ingram, J.R. An Extract of Hops (Humulus Lupulus L.) Modulates Gut Peptide Hormone Secretion and Reduces Energy Intake in Healthy-Weight Men: A Randomized, Crossover Clinical Trial. Am. J. Clin. Nutr. 2022, 115, 925–940. [CrossRef] [PubMed]
94. Reid, I.R.; Wen, J.; Mellar, A.; Liu, M.; Jabr, A.; Horne, A.M. Effect of Oral Zoledronate Administration on Bone Turnover in Older Women. Br. J. Clin. Pharmacol. 2022, 1–6. [CrossRef] [PubMed]
95. Zain, N.M.M.; Ter Linden, D.; Lilley, A.K.; Royall, P.G.; Tsoka, S.; Bruce, K.D.; Mason, A.J.; Hatton, G.B.; Allen, E.; Goldenberg, S.D.; et al. Design and Manufacture of a Lyophilised Faecal Microbiota Capsule Formulation to GMP Standards. J. Control. Release 2022, 350, 324–331. [CrossRef]
96. Reigadas, E.; Bouza, E.; Olmedo, M.; Vázquez-Cuesta, S.; Villar-Gómara, L.; Alcalá, L.; Marín, M.; Rodríguez-Fernández, S.; Valerio, M.; Muñoz, P. Faecal Microbiota Transplantation for Recurrent Clostridioides Difficile Infection: Experience with Lyophilized Oral Capsules. J. Hosp. Infect. 2020, 105, 319–324. [CrossRef]
97. Leong, K.S.W.; Jayasinghe, T.N.; Derraik, J.G.B.; Albert, B.B.; Chiavaroli, V.; Svirskis, D.M.; Beck, K.L.; Conlon, C.A.; Jiang, Y.; Schierding, W.; et al. Protocol for the Gut Bugs Trial: A Randomised Double-Blind Placebo-Controlled Trial of Gut Microbiome Transfer for the Treatment of Obesity in Adolescents. BMJ Open 2019, 9, e026174. [CrossRef]
98. Jiang, Z.-D.; Jenq, R.R.; Ajami, N.J.; Petrosino, J.F.; Alexander, A.A.; Ke, S.; Iqbal, T.; DuPont, A.W.; Muldrew, K.; Shi, Y.; et al. Safety and Preliminary Efficacy of Orally Administered Lyophilized Fecal Microbiota Product Compared with Frozen Product given by Enema for Recurrent Clostridium Difficile Infection: A Randomized Clinical Trial. PLoS ONE 2018, 13, e0205064. [CrossRef]
99. Chehri, M.; Christensen, A.H.; Halkjær, S.I.; Günther, S.; Petersen, A.M.; Helms, M. Case Series of Successful Treatment with Fecal Microbiota Transplant (FMT) Oral Capsules Mixed from Multiple Donors Even in Patients Previously Treated with FMT Enemas for Recurrent Clostridium Difficile Infection. Medicine 2018, 97, e11706. [CrossRef]
100. Halkjær, S.I.; Christensen, A.H.; Lo, B.Z.S.; Browne, P.D.; Günther, S.; Hansen, L.H.; Petersen, A.M. Faecal Microbiota Transplantation Alters Gut Microbiota in Patients with Irritable Bowel Syndrome: Results from a Randomised, Double-Blind Placebo-Controlled Study. Gut 2018, 67, 2107–2115. [CrossRef]
101. Staley, C.; Hamilton, M.J.; Vaughn, B.P.; Graiziger, C.T.; Newman, K.M.; Kabage, A.J.; Sadowsky, M.J.; Khoruts, A. Successful Resolution of Recurrent Clostridium Difficile Infection Using Freeze-Dried, Encapsulated Fecal Microbiota; Pragmatic Cohort Study. Am. J. Gastroenterol. Suppl. 2017, 112, 940–947. [CrossRef]
102. Khanna, S.; Pardi, D.S.; Kelly, C.R.; Kraft, C.S.; Dhere, T.; Henn, M.R.; Lombardo, M.-J.; Vulic, M.; Ohsumi, T.; Winkler, J.; et al. A Novel Microbiome Therapeutic Increases Gut Microbial Diversity and Prevents Recurrent Clostridium Difficile Infection. J. Infect. Dis. 2016, 214, 173–181. [CrossRef] [PubMed]
103. Hirsch, B.E.; Saraiya, N.; Poeth, K.; Schwartz, R.M.; Epstein, M.E.; Honig, G. Effectiveness of Fecal-Derived Microbiota Transfer Using Orally Administered Capsules for Recurrent Clostridium Difficile Infection. BMC Infect. Dis. 2015, 15, 191. [CrossRef] [PubMed]
104. Jones, M.L.; Martoni, C.J.; Prakash, S. Cholesterol Lowering and Inhibition of Sterol Absorption by Lactobacillus Reuteri NCIMB 30242: A Randomized Controlled Trial. Eur. J. Clin. Nutr. 2012, 66, 1234–1241. [CrossRef] [PubMed]
105. Jones, M.L.; Martoni, C.J.; di Pietro, E.; Simon, R.R.; Prakash, S. Evaluation of Clinical Safety and Tolerance of a Lactobacillus Reuteri NCIMB 30242 Supplement Capsule: A Randomized Control Trial. Regul. Toxicol. Pharmacol. 2012, 63, 313–320. [CrossRef]

106. Sonaje, K.; Chen, Y.-J.; Chen, H.-L.; Wey, S.-P.; Juang, J.-H.; Nguyen, H.-N.; Hsu, C.-W.; Lin, K.-J.; Sung, H.-W. Enteric-Coated Capsules Filled with Freeze-Dried Chitosan/Poly(γ-Glutamic Acid) Nanoparticles for Oral Insulin Delivery. *Biomaterials* **2010**, *31*, 3384–3394. [CrossRef]
107. Saphier, S.; Rosner, A.; Brandeis, R.; Karton, Y. Gastro Intestinal Tracking and Gastric Emptying of Solid Dosage Forms in Rats Using X-ray Imagining. *Int. J. Pharm.* **2010**, *388*, 190–195. [CrossRef]
108. Gómez-Lado, N.; Seoane-Viaño, I.; Matiz, S.; Madla, C.M.; Yadav, V.; Aguiar, P.; Basit, A.W.; Goyanes, A. Gastrointestinal Tracking and Gastric Emptying of Coated Capsules in Rats with or without Sedation Using CT Imaging. *Pharmaceutics* **2020**, *12*, 81. [CrossRef]

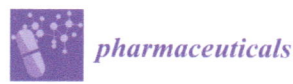 *pharmaceuticals*

Review

Digital Pills with Ingestible Sensors: Patent Landscape Analysis

Olena Litvinova [1,*], Elisabeth Klager [2], Nikolay T. Tzvetkov [3], Oliver Kimberger [2,4], Maria Kletecka-Pulker [2,5], Harald Willschke [2,4] and Atanas G. Atanasov [2,6,*]

1. Department of Management, Economy and Quality Assurance in Pharmacy, National University of Pharmacy, The Ministry of Health of Ukraine, 61002 Kharkiv, Ukraine
2. Ludwig Boltzmann Institute Digital Health and Patient Safety, Medical University of Vienna, 1180 Vienna, Austria
3. Institute of Molecular Biology "Roumen Tsanev", Department of Biochemical Pharmacology and Drug Design, Bulgarian Academy of Sciences, 1113 Sofia, Bulgaria
4. Department of Anaesthesia, Intensive Care Medicine and Pain Medicine, Medical University of Vienna, 1090 Vienna, Austria
5. Institute for Ethics and Law in Medicine, University of Vienna, 1090 Vienna, Austria
6. Institute of Genetics and Animal Biotechnology of the Polish Academy of Sciences, 05-552 Jastrzebiec, Poland
* Correspondence: hlitvinova@gmail.com (O.L.); atanas.atanasov@dhps.lbg.ac.at (A.G.A.); Tel.: +380-67-300-78-49 (O.L.); +43-1401-6036-250 (A.G.A.)

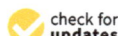

Citation: Litvinova, O.; Klager, E.; Tzvetkov, N.T.; Kimberger, O.; Kletecka-Pulker, M.; Willschke, H.; Atanasov, A.G. Digital Pills with Ingestible Sensors: Patent Landscape Analysis. *Pharmaceuticals* 2022, 15, 1025. https://doi.org/10.3390/ph15081025

Academic Editors: Silviya Petrova Zustiak and Era Jain

Received: 30 July 2022
Accepted: 18 August 2022
Published: 19 August 2022

Publisher's Note: MDPI stays neutral with regard to jurisdictional claims in published maps and institutional affiliations.

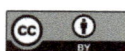

Copyright: © 2022 by the authors. Licensee MDPI, Basel, Switzerland. This article is an open access article distributed under the terms and conditions of the Creative Commons Attribution (CC BY) license (https://creativecommons.org/licenses/by/4.0/).

Abstract: The modern healthcare system is directly related to the development of digital health tools and solutions. Pills with digital sensors represent a highly innovative class of new pharmaceuticals. The aim of this work was to analyze the patent landscape and to systematize the main trends in patent protection of digital pills with ingestible sensors worldwide; accordingly, to identify the patenting leaders as well as the main prevailing areas of therapy for patent protection, and the future perspectives in the field. In July 2022, a search was conducted using Internet databases, such as the EPO, USPTO, FDA and the Lens database. The patent landscape analysis shows an increase in the number of patents related to digital pills with ingestible sensors for mobile clinical monitoring, smart drug delivery, and endoscopy diagnostics. The leaders in the number of patents issued are the United States, the European Patent Office, Canada, Australia, and China. The following main areas of patenting digital pills with ingestible sensors were identified: treatment in the field of mental health; HIV/AIDS; pain control; cardiovascular diseases; diabetes; gastroenterology (including hepatitis C); oncology; tuberculosis; and transplantology. The development of scientific and practical approaches towards the implementation of effective and safe digital pills will improve treatment outcomes, increase compliance, reduce hospital stays, provide mobile clinical monitoring, have a positive impact on treatment costs and will contribute to increased patient safety.

Keywords: digital pill; ingestible sensor; patent; clinical monitoring; medication adherence

1. Introduction

Nowadays, in the modern world the progress of the healthcare system is directly related to the development of digital health tools.

According to the WHO global strategy, digital technologies are connected to the future of world health. Digitalization has the potential to benefit health promotion, maintain global security, and provide services to the most vulnerable groups of the population [1].

Digital pills occupy an important place among the digital health solutions. Digital pills contain integrated sensors that allow monitoring of the course of pharmacotherapy through an interaction with the software of, e.g., tablets and smartphones. Such monitoring is of great importance, as low patient compliance (medication opt-out) is a major challenge for all areas of medicine.

Digital pills improve treatment adherence and efficiency in the field of mental health and behavioral modifications, such as schizophrenia, bipolar I disorder, attention deficit and hyperactivity disorder, drug abuse, smoking, pain, insomnia, and many others. The developers of the digital pills also focus on the treatment of cardiac disorders, diabetes, hepatitis C, AIDS, cancer, tuberculosis, and the monitoring of patients' use of opioid drugs after surgery, and other conditions when admission may be impaired due to the characteristics of the patient's behavior (geriatrics, neurodegenerative diseases, etc.) [2–4].

Digital pills have a significant potential for savings in healthcare costs by reducing the need for emergency medical care and the hospitalization of patients. The annual costs of non-compliance range from USD100 billion up to USD290 billion in the US, EUR1.25 billion in Europe, and approximately USD7 billion in Australia. In addition, 10% of the hospitalizations among the elderly are due to treatment noncompliance, with a typical noncompliant patient requiring three additional doctor visits per year, resulting in an annual increase of USD2000 in treatment costs. In diabetes, the estimated cost savings associated with improving noncompliance ranges from USD661 million to USD1.16 billion. Non-adherence is thus a critical clinical and economic problem [5].

Despite the progress made in this area to date, there are still a number of barriers to the widespread implementation of digital pills into medical practice. They include issues of clinical efficacy, safety, treatment costs, and confidentiality, among others. In addition, the patent landscape for the digital pill with ingestible sensors is not yet well-established. This indicates the need for further research in this area [6,7].

The development of digital pills is executed by high-tech industries that are evolving rapidly and require innovation from manufacturers. One of the sources of information reflecting the innovation process is the patent documentation.

The value of information, which is formed as a result of the work of patent offices in different countries around the world, is its universality in determining the main technological trends and building trends in market processes, and in analyzing the behavior of specific market participants, their resources, and growth prospects. The universality of patent data is ensured by the unification of standards for the presentation of data on intellectual property objects. The reliability of patent information is ensured by the procedure of the state registration of intellectual property rights. The scope of their legal protection depends on the completeness of the disclosure of information about the objects, as well as on the concretization of the features that constitute the novelty of the results of intellectual property. Therefore, in order to ensure a comprehensive protection of their own exclusive rights, the applicant is forced to detail the important technological aspects of patented development as much as possible. The examination of the patent landscape enables researchers to quantify the intellectual property characteristics.

The aim of this work was to analyze the patent landscape and systematize the main trends in the patent protection of digital pills with ingestible sensors worldwide, as well as to identify the patenting leaders, the main prevailing areas of therapy for patent protection, and future perspectives in the field.

2. Results and Discussion

By the end of June 2021, there were 137 digital therapeutic products and 122 digital care products at different stages of development, according to the IQVIA Digital Solutions database, which systematizes the different types of digital healthcare solutions [8]. Among the so-called Digital Therapeutics, 25 had secured market authorization and became available for marketing through regulatory processes. Among these 25 Digital Therapeutics with market authorization from at least one country, 9 were in the US, 19 were in Europe, and 1 was in Japan, with some overlap [8].

An analysis and systematization of the global patent protection of digital pills with ingestible sensors was completed, to identify the key developments in the sector (Figure 1).

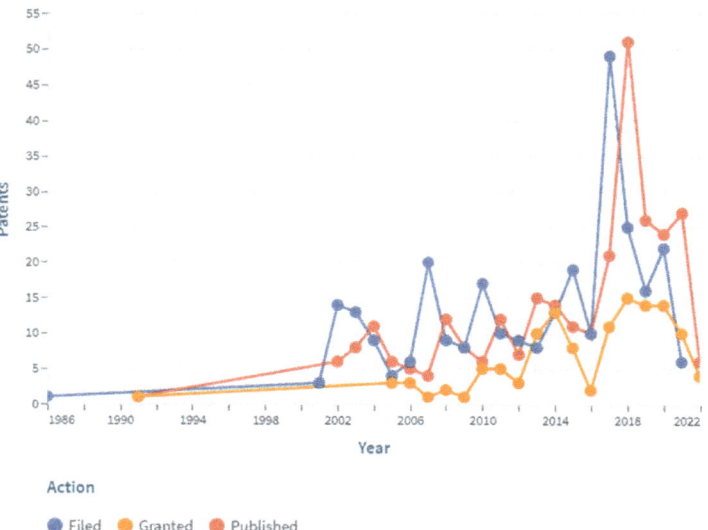

Figure 1. Dynamics of patent activity by applicants in the field of digital pills with ingestible sensor (https://www.lens.org, accessed on 30 July 2022).

A stable increase in the dynamics of applications and granted patents during the period of time between 2010 and 2018 was revealed. Most of the applications (49) were filed in 2017, and most of the patents (15) were granted in 2018. The lower patent activity in the years 2019–2022 (the first half of the year) may be associated with a focus on commercialization and the entry into the market of newly created inventions instead of the filing of new patents.

The patenting landscape presents a strong indication of the continuous efforts of scientists in the development of digital pill forms. It should be noted that some of the patents are no longer valid (Figure 2). Given the active development and replacement of technologies with newer, more modern ones, the patents are rarely kept in force for the maximum of 20 years (25 years for medicines). Most of the analyzed patents were filed during the period between 2000 and 2018.

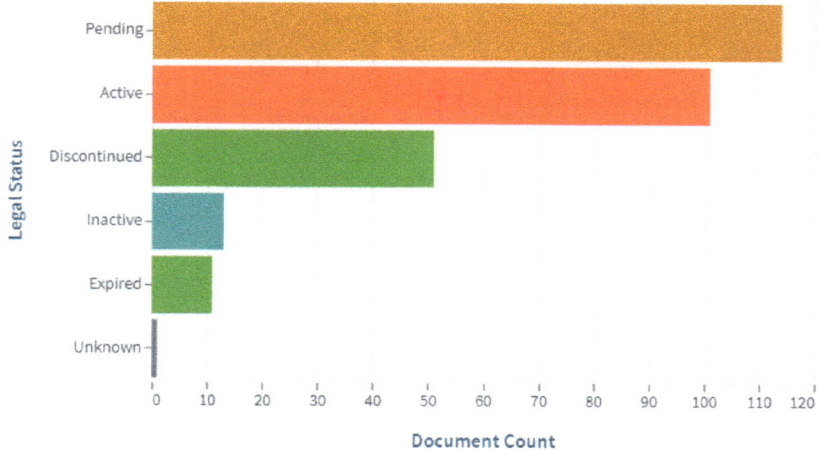

Figure 2. Patent documents by legal status (https://www.lens.org, accessed on 30 July 2022).

The leaders in the number of patents issued are the United States, the European Patent Office, Canada, Australia, and China, which together account for 72% of the total number of patents around the world.

Figure 3 shows the principal owners of the patents in the field of digital pills with an ingestible sensor. Proteus Digital Health Inc. (Redwood City, CA, USA), Otsuka Pharmaceutical Co., Ltd. (Tokyo, Japan), Given Imaging Ltd. (Yokneam, Israel), Pop Test Abuse Deterrent Technology LLC (Cliffside Park, NJ, USA), Given Imaging Inc. (Duluth, GA, USA), Innurvation Inc. (Glen Burnie, MD, USA), Otsuka America Pharmaceutical Inc. (Rockville, MD, USA), Progenity Inc. (San Diego, CA, USA), Pop Test LLC (Cliffside Park, NJ, USA), The Smart Pill Corporation (Buffalo, NY, USA), and others are among the key companies committed to expanding the digital pill market size through innovative development.

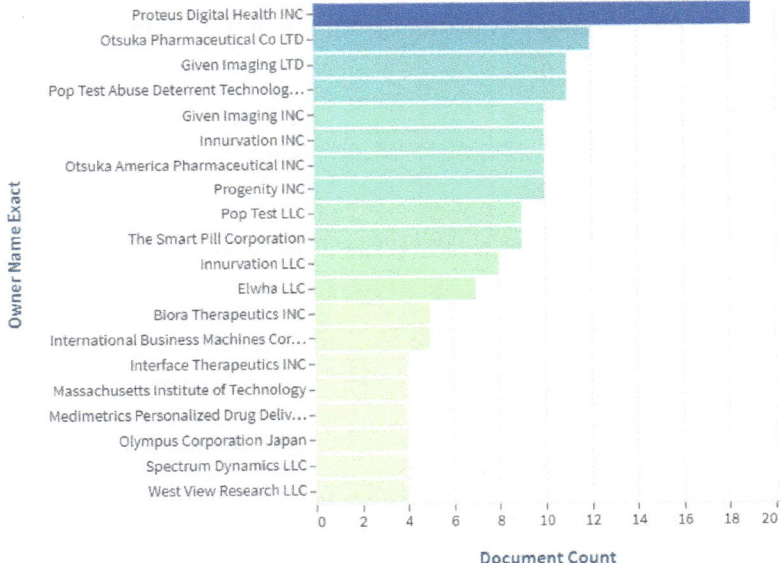

Figure 3. Top proprietors of patents in the field of digital pills with ingestible sensors (https://www.lens.org, accessed on 30 July 2022).

The top 20 inventors involved in the creation of digital pills with ingestible sensors are shown in Figure 4. Their inventions are in the fields of mobile clinical monitoring, smart drug delivery, and endoscopy diagnostics. Mobile clinical monitoring and smart drug delivery make use of digital pills with sensors, and can be applied to treat a different range of diseases in a wide range of patients. A capsule endoscopy can help to diagnose problems with gastrointestinal peristalsis, such as persistent constipation, nausea, acid reflux, gastroparesis, colon cancer, and others. It should be noted that the digital pills with ingestible sensors are currently quite expensive, and the regulations for government approval of new products are strict. Within such a framework, scientists are actively working in the domain to bring effective and safe digital pills to the healthcare market.

The analysis (Figure 3) revealed that Proteus Digital Health (Redwood City, CA, USA) is one of the leading companies creating ingestible sensor systems for medication adherence. Proteus' patented digital pill system allows for the personalization of treatment methods with wide potential benefits in various therapeutic areas. A digital ingestion tracking system—a sensor known as an "Ingestible Event Marker"—made by Proteus Digital Health was used to create the drug Abilify MyCite by Otsuka Pharmaceutical Company (Tokyo, Japan).

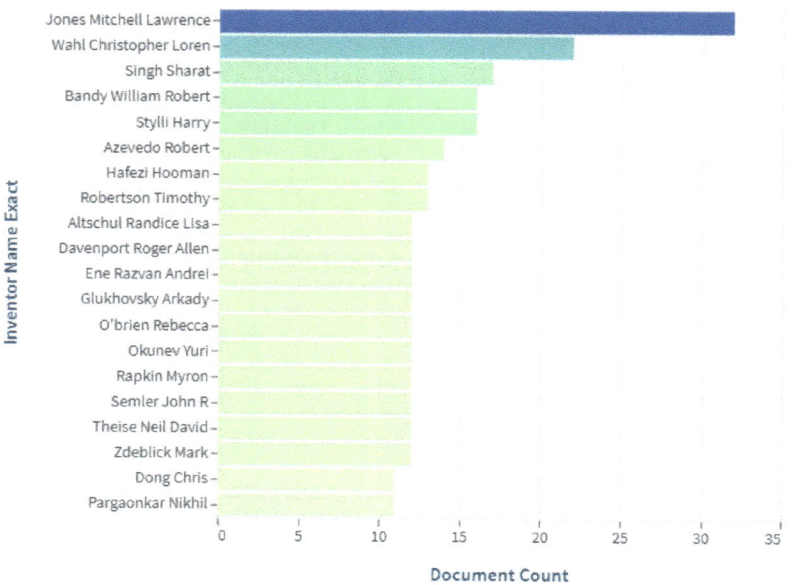

Figure 4. Top inventors of patents in the field of digital pills with ingestible sensor (https://www.lens.org, accessed on 30 July 2022).

Abilify MyCite is an atypical antipsychotic equipped with an ingestible sensor for the treatment of adults with schizophrenia, the acute treatment of adults with manic and mixed episodes associated with bipolar I disorder, and for use as an adjunctive treatment for depression in adults. A serious problem associated with psychotropic drug treatment is adherence to the treatment plan. The side effects of antipsychotics are often debilitating, including weight gain, sexual dysfunction, nausea, and vomiting, and may cause people to change their own doses or stop taking the medication.

Aripiprazole, the primary chemical component of Abilify, was discovered by Otsuka Pharmaceutical in 1988, received FDA approval as an antipsychotic in 2002, and has been accessible as a generic drug since 2015.

The Abilify My-Cite (aripiprazole tablets with sensor), a drug–device combination product of aripiprazole tablets for oral administration integrated with an Ingestible Event Marker sensor, received the FDA's first approval of a digital medicine system in 2017.

The four major components of Abilify MyCite interact using Bluetooth technology: the medication, which contains the active ingredient aripiprazole; a sensor that transmits a signal to a patch worn on the "lower edge of the rib cage"; a smartphone app; and an online portal. The 1-mm-sized sensor is built into the tablet. It is made of cuprous chloride (copper), magnesium, and silicon and releases a signal to the patch when it encounters stomach acid. When it comes in contact with the stomach acid, the magnesium and cuprous chloride within the sensor react to activate and power the device, and communicate a signal to the patch that is tracking ingestion. This information is then transmitted to the smartphone app [9].

The developed digital pills, such as Abilify MyCite, allow for the clinical monitoring of the treatment of patients with depression.

In order to improve the scientific and practical approaches to the management of scientific research in the process of digital pills with an ingestible sensor, an analysis was carried out of Proteus Digital Health and Otsuka Pharmaceutical's patent strategy for the digital pill, Abilify MyCite (Table 1).

Table 1. Analysis of Proteus Digital Health and Otsuka Pharmaceutical patent strategies for the digital pill Abilify MyCite.

US Patent No.	Patent Expiration	The Title of the Invention, the Owners
7053092	28/01/2022	5HT1a Receptor subtype agonist [10] Otsuka Pharmaceutical Co., Ltd. (Tokyo, Japan)
7978064	14/09/2026	Communication system with partial power source [11] Proteus Biomedical, Inc. (Redwood City, CA, USA)
8017615	16/06/2024	Low hygroscopic aripiprazole drug substance and processes for the preparation thereof [12] Otsuka Pharmaceutical Co., Ltd. (Tokyo, Japan)
8114021	21/06/2030	Body-associated receiver and method [13] Proteus Biomedical, Inc. (Redwood City, CA, USA)
8258962	25/11/2030	Multi-mode communication ingestible event markers and systems, and methods of using the same [14] Proteus Biomedical, Inc. (Redwood City, CA, USA)
8545402	27/04/2030	Highly reliable ingestible event markers and methods for using the same [15] Proteus Digital Health, Inc. (Redwood City, CA, USA)
8547248	18/12/2030	Implantable zero-wire communications system [16] Proteus Digital Health, Inc. (Redwood City, CA, USA)
8580796	25/09/2022	Low hygroscopic aripiprazole drug substance and processes for the preparation thereof [17] Otsuka Pharmaceutical Co., Ltd. (Tokyo, Japan)
8642760	25/09/2022	Low hygroscopic aripiprazole drug substance and processes for the preparation thereof [18] Otsuka Pharmaceutical Co., Ltd. (Tokyo, Japan)
8674825	09/04/2029	Pharma-informatics system [19] Proteus Digital Health, Inc. (Redwood City, CA, USA)
8718193	05/12/2029	Active signal processing personal health signal receivers [20] Proteus Digital Health, Inc. (Redwood City, CA, USA)
8759350	02/03/2027	Carbostyril derivatives and serotonin reuptake inhibitors for treatment of mood disorders [21] Otsuka Pharmaceutical Co., Ltd. (Tokyo, Japan)
8847766	29/03/2030	Pharma-informatics system [22] Proteus Digital Health, Inc. (Redwood City, CA, USA)
8945005	19/08/2029	Controlled activation ingestible identifier [23] Proteus Digital Health, Inc. (Redwood City, CA, USA)
8956288	06/07/2029	In-body power source having high surface area electrode [24] Proteus Digital Health, Inc. (Redwood City, CA, USA)
8961412	17/11/2030	In-body device with virtual dipole signal amplification [25] Proteus Digital Health, Inc. (Redwood City, CA, USA)
9060708	05/03/2029	Multi-mode communication ingestible event markers and systems, and methods of using the same [26] Proteus Digital Health, Inc. (Redwood City, CA, USA)
9089567	28/01/2022	Method of treating cognitive impairments and schizophrenias [27] Otsuka Pharmaceutical Co., Ltd. (Tokyo, Japan)
9119554	16/12/2028	Pharma-informatics system [28] Proteus Digital Health, Inc. (Redwood City, CA, USA)
9125939	28/07/2026	Carbostyril derivatives and mood stabilizers for treating mood disorders [29] Otsuka Pharmaceutical Co., Ltd. (Tokyo, Japan)
9149577	15/12/2029	Body-associated receiver and method [30] Proteus Digital Health, Inc. (Redwood City, CA, USA)

Table 1. *Cont.*

US Patent No.	Patent Expiration	The Title of the Invention, the Owners
9258035	05/03/2029	Multi-mode communication ingestible event markers and systems, and methods of using the same [31] Proteus Digital Health, Inc. (Redwood City, CA, USA)
9268909	15/10/2033	Apparatus, system, and method to adaptively optimize power dissipation and broadcast power in a power source for a communication device [32] Proteus Digital Health, Inc. (Redwood City, CA, USA)
9320455	15/12//2031	Highly reliable ingestible event markers and methods for using the same [33] Proteus Digital Health, Inc. (Redwood City, CA, USA)
9359302	25/09/2022	Low hygroscopic aripiprazole drug substance and processes for the preparation thereof [34] Otsuka Pharmaceutical Co., Ltd. (Tokyo, Japan)
9387182	25/12/2023	Carbostyril derivatives and serotonin reuptake inhibitors for treatment of mood disorders [35] Otsuka Pharmaceutical Co., Ltd. (Tokyo, Japan)
9433371	15/09/2029	In-body device with virtual dipole signal amplification [36] Proteus Digital Health, Inc. (Redwood City, CA, USA)
9444503	19/11/2027	Active signal processing personal health signal receivers [37] Proteus Digital Health, Inc. (Redwood City, CA, USA)
9941931	04/11/2030	System for supply chain management [38] Proteus Digital Health, Inc. (Redwood City, CA, USA)
10441194	26/07/2029	Ingestible event marker systems [39] Proteus Digital Health, Inc. (Redwood City, CA, USA)
10517507	13/06/2032	Communication system with enhanced partial power source and method of manufacturing same [40] Proteus Digital Health, Inc. (Redwood City, CA, USA)
11229378	11/07/2031	Communication system with enhanced partial power source and method of manufacturing same [41] Otsuka Pharmaceutical Co., Ltd. (Tokyo, Japan)

The performed analysis revealed that Abilify MyCite is protected by 32 US patents. This digital pill with an ingestible sensor has six hundred and seventy-one patent family members in forty-one countries.

As a result of the patent research, the patenting of a pharmacologically active ingredient aripiprazole and the technologies for its production, methods of treatment, as well as pharma-informatics systems and ingestible event marker systems, was established.

The collected data of the present review indicate the prospects and demand for digital pills with ingestible sensors in the global pharmaceutical market.

Abilify MyCite is under patent protection until 2030–2033. Licensing, which provides information about the process, is one of the ways to scale and accelerate the global long-term production of this digital drug. It is extremely important that the patent holders have the ability to control the effectiveness and quality of digital pills with ingestible sensors.

Proteus Digital Health is a company creating innovative digital health products and once had a huge valuation of USD1.5 billion. However, the company was unable to complete a USD100 million investment round in 2019. In the bankruptcy proceedings in 2020, a US affiliate of Otsuka purchased the technological assets of Proteus for USD15 million [42].

On the one hand, the rational management of intellectual human capital is extremely important in the development of digital pills. It is noted that the development of the digital pills with ingestible sensors, the Abilify MyCite technology, was expensive, and it was necessary to retain the best specialists. On the other hand, an assessment of medical technology is also very important. The average monthly cost of a generic version of Abilify is USD500 to USD800, according to GoodRx. The original digital pills with ingestible sensors, such as Abilify MyCite, cost more than USD1600.

In order to reduce the unpredictable rising costs of digital pills, it is imperative to perform comparative studies of the clinical effectiveness when discussing new treatment approaches, and to identify clear advantages over the medicines that are already used in clinical practice.

According to the ClinicalTrials.gov website, several clinical trials have been completed using the technology of digital pills with ingestible sensors. A number of digital pill clinical trials are ongoing.

The analysis of the patent landscape made it possible to identify the main therapeutic areas in which digital pills with ingestible sensors have proved themselves to be applicable. The following sections summarize the patented digital pills with ingestible sensors in the treatment of various pathological conditions.

Diseases of the nervous system.

Adherence is especially difficult in patients with serious mental illnesses, such as schizophrenia, schizophrenia-like disorders, and bipolar I disorder, with estimates of nonadherence as high as 50%. Adequate medication is essential to reduce the risk of major adverse outcomes in this population, such as psychosis, symptom recurrence, poor social functioning, hospitalizations, and suicide attempts [43].

As already mentioned above, a striking example of an active innovative strategy for creating digital pills with ingestible sensors is the tactics of Proteus Digital Health, Inc. (Redwood City, CA, USA). The inventions by this company are widely used in neurology and psychiatry. The company was formerly known as Proteus Biomedical, Inc. and changed its name to Proteus Digital Health, Inc. in July 2012.

The system, with a conductive element, an electronic component, and a partial power supply in the form of different materials, is described in patent US7978064 by Proteus Biomedical, Inc. The system is turned on when it comes into contact with a conducting liquid, since this completes the power supply and creates a voltage potential. To create a distinctive current signature, the electrical component regulates the conductance between the different materials. The system can be employed in a wide range of applications, such as ingestible event markers, ingestible identifiers, and pharmaceutical compositions with pharma-informatics capabilities.

The applicants of patent US8114021 Proteus Biomedical, Inc. disclosed a body-associated receiver, which may be external or implantable. Furthermore, the systems and procedures for using a receiver to coordinate with the dosage distribution systems are described.

The inventors of patent US8258962 (Proteus Biomedical, Inc., Redwood City, CA, USA) reported multi-mode communication ingestible event markers and systems, and the methods of using the same. The ingestible event marker consists of an integrated circuit component and upper and lower electrodes and is configured so that when it comes into contact with the stomach fluid, the current flows through the integrated circuit and causes one or more functional blocks in the circuit to emit a detectable signal. The upper and lower electrodes are made of different materials.

The pharma-informatics system is demonstrated in patent US8674825 (Proteus Digital Health, Inc., Redwood City, CA, USA). The automatic detection and identification of the pharmacological compounds actually delivered into the body is a significant new therapeutic tool provided to the clinicians by the present invention. This novel information system and device have numerous applications. Medication delivery, batch, and dose correlation to a physiological response can be achieved when employed in conjunction with other medical sensing equipment. In this way, the clinician may then create the best pharmacotherapeutic regimens. In the cases of accidental and other overdoses, the healthcare professional will be able to establish how far the intake has progressed and how many tablets are involved.

The development of a better pharma-informatics system (patent US 8945005, Proteus Digital Health, Inc., Redwood City, CA, USA) with a highly regulated identifier activation, where the signal produced by the identifier would be independent of the specific environment, such as stomach contents, the target site where activation is sought, represents another area of interest.

The effectiveness and safety of the above inventions of Proteus Digital Health were studied in clinical trials: NCT01804257 in patients (n = 28) with bipolar disorder or schizophrenia [44]; NCT03568500 in patients (n = 44) with schizophrenia, schizoaffective disorder, or first episode psychosis [45]; and NCT02091882 in patients with serious mental illness (n = 30) [46].

The clinical trials of Proteus Digital Health's digital pills with ingestible sensors confirmed their high therapeutic efficacy, favorable safety profile, and ability to significantly improve patients' quality of life. However, further post-marketing clinical trials are needed, including more patients with a high level of evidence.

HIV/AIDS.

HIV is one of the major global public health problems. Increasing access to effective HIV prevention and treatment allows patients to improve their health [47].

Proteus Digital Health inventions are widely used to monitor adherence in HIV-infected patients.

The digital health feedback system of Proteus (patents US7978064, US8114021, US8258962, US8545402, US8674825, US8718193, US8847766, etc.) was investigated in the NCT02797262 clinical trial for monitoring and increasing adherence to antiretroviral therapy in HIV-infected patients (n = 130), 18 years or older with sub-optimal adherence [48].

Moreover, the Proteus digital health feedback system is planned to be evaluated in the following clinical trials: in NCT02891720 to confirm ingestion of oral FTC/TDF as pre-exposure prophylaxis and to monitor adherence in HIV-negative YMSM (n = 100) [49]; in NCT04418037 in hospitalized individuals (n = 30) living with HIV to support ARV adherence [50]; and in NCT03693040 to collect information about patients (n = 100) taking their oral antiretroviral of TDF/FTC (Truvada) for HIV prevention [51].

The company etectRx (Gainesville, FL, USA) created an ingestible event marker (the ID-Cap^{TM} System), the technology of which is disclosed in the patent US9743880 B1 [52]. An electronic tag with an antenna and a receiver/transmitter placed on a pill capsule is part of a system and method for tracking a patient's compliance with a medication regimen. A reader placed outside the body can detect the tag's presence and location. The company will employ this technology in the NCT04065347 clinical trial to evaluate the relationship between adherence to antiretroviral therapy and HIV drug concentrations in people (n = 212) living with HIV (PLWH) who are taking tenofovir alafenamide [53].

The ID-Cap^{TM} System (made by etectRx, Gainesville, FL, USA) with Emtricitabine/Tenofovir (TDF/FTC) was investigated in an NCT03842436 clinical trial among MSM (n = 15) with substance use, to monitor PrEP adherence [54].

Since patient adherence to a medication therapy protocol is essential to preventor avoid costly consequences for the patient or the community, compliance monitoring using digital pills also offers important benefits in the prevention and treatment of HIV.

Pain control.

Another medical area with a wide use of digital pills with ingestible sensors is pain relief for various pathological conditions. Pain is a cause of passivity and depression. The somatic consequences of both acute and chronic pain are numerous, and sometimes catastrophic. Fever, while also being a protective, biologically appropriate reaction of the body, can at the same time cause a number of negative consequences [55].

The digital pills allow doctors to confirm that a patient actually took the painkillers within the predetermined time frame that they were scheduled to be delivered to them. This is a crucial tool for preventing the unintentional sale of medications that have not yet been consumed.

Tremeau Pharmaceuticals, Inc. (Concord, MA, USA) specializes in offering non-opioid pain relievers to well-defined patient populations with high unmet needs. The company has created digital pain management pills to treat pain more effectively and with fewer adverse effects.

The patent application US2021244672 A1 by Tremeau Pharmaceuticals Inc. (Concord, MA, USA) relates to digital pills in the discussed context [56]. An ingestible product, configured to be swallowed by a patient, comprises: a drug portion that requires a risk evaluation and mitigation strategy plan; and a wireless sensor portion configured to transmit sensor data concerning the drug portion to a remote device. The ingestible product is chosen from a group consisting of: a cyclooxygenase-2 Selective NSAIDs; and a D2 receptor antagonist.

Opioid analgesics are a critical treatment for those patients with advanced-stage pain from cancer. Cancer patients must have pain control as a mandatory and integral element of their treatment. Along with this, there are risks of long-term side effects, including possible abuse and addiction, which is a concern with the long-term use of opioid analgesics in patients who have had cancer.

The Proteus FDA-approved ingestible sensor (patent numbers US7978064, US8114021, US8545402, US8674825, US87181923, US8847766, etc.) was examined in the NCT04194528 clinical study on cancer patients ($n = 2$) with metastatic disease who were experiencing uncontrollable pain. Due to COVID-19's restriction on site enrollment and the extremely high difficulty in acquiring sites to participate in the study, only two participants were acquired. When the provider of the DMP and the related software filed for bankruptcy and was acquired by a business that had no interest in completing the trial, the study was terminated. Due to a lack of patient data, the investigators did not examine any of the objectives besides the telemedicine feasibility [57].

Celero Systems (Lincoln, MA, USA) is a company that developed an ingestible system to detect and reverse opioid overdose. Celero Systems, inventors of CA3149412 A1, disclosed an opioid overdose rescue device that includes an ingestible capsule [58]. A non-refillable medication dispenser containing an opioid antidote, and at least one sensor that is set up to detect at least one physiological parameter suggestive of an opioid overdose are contained within the ingestible capsule. The ingestible capsule also has a controller that is operationally connected to the medication dispenser and a minimum of one sensor. If one physiological parameter is found to be outside a threshold value or range, this indicates an opioid overdose was detected. The ingested device can release a rescue drug via a drug dispenser and send out alerts to the patient and/or a caregiver upon recognizing the physiological signs of an opioid overdose.

As a result, there are numerous significant therapeutic uses for the capacity to record with digital pills the consumption of a medicine or other actual exposure of the body to a medicine, including pain treatment. The patients are reassured that they are correctly taking their prescribed medicines, thanks to this monitoring capacity. The possibility of over-prescription of drugs is avoided by this information.

Cardiovascular diseases.

Digital pills in cardiology also provide the doctor with a precise dose–response curve that shows the patient's response to a medicine and the time at which the pill was administered. These data can be used in a variety of ways. Thus, the doctor can identify, for example, which people do not respond to the medicine in the tablet. Such patients might be excluded from a study to gauge the therapeutic effectiveness of a specific medicine. This ensures that the trial will only include the participants who have a favorable response to the medicine in question. This development will improve pharmaceuticals' efficacy and encourage patients to use less ineffective treatments. It might also be used in clinical trials to track the individuals who took their prescription and those who did not.

Arterial hypertension remains one of the most common diseases in the developed world. Arterial hypertension triggers a chain of functional and structural changes in vital organs (first of all, in the heart, kidneys, and cerebral vessels), eventually leading to end-stage disease and the death of the patient [59].

The researchers managed persistent hypertension while receiving chronic antihypertensive therapy using the Proteus digital health feedback system (patents US7978064, US8114021, US8258962, US8545402, US8718193, US8847766, etc.) in the NCT02553512 clinical trial (n = 151) [60]. The system kept track of when each tablet was taken, how many steps were taken each day, how long patients slept and how often they were up, as well as the circadian rhythm for activity and relaxation.

The invention of WO2018200691 A2 relates to lisinopril compositions with an ingestible event marker (Proteus Digital Health, Inc., Redwood City, CA, USA) [61]. The current disclosure offers a special material composition that combines electronic circuitry with battery-forming materials and particular lisinopril formulations to verify the delivery of the particular lisinopril formulations. The specific lisinopril formulations are administered orally, and the current novel composition of the matter overcomes the unpredictable nature of mixing different metals and salts with them, to create an electronic delivery system that produces its own electrical power from a partial energy source composed of different materials when exposed to a patient's bodily fluids.

Thus, digital pills make it possible for doctors to titrate to the most effective dosages of cardiac medicines by reducing the side effects, such as fatigue of the heart muscle and rebound effects, among others, and changing the dosage and time for each individual patient.

Diabetes.

Diabetes mellitus is a severe medical and societal issue worldwide. Over the past ten years, the number of diabetes mellitus patients has more than doubled, surpassing 463 million by the end of 2019. The International Diabetic Federation predicts that by 2030, 578 million people will have diabetes, and by 2045, 700 million people will be affected by this disease [62]. Digital technologies and sensors are widely used in the field of diabetes care.

The global goal of treating patients with type 2 diabetes is to reduce the cardiovascular risks. In the NCT02827630 clinical trial, scientists evaluated the efficacy of Proteus Ingestible Sensor (patents US7978064, US8114021, US8258962, US8545402, US8674825, US8718193, US8847766, etc.) to lower blood pressure and glycated hemoglobin in patients (n = 118) with uncontrolled hypertension and type 2 diabetes [63].

While the discovery of novel pharmaceuticals to treat a range of disorders has increased in recent years, many of them have restricted use because they cannot be administered orally. Numerous factors contribute to this, including poor oral toleration, which can lead to issues such as gastric irritation and bleeding; the breakdown/degradation of medicine components in the stomach; and poor, sluggish, or irregular drug absorption. Conventional alternative techniques, such as intravenous and intramuscular injection, have a number of drawbacks, such as the discomfort and risk of infection from a needle stick, the requirement and risks of maintaining an IV line in a patient for a prolonged period of time, and the need to use sterile techniques. Despite the use of a variety of drug delivery techniques, including implanted drug delivery pumps, these techniques nevertheless share many of the same problems as IV delivery because they call for the semi-permanent implantation of a device. In order to treat diabetes and other conditions that influence blood glucose homeostasis, it is necessary to develop new techniques for giving drugs and other therapeutic agents, particularly for the improved delivery of insulin and other therapeutic agents.

The inventors of patent CA 2840617 C (Rani Therapeutics LLC, San Jose, CA, USA) disclosed a therapeutic preparation comprising insulin for delivery into the lumen of the intestinal tract, using a swallowable drug delivery device. In certain implementations, the user may externally trigger the actuating mechanism to administer a medicine via RF, magnetic, or other wireless signaling means, known as an alternative to or supplement to the internally initiated drug administration [64]. Moreover, the inventors noted that a delivery device may be used to distribute a number of medications for the treatment of multiple disorders or for the treatment of a specific condition. A combination of protease inhibitors may, for example, be used to treat HIV/AIDS.

In recent years, new technologies for embedding under the skin or attaching to it for continuously measuring sugar levels have come to the market. They are systems that can be connected to other compatible medical devices and electronic interfaces, such as insulin pumps, automated insulin dosing systems, blood glucose meters, and other gadgets used in the management of diabetes.

The small intestine's glucose concentration can be measured using an ingestible device, according to the invention EP3108810 A1 (Valtronic Tech (Holding) Sa, Les Charbonnières, Switzerland) [65]. The ingestible gadget includes a retainer to keep it in place in the small intestine for a short data transmitter/receiver. The method of the invention includes the steps of activating the device, fixing the device in the small intestine via a retainer, measuring the data related to glucose concentration inside the small intestine via a glucose sensor, and transmitting the data related to the glucose concentration to a receiver located outside the small intestine, particularly for determining or predicting the glucose level in the subject's blood stream.

Thus, along with the patenting of digital pills with ingestible sensors for the treatment of diabetes, there is active patent protection of glucose sensors for indicating the blood and small intestine glucose levels of a patient with diabetes mellitus, and for smart drug delivery.

Gastroenterology.

Digital pills with ingestible sensors are widely used in gastroenterology. Better treatment regimens are still urgently needed to treat gastrointestinal disorders, such as inflammatory bowel disease. These regimens must be able to deliver therapeutics to specific areas of the gastrointestinal tract, while minimizing or avoiding the negative effects of oral or other systemic administration [66].

Several of Progenity, Inc.'s (San Diego, CA, USA) patents disclose novel therapeutic strategies for inflammatory gastrointestinal disorders.

The inventors of WO 2018/112255A1 (Progenity, Inc., San Diego, CA, USA) described a method of treating gastrointestinal disease with an immunosuppressant that is delivered through an ingestible device [67]. According to the method, the release of the medicine is triggered by data from a sensor or detector. The immunosuppressant is selected from Cyclosporine, Tacrolimus, and the generic equivalents thereof.

Application WO 2018/112240 A1 (Progenity, Inc., San Diego, CA, USA) described the use of a TNF inhibitor to treat a gastrointestinal disease [68]. An ingestible housing with a reservoir that stores a pharmaceutical composition containing a therapeutically effective amount of a TNF inhibitor is part of a TNF inhibitor delivery system. A detector is connected to the ingestible housing and is programmed to detect when the ingestible housing is close to a specific disease site.

Progenity, Inc. (San Diego, CA, USA) disclosed a targeted drug delivery system for the Il-6r inhibitor [69], an Il-12/Il-23 inhibitor [70], and an Il-1 inhibitor [71], employing one or more sensors connected to the ingestible housing.

When treating or reducing the symptoms of various medical illnesses, the therapeutic medications may occasionally need to be injected into specific regions of the small or large intestine. This is more effective than giving the medicine orally. The therapeutic drugs, for instance, may bypass the stomach's gastrointestinal tract entirely and be delivered directly to the small intestine. This would make it possible to deliver a higher dose at a specific location inside the small intestine.

Along this line, the Drug Delivery System (DDS), developed by the biotechnology company Progenity, Inc. (San Diego, CA, USA), is of interest for the treatment of the gastrointestinal (GI) tract-related conditions. The applicants of EP3197336 B1 (Progenity, Inc., San Diego, CA, USA) disclosed an electromechanical pill device with localization capabilities [72]. By utilizing the reflection characteristics of organ tissue and sporadic particles, the ingestible device, which contains optical illumination sources and detectors that work at a variety of different wavelengths, may distinguish the areas of the gastrointestinal tract. Based on a detected device position, the ingestible device may sample fluid or release medication. The DDS will be used to target disease in the GI tract in order to improve efficacy by raising localized medicine concentration and lowering systemic adverse effects.

The inventors (Olympus Corporation, Tokyo, Japan) of patent US 8021356 B2 reported a capsule medication administration system [73]. This capsule medication administration system consists of an external device, a capsule-type medical device, a drug retention section, a drug release section, and a communication section. The external device has an external communication section that transmits and receives signals with the capsule-type medical device.

It should be noted that the ingestible sensors also allow for the collection of images and the tracking of luminal fluid and each gut segment's contents, including electrolytes, enzymes, metabolites, hormones, and microbial populations. Due to the increasing usage of smart phones with Internet connectivity, the users and physicians can readily view and assess online the data produced by this technology.

Many ingestible capsules with sensors have been created and are set up to take pictures from inside passages and cavities within a body, such as those passageways and cavities within the GI tract. These gadgets often have an enclosed digital camera along with illumination light sources. Batteries or an external inductive power transfer may be used to power the capsule. Furthermore, the capsule might have a radio transmitter and/or memory for transferring data to an external receiver outside the body [66].

For instance, the inventors (Given Imaging Inc. (Duluth, GA, USA)and The Smart Pill Corporation (Buffalo, NY, USA)) of application US 2012/0209083 A1 explored the method of using, and determining the location of, an ingestible capsule [74]. An extracorporeal receiver can receive signals from an ingestible capsule that senses and transmits physiological parameters from patients. When in operation, the capsule and receiver carry out the process of locating the capsule in real time inside a mammal tract. This process involves supplying the capsule, which has one or more sensors, ingesting the capsule, having the capsule transmit a signal, having the capsule receive a transmitted signal, and then locating where the capsule is in the tract in real time, based on the received signal. The value of one or more sensed parameters may also be indicated by the received signal.

Hepatitis C.

Due to scientific breakthroughs in the treatment of HCV infection, it has been possible to make significant progress in the therapy of this pathology and to actually translate chronic hepatitis C into the category of diseases that are completely cured [75].

Thus, the NCT03164902 clinical trial will evaluate the ability of Proteus digital pills to promote adherence and thus achieve a cure for hepatitis C in the patients ($n = 253$) at a high risk of not adhering to their hepatitis C therapy [76].

The Proteus digital health feedback system (patents US7978064, US8114021, US8258962, US8545402, US8674825, US8718193, US8847766, etc.) is multi-fold.

An effective antiviral therapy with digital pills, leading to the eradication of HCV infection, reduces the risk of progression of the hepatic and extrahepatic manifestations of HCV infection, especially if treatment is carried out before the formation of liver cirrhosis.

Without a doubt, digital pills with ingestible sensors have the potential to provide enormous amounts of information in the field of gastroenterology, along with imaging capsules. The dosing devices for releasing medicines into the gastrointestinal tract via one or more sensors are also promising to improve the effectiveness of treatment.

Oncology.

Health care costs pose a major challenge to national economic welfare. As a result of the aging of the population, the implementation of expensive innovative medicines, methods of radiation therapy and surgery, and diagnostic tests, the cost of treating oncopathologies increases, which is not always justified.

In some cases, the effectiveness of innovative, more expensive pills may not be supported by medical evidence, resulting in increased costs without improving outcomes. In the US, the term "financial toxicity" has come into use as a means of describing the financial stress that now often accompanies cancer treatment and reduces quality of life [77].

The researchers conducting the NCT04088955 clinical trial will collect and analyze data on the use of ingestible sensors with capecitabine or supportive medications (Proteus patents US7978064, US8114021, US8258962, US8545402, US8674825, US8718193, US8847766, etc.) and a digital feedback system on medication adherence and data-driven optimization of therapy for cancer patients ($n = 500$) [78].

Thus, further research is needed that aims to confirm that digital pills are not only clinically effective and relatively safe for the treatment of oncopathologies, but will also reveal their cost-effectiveness and possess additional benefits compared to other medicines.

Tuberculosis.

Multi-resistant tuberculosis is still a significant problem in the field of public health. Without the emergence of new pills, which in combination with other medicines could be used to create shorter, more effective, and less toxic treatment regimens, the global epidemic of multi-drug resistant tuberculosis will continue to grow [79].

The Proteus digital health feedback system (patents US7978064, US8114021, US8258962, US8545402, US8674825, US8718193, US8847766, etc.) was used in the NCT01960257 study to collect information about patients ($n = 92$) taking their tuberculosis medications [80]. The participants favored the digital health feedback system over the directly observed therapy for supporting confirmed daily adherence to tuberculosis drugs during the continuation phase of the tuberculosis treatment.

Therefore, taking digital pills can crucially contribute to avoiding the development of drug-resistant infectious disease strains, which can happen when proper dosing regimens are not adhered to. These resistant strains enhance the transmission, morbidity, and mortality, while costing significantly more to treat or eradicate, sometimes by orders of magnitude.

Transplantology.

Organ transplantation is associated with numerous concomitant conditions that affect the cardiovascular and other body systems. Careful follow-up of patients throughout transplantation is necessary. These patients need long-term rehabilitation with the participation of many specialists. Nonadherence to immunosuppressants leads to worse outcomes [81,82].

The investigations focused on the efficiency of the Ingestible Event Marker (Proteus patents US7978064, US8114021, US8258962, US8545402, US8674825, US8718193, US8847766, etc.) combined with Myfortic (360 mg) in adult kidney transplant patients ($n = 30$) are conducted within the NCT01320358 study [83].

The Ingestible Event Marker, according to the participating scientists, is a promising new device that offers incredibly accurate assessments of drug intake and timing in the clinical care of kidney transplant patients.

The above-described digital pill patents are presented for the purposes of illustration and not of limitation. There are a number of other inventions in the field of digital pills. In the last two decades, the scientists, in collaboration with industrial companies, have been activated in the search for effective and safe digital pills with ingestible sensors.

An analysis of the patent landscape showed that mobile clinical monitoring is widely used for treatment in the fields of mental health, HIV/AIDS, pain control, cardiovascular diseases, diabetes, oncology, tuberculosis, and transplantology. The devices for smart drug delivery and endoscopy diagnostics are patented in the field of gastroenterology to a greater degree. A detailed digital pill technology is presented in the descriptions of the patents. The description of the patent discloses the essence of the invention clearly and completely, so that it can be carried out by a person skilled in the art. However, the patent owner may also protect the technology as a trade secret.

It should be noted that digital pills are a new development both for pharmacy and medicine, which will be widely used in the future due to their advantages and in line with the global general digitalization trends. The key to their successful implementation is to ensure efficiency and safety, quality, and affordability, as well as compliance with ethical aspects in medical practice. Ensuring the continuous monitoring of the safety use of digital pills and identifying the potential side effects will help reduce and manage the risks associated with their use.

There is no doubt that the implementation of digital pills with ingestible sensors into the healthcare system is promising. Further large-scale comparative randomized clinical trials evaluating the efficacy and safety of digital and non-digital forms and meta-analysis data are needed. Nevertheless, it can be confidently predicted that soon all of these developments will come to fruition; progress cannot be stopped.

3. Materials and Methods

By the end of July 2022, search studies were conducted using Internet databases, such as the European Patent Office, the United States Patent Office, the United States Food and Drug Administration (FDA, Orange Book), the Lens database, Google Scholar, and ClinicalTrials.gov (accessed on 30 July 2022).

The following keywords were used in the patent search: ingestible sensor; digital pill; smart pill; and their combinations.

The International Patent Classification and Cooperative Patent Classification were utilized in conjunction with the title, abstract, and claims fields as search terms. When looking for information about patents, keywords are helpful. However, a lot of information is linked to many keywords and their synonyms, which makes analysis time-consuming and challenging. The use of language-neutral patent classification enables focusing the search, making it clearer and faster. Thus, the combined method using the keywords and codes of the International Patent Classification and the Cooperative Patent Classification improves the results of studies examining the patent landscape.

Digital products, such as subcutaneous and implantable sensors for continuous glucose monitoring systems, were considered to be outside the scope of this work and are not included in this study.

The analysis and systematization of the data made it possible to create the following search query: ((Q1 OR Q2 OR Q3) AND Q4). Q1, Q2, and Q3 are combinations of the keywords, and Q4 uses the International Patent Classification and Cooperative Patent Classification codes that match the digital pills.

The patent search results using the keywords: ingestible sensor; digital pill; smart pill; and their combinations, revealed 3101 patents and 1655 simple families.

Then, the 3101 patents were analyzed using the International Patent Classification and Cooperative Patent Classification codes (query Q4) to further filter and obtain relevant information. Their codes used in the search are shown in Table 2.

Table 2. The International Patent Classification and Cooperative Patent Classification codes are used in the patent search.

Code	Meaning
	International Patent Classification
A61B5/00	Measuring for diagnostic purposes radiation diagnosis by ultrasonic, sonic, or infrasonic waves. Identification of persons
A61B5/07	Endoradiosondes
A61B5/145	Measuring characteristics of blood in vivo, e.g., gas concentration, pH-value measuring of blood pressure or blood flow non-radiation detecting or locating of foreign bodies in blood
A61K9/00	Medicinal preparations characterized by special physical form
	Cooperative Patent Classification
A61B5/073	Intestinal transmitters

As result, the study altogether ultimately covered 291 patents, including 132 families. The yearly trends of the patent publications, the top 20 owners, the countries participating in innovations, and the key inventors were all studied. The most significant therapeutic application of digital tablets in medicine was identified.

Retrospective, logical, and graphic research methods and content analysis were used.

4. Conclusions

The patent landscape analysis shows an increase in the number of patents related to digital pills with ingestible sensors, which indicates the rapid progress and highly dynamic field of digital medicine technologies. The leaders in the number of patents issued are the United States, the European Patent Office, Canada, Australia, and China, which account for 72% of the total number of patents worldwide. The top 20 leading applicants were identified, whose inventions are related to the developments in the fields of mobile clinical monitoring, smart drug delivery, and endoscopy diagnostics.

The analysis revealed powerful patent protection for digital pills with an ingestible sensor, with often protection afforded by several patents in some countries, e.g., Abilify MyCite is protected by 32 US patents. This digital pill has six hundred and seventy-one patent family members in forty-one countries.

The following main areas of patenting digital pills with ingestible sensors were identified: treatment in the areas of mental health; HIV/AIDS; pain control; cardiovascular diseases; diabetes; gastroenterology (including hepatitis C); oncology; tuberculosis; and transplantology. The problems associated with the rapid implementation into medical practice are technical limitations, medical ethics, the legal framework, and thorough clinical trials of efficacy and safety.

Thus, the development of further scientific and practical approaches to the implementation of effective and safe digital pills will improve treatment outcomes, increase compliance, reduce hospital stays, provide mobile clinical monitoring, have a positive impact on treatment costs, and most likely become mainstream for most of the companies in the healthcare sector.

Author Contributions: Conceptualization, O.L. and A.G.A.; methodology, O.L. and A.G.A.; formal analysis, O.L.; writing—original draft preparation, O.L.; writing—review and editing, O.L., E.K., N.T.T., O.K., M.K.-P., H.W. and A.G.A. All authors have read and agreed to the published version of the manuscript.

Funding: This study was supported by a grant from the Austrian Academy of Sciences through the academic mobility program "Joint Excellence in Science and Humanities" (JESH) for applications from Ukrainian researchers (O.L. is a fellowship recipient).

Institutional Review Board Statement: Not applicable.

Informed Consent Statement: Not applicable.

Data Availability Statement: Data is contained within the article. Further queries addressed to the corresponding authors are welcome.

Acknowledgments: The Ukrainian researcher acknowledge support from the Austrian Academy of Sciences and the Ludwig Boltzmann Institute for Digital Health and Patient Safety.

Conflicts of Interest: The authors declare no conflict of interest.

References

1. *Global Strategy on Digital Health 2020–2025*; World Health Organization: Geneva, Switzerland, 2021.
2. Knights, J.; Heidary, Z.; Cochran, J.M. Detection of Behavioral Anomalies in Medication Adherence Patterns Among Patients With Serious Mental Illness Engaged With a Digital Medicine System. *JMIR Ment. Health* **2020**, *7*, e21378. [CrossRef]
3. Chai, P.R.; Carreiro, S.; Innes, B.J.; Rosen, R.K.; O'Cleirigh, C.; Mayer, K.H.; Boyer, E.W. Digital Pills to Measure Opioid Ingestion Patterns in Emergency Department Patients With Acute Fracture Pain: A Pilot Study. *J. Med. Internet Res.* **2017**, *19*, e19. [CrossRef] [PubMed]
4. Chai, P.R.; Vaz, C.; Goodman, G.R.; Albrechta, H.; Huang, H.; Rosen, R.K.; Boyer, E.W.; Mayer, K.H.; O'Cleirigh, C. Ingestible electronic sensors to measure instantaneous medication adherence: A narrative review. *Digit. Health* **2022**, *8*, 205520762210831. [CrossRef] [PubMed]
5. Cutler, R.L.; Fernandez-Llimos, F.; Frommer, M.; Benrimoj, C.; Garcia-Cardenas, V. Economic impact of medication non-adherence by disease groups: A systematic review. *BMJ Open* **2018**, *8*, e016982. [CrossRef] [PubMed]
6. Martani, A.; Geneviève, L.D.; Poppe, C.; Casonato, C.; Wangmo, T. Digital pills: A scoping review of the empirical literature and analysis of the ethical aspects. *BMC Med. Ethics* **2020**, *21*, 3. [CrossRef] [PubMed]

7. Alipour, A.; Gabrielson, S.; Patel, P.B. Ingestible Sensors and Medication Adherence: Focus on Use in Serious Mental Illness. *Pharmacy* **2020**, *8*, 103. [CrossRef] [PubMed]
8. *Digital Health Trends 2021. Innovation, Evidence, Regulation, and Adoption*; IQVIA Institute for Human Data Science: Durham, NC, USA, 2021.
9. Flore, J. Ingestible sensors, data, and pharmaceuticals: Subjectivity in the era of digital mental health. *New Media Soc.* **2021**, *23*, 2034–2051. [CrossRef]
10. Shaun, J.; Tetsuro, K.; Katsura, T.; Tsuyoshi, H.; Yasufumi, U. 5-HT1a Receptor Subtype Agonist. U.S. Patent 7,053,092 B2, 30 May 2006.
11. Mark, Z.; Timothy, R.; Aleksandr, P.; Hooman, H. Communication System with Partial Power Source. U.S. Patent 7,978,064 B2, 12 July 2011.
12. Takuji, B.; Satoshi, A.; Junichi, K.; Makoto, I.; Youichi, T.; Tsuyoshi, Y.; Kiyoshi, F.; Yoshihiro, N.; Noriyuki, K.; Tsutomu, F.; et al. Low Hygroscopic Aripiprazole Drug Substance and Processes for the Preparation Thereof. U.S. Patent 8,017,615 B2, 13 September 2011.
13. Timothy, R.; Fataneh, O.; Yashar, B.; Lawrence, A.; Kenneth, R.; James, H.; Robert, L.; George, S.; Andrew, T.; Mark, Z.; et al. Body-Associated Receiver and Method. U.S. Patent 8,114,021 B2, 14 February 2012.
14. Robertson, T.; Zdeblick, M.J. Multi-Mode Communication Ingestible Event Markers and Systems, and Methods of Using the Same. U.S. Patent 8,258,962 B2, 4 September 2012.
15. Hooman, H.; Kityee, A.-Y.; Robert, D.; Maria, H.; Timothy, R.; Benedict, C. Highly Reliable Ingestible Event Markers and Methods for Using the Same. U.S. Patent 8,545,402 B2, 1 October 2013.
16. Mark, Z.; Timothy, R. Implantable Zero-Wire Communications System. U.S. Patent 8,547,248 B2, 1 October 2013.
17. Takuji, B.; Satoshi, A.; Junichi, K.; Makoto, I.; Youichi, T.; Tsuyoshi, Y.; Kiyoshi, F.; Yoshihiro, N.; Noriyuki, K.; Tsutomu, F.; et al. Low Hygroscopic Aripiprazole Drug Substance and Processes for the Preparation Thereof. U.S. Patent 8,580,796 B2, 12 November 2013.
18. Takuji, B.; Satoshi, A.; Junichi, K.; Makoto, I.; Youichi, T.; Tsuyoshi, Y.; Kiyoshi, F.; Yoshihiro, N.; Noriyuki, K.; Tsutomu, F.; et al. Low Hygroscopic Aripiprazole Drug Substance and Processes for the Preparation Thereof. U.S. Patent 8,642,760 B2, 4 February 2014.
19. Mark, Z.; Andrew, T.; Aleksandr, P.; Timothy, R. Pharma-Informatics System. U.S. Patent 8,674,825 B2, 4 February 2014.
20. Lawrence, A.; Kityee, A.-Y.; Kenneth, C.; Timothy, R. Active Signal Processing Personal Health Signal Receivers. U.S. Patent 8,718,193 B2, 6 May 2014.
21. Tetsuro, K.; Taro, I.; Tsuyoshi, H. Carbostyril Derivatives and Serotonin Reuptake Inhibitors for Treatment of Mood Disorders. U.S. Patent 8,759,350 B2, 24 June 2014.
22. Mark, Z.; Andrew, T.; Aleksandr, P.; Timothy, R.; Hooman, H. Pharma-Informatics System. U.S. Patent 8,847,766 B2, 30 September 2014.
23. Hooman, H.; Timothy, R.; Olivier, C.; Mark, Z. Controlled Activation Ingestible Identifier. U.S. Patent 8,945,005 B2, 3 February 2015.
24. Hooman, H.; Timothy, R.; Eric, S.; Brad, C. In-Body Power Source Having High Surface Area Electrode. U.S. Patent 8,956,288 B2, 17 February 2015.
25. Hooman, H.; James, C.B.; Timothy, R.; Maria, C.H. In-Body Device with Virtual Dipole Signal Amplification. U.S. Patent 8,961,412 B2, 24 February 2015.
26. Timothy, R.; Mark, Z. Multi-Mode Communication Ingestible Event Markers and Systems, and Methods of Using the Same. U.S. Patent 9,060,708 B2, 23 June 2015.
27. Shaun, J.; Tetsuro, K.; Katsura, T.; Tsuyoshi, H.; Yasufumi, U. Method of Treating Cognitive Impairments and Schizophrenias. U.S. Patent 9,089,567 B2, 28 July 2015.
28. Mark, Z.; Aleksandr, P.; Timothy, R.; Hooman, H. Pharma-Informatics System. U.S. Patent 9,119,554 B2, 1 September 2015.
29. Tetsuro, K.; Taro, I.; Tsuyoshi, H. Carbostyril Derivatives and Mood Stabilizers for Treating Mood Disorders. U.S. Patent 9,125,939 B2, 8 September 2015.
30. Timothy, R.; Fataneh, O.; Yashar, B.; Lawrence, A.; Kenneth, R.; James, H.; Robert, L.; George, S.; Andrew, T.; Mark, Z.; et al. Body-Associated Receiver and Method. U.S. Patent 9,149,577 B2, 6 October 2015.
31. Timothy, R.; Mark, Z. Multi-Mode Communication Ingestible Event Markers and Systems, and Methods of Using the Same. U.S. Patent 9,258,035 B2, 9 February 2016.
32. Nilay, J.; Douglas, W.; Jonathan, W.; Jeffrey, B.; Haifeng, L. Apparatus, System, and Method to Adaptively Optimize Power Dissipation and Broadcast Power in a Power Source for a Communication Device. U.S. Patent 9,268,909 B2, 23 February 2016.
33. Hooman, H.; Kityee, A.-Y.; Robert, D.; Casillas, H.M.; Timothy, R.; James, C.B. Highly Reliable Ingestible Event Markers and Methods for Using the Same. U.S. Patent 9,320,455 B2, 26 April 2016.
34. Takuji, B.; Satoshi, A.; Junichi, K.; Makoto, I.; Youichi, T.; Tsuyoshi, Y.; Kiyoshi, F.; Yoshihiro, N.; Noriyuki, K.; Tsutomu, F.; et al. Low Hygroscopic Aripiprazole Drug Substance and Processes for the Preparation Thereof. U.S. Patent 9,359,302 B2, 7 June 2016.
35. Tetsuro, K.; Taro, I.; Tsuyoshi, H. Carbostyril Derivatives and Serotonin Reuptake Inhibitors for Treatment of Mood disorders. U.S. Patent 9,387,182 B2, 12 July 2016.
36. Hooman, H.; Benedict, C.; Timothy, R.; Casillas, H.M. In-Body Device with Virtual Dipole Signal Amplification. U.S. Patent 9,433,371 B2, 9 September 2016.
37. Lawrence, A.; Yee, A.-Y.K.; Kenneth, C.; Timothy, R. Active Signal Processing Personal Health Signal Receivers. U.S. Patent 9,444,503 B2, 13 September 2016.
38. Mark, Z. System for Supply Chain Management. U.S. Patent 9,941,931 B2, 10 April 2018.

39. Timothy, R.; George, S.; Mark, Z.; Yashar, B.; Benedict, C.; Jeremy, F.; Hooman, H.; Tariq, H.; David, O. Ingestible Event Marker Systems. U.S. Patent 10,441,194 B2, 15 October 2019.
40. Jeremy, F.; Peter, B.; Hooman, H.; Robert, A.; Robert, D.; Iliya, P.; Benedict, C.; Eric, S. Communication System with Enhanced Partial Power Source and Method of Manufacturing Same. U.S. Patent 10,517,507 B2, 31 December 2019.
41. Jeremy, F.; Peter, B.; Hooman, H.; Robert, A.; Robert, D.; Iliya, P.; Benedict, C.; Eric, S. Communication System with Enhanced Partial Power Source and Method of Manufacturing Same. U.S. Patent 11,229,378 B2, 25 January 2022.
42. From Big Deals to Bankruptcy, a Digital Health Unicorn Falls Short. Here's What Other Startups Can Learn from Proteus. Available online: https://www.fiercehealthcare.com/tech/from-billions-to-bankruptcy-proteus-digital-health-fell-short-its-promise-here-s-what-other (accessed on 4 July 2022).
43. Velligan, D.I.; Sajatovic, M.; Hatch, A.; Kramata, P.; Docherty, J. Why do psychiatric patients stop antipsychotic medication? A systematic review of reasons for nonadherence to medication in patients with serious mental illness. *Patient Prefer. Adherence* **2017**, *11*, 449–468. [CrossRef]
44. Kane, J.M.; Perlis, R.H.; DiCarlo, L.A.; Au-Yeung, K.; Duong, J.; Petrides, G. First experience with a wireless system incorporating physiologic assessments and direct confirmation of digital tablet ingestions in ambulatory patients with schizophrenia or bipolar disorder. *J. Clin. Psychiatry* **2013**, *74*, e533–e540. [CrossRef]
45. Fowler, J.C.; Cope, N.; Knights, J.; Phiri, P.; Makin, A.; Peters-Strickland, T.; Rathod, S. Hummingbird Study: A study protocol for a multicentre exploratory trial to assess the acceptance and performance of a digital medicine system in adults with schizophrenia, schizoaffective disorder or first-episode psychosis. *BMJ Open* **2019**, *9*, e025952. [CrossRef]
46. Rohatagi, S.; Profit, D.; Hatch, A.; Zhao, C.; Docherty, J.P.; Peters-Strickland, T.S. Optimization of a Digital Medicine System in Psychiatry. *J. Clin. Psychiatry* **2016**, *77*, e1101–e1107. [CrossRef] [PubMed]
47. Delpech, V. The HIV epidemic: Global and United Kingdom trends. *Medicine* **2022**, *50*, 202–204. [CrossRef] [PubMed]
48. Measuring and Monitoring Adherence to ART with Pill Ingestible Sensor System. ClinicalTrials.gov Identifier: NCT02797262. Updated 20 December 2021. Available online: https://clinicaltrials.gov/ct2/show/results/NCT02797262?term=NCT02797262&draw=2&rank=1 (accessed on 4 July 2022).
49. Feasibility of an Ingestible Sensor System to Measure PrEP Adherence in YMSM. ClinicalTrials.gov Identifier: NCT02891720. Updated 7 September 2016. Available online: https://clinicaltrials.gov/ct2/show/NCT02891720?term=NCT02891720&draw=2&rank=1 (accessed on 4 July 2022).
50. DHFS for Medication Adherence Support During Hospital Admissions for Person Living with HIV. ClinicalTrials.gov Identifier: NCT04418037. Updated 25 August 2021. Available online: https://clinicaltrials.gov/ct2/show/NCT04418037?term=NCT04418037&draw=2&rank=1 (accessed on 4 July 2022).
51. Digital Health Feedback System (DHFS) for Longitudinal Monitoring of ARVs Used in HIV Pre-Exposure Prophylaxis (PrEP). ClinicalTrials.gov Identifier: NCT03693040. Updated 25 August 2021. Available online: https://clinicaltrials.gov/ct2/show/NCT03693040?term=NCT03693040&draw=2&rank=1 (accessed on 4 July 2022).
52. Euliano Neil, W.; Myers Brent, A.; Principe Jose, C.; Meka Venkata, V.; Flores, G. Electronic Medication Compliance Monitoring System and Associated Methods. U.S. Patent 9,743,880 B1, 29 August 2017.
53. Quantification of Tenofovir Alafenamide Adherence (QUANTI-TAF). ClinicalTrials.gov Identifier: NCT04065347. Updated 25 April 2022. Available online: https://clinicaltrials.gov/ct2/show/NCT04065347?term=NCT04065347&draw=2&rank=1 (accessed on 4 July 2022).
54. Chai, P.R.; Goodman, G.R.; Bronzi, O.; Gonzales, G.; Baez, A.; Bustamante, M.J.; Najarro, J.; Mohamed, Y.; Sullivan, M.C.; Mayer, K.H.; et al. Real-World User Experiences with a Digital Pill System to Measure PrEP Adherence: Perspectives from MSM with Substance Use. *AIDS Behav.* **2022**, *26*, 2459–2468. [CrossRef]
55. Mills, S.E.E.; Nicolson, K.P.; Smith, B.H. Chronic pain: A review of its epidemiology and associated factors in population-based studies. *Br. J. Anaesth.* **2019**, *123*, e273–e283. [CrossRef]
56. Sippy, B.C. Ingestible Product and a Method of Using the Same. U.S. Patent 20210244672 A1, 28 April 2021.
57. S1916 Digital Medicine Program for Pain Control in Cancer Patients. ClinicalTrials.gov identifier: NCT04194528. Updated 10 December 2021. Available online: https://clinicaltrials.gov/ct2/show/NCT04194528?term=NCT04194528&draw=2&rank=1 (accessed on 4 July 2022).
58. Pless Benjamin, D.; Bacher, D. Opioid Overdose Rescue Device. CA Patent 3149412 A1, 4 March 2021.
59. Brouwers, S.; Sudano, I.; Kokubo, Y.; Sulaica, E.M. Arterial hypertension. *Lancet* **2021**, *398*, 249–261. [CrossRef]
60. Godbehere, P.; Wareing, P. Hypertension assessment and management: Role for digital medicine. *J. Clin. Hypertens.* **2014**, *16*, 235. [CrossRef]
61. Kurt, S.; Nikhil, P.; Chris, D.; Ling, C.A.; Dawn, A. Lisinopril Compositions with an Ingestible Event Marker. WO Patent 2018200691 A3, 3 January 2018.
62. Saeedi, P.; Petersohn, I.; Salpea, P.; Malanda, B.; Karuranga, S.; Unwin, N.; Colagiuri, S.; Guariguata, L.; Motala, A.A.; Ogurtsova, K.; et al. Global and regional diabetes prevalence estimates for 2019 and projections for 2030 and 2045: Results from the International Diabetes Federation Diabetes Atlas, 9th edition. *Diabetes Res. Clin. Pract.* **2019**, *157*, 107843. [CrossRef]
63. Frias, J.; Virdi, N.; Raja, P.; Kim, Y.; Savage, G.; Osterberg, L. Effectiveness of Digital Medicines to Improve Clinical Outcomes in Patients with Uncontrolled Hypertension and Type 2 Diabetes: Prospective, Open-Label, Cluster-Randomized Pilot Clinical Trial. *J. Med. Internet Res.* **2017**, *19*, e246. [CrossRef]

64. Mir, I. Therapeutic Agent Preparations for Delivery into a Lumen of the Intestinal Tract Using a Swallowable Drug Delivery Device. CA Patent 2840617 C, 24 March 2020.
65. Albrecht, L.-W. Ingestible Device for Measuring Glucose Concentration. EP Patent 3108810 A1, 28 December 2016.
66. Kalantar-zadeh, K.; Ha, N.; Ou, J.Z.; Berean, K.J. Ingestible Sensors. *ACS Sens.* **2017**, *2*, 468–483. [CrossRef]
67. Lawrence, J.M.; Sharat, S.; Loren, W.C.; Harry, S. Treatment of a Disease of the Gastrointestinal Tract with an Immunosuppressant. WO Patent 2018112255 A1, 21 June 2018.
68. Lawrence, J.M.; Sharat, S.; Loren, W.C.; Harry, S. Treatment of a Disease of the Gastrointestinal Tract with a TNF Inhibitor. WO Patent 2018112240 A1, 21 June 2018.
69. Lawrence, J.M.; Sharat, S.; Loren, W.C.; Harry, S. Treatment of a Disease of the Gastrointestinal Tract with an IL-6R Inhibitor. WO Patent 2018/112237 A1, 21 June 2018.
70. Lawrence, J.M.; Sharat, S.; Loren, W.C.; Harry, S. Treatment of a Disease of the Gastrointestinal Tract with an Il-12/Il-23 Inhibitor Released Using an Ingestible Device. WO Patent 2018112232 A1, 21 June 2018.
71. Lawrence, J.M.; Sharat, S.; Loren, W.C.; Harry, S. Methods and Ingestible Devices for the Regio-Specific Release of IL-1 Inhibitors at the Site of Gastrointestinal Tract Disease. WO Patent 2018111329 A1, 21 June 2018.
72. Lawrence, J.M.; Alain, L.; Sasha, D.M.; Terry, P.M.C. Electromechanical Pill Device with Localization Capabilities. EP Patent 3197336 B1, 23 December 2020.
73. Akio, U.; Hironobu, T.; Hidetake, S.; Hironao, K. Capsule Medication Administration System, Medication Administration Method Using Capsule Medication Administration System, Control Method for Capsule Medication administration System. U.S. Patent 8,021,356 B2, 20 September 2011.
74. Semler, J.R. Method of Locating an Ingested Capsule. U.S. Patent 20120209083 A1, 16 August 2012.
75. Lynch, S.M.; Wu, G.Y. Hepatitis C Virus: A Review of Treatment Guidelines, Cost-effectiveness, and Access to Therapy. *J. Clin. Transl. Hepatol.* **2016**, *4*, 310–319. [CrossRef]
76. Digimeds to Optimize Adherence in Patients with Hepatitis C and Increased Risk for Nonadherence. ClinicalTrials.gov Identifier: NCT03164902. Updated 13 December 2018. Available online: https://www.clinicaltrials.gov/ct2/show/NCT03164902?term=NCT03164902&draw=2&rank=1 (accessed on 4 July 2022).
77. Desai, A.; Gyawali, B. Financial toxicity of cancer treatment: Moving the discussion from acknowledgement of the problem to identifying solutions. *EClinicalMedicine* **2020**, *20*, 100269. [CrossRef]
78. A Digimed Oncology PharmacoTherapy Registry (ADOPTR). ClinicalTrials.gov Identifier: NCT04088955. Updated 11 March 2020. Available online: https://www.clinicaltrials.gov/ct2/show/NCT04088955?term=NCT04088955&draw=2&rank=1 (accessed on 4 July 2022).
79. Singh Dewhare, S. Drug resistant tuberculosis: Current scenario and impending challenges. *Indian J. Tuberc.* **2022**, *69*, 227–233. [CrossRef] [PubMed]
80. Browne, S.H.; Umlauf, A.; Tucker, A.J.; Low, J.; Moser, K.; Gonzalez Garcia, J.; Peloquin, C.A.; Blaschke, T.; Vaida, F.; Benson, C.A. Wirelessly observed therapy compared to directly observed therapy to confirm and support tuberculosis treatment adherence: A randomized controlled trial. *PLoS Med.* **2019**, *16*, e1002891. [CrossRef] [PubMed]
81. Hussain, T.; Nassetta, K.; O'Dwyer, L.C.; Wilcox, J.E.; Badawy, S.M. Adherence to immunosuppression in adult heart transplant recipients: A systematic review. *Transplant. Rev.* **2021**, *35*, 100651. [CrossRef]
82. Gandolfini, I.; Palmisano, A.; Fiaccadori, E.; Cravedi, P.; Maggiore, U. Detecting, preventing and treating non-adherence to immunosuppression after kidney transplantation. *Clin. Kidney J.* **2022**, *15*, 1253–1274. [CrossRef] [PubMed]
83. Eisenberger, U.; Wüthrich, R.P.; Bock, A.; Ambühl, P.; Steiger, J.; Intondi, A.; Kuranoff, S.; Maier, T.; Green, D.; DiCarlo, L.; et al. Medication adherence assessment: High accuracy of the new Ingestible Sensor System in kidney transplants. *Transplantation* **2013**, *96*, 245–250. [CrossRef]

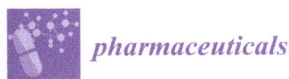

Review

Application of Design of Experiments in the Development of Self-Microemulsifying Drug Delivery Systems

Chien-Ming Hsieh [1,2], Ting-Lun Yang [3], Athika Darumas Putri [1,4] and Chin-Tin Chen [3,*]

1. School of Pharmacy, College of Pharmacy, Taipei Medical University, Taipei 110, Taiwan
2. Ph.D. Program in Drug Discovery and Development Industry, College of Pharmacy, Taipei Medical University, Taipei 110, Taiwan
3. Department of Biochemical Science and Technology, National Taiwan University, Taipei 106, Taiwan
4. Department of Pharmaceutical Chemistry, Semarang College of Pharmaceutical Sciences (STIFAR), Semarang City 50192, Indonesia
* Correspondence: chintin@ntu.edu.tw; Tel.: +886-02-3366-9487

Abstract: Oral delivery has become the route of choice among all other types of drug administrations. However, typical chronic disease drugs are often poorly water-soluble, have low dissolution rates, and undergo first-pass metabolism, ultimately leading to low bioavailability and lack of efficacy. The lipid-based formulation offers tremendous benefits of using versatile excipients and has great compatibility with all types of dosage forms. Self-microemulsifying drug delivery system (SMEDDS) promotes drug self-emulsification in a combination of oil, surfactant, and co-surfactant, thereby facilitating better drug solubility and absorption. The feasible preparation of SMEDDS creates a promising strategy to improve the drawbacks of lipophilic drugs administered orally. Selecting a decent mixing among these components is, therefore, of importance for successful SMEDDS. Quality by Design (QbD) brings a systematic approach to drug development, and it offers promise to significantly improve the manufacturing quality performance of SMEDDS. Furthermore, it could be benefited efficiently by conducting pre-formulation studies integrated with the statistical design of experiment (DoE). In this review, we highlight the recent findings for the development of microemulsions and SMEDDS by using DoE methods to optimize the formulations for drugs in different excipients with controllable ratios. A brief overview of DoE concepts is discussed, along with its technical benefits in improving SMEDDS formulations.

Keywords: oral delivery; self-microemulsifying drug delivery system (SMEDDS); quality by design (QbD); design of experiments (DoE)

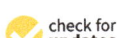

Citation: Hsieh, C.-M.; Yang, T.-L.; Putri, A.D.; Chen, C.-T. Application of Design of Experiments in the Development of Self-Microemulsifying Drug Delivery Systems. *Pharmaceuticals* 2023, 16, 283. https://doi.org/10.3390/ph16020283

Academic Editors: Silviya Petrova Zustiak and Era Jain

Received: 29 December 2022
Revised: 10 February 2023
Accepted: 10 February 2023
Published: 13 February 2023

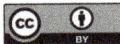

Copyright: © 2023 by the authors. Licensee MDPI, Basel, Switzerland. This article is an open access article distributed under the terms and conditions of the Creative Commons Attribution (CC BY) license (https:// creativecommons.org/licenses/by/ 4.0/).

1. Introduction

Numerous compounds are selected as potential drug candidates by employing high-throughput screening tools. However, >75% of the compounds under current development have poor aqueous solubility [1,2]. In addition, due to the difficulty in disintegrating and dissolving in the gastrointestinal tract, the bioavailability of poorly soluble drugs after oral administration is prone to be low. Physical and chemical modifications of poorly water-soluble drugs have been used to increase their solubility and bioavailability, but there are still some limitations [3,4]. For example, salt form and derivatization may alter the physiochemical properties; however, the change of pH in the physiological environment may lead to drug aggregation or precipitation [5]. Size reduction by micronization could be used to increase the bioavailability of poorly soluble drugs; however, the increased electrostatic interaction between particles may result in difficulties for further compounding and packaging [6]. Recently, lipid-based drug delivery systems, including emulsions [7], microemulsions, self-microemulsifying drug delivery systems (SMEDDS) [8], solid lipid nanoparticle (SLN) [9], nanostructured lipid carrier (NLC) [10,11], and liposome [12], have gained increasing attention for the past decade by virtue of improving the oral bioavailability of poor water-soluble or lipophilic compounds.

2. Lipid-Based Formulation for Oral Administration

2.1. Lipid Formulation Classification System

The concept of the lipid formulation classification system (LFCS) was introduced by Pouton in 2000 [13] and further well-defined in 2006 [14]. The designation of LFCS depends on the amount of oil (triglycerides or mixed glycerides), surfactant (lipophilic or hydrophilic surfactants), and co-solvent phase. Table 1 shows the four types of compositions and properties of LFCS, which could be used to simulate or interpret different lipid formulations in vivo. Briefly, type I formulations have oils requiring further digestion and emulsification by lipase and endogenous surfactant. This system is suitable for drugs with higher solubility in oils, forming coarse dispersions on dilution. To improve the emulsification and solvent capacities, lipophilic surfactants with hydrophilic-hydrophobic balance (HLB) values of less than 12 are included in type II formulations. However, a continuous phase or coarse emulsion might be found once the content of lipophilic surfactants extends beyond the threshold of 25% (w/w). In type III formulations, co-solvents are included to blend with oil and surfactants to form a self-emulsifying system. The water-soluble components tend to separate from the oil during dispersion and further dissolve in the water [13]. Moreover, the size of type III formulations easily reaches the nanoscale level after self-emulsification; therefore, these delivery systems are commonly referred to as SMEDDS. Type III formulations are classified into type IIIa and type IIIb. In type IIIa formulations, more amounts of lipids are blended with lipophilic surfactants (HLB < 12) and co-solvents to stabilize the emulsion. In contrast, less amount of lipids are mixed with hydrophilic surfactants (HLB > 12) and/or co-solvents in type IIIb formulations. It has been reported that a fine dispersion with a small particle size (<100 nm) could be produced in the formulations when the amounts of hydrophilic surfactants are over 40% (w/w) or combined with co-solvents [13]. In this regard, type IIIb can achieve greater dispersion rates with small particle sizes compared to type IIIa formulations. However, drug precipitation might appear in the dispersion process due to the lower lipid content. Type IV formulations do not contain any oil and constitute lipophilic and hydrophilic surfactants. These formulations are suitable for a drug that is hydrophobic but not lipophilic [14]. Since surfactant is mixed with co-solvent in type IV formulations, it provides better solvent capacity on dilution than using co-solvent alone.

Table 1. The features of four essential lipid formulation types in the lipid formulation classification system [14–17].

		Type I	Type II	Type IIIa	Type IIIb	Type IV
Composition (w/w %)	Glycerides (mono-, di-, tri-glycerides)	100	40–80	40–80	<20	0
	Lipophilic surfactants (HLB < 12)	–	20–60	20–40	0	0–20
	Hydrophilic surfactants (HLB > 12)	–	–	0	20–50	20–80
	Co-solvents	–	–	0–40	20–50	0–80
Characteristic features		Oil solution	Self-emulsification	Self-emulsification	Self-micro-emulsification	Spontaneous micelle dispersion
Droplet size		Coarse	0.25–2 μm	100–250 nm	50–100 nm	<50 nm

Table 1. Cont.

	Type I	Type II	Type IIIa	Type IIIb	Type IV
Lipase digestion	Crucial	Not crucial, but likely	Not crucial, but may occur	Not important	Not important
Disadvantages	Poor solvent capacity for the drugs with log p < 2	Coarser emulsion	Possible loss of solvent capacity on dispersion	May cause partial drug precipitation	Risk of drug precipitation upon dispersion

2.2. The Compositions of Lipid-Based Formulations and Their Role in Enhancement of Bioavailability

2.2.1. Triglycerides and Mixed Glycerides Used as Lipid Phase in Lipid-Based Formulations

Triglyceride is an ester in which three molecules of fatty acid are linked to the alcohol glycerol. Since triglyceride can be completely digested and absorbed after oral administration, the safety concerns are minimized for further pharmaceutical development. Common oils used in the preparation of lipid-based formulation for oral administration are shown in Table 2. Current triglycerides approved by the US Food and Drug Administration (FDA) are mainly derived from plants. According to the length of the fatty acid chain, it could be divided into medium-chain triglycerides (MCT) and long-chain triglycerides (LCT). Basically, MCT is the preferred oil phase used for the preparation of lipid formulations [15,18,19] due to their less suspected oxidative damage [20] and greater solvent capacity compared to LCT [21].

Table 2. The characterizations of different types of glycerides used in lipid-based formulations [22].

Class	Example	Characteristics
Medium chain triglycerides (MCT)	Coconut oil Palm seed oil, Miglyol® 812 Captex® 355	Good solubilizing capacity for less lipophilic drugs Higher self-dispersing ability
Long chain triglycerides (LCT)	Corn oil Soybean oil Olive oil Peanut oil Sesame oil Sunflower oil Castor oil	GRAS status Easily ingested, digested, and absorbed Poor self-dispersing properties Lower loading capacity for drugs with intermediate log p values Higher solubilizing capacity after dispersion and digestion of the formulation
Mixed mono-, di- and triglycerides	Imwitor® 988 Imwitor® 308 Maisine® 35-1 Peceol® Plurol Oleique® CC49 Capryol® Myrj®	Higher self-dispersing ability Higher solubilizing capacity for poorly water-soluble drugs

2.2.2. Surfactants

Surfactants are included as an emulsifying agent to avoid phase separation, reduce the interfacial tension and protect the droplets from agglomeration [23]. Presently, the choice of surfactants is still limited due to the safety concern for oral administration. Compared to synthetic surfactants, emulsifiers of natural origin, such as lecithin, have priority for use since they are considered to be safer. Nonionic surfactants are widely used due to the advantages of lower toxicity and irritancy to the GI tract [24], a greater degree of mixing compatibility [25], and maintaining the stability of emulsified vesicles over a wide range of pH or electrolyte [22]. The role of surfactants in these systems is to reduce the interfacial tension and provide sufficient interfacial coverage for microemulsifying the entire oil and water phases [26]. As nonionic surfactants are often used in microemulsions, their selection is very critical, considering the undesirable side effects such as allergy, irritation, or potential intoxication. However, limited references discuss the threshold or maximum dose of nonionic surfactants used in clinicals. Table 3 shows the latest FDA-approved nonionic surfactants with recommended threshold values for lipid-based formulation.

Table 3. Approved nonionic surfactants by the FDA and their descriptions, along with each latest maximum potency per dosage unit per 20 October 2022 [27]. The n/a refers to data not available for the corresponding surfactant.

Surfactants		HLB	Description	Oral	Topical	Injection	Maximum Potency per Dosage Unit
Polyoxylglycerides	Caprylocaproyl polyoxylglycerides (Labrasol®)	12	Pale-yellow oily liquids	✓	✓	–	Oral = 61.2 mg/mL
	Lauroyl polyoxylglyceride (Gelucire 44/14®)	11	Pale-yellow waxy solids	✓	–	–	Oral = 0.15–218 mg
	Stearoyl polyoxylglycerides (Gelucire 50/13®)	11	Pale-yellow waxy solids	✓	–	–	Oral = 23.34 mg
Polyoxyethylene Stearates	Polyoxyl 8 stearate	11.1	Waxy cream	✓	✓	✓	Oral = 25 mg/5 mL
	Polyoxyl 12 stearate	13.6	Pasty solid	✓	✓	✓	n/a
	Polyoxyl 20 stearate	14	Waxy solid	✓	✓	✓	n/a
	Polyoxyl 40 stearate	16.9	Waxy solid	✓	✓	✓	Oral = 2–8.48 mg; Topical = 3–8.8% w/w
	Polyoxyl 50 stearate	17.9	Solid	✓	✓	✓	n/a
	Polyoxyl 100 stearate	18.8	Solid	✓	✓	✓	Topical = 0.5–2.1% w/w
	Polyoxyl 12 distearate	10.6	Paste	✓	✓	✓	n/a
Polyoxyethylene Sorbitan Fatty Acid Esters	Polyoxyethylene 20 sorbitan monolaurate (Tween 20)	16.7	Yellow oily liquid	✓	✓	✓	Oral = 0.35–4.2 mg; Topical = 0.02–8% w/w
	Polyoxyethylene 20 sorbitan monopalmitate (Tween 40)	15.6	Yellow oily liquid	✓	✓	✓	Oral = 0.05 mg/5 mL; Topical = 2–3% w/w
	Polyoxyethylene 20 sorbitan monostearate (Tween 60)	14.9	Yellow oily liquid	✓	✓	✓	Oral = 5–20 mg/mL; Topical = 0.42–14.55% w/w
	Polyoxyethylene 20 sorbitan tristearate (Tween 65)	10.5	Tan solid	✓	✓	✓	Topical = 0.5% w/w
	Polyoxyethylene 20 sorbitan monooleate (Tween 80)	15	Yellow oily liquid	✓	✓	✓	Oral = 0.04–418.37 mg; Topical = 0.1–15% w/w
	Polyoxyethylene 20 sorbitan trioleate (Tween 85)	11	Amber liquid	✓	✓	✓	Oral = 1.5 mg/5 mL
	Polyoxyethylene 20 sorbitan monoisostearate	14.9	Yellow oily liquid	✓	✓	✓	n/a
Polyoxyethylene Alkyl Ethers	Polyoxyl 23 lauryl ether (Brij 35®)	16.9	White waxy solid	✓	✓	–	Topical = 0.45–1.08% w/w
	Polyoxyl 10 cetyl ether (Brij 56®)	12.9	White waxy solid	✓	✓	–	Topical = 2.5% w/w
	Polyoxyl 20 cetyl ether (Brij 58®)	15.7	Waxy solid	✓	✓	–	Topical = 2–6% w/w
	Polyoxyl 10 stearyl ether (Brij 76®)	12.4	White waxy solid	✓	✓	–	n/a

Table 3. Cont.

Surfactants		HLB	Description	Oral	Topical	Injection	Maximum Potency per Dosage Unit
Polyoxyethylene Castor Oil Derivatives	Polyoxyl 35 castoroil (Cremophor EL®)	12–14	Pale yellow oily liquid Clear above 26 °C with faint characteristic odor	√	√	√	Oral = 0.4–515 mg/mL Topical = 4% w/w
	Poloxyl 35 castoroil, purified (Cremophor ELP®)	12–14	White to slightly yellowish paste or cloudy liquid with weak characteristic odor	√	√	√	n/a
	Polyoxyl 40 hydrogenated castoroil (Cremophor RH40®)	14–16	Viscous liquid or soft paste with very little odor in aqueous solutions, almost tasteless	√	√	√	Oral coated capsule = 101.25 mg Oral solution = 450 mg/mL Topical = 1% w/w
	Polyoxyl 60 hydrogenated castor oil	15–17	White to yellowish soft or flowing paste with faint odor or taste in aqueous solutions	√	√	√	Topical = 1.9% w/w
D-α-Tocopherol polyethylene glycol 1000 succinate (TPGS)		13.2	White to light-brown, waxy solid	√	√	–	n/a

2.2.3. Co-Surfactants/Co-Solvents

Like co-surfactants, co-solvents could regulate the partition of surfactant between the aqueous and oil phases, thereby stabilizing microemulsions to exclude unbounded structures such as liquid crystals, gels, or precipitates [28]. Although both co-surfactants and co-solvents can affect the partition of surfactants, the main role of co-solvents is to accelerate the process of emulsification [29], while co-surfactants is to enhance the interface flexibility of the emulsified vesicle [30]. In general, short to medium-chain length alcohols (C2–C12), ethylene glycol, glycerol, propylene glycol, and other above derivations are adequate co-solvents [22]. Among them, ethanol has been used traditionally as a co-solvent in oral solutions, but it may not be suitable for pediatric or other patients who cannot tolerate alcohol.

2.3. Macroemulsions, Microemulsions and Nanoemulsions

Macroemulsion is a thermodynamically unstable state; therefore, oil-water separation often occurs after storage. If co-solvents such as short-chain alcohols are added during high-speed homogenization, nanoemulsions with particle sizes ranging from 100 nm to 1000 nm can be obtained. When a large amount of surfactant is presented in the oil and water phases, microemulsions with particle sizes ranging from 10 to 100 nm can be formed spontaneously [31,32]. Microemulsions and nanoemulsions are all prepared by oil, water, and surfactant, having relatively similar structures (Figure 1). Owing to the small light scattering of microemulsions and nanoemulsions, the appearance of both is mostly transparent or translucent. However, these two types of emulsions have different composition ratios and formation mechanisms. Microemulsions are formed due to the saturated state of surfactant micelles after a large amount of oil is introduced into them. The free energy of colloidal dispersion is smaller than the separate phase. Therefore, when oil, surfactant, and co-surfactant are blended all together, the microemulsions occur rather spontaneously and involve almost no external energy, further indicating a favorable or stable thermodynamic state. In contrast, the nanoemulsions themselves are usually produced by applying shear stress to induce the formation of nano-sized droplets, resulting in an increase in the interfacial surface free energy. In this regard, nanoemulsions are regarded as thermodynamically unstable because they might further decompose into separate phases over time. However, this mechanism might also offer the nanodroplets to be kinetically stable, which is beneficial for long-term storage. The greater the energy barrier between the initial phase state and the emulsion state, the longer the nanoemulsions last before reverting to their original phase [33].

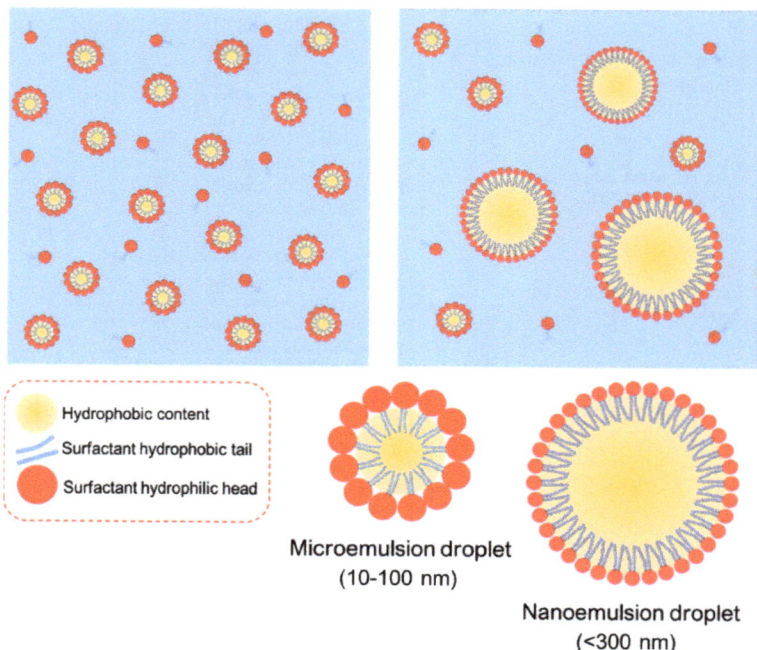

Figure 1. Illustration of microemulsions and nanoemulsions prepared from the similar elements of oil, water, and surfactant, giving the relatively similar structures with each other.

Particle size is first used to differentiate microemulsions and nanoemulsions. The narrow and sharp peaks refer to microemulsions, whereas the broad or multi-peaks belong to nanoemulsions, suggesting unstable thermodynamics during the nanoemulsion process [33]. Another method for identifying the microemulsions or nanoemulsions is to observe the behavior upon the addition of excess water. In general, a microemulsion is a thermodynamically stable system under a particular range of conditions. However, the system would become unstable during the dilution, and the droplets may break down. Conversely, nanoemulsions are kinetically stable and dilutable with water, which keep the size distribution unchanged with no sign of phase inversion [33].

The advantage of microemulsions and nanoemulsions is their ability to encapsulate lipophilic drugs to enhance their solubility, dissolution (or dispersion) rate, and bioavailability. However, the number of clinical trials related to microemulsions and nanoemulsions decreased over the years [34] due to the large volume and a high proportion of surfactants used in these systems [35]. Table 4 shows the comparison of microemulsions and nanoemulsions.

Table 4. The comparison of nanoemulsions and microemulsions [22,32].

	Nanoemulsions	Microemulsions
Stability	Kinetic stable system	Thermodynamic stable system
Compositions	Oil, Surfactants, Water	Oil, Surfactants, Water
Order of mixing	The surfactant should first be mixed with the oil phase, and then titrated with the aqueous	The order of mixing does not affect the size of particle
Particle size	50–300 nm	10–100 nm
Manufacturing process	Specific equipment is required to provide sufficient energy to increase the interfacial area	Spontaneous formation

2.4. Self-Microemulsifying Drug Delivery System (SMEDDS)

Emulsion systems are associated with their own set of complexities, including stability and manufacturing problems associated with their commercial production. SMEDDS belongs to lipid-based self-emulsification systems with isotropic appearance. They are promising formulations for delivering poorly water-soluble lipophilic drugs and can spontaneously generate oil-in-water (w/o) nanosized droplets under gentle blending after dilution in an aqueous medium. Their self-dispersion behavior and small droplet sizes upon dispersion have been shown to improve drug absorption from the large interfacial area. Recently, much attention has been focused on this formulation owing to the ease of manufacture [29], higher drug loading capacity [36,37], and the reduction in food effect [38,39]. Compared to microemulsions and nanoemulsions, SMEDDS can significantly reduce the dose volume, which results in attractive commercial viability and patient compliance. In general, a water-free system not only bears lower solvent effects but also diminishes the dosing volume and increases drug stability. Another advantage of SMEDDS is that drug absorption is less affected by food. Dronedarone is a famous example. Dronedarone is an anti-arrhythmic agent with different bioavailability in fed and fast states [40]. Compared to the fasted state, the $AUC_{0-24\,h}$ and C_{max} of the fed state were approximately 10-fold and 8-fold higher, respectively, after oral administration of marketed dronedarone product (Multaq®) to beagle dogs [39]. However, SMEDDS formulation significantly mitigated the food effect as $AUC_{0-24\,h}$ and C_{max} in the fed state were only 2.9-fold and 2.6-fold higher, respectively. In this regard, it is speculated that SMEDDS may reduce the variability of drug absorption between pre- and post-prandial state, thereby improving therapeutic efficacy and patient compliance.

2.4.1. Formulation Design and Factors Affecting SMEDDS Formulations

SMEDDS formulations consist of mixing aqueous and oily phases in the presence of surfactants and/or co-solvents. Except for the excipient's selection, several factors are known to influence the formation of a stable SMEDD, such as preparation conditions, equipment conditions, and preparation temperature. Therefore, to develop a successful formulation, it is critical to understand the scientific information behind the system compositions and preparation conditions, which will affect the phase behavior in each excipient.

Screening of Excipients

In general, SMEDDS formulations are prepared by mixing different proportions of oil, surfactant, and co-solvent selected by ternary phase diagrams. Construction of ternary phase diagrams is frequently used to determine the types of structures resulting from emulsification and to characterize the behavior of a formulation along a dilution process. After equilibration at atmospheric temperature for a period of time, the drugs are added to the mixture and agitated gently to reach the expected concentration. The appearance of formulations should be transparent and clear without any precipitation. Since external forces are added to accelerate the equilibration during SMEDDS preparation, it is necessary to figure out the sequence of adding the excipients and drugs because it will affect the final appearance. In addition, as the solvent capacity of surfactants in SMEDDS will decrease after solubilizing the drug in co-surfactant [41], the sequence in adding the excipients and drugs not only affect the equilibration of formulation but also the drug solubility.

Active Pharmaceutical Ingredient (API) Dose

The SMEDDS is a suitable template for highly hydrophobic APIs, which could dissolve in the oil of formulation. In general, APIs with log p larger than five are more suitable to encapsulate in the SMEDDS with high-loading doses [29]. Since SMEDDS belongs to type IIIb lipid-based formulation, more drugs can be loaded into the formulation when higher amounts of surfactant are used. However, if water-soluble constituents are present in SMEDDS, formulation development requires further consideration because it can initiate precipitation of the drug from the formulation into the GI tract medium.

Polarity of the Lipid Phase

The digestion of lipid excipients and drug partitioning in SMEDDS begins in the GI tract, involving lipid emulsification and solubilization. During this period, some changes in the properties of the protected APIs in oil droplets could be found [42]. Once the lipase catalyzes the oil droplets, there are differences in the absorption quality and biodistribution of the drug, depending on the lipids sealing it. Then, the drug will be fractionated, dissolved in intestinal fluid, and facilitated by the lipoproteins to transport from the lymphatic system to the blood. Therefore, it is necessary to consider the criterion of lipid selection during SMEDDS formulation.

Caliph and co-workers have compared the triglyceride chains used in SMEDDS. They demonstrated that the combination of medium and long-chain fatty acids improved the droplet formation of microemulsions and increased the bioavailability in 12 h compared to that of using long-chain fatty acid only [43]. Lipids and/or glycerides with longer chains are preferable to act as the oil phase for SMEDDS because they can transform to triglycerides which is more favorable to associate with the chylomicron [44].

2.4.2. Characterization and Evaluation Methods for SMEDDS Formulations

Droplet size is an important parameter in the assessment of SMEDDS since it influences the lipolysis process, drug release, and, consequently, absorption. The droplet size distribution of microemulsion vesicles can be determined by either electron microscopy or light-scattering techniques. The surface charge is determined using a zeta potential analyzer by measuring the zeta potential of the preparations. Zeta potential is the electrical potential in the interfacial double layer of a dispersed particle or droplet versus a point in the continuous phase away from the interface. It is often used as an indicator of droplet stability, where values more positive than +30 mV and more negative than −30 mV indicate good stability against coalescence [45].

The characteristics of SMEDDS not only include droplet size and z-potential but also self-emulsification time, which can generally be evaluated using a USP Type II dissolution apparatus. Briefly, the formulation was added into distilled water maintained at 37 °C, and the time to form a clear solution was recorded with gentle agitation provided at 100 rpm [38]. If the emulsion rapidly forms a clear appearance in less than 1 min, it can be considered as grade I. Grade II indicates the opacity of the emulsion is slightly foggy within 2 min. If a bright white emulsion forms within 3 min, it can be regarded as grade III. Grade IV shows the appearance of dull and grayish-white emulsion with a slightly oily appearance for more than 3 min. In contrast, grade V exhibits poor emulsification with large oil droplets present on the surface [46].

The degree of lipolysis in vitro is also used to evaluate the pre-formulations of SMEDDS. The degradation rate affects the toxicological acceptability and the matrix-controlled release of drugs. In general, lipids digested by lipases to form amphiphilic products are a key process in controlling the utility of most lipid-based formulations. The interaction of these digested products with endogenous amphiphilic components such as bile salts, phospholipids, and cholesterol results in the formation of colloidal structures (e.g., droplet vesicles and micelles). These colloidal structures act as a lipophilic reservoir, enabling the partitioning of drugs into colloidal phases during the gastrointestinal transition. Moreover, exogenous lipids may insert into the bile salts or phospholipid structure, promoting micelle expansion and solubility enhancement. The experimental device consisting of a thermally stable reaction vessel under continuous agitation and a pH-stat with an automated burette to add NaOH solution is used to mimic the in vivo situation of lipolysis. FaSSIF or FeSSIF solution is commonly used as the experimental medium. After lipolysis, the digested mixture is ultra-centrifuged to separate the aqueous phase and sedimentation phase. It is believed that an aqueous phase contains the colloidal structure and dissolved drug, which is imperative for absorption. The sedimentation phase usually contains calcium soap of fatty acid and precipitated drugs, which can be used to evaluate the sedimentation velocity of the lipid-based formulation.

The stability assessment of SMEDDS under different stress can be used to predict their shelf life. As the extra force is included in the SMEDDS manufacturing process, the stability of these formulations depends on the thermodynamic equilibrium. Commonly used experimental tests for stability evaluation include centrifugation tests, freeze-thaw cycle tests, thermal stress tests, and dilution stability [47]. Basically, a SMEDDS pre-formulation is centrifuged for more than 20 min at 3000–13,000 rpm. The appearance of the post-centrifugated suspension was observed and correlated with the size distribution upon self-emulsification in the aqueous. Freeze-thaw cycles are regarded as an experiment to determine the thermal stability of SMEDDS. Some APIs or excipients might be sedimented when SMEDDS is stored at low temperatures. For a stable formulation, the sedimentation should rapidly re-dissolve in SMEDDS as the temperature rises to room temperature. Three freeze-thaw cycles are usually performed on the SMEDDS suspension, including freezing at −20 °C for 48 h and followed by thawing at 40 °C for 48 h. For thermal stress testing, the samples will be placed in a certain temperature range (45 °C to 80 °C) for a period of time to observe whether phase separation occurs. Dilution stability is to evaluate the thermodynamic stability of SMEDDS upon dilution in water. For this purpose, various dilution ratios of the dispersive medium should be tested to determine the consistency of droplet size.

2.4.3. New Strategy for SMEDDS Development

As mentioned above, SMEDDS formulations are used to increase the bioavailability of APIs that are difficult to dissolve and have low bioavailability. Although they are regarded as the most appropriate method to increase drug solubility and bioavailability in oral drug administration, there are still few available products on the pharmaceutical market formulated as SMEDDS. This is associated with the several challenges and difficulties that may be encountered during the SMEDDS preparation and administration process.

API deposition from SMEDDS is one of the most common factors. It is known that drugs encapsulated in SMEDDS must be presented in a dissolved state during transit in the GIT. However, some of the encapsulated drugs are strongly affected by the change of pH values upon contact with GI fluids, resulting in ionization and cancellation of absorption [48,49]. The use of water-soluble solvents or volatile oils may interfere with drug solubility (which increases drug precipitation) when further dilution or high-temperature tests are performed. It is essential for drugs to present in a well-dissolved state in lipid-based delivery. The combined surfactant/co-surfactant and lipid imbalance also increase the possibility of drug precipitation if a greater amount of surfactant/co-surfactant was added than the lipid used in the formulation [50]. The incorporation of polymers to SMEDDS is possible to minimize drug precipitation in vivo [51].

Most of the marketed SMEDDS formulations are in soft gelatin capsules, which causes handling issues and also increases the cost of the product. However, gelatin capsules are associated with few drawbacks. Immature stability can be detrimental from this endeavor as the liquid form is susceptible to possible exposure from hydrolysis, temperature/pH changes, and light, which induce drug/excipient degradation, especially unsaturated lipids as they tend to be oxidized by impurities originating from the gelatin capsule [52,53]. Volatile excipients such as co-solvents in SMEDDS formulations are known to migrate into the shells of soft or hard gelatin capsules, resulting in the precipitation of the lipophilic drugs. Thus, combined polymers and the preparation of solid SMEDDS seems to be a logical solution to address these [54].

The efficiency of oral absorption of the hydrophobic drug from the SMEDDS depends on many formulation-related parameters, such as surfactant concentration, oil/surfactant ratios, the polarity of the emulsion, droplet size, and charge, all of which, in essence, determine the self-emulsification ability. Small changes in material attributes could cause poor product performance in SMEDDS development. The ratio of the oil, surfactant, and co-solvent phases is a key factor in producing a suitable SMEDDS formulation. It has been shown that the formulation efficiency of drugs is affected by the oil/surfactant pairing properties, surfactant concentration, oil/surfactant ratio, and the temperature at which self-emulsification occurs. Therefore, in order to obtain the most efficient self-emulsification zone, the selection of the pharmaceutical excipients is very critical to produce an effective delivery system with better bioavailability. Once a list of suitable excipients is determined, screening of binary drug excipients for solubility, compatibility, and stability will be followed to identify the most appropriate lipid system for the drug in question. According to the LFCS category, SMEDDS can be obtained when the proportions of oil, hydrophilic surfactant, and co-solvent are within <20%, 20–50%, and 20–50%, respectively. However, the range of individual ratios suggested in the LFCS is too wide to find a suitable pre-formulation in a limited time period. Moreover, it can be time-consuming for a formulations scientist to determine the optimal composition of the formulation by a traditional approach.

Quality by design (QbD) is a regulatory-driven approach that adopts a multitude of techniques in product development. This approach can help us to choose the most appropriate component and systemically optimize the formulations. With a controlled and reproducible result, a formulation may meet the specific therapeutic goals. Design of experiment (DoE) and risk assessment techniques based on QbD methodologies are increasingly used in the formulation development of SMEDDS. DoE is a rational and scientific approach for understanding how various formulation/process parameters individually and synergically influence the pivotal product characteristics.

3. Overview of the Quality by Design (QbD) and Design of Experiment (DoE) for Pharmaceutical Development

To achieve consistent formulation effects and better quality control, QbD supports parametric options for strong critical attributes. Since reproducibility is a major concern, it is essential to take into account appropriate experimental factors during the variability processing and control or necessarily eliminate a contradictory factor. In other words, it is preferred to ensure the high quality of a product, even though the greater risks are involved, rather than increasing the run quantities [55,56]. Herein, the experiments are not only statistically evaluated (e.g., t-test) but also have all the studied parameters analyzed, and the outcomes of those are validated.

3.1. Quality by Design (QbD)

QbD in pharmaceuticals involves a systematic methodology incorporated into a series of studies with predetermined objectives, emphasizing the controlled quality of the entire process to produce quality products. Here, risk management is more about how to strategically design and mix inputs and outputs to reduce failure rates. In detail, below are some of the issues in performing pharmaceutical QbD that need to be addressed with reference to the FDA regulations [55,56]: (1) the capability of the selected processes to meet the critical quality attributes, (2) low/minimized product variability amongst the batches, (3) clinical relevance of the developed product specification, (4) efficiency of product manufacture and robustness, and (5) the capability in identifying the problem and management of post-approval change of product.

Several components in QbD include: (1) determining the quality target product profile (QTPP) as critical quality attributes (CQAs) of the developed product, (2) determining the critical material attributes (CMAs) through the design of the product, (3) identifying the critical process parameters (CPPs) through the design of the process and correlating the scale-up principles, CMAs, and CPPs to CQAs, and (4) process capability and continual improvement. By including QbD during the pharmaceutical manufacturing, it is expected that product development could be accelerated with a controlled and measurable risk.

3.2. Design of Experiment (DoE)

As mentioned earlier, product and process understanding are key elements of QbD. To best achieve these objectives, in addition to mechanistic models, DoE is an excellent tool that allows pharmaceutical scientists to systematically manipulate factors according to a prespecified design. Traditionally, common experimentation was designed using OFAT (one-factor-at-a-time), which worked by keeping all other variables constant while varying one variable at the same time [57]. Since each experiment must be performed one at a time, numerous runs would be required to achieve adequate information regarding the condition causing the particular problem. Besides being resource (cost, experiments, time, manpower)-intensive, the OFAT method cannot estimate interactions between the variables. DoE, first coined by Ronald A. Fisher in 1935 [58], however, includes all the factors simultaneously by systematic experiments. It has become increasingly prevalent in the formulation arena over the past few years. DoE is a statistical approach to help establish statistical relationships between a set of input and output variables designated by the system/process being studied. Several terms commonly used to describe the flow of DoE include (1) input/independent variables ($x_1, x_2, x_3, \ldots$), (2) output/dependent variables ($y_1, y_2, y_3, \ldots$), (3) uncontrollable inputs ($z_1, z_2, z_3, \ldots$) [59]. Unlike the trial-error method (OFAT), DoE is more efficient and helps structure experiments rationally. The model built by DoE is not only a mathematical model but rather a formal statistical or correlation model that can be derived between input and output variables, wherein each of which is independent.

3.3. Screening Experiment and Factorial Design

Many experiments contain various types of parameters/factors with different levels that need to be investigated. Therefore, to make use of DoE involved in the experiments, the possible factors are sorted through the screening experiment, leaving only a few factors having a large effect. The screening stage usually occurs in the early stages of the experiment, where all factors are first considered as likely to have little or no effect on the response. Furthermore, it is important to ensure that the selected factors are presented within their upper and lower limits [57].

To determine the limits, researchers usually use a certain background of the factors studied, for example, based on literature studies or empirical data. The studied factors should then meet factor compatibility, where all the selected factors, any combination amongst, or their upper/lower limits are physically recognized by the system. The determined combinations of the selected factors are expressed as zero points and presented as coordinates in a multi-dimensional factorial space, which is referred to as the zero level [57].

The term 'interval of factor variation' refers to the number that will become the upper limit when added to the zero level and will become the lower limit when subtracted from the zero level. In a numerical way, this is usually expressed as +1 as the upper limit (high), −1 as the lower limit (low), and 0 as the central/zero level. These terms later would be used in a factorial design, which is one of the screening methods of DoE to study the effects due to a variable or combination of some factors simultaneously on a response being examined. Geometrically, factorial design collects the data at the vertices of a cube in k-dimensions, wherein **k** is the amount of the studied factors. In full-factorial design (FFD), the data are collected from all the vertices [57,59]. Since this method investigates each factor at 2 levels (i.e., high and low, +1 and −1), therefore it requires 2^k experimental runs.

There are circumstances that a particular experiment requires many factors to study. In this case, the fractional factorial design (FrFD) is often used as a strategy against the FFD to deliberately cut the FFD in half [57]. FrFD allows to collect data from specific sub-part of all possible factors, which requires 2^{k-q} runs with -q as the number selected to fractionate the FFD. The most important variable could be identified with this FrFD, allowing for more in-depth tests in the future. FrFD contains several resolutions, and the most important ones are III, IV, and V (regarding the description of each, it has been extensively discussed in another review [60]). FrFD strategy works well in basic designs, such as the most regular fractions, but not in complicated situations, such as some irregular fractions and partial fold designs [59].

In addition, certain fractional factorials have no defining interaction between the factors, such as the Plackett–Burman design (PBD) [59]. PBD is a two-level orthogonal type and is used to develop a proximity fuse [61,62]. The total runs of experiment (N) can be investigated up to N-1 factors with N of multiples of 4 [63,64]. This tool only estimates the main effect of the factors during the process and could not be utilized to obtain surface responses during any optimization [65]. It is recommended to choose a matrix with four or more tests from the selected factors being studied, with three replicates included in the center point of the PBD matrix [64]. Another orthogonal array is the so-called Taguchi method, which is generally similar to fractional factorial experiments. The main objective of this method is to use a standardized method to conduct an experiment and to analyze the results [57,59].

3.4. Response Surface Methodology

Response surface methodology (RSM) is a statistical approach used to generate empirical models that typically correlate responses with multiple input factors. It is possible to study the optimization process using the data gathered in this way from the experiments. The y response is a continuous function of several input variables $x_1, x_2, x_3, \ldots$ where the screening design is basically used sequentially to obtain the shape of the response surface [59]. Since the goal of RSM is to find the optimal response, some factors are utilized to obtain the process yield. For instance, in order to find the temperature (x_1) and pH (x_2) which has an acceptable particle size of SMEDDS (y), the approximation can be denoted as follow:

$$y = f(x_1, x_2) + \epsilon \quad (1)$$

ϵ is the noise observed in the response y. If the expected response is used herein (i.e., $E(y) = f(x_1, x_2) = \eta$), so the surface will be known as the surface of the response:

$$\eta = f(x_1, x_2) \quad (2)$$

A screening design performed initially is useful herein to quickly identify which input factors affect the response the most [59]. For example, regarding the maximum drug loading response on SMEDDS parameters such as surface morphology, particle size, and zeta potential can be the most influencing input factors. Analysis of variance (ANOVA) is further used to assess the significance of the combined factors or the influence of their individuals on the response [59].

In RSM, the relationship between response and the factors is apparently not identified yet. Therefore, the steps in doing the RSM begin with finding an appropriate approximation to determine the correct relationship between the response *y* and a set of factors *x* [57,59]. Most of the time, it starts with the low-order polynomial. The first-order model is attributed to a well-modeled response with the factors by linear correlation of the factors:

$$y = \beta_0 + \beta_1 x_1 + \beta_2 x_2 + \cdots + \beta_k x_k + \epsilon \quad (3)$$

The second-order model is a polynomial of higher degree which is defined for the system which has curvature:

$$y = \beta_0 + \sum_{i=1}^{k} \beta_i x_i + \sum_{i=1}^{k} \beta_{ii} x_i^2 + \sum\sum_{i<j} \beta_{ij} x_i x_j + \epsilon \qquad (4)$$

The β_0, β_i, β_{ii}, ϵ represent the model constant term, coefficient of the linear term, and coefficient of the quadratic term, respectively. Most of the RSM problems use one or both models to construct the relationship [59,64]. The least squares method is usually then used to estimate the parameters in the polynomial equation. The mathematical model can be considered relevant if the regression is statistically significant and DoEs do not have a meaningful error (lack of fit; usually indicated as $p > 0.05$). Regarding the coefficient of determination (R^2), it is indicated to be data representative if the coefficient value is closer to 1 [59,64].

3.5. Optimization Methodology

RSM is normally employed in the optimization stage of formulation development. Two of the mostly used RSM methods are known as central composite design (CCD) and Box-Behnken design (BBD) (Figure 2). Three-level full factorial design is another type of optimization that is used if two or three input factors are investigated. The number of experiments is set using 3^k; for example, if there are three input factors, the total runs will be 3^3, 27 experiments [59]. CCD is one of the examples for fitting a second-order model. It has two level (-1 and $+1$) factorials with an additional point (axial point or star and center point), which allows for the estimation of the effect of pure squares [59,64]. Mathematically, it consists of 2^k factorial with factorial runs of 2^k axial or star runs and n_C as center runs. The CCD is often used in sequential experimentation, wherein the 2^k will be used to fit the first-order model, followed by the axial runs to allow the quadratic terms to be incorporated into the model. Mathematically, it is a selected design to fit the second-order model with the distance α of the axial runs from the design center and the number of center point n_C. The difference between this design and the factorial design is the presence of a single factor with a coded value in CCD, $\pm\alpha$, varied from 1 to $k^{\frac{1}{2}}$. The α involves rotatability, which depends on the factorial portion of the design. Rotatability is important in RSM. This is because when the optimal location is unknown during optimization, the rotatability acts as the basis for selecting an appropriate design that has the same precision for estimation in all directions [59].

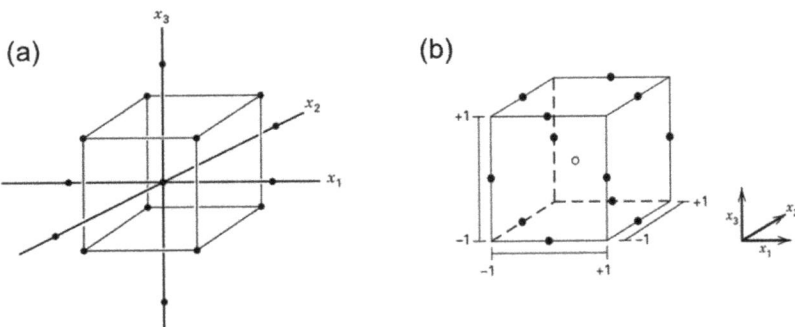

Figure 2. The central composite design (a) and Box-Behnken design (b) of three factors ($k = 3$). Adapted from Montgomery [59].

BBD combines 2^k factorials with an incomplete block design. It is the three-level design used to fit the response surface. The design is suitable for most of the experiments due to its efficiency and rotatable characteristics. Mathematically, BBD belongs to a spherical design where all the points are on the sphere of radius $2^{\frac{1}{2}}$ [59]. The points are not available at the vertices of the cubic area formed by the upper and lower limits for each variable in the BBD. The number of the experiments is usually counted as $N = 2k(k-1) + Co$ with Co as the number of central points [64].

4. Advantages of Applying DoE Techniques for the Development of SMEDDS Formulations

Numerous important parameters need to be involved during the development of SMEDDS formulations, while resources and time are nearly limited. Beyond all that, DoE is one of the effective tools to optimize SMEDDS composition. It offers an efficient experimental formulation that is more rational, ranging from the solubility of the active compound in the combination of excipients, construction of phase diagrams to obtain the most optimal formulation for SMEDDS, all characterizations, and the final responses [66–68]. Briefly, an overview of the DoE application in its role in SMEDDS development is presented in Figure 3, wherein it starts from the beginning of the experiments until the evaluation stages.

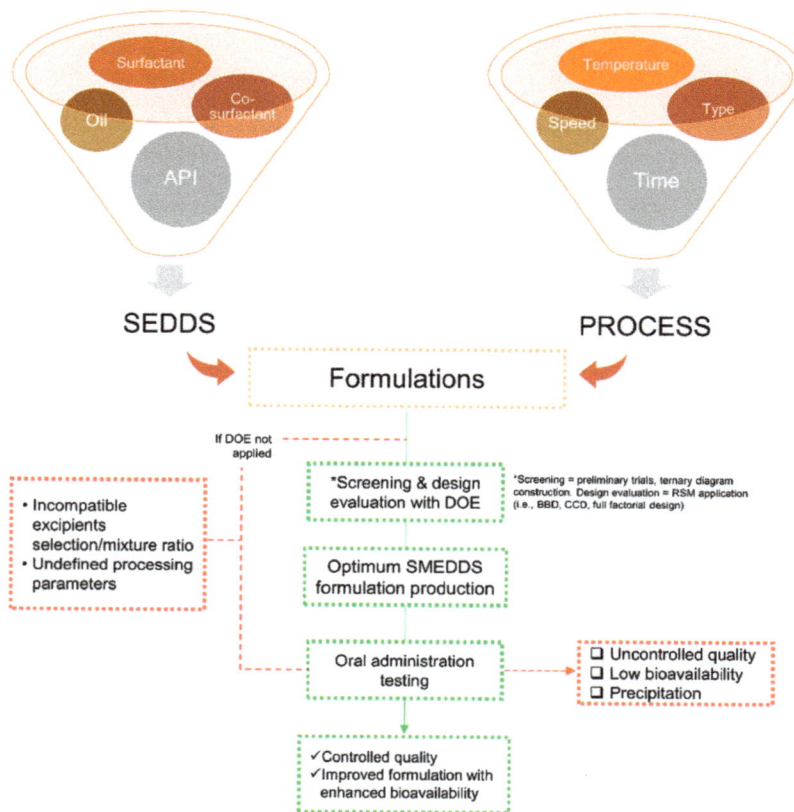

Figure 3. Scheme of the design of experiment (DoE) application in SMEDDS flow-work starting from the selection of materials and processing attributes in a statistical manner to obtain an optimized SMEDDS formulation/parameter. The mentioned abbreviations include self-emulsifying drug delivery (SEDDS), Box-Behnken design (BBD), and central composite design (CCD).

The following sections are several studies in SMEDDS development using DoE to optimize the variables employed to produce an optimum formulation.

4.1. Box-Behnken Design (BBD)

Marasini and coworkers used BBD to investigate the optimum conditions of spray drying parameters for the solid-SMEDDS flurbiprofen formulation [69]. First, the authors conducted a screening study using a spray drying method with dextran as the solid carrier to obtain a range of independent parameter values, including inlet temperature, feed rate, and carrier concentration. Three levels of three-factors (3^3) BBD were used thereafter to generate a factorial combination of these independent parameters on responses to evaluate powder characteristics, including %moisture, %yield, drug content, and particle size. All parametric factors contributed to influencing the final product characteristics of SMEDDS with a significance value of $p < 0.05$. The most critical factor is the concentration of dextran which has a negative effect on the drug content. The authors showed that the optimized parameter validation of the independent variables was close to the predicted value and could reproduce solid SMEDDS with higher yield (58.5%) and drug content (70.1 mg/g) with minimum moisture content (0.72%) and particle size (166.8 nm).

More recently, Dalvadi and coworkers developed zotepine-solid SMEDDS to improve their dissolution rate [68]. Initial screening was performed for the solubility of zotepine in various oil, surfactant, and co-surfactant, which was followed by the construction of pseudo-ternary diagrams to determine the amounts of the selected element. Various solid carriers in different ratios were examined, and Aerosil 200 was chosen as the best one. Three-factor, three-level (3^3) BBD was then employed to characterize the effect of independent variables (i.e., oleic acid (oil), Tween 80 (surfactant), and PEG400 (co-surfactant)) in the formulation. The % microemulsions transparency and % cumulative drug release were selected based on the principal component analysis as the critical responses used in the BBD. Other variables were also examined, such as the cloud point, emulsification time, and drug content. Irrespective of other variables, the oil content showed an antagonist effect toward both responses significantly, which decreased the % microemulsions transparency and % cumulative drug release (Figure 4a,b). As compared to the conventional zotepine, all optimized parameters produced a higher % transmittance and an improved 30 min-in vitro drug release as final properties of the solid-SMEDDS, which were 98.75% and 86.57%, respectively.

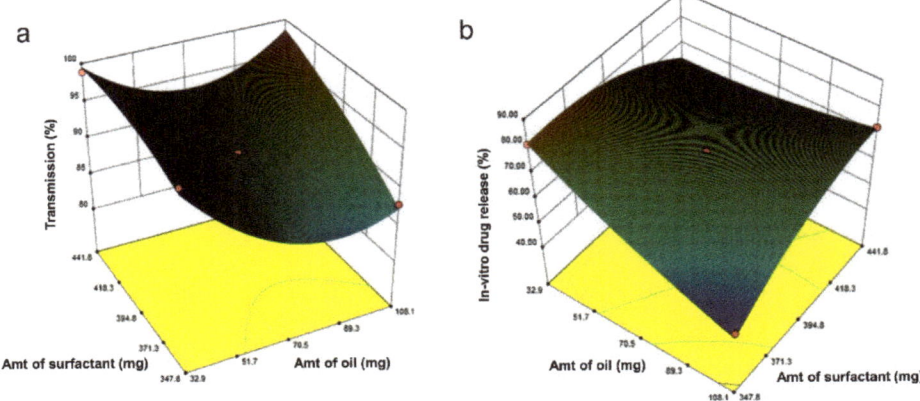

Figure 4. Response surface plot in three dimensions for BBD showing interaction effects between surfactant and oil on % transmission (**a**) and % cumulative drug release (**b**), from the study of zotepine in solid SMEDDS by Dalvadi and coworkers. Adapted from Dalvadi and coworkers [68].

Silva and coworkers developed solid SMEDDS for carvedilol using hot-melt extrusion [70]. Preliminary experiments were done to determine the optimized operating parameters of the extruder with an emphasis on obtaining recirculation time parameters for a homogenous mixing process. BBD was then utilized to evaluate several independent factors, including recirculation time, temperature, and carvedilol concentration, in affecting the cumulative releases in pH 1.2 and pH 6.8. As a result, the increases in recirculation time and temperature significantly lowered the drug release at pH 1.2, while the reduction of both factors increased the release at pH 6.8. In addition, the limited carvedilol solubility significantly affected drug release at pH 6.8, wherein the release was induced if the drug amount decreased. These results underlined another applicability of RSM in constructing efficient and rational variables for system performance used to produce SMEDDS.

Čerpnjak and coworkers evaluated several solidification methods to produce naproxen solid SMEDDS (tablet), including adsorption, spray-drying, high-shear, and fluid-bed granulation methods [71]. Various carriers were also tested depending on the type of technique to obtain the best solid carrier in transforming the liquid naproxen to a solid state. After obtaining the preliminary results, the spray-drying technique with maltodextrin was selected as the best condition and further used for DoE implementation. The three-factor, two-level (2^3) factorial design was employed to examine the selected variables, which were inlet temperature, pressure, and pump, on their influences on droplet size, polydispersity index (PDI), and yield. According to the weighted regression coefficients, the antagonistic effects were only indicated in the change of pressure toward the droplet size and the pump speed toward the PDI, whereas the interaction of the three responses had synergistic values. These combined parameters were thus selected to produce the most optimized solid SMEDDS with an inlet temperature of 120 °C, pressure of 50 mmHg, and pump speed of 15 mL/min. Further recent SMEDDS developments governing BBD application are listed in Table 5.

Table 5. List of the SMEDDS developments along with the applied response surface methodology (RSM) of central composite design (CCD).

Compound	Screening	RSM	Experiments	Independent Variables	Responses	Program	Optimized Conditions	Reference
6-Shogaol (purified alkylphenol from ginger root)	n/a	CCD	$p < 0.05$	Ethyl oleate (18.62% w/w), tween 80:PEG 400 (1.73:1 w/w)	Particle size, PDI, cumulative drug release	Design-Expert®, version 8.0.6	Particle size (20.00 ± 0.26 nm), PDI (0.18 ± 0.02), increased cumulative release compared to free 6-shogaol, oral bioavailability	[72]
Lornoxicam	Regular experiment	CCD	$p < 0.05$	Labrafil M 1944 CS (25%), Kolliphor HS 15 (56.25%), Transcutol HP (18.75%)	Particle size, PDI, self-emulsifying time	Design-Expert® n/a version	Particle size (70.14 ± 1.06 nm), PDI (0.193 ± 0.010), self-emulsifying time (68 ± 2 s)	[73]
Chrysin	Compatibility tests and pseudo-ternary phase diagram studies	CCD	$p < 0.05$	Surface morphology, pH, diameter, PDI, zeta potential, and phase type	Maximum drug loading and optimize SMEDDS formation	Design-Expert® n/a version	Medium chain triglyceride:oleic acid:Cremophor RH40: Transcutol HP w/w (12%:12%:32%:44%), with a drug loading capacity of 5 mg/g	[74]
Phillygenin	Compatibility tests and pseudo-ternary phase diagram studies	CCD	$p < 0.05$	Oil phase mass% and surfactant/co-surfactant mixture weight ratio	Equilibrium solubility, particle size, PDI	Design-Expert® version 8.0.6	Optimized Labrafil M1944CS:Cremophor EL:PEG400 = 27.8:33.6:38.6% wt produced 10.2 mg/g equilibrium solubility, 40.11 ± 0.74 nm particle size, and 0.243 ± 0.01 PDI	[75]

Table 5. Cont.

Compound	Screening	RSM	Experiments	Independent Variables	Responses	Program	Optimized Conditions	Reference
Luteolin	Compatibility tests and pseudo-ternary phase diagram studies	CCD	$p < 0.05$	Weight percent of oil and the mass ratio	Particle size, PDI, self-emulsifying time	Design-Expert® version 8.0	Optimized Crodamol GTCC:Kolliphor EL:PEG400 = 20.1:48.2:31.7% wt produced LUT loading capacity = 24.66 mg/g; S-SNEDDS showed 2.2-fold increase of bioavailability compared to conventional SNEDDS.	[76]
Triptolide	n/a	CCD	n/a	Oil phase mass% and surfactant/co-surfactant mixture weight ratio	Particle size and drug content	Design-Expert® version 8.0.6	Optimized MCT:EL:PEG400 = 25.3:49.6:25.1 with particle size of 30.46 nm and drug content of 2.91 mg/g. These optimized parameters produced SMEDDS with complete release in 6 h, increased oral bioavailability, and enhanced the tumor inhibitory effect.	[77]
Ellagic acid	Ternary phase diagram studies	CCD	$p < 0.01$	Oil phase mass% and surfactant/co-surfactant mixture weight ratio	Particle size and solubility	Design-Expert® version 8.0.5	10% ethyl oleate, 67.5% Tween 80, 22.5% PEG 400, 0.5% PVP K30 and 4 mg/g ellagic acid. The presence of PVP K30 in the optimized excipients inhibited the precipitation. The in vitro and in vivo showed an improved antioxidant ability of eligilic acid.	[78]
Rhubarb free-anthraquinone	n/a	CCD	$p < 0.05$	Mass ratio of Neusilin US2/preconcentrated RhA nanoemulsions and contents of PVPP % w/w	Friability, disintegration time, and 4 h cumulative dissolution rate of RhA in SNEDDS tablets	Design-Expert® version 8.0.6	Optimized 1:1(w/w) Neusilin US2/pre-concentrated RhA nanoemulsions, 5.0% w/w PVPP, 1% w/w Mg stearate produced friability of 0.389 ± 0.007%, disintegration time of 5.13 ± 0.14 min, and 4 h-dissolution rate of 87.91 ± 1.89%.	[79]

4.2. Central Composite Design (CCD)

The central composite design (CCD) is the most commonly used fractional factorial design used in the RSM. It is highly applied in constructing the SMEDDS formulations. The CCD was employed in determining the optimized factors for the osmotic pump capsule developed for SMEDDS [80]. The authors constructed the pseudo-ternary phase diagrams to help examine self-emulsifying regions from various types of oils, surfactants, and co-surfactants, followed by a series of characterizations and analyses. To obtain the optimally controlled release properties, the CCD was done on the elements used in capsule coating, including PEG 400, coating weight, and drug release orifice size. The effect of the independent variables resulted in 81.22% cumulative drug release in 12 with the final formulation of 3% PEG 400, 7.5% coating weight, and 0.5 mm of orifice size. The authors also emphasized the use of lack-of-fit analysis to evaluate critical parameters from the pure error in the replicates ($p > 0.05$).

Zheng and coworkers demonstrated supersaturable-SMEDDS for ellagic acid to improve its solubility [78]. The screening process was done using ternary phase diagram studies which were then followed by the CCD to find the best formulation. Oil phase and surfactant/co-surfactant mixture masses ratio were investigated as the independent factors toward the responses, including particle size and solubility (Figure 5). The decrease of oil mass has an effect on the decrease of particle size, yet reversely for the surfactant mixture (K_m). In contrast, the oil gives an inverse relationship toward the solubility. Further, the optimized conditions of supersaturable SMEDDS were revealed to be 10% ethyl oleate, 67.5% Tween 80, 22.5% PEG 400, 0.5% PVP K30, and 4 mg/g ellagic acid. The presence of PVP K30 incorporated in the optimized excipients inhibited the precipitation of the drug due to the nucleation effect. The in vitro and in vivo results showed an improved antioxidant ability of ellagic acid in supersaturable SMEDDS formulation.

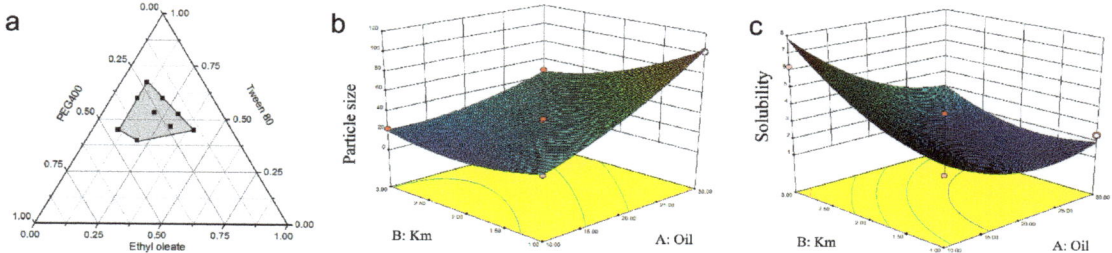

Figure 5. Tertiary-phase diagram showing emulsion areas (in grey color) of the selected masses of the independent variables containing surfactants (i.e., PEG400 and Tween 80 (K_m)) and oil phases (i.e., ethyl oleate) (**a**). Interaction effects in three-dimensional response surface plots for CCD between K_m and oil on particle size (**b**) as well as on solubility (**c**). Adapted from Zheng and coworkers [78].

In addition, Tung and coworkers demonstrated DoE on the selection of excipients to produce pellet SMEDDS containing l-tetrahydropalmatine (l-THP) [81]. The pseudo-ternary diagram was made based on water titration to define the optimum range of Capryol 90, Cremophor RH40, and Transcutol HP as excipients in the selected formulations. The solid carrier employed for pellet SMEDDS was Avicel or Aerosil through extrusion and spheronization techniques. After determining Capryol 90 and the S_{mix} (Cremophor RH40 and Transcutol HP; 3:1) in their best ratio, the central composite face (CCF) design was employed to assess the droplet size, PDI, and dissolution efficiency upon them. As a result, the S_{mix} was indicated to be an antagonist affecting the droplet size and PDI significantly, whereas the Capryol 90 showed a synergistic effect. All responses were well defined according to the optimized parameters with dissolution efficiency of 50%, droplet size of <50 nm, and PDI < 0.3 when using 39.5% capryol 90, 59.2% S_{mix}, and 1.3% l-THP to proceed the liquid SMEDDS to the pellet form. Another CCD strategy was used by Yan and coworkers to examine the similar responses (droplet size, PDI, and dissolution efficiency) toward SMEDDS for β-elemene formulation composing poly (acrylic acid) (PAA) entailed on mesoporous silica nanoparticles (MSNPs). The authors emphasized the use of the PAA/MSNPs loaded in SMEDDS to increase the drug loading and to act as the pH triggers in improving a controlled release behavior in an acidic environment [82]. Several reports of CCD applications that have been incorporated in SMEDDS are listed in Table 6.

4.3. The Mixture Design

There are other design methods in DoE apart from RSM, which are also widely used in optimizing parameters to be selected in SMEDDS studies, such as the simplex lattice. In contrast to the previous explanation that the levels of the factors are independent, in the simplex lattice, the factors are seen as mixed elements that are not independent. Thus, the simple lattice is categorized as a mixture experiment. Another type of mixture experiment design is a D-optimal mixture, which belongs to the optimality criterion design of the 2k factorial. D-optimal mixture design is available in many commercial software packages and is normally selected if there are design points that need to be further minimized so as to reduce the total time required to produce an optimal design [59]. The applications of these methods also provide key information throughout their results, such as described in Table 7.

Table 6. List of the SMEDDS developments along with the applied response surface methodology (RSM) of Box-Behnken design (BBD).

Compound	Screening	RSM	Experiments	Independent Variables	Responses	Program	Optimized Conditions	Reference
Furbiprofen	Regular experiment	BBD (3^3)	$p < 0.05$	Inlet temperature, feed rate, and carrier concentration	%moisture, %yield, drug content, and particle size	Design-Expert® version 8.0.5	%yield (58.5%) and drug content (70.1 mg/g) with minimum moisture content (0.72%) and particle size (166.8 nm).	[69]
Zotepine	Pseudo-ternary diagrams studies	BBD (3^3)	$p < 0.05$	Oleic acid (oil), Tween 80 (surfactant), and PEG400 (co-surfactant)	%microemulsions transparency and %cumulative drug release	Design-Expert® version 8.0.5	%transmittance of 98.75% and an improved 30 min-in vitro drug release of 86.57%.	[68]
Dapsone	Pseudo-ternary diagrams studies	BBD (3^3)	$p < 0.05$	Inlet temperature, feed flow rate, carrier concentration	Particle size and %yield	Design-Expert® version 11.0	The optimized solid SMEDDS with inlet temperature of 130 °C, flow rate of 6 mL/min, and carrier conc. (i.e., neusilin US2) of 0.25% resulted in 87.5 ± 4.95 nm of particle size and yielded 34.06 ± 1.70%.	[83]
Carvedilol	Regular experiments on formulation compositions and hot melt extruder conditions	BBD (3^3)	$p < 0.05$	Recirculation time, first heating zone temperature, API concentration	%drug releases (in 0.1 M HCl and 0.4 M phosphate buffer), %efficiency, and particle size	Statistica® version 7.0	The optimized formulation of carvedilol in solid SMEDDS using hot-melt extrusion resulted in max. 25.54 ± 0.77% release in HCl followed by max. 85.54 ± 1.79% release in phosphate buffer.	[70]
Fenofibrate	Pseudo-ternary diagrams studies	BBD (3^3)	$p < 0.05$	Amount of Labrafil M 1944 (oil), Labrasol (surfactant), and Capryol (co-surfactant)	Particle size, %cumulative release in 30 min, and equilibrium solubility	Design-Expert® version 8.0.4	The optimized formulation of fenofibrate in solid SMEDDS resulted in 113.13 ± 1.63 mg/g solubility with particle size of 171.4 ± 2.5 nm, %cumulative release of 87.7 ± 1.6%, and 3.6-fold higher bioavailability than its free-form suspension.	[84]
Ezetimibe	Pseudo-ternary diagrams studies	BBD (3^3)	$p < 0.05$	Amount of Peceol (oil), Tween 80 (surfactant), Transcutol P (co-surfactant)	Particle size, %transmittance, self-emulsification time, %cumulative releases in 5 and 40 min	Design-Expert® version 11.0	The optimized ezetimibe in solid SMEDDS resulted in 26.31 ± 2.64 nm particle size, 69.26 ± 2.56 self-emulsification time, and 95.38 ± 3.67% cumulative release in 40 min.	[85]
Naproxen	Regular experiment	FFD	$p < 0.05$, except %yield	Inlet temperature, pressure, and pump speed	Droplet size, PDI, and %yield	Unscrambler1 software (version 10.1, CAMO software)	The inlet temperature of 120 °C, pressure of 50 mmHg, and pump speed of 15 mL/min resulted the optimized solid SMEDDS.	[71]

Table 7. List of the SMEDDS developments along with the applied response surface methodology (RSM) of D-optimal mixture design.

Compound	Screening	RSM	Experiments	Independent Variables	Responses	Program	Optimized Conditions	Reference
HL235 (i.e., Cathepsin K inhibitor)	Pseudo-ternary diagrams studies	D-optimal mixture	$p < 0.05$	Capmul MCM (oil), Tween-20 (surfactant), Carbitol (co-surfactant)	Cumulative drug release in 15 min and solubilization capacity	Design-Expert® version 7.0	The optimized SMEDDs formulation resulting in 2.34 ± 0.21 µg/mL and solubilization capacity of 6.164 ± 0.06 mg/mL.	[86]
Blonanserin	Pseudo-ternary diagrams studies	D-optimal mixture	n/a	Captex 200P: Capmul MCM (1:1) (oil), Tween-20 (surfactant), and ethanol (co-surfactant)	Drug loading, percentage cumulative drug release, particle size	n/a	The optimized Blonanserin in SMEDDS with 1:1 (23% v/v) Captex 200P:Capmul MCM mixture, Tween-80 (57% v/v), and ethanol (20% v/v) produced cumulative drug release of 94.72% in 30 min and particle size of 21 nm	[87]
Olmesartan medoxomil	Pseudo-ternary diagrams studies	D-optimal mixture	$p < 0.05$	Capmul MCM EP (oil), Kolliphore EL (surfactant), Transcutol P (co-surfactant)	Cumulative drug release and particle size	JMP ver.9.0.0 software	The optimized formulation with Capmul MCM EP (23% v/v), Kolliphore EL (49% v/v) and Transcutol P (28% v/v) resulted in 94.7% of drug release and 105 nm of particle size.	[88]
Telmisartan (loaded with phospholipid complex)	Pseudo-ternary diagrams studies	D-optimal mixture	$p < 0.05$	Capryol 90 (oil), Tween 80 (surfactant), and tetraglycol (co-surfactant)	Drug loading, drug release, and particle size	Minitab ver.17.0 software	The optimized SMEDDS formulation of telmisartan loaded phospholipid complex resulted in 22.17 nm of globular size, 4.06 mg/mL of solubilization, and 99.4% of drug release in 15 min.	[89]
Curcumin and artemisin	Pseudo-ternary diagrams studies	D-optimal mixture	$p < 0.05$	Oleic acid (oil), Tween-80 (surfactant), and PEG400 (co-surfactant)	%transmittance, particle size, and polydispersity index	Design-Expert® version 10.0	The optimized SMEDDS containing curcumin and artemisin produced 98.27% of transmittance, 150.7 nm of particle size, and 0.118 of polydispersity index.	[90]
Ziyuglycoside I	Solubility and pseudo-ternary diagrams studies	D-optimal mixture	$p < 0.05$	Obleique CC497 (oil), Tween-20 (surfactant), Transcutol HP (co-surfactant)	Drug loading and particle size	Design Expert version 8.0.4.1	An enhanced solubility up to 23.93 mg/g and particle size of 207.92 ± 2.13 nm, along with an improved bioavailability (21.94%) as compared to the free drug (3.16%)	[91]
Insulin	Solubility and pseudo-ternary diagrams studies	D-optimal mixture	$p < 0.05$	Capmul MCM (oil), Labrasol (surfactant), Tetraglycol (co-surfactant)	Particle size, stability, and leakage	Design-Expert version 11.0	The optimized insulin in SMEDDS formulation resulted in particle size of 115.2 nm, enhanced stability up to 46.75%, and lessened leakage down to 17.67%	[92]

Jain and coworkers developed solid SMEDDS for raltegravir potassium, the first line of HIV treatment, by formulating all the selected components within a tablet excipient to improve better stability and dissolution properties of SMEDDS [93]. The simplex lattice method was then employed to rationally design the optimized amounts of independent variables, Labrasol (as oil), Tween-20 (as surfactant), and PEG400 (as co-surfactant). The cumulative percentage of drug release and globular size were examined afterward as the dependent variables. The optimized formulations of SMEDDS were then proceeded with the selected adsorbents to create solid SMEDDS. As a result, the formation of transparent microemulsions of these variables were 50–60% of Labrasol, 20–30% of Tween-20, and 10–30% of PEG400. The presence of either lipid or lipid with co-surfactant interaction greatly affected the cumulative drug release, as shown by the highest coefficient, suggesting that the greater amount of drug was accordingly increased. Meanwhile, lipids with surfactant or lipids with co-surfactant interaction showed a negative coefficient for the globular size, indicating that the increase of either one proportion decreases the globular size of solid SMEDDS to less than 50 nm.

Another simplex lattice design was also employed by Dhaval and coworkers to investigate seven batches of clofazimine formulations in solid SMEDDS. To do this, the authors used the simplex lattice method to obtain critical parameters toward the responses (particle size and cumulative drug releases in pH 1.2 and pH 6.8) from the screened regions of ternary diagram of the independent variables (Capmul MCM, Tween20, and Labrasol). According to the regression analysis of particle size, the coefficient value of oil was much higher than the other variables, suggesting that the change in Capmul MCM proportion significantly influenced particle size microemulsions. In contrast, the increase of the surfactant (Tween 20) showed a significant decrease of the particle size, as depicted in the 3D response surface and contour plots (Figure 6a). Meanwhile, a lower surfactant level with more oil in pH 1.2 media suggested a decrease in drug release percentage from ~90% to 60% (Figure 6b). A similar trend was found in drug release of pH 6.8 results. Therefore, the authors then concluded to use a high proportion of surfactant to later obtain greater cumulative drug release in the batches studies. The desirability function was then employed to evaluate the closeness of the predicted and actual values obtained from the simplex lattice results. All the designed batches demonstrated acceptable results between the predicted and experimental values (with a bias of <5%), showing the effectiveness of the models. From the optimized parameters, the final cumulative drug release obtained was 85% in less than 60 min at two different dissolution media with a globular size of less than 70 nm.

Lee and coworkers investigated SMEDDS formulations for the BCS IV compound, tolvaptan, through the D-optimal mixture design of DoE [66]. Capryol 90, Tween 20, and Transcutol (or PEG200) were selected for the optimized compositions based on tolvaptan solubility studies. Small particle sizes of <250 nm and an increased cumulative drug release of up to 90% in 60 min were obtained in the formulations involving the oil, surfactant, and co-surfactant with a ratio of 10%, 70%, and 20%, respectively. Their results demonstrate that the successful use of a D-optimal mixture design during the development of tolvaptan-loaded SMEDDS improved the dissolution rate and oral drug bioavailability.

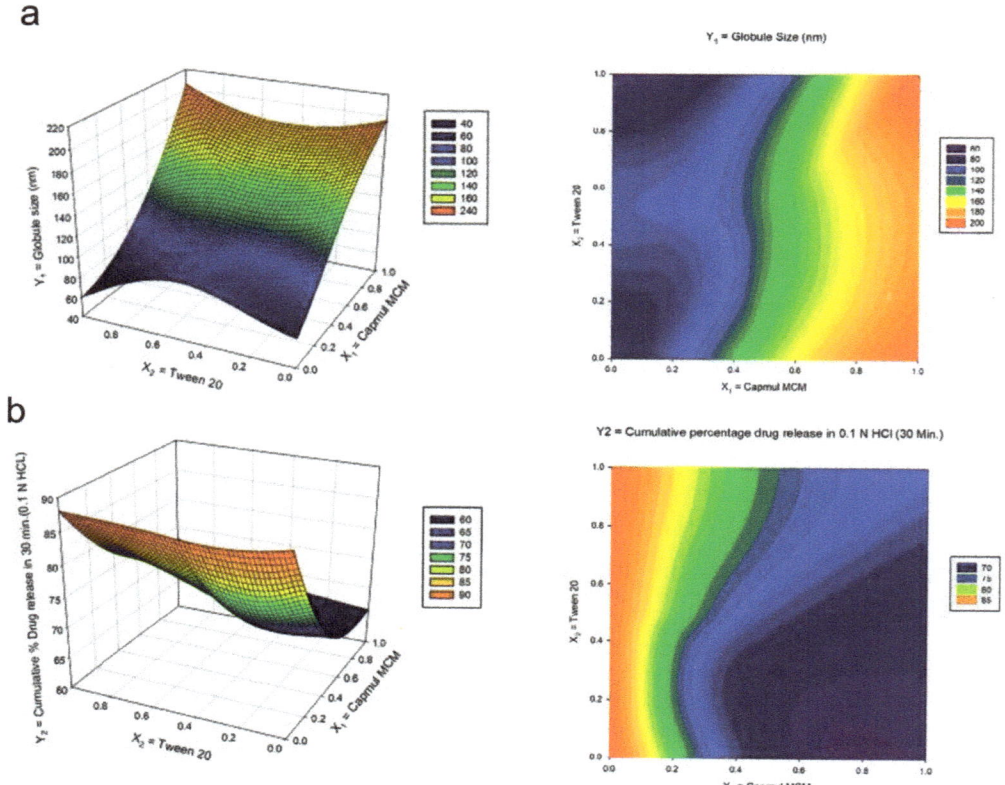

Figure 6. Response surface plot in three-dimension (3D) (left) and the contour plot (right) for the mixture design of the (**a**) globule size and (**b**) cumulative drug release in pH 1.2 media from the study of clofazimine in solid SMEDDS by Dhaval and coworkers. Adapted from Dhaval and coworkers [94].

More recently, Na and coworkers carried out SMEDDS to improve the bioavailability of platelet inhibitor, ticagrelor. The authors first performed a preliminary screening to select the optimum excipients from various oils, surfactants, and co-surfactants through solubility and emulsification studies, where the drug in each excipient resulting in greater solubility would be selected. The variables were then selected according to the optimized regions in the pseudo-ternary diagram, including Capmul MCM (oil), Tween 20, or Cremophor EL (surfactant), and Transcutol P (co-surfactant). Scheffe's mixture design was employed to examine the excipients percentages used with the drug in microemulsions formation toward its solubility, particle size, % transmittance, and % precipitation. As a result, the optimized formulation of ticagrelor in SMEDDS consisting of 10% Capmul MCM, 53.8% Cremophor EL, and 36.2% Transcutol P resulted in maximum values of solubility and % transmittance and minimum values of % precipitation and particle size, along with an exhibited oral bioavailability up to 637.1% as compared to the ticagrelor suspension [95].

There are some reports that only performed the screening process throughout the SMEDDS studies. For instance, Kim and coworkers developed methotreaxate-containing solid SMEDDS [37]. The formulations were done using a spray-drying technique with calcium silicate as the solid carrier. The optimized ratio for castor oil (oil), Tween 80 (surfactant), and Plurol (co-surfactant) were 27:63:10, respectively. The pseudo-ternary diagram was made to assess which formulation could form emulsion simultaneously with a high dissolution rate. As a result, the use of more than 55% surfactant/co-surfactant showed high emulsification efficiency. The methotrexate-containing solid SMEDDS absorption also demonstrated a greater AUC and C_{max} of 2.04 and 3.41 fold, respectively, than the free methotrexate [37].

5. Conclusions

SMEDDS have been a popular lipid-based formulation system for the delivery of poorly soluble drugs due to their potential to improve the bioavailability of these active compounds. However, the process of structure formation can be complicated for a complex lipid-based system due to the presence of surfactant, co-surfactant, co-solvent, and carrier that can significantly influence the processing. Using the DoE approach allows formulation scientists to quickly identify interactions between ingredients and reduce the number of experiments required to optimize formulations. As the consequence, scientists have dramatically reduced the time required for formulation development by utilizing this statistical tool. This review illustrates the principles and applications of the most common screening designs applied to SMEDDS development. Furthermore, the use of DoE can be an efficient and fundamental tool to identify and control the variables involved in this scaling-up process to guarantee large-scale production of SMEDDS with the same pharmaceutical activity obtained on the laboratory scale. Finally, the development of SMEDDS by the application of the DoE concept could be a desirable approach to attaining therapeutic and formulary goals.

Author Contributions: C.-M.H. participated in the conceptualization of this manuscript, writing and editing the manuscript. T.-L.Y. participated in preparing the review structure and writing the original draft. A.D.P. participated in preparing the review structure and writing the original draft. C.-T.C. conceived and conceptualized the manuscript writing, editing, and finalization. All authors have read and agreed to the published version of the manuscript.

Funding: This work was mainly supported by the Ministry of Education, Taiwan, and the Ministry of Science and Technology, Taiwan (MOST-111-2314-B-002-152-M3 & MOST-109-2221-E-038-001-MY3).

Institutional Review Board Statement: Not applicable.

Informed Consent Statement: Not applicable.

Data Availability Statement: Data sharing is not applicable.

Conflicts of Interest: The authors declare no conflict of interest.

References

1. Ghadi, R.; Dand, N. BCS class IV drugs: Highly notorious candidates for formulation development. *J. Control. Release* **2017**, *248*, 71–95. [CrossRef] [PubMed]
2. Kawabata, Y.; Wada, K.; Nakatani, M.; Yamada, S.; Onoue, S. Formulation design for poorly water-soluble drugs based on biopharmaceutics classification system: Basic approaches and practical applications. *Int. J. Pharm.* **2011**, *420*, 1–10. [CrossRef] [PubMed]
3. Savjani, K.T.; Gajjar, A.K.; Savjani, J.K. Drug solubility: Importance and enhancement techniques. *ISRN Pharm* **2012**, *2012*, 195727. [CrossRef] [PubMed]
4. Bhalani, D.V.; Nutan, B.; Kumar, A.; Singh Chandel, A.K. Bioavailability Enhancement Techniques for Poorly Aqueous Soluble Drugs and Therapeutics. *Biomedicines* **2022**, *10*, 2055. [CrossRef]
5. Sharma, V.K.; Koka, A.; Yadav, J.; Sharma, A.K.; Keservani, R.K. Self-micro emulsifying drug delivery systems: A strategy to improve oral bioavailability. *Ars Pharm.* **2016**, *57*, 97–109. [CrossRef]
6. Desai, P.M.; Tan, B.M.; Liew, C.V.; Chan, L.W.; Heng, P.W. Impact of Electrostatics on Processing and Product Performance of Pharmaceutical Solids. *Curr. Pharm. Des.* **2015**, *21*, 5923–5929. [CrossRef]
7. Pedrosa, V.M.; Sanches, A.G.; da Silva, M.B.; Gratao, P.L.; Isaac, V.L.; Gindri, M.; Teixeira, G.H. Production of mycosporine-like amino acid (MAA)-loaded emulsions as chemical barriers to control sunscald in fruits and vegetables. *J. Sci. Food Agric.* **2022**, *102*, 801–812. [CrossRef]
8. Koli, A.R.; Ranch, K.M.; Patel, H.P.; Parikh, R.K.; Shah, D.O.; Maulvi, F.A. Oral bioavailability improvement of felodipine using tailored microemulsion: Surface science, ex vivo and in vivo studies. *Int. J. Pharm.* **2021**, *596*, 120202. [CrossRef]
9. Baek, J.S.; Cho, C.W. Surface modification of solid lipid nanoparticles for oral delivery of curcumin: Improvement of bioavailability through enhanced cellular uptake, and lymphatic uptake. *Eur. J. Pharm. Biopharm.* **2017**, *117*, 132–140. [CrossRef]

10. Murthy, A.; Ravi, P.R.; Kathuria, H.; Malekar, S. Oral Bioavailability Enhancement of Raloxifene with Nanostructured Lipid Carriers. *Nanomaterials* **2020**, *10*, 1085. [CrossRef]
11. Sharma, A.; Streets, J.; Bhatt, P.; Patel, P.; Sutariya, V.; Varghese Gupta, S. Formulation and Characterization of Raloxifene Nanostructured Lipid Carriers for Permeability and Uptake Enhancement Applications. *Assay Drug. Dev. Technol.* **2022**, *20*, 164–174. [CrossRef] [PubMed]
12. Yamazoe, E.; Fang, J.Y.; Tahara, K. Oral mucus-penetrating PEGylated liposomes to improve drug absorption: Differences in the interaction mechanisms of a mucoadhesive liposome. *Int. J. Pharm.* **2021**, *593*, 120148. [CrossRef] [PubMed]
13. Pouton, C.W. Lipid formulations for oral administration of drugs: Non-emulsifying, self-emulsifying and 'self-microemulsifying' drug delivery systems. *Eur. J. Pharm. Sci.* **2000**, *11* (Suppl. 2), S93–S98. [CrossRef]
14. Pouton, C.W. Formulation of poorly water-soluble drugs for oral administration: Physicochemical and physiological issues and the lipid formulation classification system. *Eur. J. Pharm. Sci.* **2006**, *29*, 278–287. [CrossRef]
15. Huang, Y.; Yu, Q.; Chen, Z.; Wu, W.; Zhu, Q.; Lu, Y. In vitro and in vivo correlation for lipid-based formulations: Current status and future perspectives. *Acta Pharm. Sin. B* **2021**, *11*, 2469–2487. [CrossRef] [PubMed]
16. Tay, E.; Nguyen, T.H.; Ford, L.; Williams, H.D.; Benameur, H.; Scammells, P.J.; Porter, C.J.H. Ionic Liquid Forms of the Antimalarial Lumefantrine in Combination with LFCS Type IIIB Lipid-Based Formulations Preferentially Increase Lipid Solubility, In Vitro Solubilization Behavior and In Vivo Exposure. *Pharmaceutics* **2019**, *12*, 17. [CrossRef] [PubMed]
17. Rahman, M.A.; Harwansh, R.; Mirza, M.A.; Hussain, S.; Hussain, A. Oral lipid based drug delivery system (LBDDS): Formulation, characterization and application: A review. *Curr. Drug Deliv.* **2011**, *8*, 330–345. [CrossRef]
18. Feng, W.; Qin, C.; Cipolla, E.; Lee, J.B.; Zgair, A.; Chu, Y.; Ortori, C.A.; Stocks, M.J.; Constantinescu, C.S.; Barrett, D.A.; et al. Inclusion of Medium-Chain Triglyceride in Lipid-Based Formulation of Cannabidiol Facilitates Micellar Solubilization In Vitro, but In Vivo Performance Remains Superior with Pure Sesame Oil Vehicle. *Pharmaceutics* **2021**, *13*, 1349. [CrossRef]
19. Gao, H.; Jia, H.; Dong, J.; Yang, X.; Li, H.; Ouyang, D. Integrated in silico formulation design of self-emulsifying drug delivery systems. *Acta Pharm. Sin. B* **2021**, *11*, 3585–3594. [CrossRef]
20. Jadhav, H.; Waghmare, J.; Annapure, U. Study on oxidative stability of deep fat fried food in Canola oil blended with medium chain triglyceride. *Indian J. Chem. Technol.* **2022**, *29*, 95–98.
21. Kaukonen, A.M.; Boyd, B.J.; Porter, C.J.; Charman, W.N. Drug solubilization behavior during in vitro digestion of simple triglyceride lipid solution formulations. *Pharm. Res.* **2004**, *21*, 245–253. [CrossRef] [PubMed]
22. Cerpnjak, K.; Zvonar, A.; Gasperlin, M.; Vrecer, F. Lipid-based systems as a promising approach for enhancing the bioavailability of poorly water-soluble drugs. *Acta Pharm.* **2013**, *63*, 427–445. [CrossRef]
23. Rosen, M.J.; Kunjappu, J.T. *Surfactants and Interfacial Phenomena*; John Wiley & Sons: Hoboken, NJ, USA, 2012.
24. Wilson, C.G.; Halbert, G.W.; Mains, J. The gut in the beaker: Missing the surfactants? *Int. J. Pharm.* **2016**, *514*, 73–80. [CrossRef] [PubMed]
25. Gelardi, G.; Mantellato, S.; Marchon, D.; Palacios, M.; Eberhardt, A.B.; Flatt, R.J. admixtures. In *Science and Technology of Concrete Admixtures*; Aïtcin, P.-C., Flatt, R.J., Eds.; Woodhead Publishing: Cambridge, UK, 2016; pp. 149–218. [CrossRef]
26. Zhu, Y.; Ye, J.; Zhang, Q. Self-emulsifying Drug Delivery System Improve Oral Bioavailability: Role of Excipients and Physico-chemical Characterization. *Pharm. Nanotechnol.* **2020**, *8*, 290–301. [CrossRef]
27. Rowe, R.C.; Sheskey, P.J.; Cook, W.G.; Fenton, M.E. *Handbook of Pharmaceutical Excipients*, 6th ed.; APhA/Pharmaceutical Press: London, UK, 2012; p. 1033.
28. Lalanne-Cassou, C.; Carmona, I.; Fortney, L.; Samii, A.; Schechter, R.; Wade, W.; Weerasooriya, U.; Weerasooriya, V.; Yiv, S. Minimizing cosolvent requirements for microemulsion formed with binary surfactant mixtures. *J. Dispers. Sci. Technol.* **1987**, *8*, 137–156. [CrossRef]
29. Dokania, S.; Joshi, A.K. Self-microemulsifying drug delivery system (SMEDDS)—Challenges and road ahead. *Drug Deliv.* **2015**, *22*, 675–690. [CrossRef]
30. Jorgensen, A.M.; Friedl, J.D.; Wibel, R.; Chamieh, J.; Cottet, H.; Bernkop-Schnurch, A. Cosolvents in Self-Emulsifying Drug Delivery Systems (SEDDS): Do They Really Solve Our Solubility Problems? *Mol. Pharm.* **2020**, *17*, 3236–3245. [CrossRef]
31. Prince, L.M. *Microemulsions: Theory and Practice*; Academic Press: New York, NY, USA, 1977; p. 179.
32. Anton, N.; Vandamme, T.F. Nano-emulsions and micro-emulsions: Clarifications of the critical differences. *Pharm Res.* **2011**, *28*, 978–985. [CrossRef] [PubMed]
33. McClements, D.J. Nanoemulsions versus microemulsions: Terminology, differences, and similarities. *Soft Matter.* **2012**, *8*, 1719–1729. [CrossRef]
34. Tiwari, P.; Ranjan Sinha, V.; Kaur, R. Chapter 4—Clinical considerations on micro- and nanodrug delivery systems. In *Drug Delivery Trends*; Shegokar, R., Ed.; Elsevier: Amsterdam, The Netherlands, 2020; pp. 77–101. [CrossRef]
35. Callender, S.P.; Mathews, J.A.; Kobernyk, K.; Wettig, S.D. Microemulsion utility in pharmaceuticals: Implications for multi-drug delivery. *Int. J. Pharm.* **2017**, *526*, 425–442. [CrossRef]
36. Yang, T.L.; Hsieh, C.M.; Meng, L.J.; Tsai, T.; Chen, C.T. Oleic Acid-Based Self Micro-Emulsifying Delivery System for Enhancing Antifungal Activities of Clotrimazole. *Pharmaceutics* **2022**, *14*, 478. [CrossRef] [PubMed]
37. Kim, D.S.; Cho, J.H.; Park, J.H.; Kim, J.S.; Song, E.S.; Kwon, J.; Giri, B.R.; Jin, S.G.; Kim, K.S.; Choi, H.G.; et al. Self-microemulsifying drug delivery system (SMEDDS) for improved oral delivery and photostability of methotrexate. *Int. J. Nanomed.* **2019**, *14*, 4949–4960. [CrossRef]

38. Kamboj, S.; Rana, V. Quality-by-design based development of a self-microemulsifying drug delivery system to reduce the effect of food on Nelfinavir mesylate. *Int. J. Pharm.* **2016**, *501*, 311–325. [CrossRef] [PubMed]
39. Han, S.D.; Jung, S.W.; Jang, S.W.; Son, M.; Kim, B.M.; Kang, M.J. Reduced Food-Effect on Intestinal Absorption of Dronedarone by Self-microemulsifying Drug Delivery System (SMEDDS). *Biol. Pharm. Bull.* **2015**, *38*, 1026–1032. [CrossRef] [PubMed]
40. Naccarelli, G.V.; Wolbrette, D.L.; Levin, V.; Samii, S.; Banchs, J.E.; Penny-Peterson, E.; Gonzalez, M.D. Safety and efficacy of dronedarone in the treatment of atrial fibrillation/flutter. *Clin. Med. Insights Cardiol.* **2011**, *5*, 103–119. [CrossRef]
41. Renugopal, P.; Sangeetha, S.; Damodharan, N. An Emerging Trend in Solid Self Micro Emulsifying Drug Delivery System. *Res. J. Pharm. Technol.* **2020**, *13*, 3028–3034. [CrossRef]
42. Salawi, A. Self-emulsifying drug delivery systems: A novel approach to deliver drugs. *Drug Deliv.* **2022**, *29*, 1811–1823. [CrossRef]
43. Caliph, S.M.; Charman, W.N.; Porter, C.J.H. Effect of Short-, Medium-, and Long-Chain Fatty Acid-Based Vehicles on the Absolute Oral Bioavailability and Intestinal Lymphatic Transport of Halofantrine and Assessment of Mass Balance in Lymph-Cannulated and Non-cannulated Rats. *J. Pharm. Sci.* **2000**, *89*, 1073–1084. [CrossRef]
44. Rahman, M.A.; Hussain, A.; Hussain, M.S.; Mirza, M.A.; Iqbal, Z. Role of excipients in successful development of self-emulsifying/microemulsifying drug delivery system (SEDDS/SMEDDS). *Drug Dev. Ind. Pharm.* **2013**, *39*, 1–19. [CrossRef]
45. Kadu, P.J.; Kushare, S.S.; Thacker, D.D.; Gattani, S.G. Enhancement of oral bioavailability of atorvastatin calcium by self-emulsifying drug delivery systems (SEDDS). *Pharm. Dev. Technol.* **2011**, *16*, 65–74. [CrossRef]
46. Heshmati, N.; Cheng, X.; Eisenbrand, G.; Fricker, G. Enhancement of oral bioavailability of E804 by self-nanoemulsifying drug delivery system (SNEDDS) in rats. *J. Pharm. Sci.* **2013**, *102*, 3792–3799. [CrossRef] [PubMed]
47. Li, L.; Hui Zhou, C.; Ping Xu, Z. Chapter 14—Self-Nanoemulsifying Drug-Delivery System. In *Nanocarriers for Drug Delivery*; Mohapatra, S.S., Ranjan, S., Dasgupta, N., Mishra, R.K., Thomas, S., Eds.; Elsevier: Amsterdam, The Netherlands, 2019; pp. 421–449. [CrossRef]
48. Hamed, R.; Awadallah, A.; Sunoqrot, S.; Tarawneh, O.; Nazzal, S.; AlBaraghthi, T.; Al Sayyad, J.; Abbas, A. pH-Dependent Solubility and Dissolution Behavior of Carvedilol–Case Example of a Weakly Basic BCS Class II Drug. *AAPS PharmSciTech* **2016**, *17*, 418–426. [CrossRef]
49. Abuhelwa, A.Y.; Williams, D.B.; Upton, R.N.; Foster, D.J. Food, gastrointestinal pH, and models of oral drug absorption. *Eur. J. Pharm. Biopharm.* **2017**, *112*, 234–248. [CrossRef] [PubMed]
50. Akula, S.; Gurram, A.K.; Devireddy, S.R. Self-Microemulsifying Drug Delivery Systems: An Attractive Strategy for Enhanced Therapeutic Profile. *Int. Sch. Res. Not.* **2014**, *2014*, 964051. [CrossRef] [PubMed]
51. Yang, Z.; Wang, Y.; Cheng, J.; Shan, B.; Wang, Y.; Wang, R.; Hou, L. Solid self-microemulsifying drug delivery system of Sophoraflavanone G: Prescription optimization and pharmacokinetic evaluation. *Eur. J. Pharm. Sci* **2019**, *136*, 104953. [CrossRef]
52. Musakhanian, J.; Rodier, J.D.; Dave, M. Oxidative Stability in Lipid Formulations: A Review of the Mechanisms, Drivers, and Inhibitors of Oxidation. *AAPS PharmSciTech* **2022**, *23*, 151. [CrossRef]
53. Gabric, A.; Hodnik, Z.; Pajk, S. Oxidation of Drugs during Drug Product Development: Problems and Solutions. *Pharmaceutics* **2022**, *14*, 325. [CrossRef]
54. Yeom, D.W.; Chae, B.R.; Son, H.Y.; Kim, J.H.; Chae, J.S.; Song, S.H.; Oh, D.; Choi, Y.W. Enhanced oral bioavailability of valsartan using a polymer-based supersaturable self-microemulsifying drug delivery system. *Int. J. Nanomed.* **2017**, *12*, 3533–3545. [CrossRef] [PubMed]
55. ICH. *ICH Harmonised Tripartite Guideline*; Q8 (R2) Pharmaceutical Development; ICH: London, UK, 2009.
56. Yu, L.X.; Amidon, G.; Khan, M.A.; Hoag, S.W.; Polli, J.; Raju, G.; Woodcock, J.J.T.A.j. Understanding pharmaceutical quality by design. *AAPS J.* **2014**, *16*, 771–783. [CrossRef]
57. Astakhov, V.P. Design of experiment methods in manufacturing: Basics and practical applications. In *Statistical and Computational Techniques in Manufacturing*; Springer: Berlin/Heidelberg, Germany, 2012; pp. 1–54.
58. Fisher, R.A. Design of experiments. *Br. Med. J.* **1936**, *1*, 554. [CrossRef]
59. Montgomery, D.C. *Design and Analysis of Experiments*; John Wiley & Sons: Hoboken, NJ, USA, 2017.
60. Beg, S.; Raza, K. Full Factorial and Fractional Factorial Design Applications in Pharmaceutical Product Development. In *Design of Experiments for Pharmaceutical Product Development: Volume I: Basics and Fundamental Principles*; Beg, S., Ed.; Springer: Singapore, 2021; pp. 43–53. [CrossRef]
61. Box, G.E.; Hunter, W.H.; Hunter, S. *Statistics for Experimenters*; John Wiley and Sons: New York, NY, USA, 1978; Volume 664.
62. Plackett, R.L.; Burman, J.P. The design of optimum multifactorial experiments. *Biometrika* **1946**, *33*, 305–325. [CrossRef]
63. Mousavi, L.; Tamiji, Z.; Khoshayand, M.R. Applications and opportunities of experimental design for the dispersive liquid–liquid microextraction method—A review. *Talanta* **2018**, *190*, 335–356. [CrossRef]
64. Luiz, M.T.; Viegas, J.S.R.; Abriata, J.P.; Viegas, F.; de Carvalho Vicentini, F.T.M.; Bentley, M.V.L.B.; Chorilli, M.; Marchetti, J.M.; Tapia-Blacido, D.R. Design of experiments (DoE) to develop and to optimize nanoparticles as drug delivery systems. *Eur. J. Pharm. Biopharm.* **2021**, *165*, 127–148. [CrossRef] [PubMed]
65. Sy Mohamad, S.F.; Mohd Said, F.; Abdul Munaim, M.S.; Mohamad, S.; Azizi Wan Sulaiman, W.M.J.C.r.i.b. Application of experimental designs and response surface methods in screening and optimization of reverse micellar extraction. *Crit. Rev. Biotechnol.* **2020**, *40*, 341–356. [CrossRef]
66. Lee, J.H.; Lee, G.W. Formulation Approaches for Improving the Dissolution Behavior and Bioavailability of Tolvaptan Using SMEDDS. *Pharmaceutics* **2022**, *14*, 415. [CrossRef] [PubMed]

67. Na, Y.G.; Byeon, J.J.; Wang, M.; Huh, H.W.; Kim, M.K.; Bang, K.H.; Han, M.G.; Lee, H.K.; Cho, C.W. Statistical approach for solidifying ticagrelor loaded self-microemulsifying drug delivery system with enhanced dissolution and oral bioavailability. *Mater. Sci. Eng. C Mater. Biol. Appl.* **2019**, *104*, 109980. [CrossRef]
68. Dalvadi, H.; Patel, N.; Parmar, K. Systematic development of design of experiments (DoE) optimised self-microemulsifying drug delivery system of Zotepine. *J. Microencapsul.* **2017**, *34*, 308–318. [CrossRef]
69. Marasini, N.; Tran, T.H.; Poudel, B.K.; Choi, H.-G.; Yong, C.S.; Kim, J.O.J.C.; Bulletin, P. Statistical modeling, optimization and characterization of spray-dried solid self-microemulsifying drug delivery system using design of experiments. *Chem. Pharm. Bull.* **2013**, *61*, 184–193. [CrossRef] [PubMed]
70. Silva, L.A.D.; Almeida, S.L.; Alonso, E.C.P.; Rocha, P.B.R.; Martins, F.T.; Freitas, L.A.P.; Taveira, S.F.; Cunha-Filho, M.S.S.; Marreto, R.N. Preparation of a solid self-microemulsifying drug delivery system by hot-melt extrusion. *Int. J. Pharm.* **2018**, *541*, 1–10. [CrossRef]
71. Čerpnjak, K.; Pobirk, A.Z.; Vrečer, F.; Gašperlin, M. Tablets and minitablets prepared from spray-dried SMEDDS containing naproxen. *Int. J. Pharm.* **2015**, *495*, 336–346. [CrossRef]
72. Huang, Y.; Zhang, S.; Shen, H.; Li, J.; Gao, C.J.A.P. Controlled release of the Nimodipine-loaded self-microemulsion osmotic pump capsules: Development and characterization. *AAPS PharmSciTech* **2018**, *19*, 1308–1319. [CrossRef] [PubMed]
73. Zheng, D.; Lv, C.; Sun, X.; Wang, J.; Zhao, Z. Preparation of a supersaturatable self-microemulsion as drug delivery system for ellagic acid and evaluation of its antioxidant activities. *J. Drug Deliv. Sci. Technol.* **2019**, *53*, 101209. [CrossRef]
74. Tung, N.-T.; Tran, C.-S.; Nguyen, H.-A.; Nguyen, T.-L.; Chi, S.-C.; Nguyen, D.-D.J.I.j.o.p. Development of solidified self-microemulsifying drug delivery systems containing l-tetrahydropalmatine: Design of experiment approach and bioavailability comparison. *Int. J. Pharm.* **2018**, *537*, 9–21. [CrossRef] [PubMed]
75. Yan, B.; Wang, Y.; Ma, Y.; Zhao, J.; Liu, Y.; Wang, L. In vitro and in vivo evaluation of poly (acrylic acid) modified mesoporous silica nanoparticles as pH response carrier for β-elemene self-micro emulsifying. *Int. J. Pharm.* **2019**, *572*, 118768. [CrossRef] [PubMed]
76. Jain, S.; Dudhat, K.; Soniwala, M.; Kotadiya, N.; Mori, D.J.J.o.P.I. DoE-Based Solid Self-microemulsifying Drug Delivery System (S-SMEDDS) Approach for Improving the Dissolution Properties of Raltegravir Potassium. *J. Pharm. Innov.* **2022**. [CrossRef]
77. Dhaval, M.; Panjwani, M.; Parmar, R.; Soniwala, M.M.; Dudhat, K.; Chavda, J. Application of Simple Lattice Design and Desirability Function for Formulating and Optimizing SMEDDS of Clofazimine. *J. Pharm. Innov.* **2021**, *16*, 504–515. [CrossRef]
78. Na, Y.G.; Byeon, J.J.; Wang, M.; Huh, H.W.; Son, G.H.; Jeon, S.H.; Bang, K.H.; Kim, S.J.; Lee, H.J.; Lee, H.K.; et al. Strategic approach to developing a self-microemulsifying drug delivery system to enhance antiplatelet activity and bioavailability of ticagrelor. *Int. J. Nanomed.* **2019**, *14*, 1193–1212. [CrossRef]
79. Yang, Q.; Wang, Q.; Feng, Y.; Wei, Q.; Sun, C.; Firempong, C.K.; Adu-Frimpong, M.; Li, R.; Bao, R.; Toreniyazov, E.; et al. Anti-hyperuricemic property of 6-shogaol via self-micro emulsifying drug delivery system in model rats: Formulation design, in vitro and in vivo evaluation. *Drug Dev. Ind. Pharm.* **2019**, *45*, 1265–1276. [CrossRef]
80. Li, F.; Song, S.; Guo, Y.; Zhao, Q.; Zhang, X.; Pan, W.; Yang, X. Preparation and pharmacokinetics evaluation of oral self-emulsifying system for poorly water-soluble drug Lornoxicam. *Drug Deliv.* **2015**, *22*, 487–498. [CrossRef]
81. Qu, Y.; Mu, S.; Song, C.; Zheng, G. Preparation and in vitro/in vivo evaluation of a self-microemulsifying drug delivery system containing chrysin. *Drug Dev. Ind. Pharm.* **2021**, *47*, 1127–1139. [CrossRef]
82. Wang, L.; Yan, W.; Tian, Y.; Xue, H.; Tang, J.; Zhang, L. Self-microemulsifying drug delivery system of phillygenin: Formulation development, characterization and pharmacokinetic evaluation. *Pharmaceutics* **2020**, *12*, 130. [CrossRef]
83. Zhang, N.; Zhang, F.; Xu, S.; Yun, K.; Wu, W.; Pan, W. Formulation and evaluation of luteolin supersaturatable self-nanoemulsifying drug delivery system (S-SNEDDS) for enhanced oral bioavailability. *J. Drug Deliv. Sci. Technol.* **2020**, *58*, 101783. [CrossRef]
84. Xie, M.; Wu, J.; Ji, L.; Jiang, X.; Zhang, J.; Ge, M.; Cai, X. Development of triptolide self-microemulsifying drug delivery system and its anti-tumor effect on gastric cancer xenografts. *Front. Oncol.* **2019**, *9*, 978. [CrossRef] [PubMed]
85. Niu, J.e.; Xu, Z.; Li, X.; Wang, Z.; Li, J.; Yang, Z.; Khattak, S.U.; Liu, Y.; Shi, Y. Development and evaluation of rhubarb free anthraquinones loaded self-nanoemulsifying tablets. *J. Drug Deliv. Sci. Technol.* **2020**, *57*, 101737. [CrossRef]
86. Mahore, J.; Shelar, A.; Deshkar, S.; More, G.J.J.R.P. Conceptual design and optimization of self microemulsifying drug delivery systems for dapsone by using Box-Behnken design. *J. Res. Pharm.* **2021**, *25*, 179–195.
87. Lee, D.W.; Marasini, N.; Poudel, B.K.; Kim, J.H.; Cho, H.J.; Moon, B.K.; Choi, H.-G.; Yong, C.S.; Kim, J.O.J.J.o.m. Application of Box–Behnken design in the preparation and optimization of fenofibrate-loaded self-microemulsifying drug delivery system (SMEDDS). *J. Microencapsul.* **2014**, *31*, 31–40. [CrossRef]
88. Yadav, P.; Rastogi, V.; Verma, A. Application of Box–Behnken design and desirability function in the development and optimization of self-nanoemulsifying drug delivery system for enhanced dissolution of ezetimibe. *Future J. Pharm. Sci.* **2020**, *6*, 7. [CrossRef]
89. Visetvichaporn, V.; Kim, K.-H.; Jung, K.; Cho, Y.-S.; Kim, D.-D. Formulation of self-microemulsifying drug delivery system (SMEDDS) by D-optimal mixture design to enhance the oral bioavailability of a new cathepsin K inhibitor (HL235). *Int. J. Pharm.* **2020**, *573*, 118772. [CrossRef] [PubMed]
90. Vaghela, S.; Chaudhary, S.; Chaudhary, A. Formulation Development and Optimization of Blonanserin Liquid SMEDDS using D-Optimal Mixture Design. *Curr. Drug Ther.* **2022**, *17*, 266–280. [CrossRef]

91. Gahlawat, N.; Verma, R.; Kaushik, D. Application of D-optimal Mixture Design for Development and Optimization of Olmesartan Medoxomil Loaded SMEDDS. *Curr. Drug Ther.* **2020**, *15*, 548–560. [CrossRef]
92. Son, H.Y.; Chae, B.R.; Choi, J.Y.; Shin, D.J.; Goo, Y.T.; Lee, E.S.; Kang, T.H.; Kim, C.H.; Yoon, H.Y.; Choi, Y.W. Optimization of self-microemulsifying drug delivery system for phospholipid complex of telmisartan using D-optimal mixture design. *PLoS ONE* **2018**, *13*, e0208339. [CrossRef] [PubMed]
93. Shah, A.; Thakkar, V.; Gohel, M.; Baldaniya, L.; Gandhi, T. Optimization of Self Micro Emulsifying Drug Delivery System Containing Curcumin and Artemisinin Using D-Optimal Mixture Design. *J Saudi J. Med. Pharm. Sci* **2017**, *3*, 388–398.
94. Xiong, Y.; Zou, Y.; Chen, L.; Xu, Y.; Wang, S.J.A.P. Development and in vivo evaluation of ziyuglycoside i–loaded self-microemulsifying formulation for activity of increasing leukocyte. *AAPS PharmSciTech* **2019**, *20*, 101. [CrossRef] [PubMed]
95. Goo, Y.T.; Lee, S.; Choi, J.Y.; Kim, M.S.; Sin, G.H.; Hong, S.H.; Kim, C.H.; Song, S.H.; Choi, Y.W. Enhanced oral absorption of insulin: Hydrophobic ion pairing and a self-microemulsifying drug delivery system using a D-optimal mixture design. *Drug Deliv.* **2022**, *29*, 2831–2845. [CrossRef] [PubMed]

Disclaimer/Publisher's Note: The statements, opinions and data contained in all publications are solely those of the individual author(s) and contributor(s) and not of MDPI and/or the editor(s). MDPI and/or the editor(s) disclaim responsibility for any injury to people or property resulting from any ideas, methods, instructions or products referred to in the content.

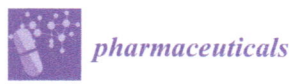

Review

Gastrointestinal Permeation Enhancers for the Development of Oral Peptide Pharmaceuticals

Jae Cheon Kim [1], Eun Ji Park [2,*] and Dong Hee Na [1,*]

[1] College of Pharmacy, Chung-Ang University, Seoul 06974, Republic of Korea
[2] D&D Pharmatech, Seongnam 13486, Republic of Korea
* Correspondence: ejpark@ddpharmatech.com (E.J.P.); dhna@cau.ac.kr (D.H.N.)

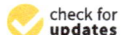

Citation: Kim, J.C.; Park, E.J.; Na, D.H. Gastrointestinal Permeation Enhancers for the Development of Oral Peptide Pharmaceuticals. *Pharmaceuticals* 2022, 15, 1585. https://doi.org/10.3390/ph15121585

Academic Editors: Silviya Petrova Zustiak and Era Jain

Received: 7 November 2022
Accepted: 16 December 2022
Published: 19 December 2022

Publisher's Note: MDPI stays neutral with regard to jurisdictional claims in published maps and institutional affiliations.

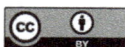

Copyright: © 2022 by the authors. Licensee MDPI, Basel, Switzerland. This article is an open access article distributed under the terms and conditions of the Creative Commons Attribution (CC BY) license (https://creativecommons.org/licenses/by/4.0/).

Abstract: Recently, two oral-administered peptide pharmaceuticals, semaglutide and octreotide, have been developed and are considered as a breakthrough in peptide and protein drug delivery system development. In 2019, the Food and Drug Administration (FDA) approved an oral dosage form of semaglutide developed by Novo Nordisk (Rybelsus®) for the treatment of type 2 diabetes. Subsequently, the octreotide capsule (Mycapssa®), developed through Chiasma's Transient Permeation Enhancer (TPE) technology, also received FDA approval in 2020 for the treatment of acromegaly. These two oral peptide products have been a significant success; however, a major obstacle to their oral delivery remains the poor permeability of peptides through the intestinal epithelium. Therefore, gastrointestinal permeation enhancers are of great relevance for the development of subsequent oral peptide products. Sodium salcaprozate (SNAC) and sodium caprylate (C8) have been used as gastrointestinal permeation enhancers for semaglutide and octreotide, respectively. Herein, we briefly review two approved products, Rybelsus® and Mycapssa®, and discuss the permeation properties of SNAC and medium chain fatty acids, sodium caprate (C10) and C8, focusing on Eligen technology using SNAC, TPE technology using C8, and gastrointestinal permeation enhancement technology (GIPET) using C10.

Keywords: peptides; oral delivery; permeation enhancers; medium chain fatty acids; sodium salcaprozate

1. Introduction

Significant attention in the pharmaceutical industry is being given to therapeutic peptides; an increasingly important group of pharmaceuticals [1]. There are currently over 80 peptide drugs in the global market, and research on new peptide therapeutics is ongoing, including over 150 peptides in clinical development and about 600 peptides in preclinical studies [2]. Peptides are a therapeutically unique class of pharmaceuticals poised between small organic molecules and large proteins, with potential as medium-sized therapeutics with properties that differ from those of small chemicals and large biomolecules [3]. Compared with small chemical drugs, peptides can cover a wider area of the target site and thus have superior potency and lower toxicity due to the specificity of interaction with target receptors. Moreover, peptides are often superior to proteins as drug candidates because of their lower cost of production and higher tissue permeability [4,5]. However, a therapeutic drawback of peptide drugs exists; their administration is mainly limited to injectable routes for two major reasons: low gastrointestinal permeability and high enzymatic degradation [6–8].

Since injectable peptide drugs require continuous and repeated administration, which causes patient discomfort and has a great effect on medication compliance, pharmaceutical efforts have been directed at improving the invasive administration of injectable formulations [9,10].

The first representative example is the adjustment of the dosing interval through glucagon-like peptide-1 (GLP-1) receptor agonist half-life improvement. Exenatide, first developed in 2005, requires injection twice daily [11]. Since then, products that are administered once daily (lixisenatide and liraglutide) and once a week (dulaglutide, albiglutide, and semaglutide) have been developed by improving the half-life of the peptide. More recently, a daily oral administration product (oral semaglutide, Rybelsus®) has been developed [12].

Furthermore, octreotide has also undergone a flow of formulation development to improve dosing convenience. Since the endogenous hormone somatostatin has a short half-life of less than 3 min, octreotide, a synthetic somatostatin receptor ligand with an improved half-life (90–120 min), was developed in the 1980s [13]. Octreotide was initially developed as a subcutaneous injectable formulation administered 2–3 times daily. The frequent administration caused patient discomfort, and in the 1990s, octreotide LAR (long-acting release) product, administered once a month, was developed to improve the dosing interval [14]. Notwithstanding this dramatic dosing interval improvement, the intramuscular injectable form of octreotide LAR required a fairly thick 19-gauge (diameter: 1.1 mm) needle, which caused pain during administration and posed several pharmaceutical problems [15–17]. In order to improve the disadvantages of the octreotide injectable administration, an octreotide subcutaneous depot formulation (CAM2029)—with the advantages of being administered once a month, being less painful because of a thinner needle, and its self-administration option by subcutaneous injection—is being developed and is undergoing phase 3 clinical trials [18,19]. Finally, in 2020, the FDA approved an oral octreotide product (Mycapssa®) that goes beyond the limits of injectable products (Figure 1).

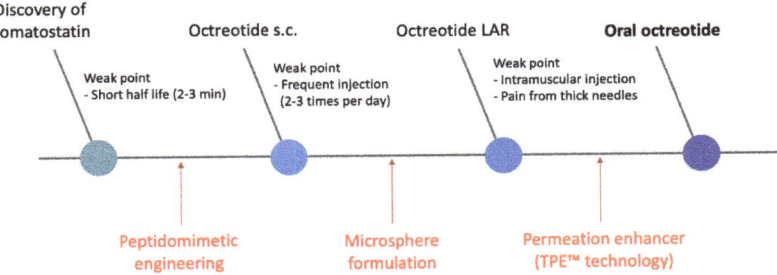

Figure 1. The historical chart of the octreotide formulation development process.

As seen in the development flow of two peptide drugs, injectable peptide drugs have a history of improved injectable formulations with longer administration intervals and better convenience. Recently, research is ongoing to achieve the final goal of developing oral formulations. Strategies for oral administration of peptides are broadly divided into four methods: (1) permeation enhancers (PEs), (2) nanoparticles [20–23], (3) lipid-based drug delivery systems (self-emulsifying drug delivery systems (SEDDS) or hydrophobic ion-pairing [24,25], and (4) microneedle devices [26–28]. Among these, PEs are the leading strategy. Two hitherto approved oral peptide drugs, Rybelsus® and Mycapssa®, have been successfully converted to oral dosage forms using the PE strategy, and research is underway for the development of oral dosage forms of many peptide drugs through a similar strategy.

There are several substances expected to be used as PEs that can be classified into chemical and peptide PEs as per the material standard, and into paracellular and transcellular PEs as per the mechanism standard. Representative examples of chemical PEs that are being applied to various peptides and currently being studied include medium chain fatty acids (MCFAs), Eligen™ technology-based PEs (SNAC, 5-CNAC, 4-CNAB), EDTA, bile salt [29,30], acyl carnitine [30,31], and alkylmaltoside [32] (Table 1). Peptide PEs include peptide-derived microbial toxins like C-CPE [33], AT1002 [34], and angubindin-1 [35], and PN159 [36], an artificial peptide developed using phage display technology. These have clearer mechanisms due to the nature of their origin, albeit with several impending challenges to their practical application, including safety concerns and a sense of greater distance from the classical excipient concept.

Table 1. Summary of chemical permeation enhancers.

Permeation Enhancer	Proposed Mechanism
MCFAs (C8, C10)	Paracellular - Direct or indirect tight junction modulation Transcellular - Membrane perturbation and fluidization
Eligen™ technology-based PE (SNAC, 4-CNAB, 5-CNAC)	Transcellular - Carrier mechanism - Local pH elevating and inhibition of gastric enzyme, peptide monomerization, membrane fluidization (SNAC-Semaglutide)
EDTA	Paracellular - Decreased tight junction integrity by chelation of Ca^{2+} [37,38]
Bile salt	Transcellular - Hydrophobic ion pairing, membrane fluidization [39–41]
Acyl-carnitine	Transcellular - Membrane perturbation [42] Paracellular - Tight junction modulation inferred from the decrease in TEER [43,44]
Alkyl-maltoside	Combined transcellular, paracellular action - A complex and colon-specific mechanism expected mild surfactant characteristics [32,45]
Sodium docusate	Transcellular - Hydrophobic ion pairing [46]
Sucrose laurate	Combined transcellular, paracellular action - Tight junction opening after membrane fluidization [47]
Choline geranate (CAGE, Ionic liquid)	Paracellular - Tight junction opening, protection from enzymatic degradation, decrease in mucus viscosity [48]

Most of the PEs that have entered the clinical trial stage are chemical PEs, and among them MCFAs (C8 and C10) and SNAC, which have secured safety status as a food additive and are generally recognized as safe (GRAS), respectively, and are forefront PEs. In this paper, a brief introduction to the oral peptide drugs (Mycapssa® and Rybelsus®) developed using the PE strategy and the development process of PE (MCFA and Eligen™ technology-based PE) applied to each is given, the studies of mechanisms and permeability enhancement are reviewed, and the results of the clinical trial stage are discussed.

2. Approved Oral Peptide Drugs

2.1. Mycapssa® (Oral Octreotide)

In 2020, the FDA approved Mycapssa®, an oral formulation of octreotide used in acromegaly. Chiasma's Transient Permeation Enhancer (TPE™) technology was used to develop this formulation. Octreotide, a cyclic peptide with a relatively low molecular weight

(1019.2 g/mol), was selected as the first candidate for the TPE™ technology application due to its high stability compared to other linear peptides [49,50]. Sodium caprylate (C8) is the key component that acts as a PE in the technology; however, its mechanism as a PE is not clearly elucidated. According to Chiasma, C8 exhibits temporary and reversible permeation enhancement action and induces the reorganization of tight junction (TJ) proteins such as ZO-1 and Claudin, which is presumed to be a paracellular mechanism through TJ modulation [51].

Unlike the unusual case of Rybelsus®, which targets absorption in the stomach, Mycapssa® targets drug absorption in the small intestine. Mycapssa® was designed to use an enteric capsule to prevent the breakdown of octreotide in the stomach, otherwise known as drug dissolution, by coating Acryl-EZE® (methacrylate) on gelatin capsules. This capsule contains an oily suspension in which hydrophilic fine particles of octreotide, C8, and polyvinylpyrrolidone (PVP) are suspended in an oil blend containing glycerol monocaprylate and glycerol tricaprylate. Furthermore, to prevent particle aggregation in the suspension, polysorbate 80 in the oil phase was used as a non-ionic surfactant [52]. The dominant PE in this composition is C8; however, it is known that additional PE effects can be expected by using high concentrations of additional additives such as PVP, glycerol monocaprylate, and polysorbate 80 [49].

2.2. Rybelsus® (Oral Semaglutide)

Rybelsus® was the first oral peptide drug based on the PE strategy and was approved by the FDA and EMA in September 2019 and March 2020, respectively. Rybelsus, indicated for type 2 diabetes mellitus (T2DM), is an oral formulation of semaglutide with sodium salcaprozate (SNAC) as the PE. SNAC is a synthetic N-acylated amino acid derivative of salicylic acid, developed by Emisphere's Eligen™ technology [53]. This technology conducted carrier libraries to develop carriers that increase hydrophobicity through non-covalent interactions with the payload (drug), which aims to increase transcellular absorption [54]. Eligen B12 (vitamin B12), approved as an FDA medical food in 2015, was the first product to be commercialized using SNAC. Subsequently, Novo Nordisk transferred Eligen™ technology from Emisphere and applied it to the development of an oral GLP-1 receptor agonist. The precedent approval of Eligen B12 and the safety status of FDA GRAS of SNAC secured in the process made the development of the current Rybelsus® product easier [55].

The contribution to the birth of oral semaglutide products has two main categories, the first of which is chemical modification of peptides. Novo Nordisk successfully launched Victoza® (Liraglutide) by improving the short half-life, which was a significant drawback of GLP-1 and exendin-4 [56–58]. This was made possible by acylation (palmitoylation (C16) to Lys-28), and the half-life was improved through enhanced binding with albumin and resistance by dipeptidyl peptidase-4 (DPP-4) [59]. Semaglutide (a peptide) further improved the half-life of liraglutide. In the liraglutide structure, octadecanoic (C18) diacid was added to the acylation of Lys-28 by a bis-aminodiethoxyacetyl linker to acylate it. Moreover, Ala-8 was substituted with an artificial amino acid, 2-amino-isobutyric acid (Aib), preventing decomposition by DPP-4. Through this, it was possible to develop oral formulations (Rybelsus®) as well as subcutaneous injectable formulations, which are given once a week (Wegovy®, Ozempic®) [60].

The second contribution is the improvement of oral absorption by SNAC. Unlike SNAC's mechanism presented by the existing Eligen™ technology, Novo Nordisk asserts that SNAC increases the transcellular absorption of semaglutide by elevating the local pH around the tablet in the stomach. In other words, it protects against pepsin by increasing the pH near the semaglutide that is eluted after the tablet sinks near the lower mucous membrane of the stomach, improves the solubility of the semaglutide, and induces monomerization in the local environment [61]. According to Novo Nordisk, these PE mechanisms of SNAC work specifically for semaglutide [55].

3. Permeation Enhancers–MCFAs (Medium Chain Fatty Acids)

Medium chain fatty acid (MCFA) is a naturally derived fatty acid with a length of about C6 to C12. For about 30 years now, active research has been performed on MCFA as a PE for hydrophilic, impermeable drugs. The Japanese Nishmura and Kitao research team, who obtained patents in the United States in early 1980, devised the application of this series of compounds to PEs [62]. They tried to find a PE that improves drug absorption in suppository form in the rectum by screening carboxyl group derivatives, with the main drug target being beta-lactam antibiotics. Their proposed mechanism was carboxylic acid derivatives increasing drug permeation by opening TJs while temporarily removing calcium ions necessary for maintaining TJs. During this study, sodium caprate (C10) and C8 were selected as the most potent PEs (particularly C10) [63] (Figure 2). Based on this study, ampicillin suppositories using C10 as a PE were approved in Japan and Sweden (Doktacillin™) [64].

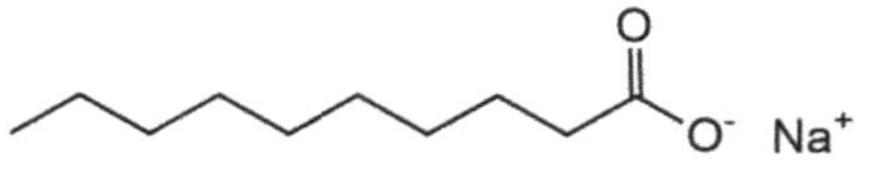

(a) sodium caprate (C10)

MW 194.25 g/mol, pKa = 4.95

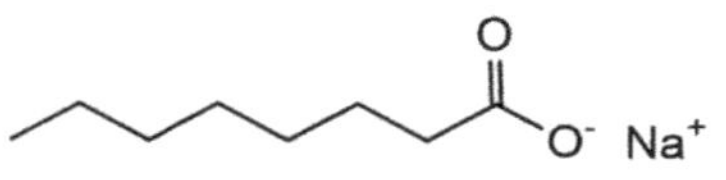

(b) sodium caprylate (C8)

MW 166.19 g/mol, pKa = 5.19

Figure 2. Structures of sodium caprate (C10) and sodium caprylate (C8).

Beyond the application of suppositories, MCFA PE studies centered on C8 and C10 have led to oral administration studies of low permeable drugs. Until now, the mechanism of action of C8 and C10 remains poorly defined. However, C8 and C10 are known to act as PEs through a common pathway; they act mainly in the form of a monomer because their action is based on a surfactant-like action. Therefore, the point of focus in these MCFAs is their critical micelle concentration (CMC) [65], because a high CMC ensures the existence of a high concentration of monomeric surfactant that can act as a PE. It is challenging to characterize the CMC of surfactant because it is greatly affected by temperature, ionic strength, pH, and the measurement method [66]. Among MCFAs, C8 and C10 are PEs with high CMC values. Hossain MS et al. conducted a study to determine the CMC of MCFA in various solvent environments through the classical surface tension measurement method (Wilhelmy method) and coarse-grained molecular dynamics (CG-MD) simulation [66]. The experimental results in the environment most similar to the physiological buffer (pH 7, 140 mM NaCl) are as follows. In the Wilhelmy method, C8 and C10 showed CMC values of 42.1 mM and 15.5 mM, respectively. In CG-MD simulation, it was predicted that C8 and C10 have CMC values of 13.88 mM and 8.27 mM, respectively. On the other hand, the calculated CMC values of C12 and C14 with longer carbon chains were 1.09 mM and 0.83 mM, respectively.

The relatively low regulatory hurdles based on the accumulated safety data of MCFAs make them desirable PEs. Both C8 and C10 are FDA-approved food additives [67]. The European Food Safety Authority (EFSA) also concluded that there are no safety problems in using fatty acids ranging from C8 to C18 as food additives. Their rationale is that fatty acids used as food additives are absorbed and metabolized in the same way as free fatty acids from lipid molecules present in the general diet, and although the toxicity database is limited, no sub-chronic toxicity and no genotoxicity have been observed [68].

3.1. Sodium Caprylate (C8)

C8 is an eight-carbon saturated fatty acid belonging to the class of MCFAs with a molecular weight of 166.19 g/mol and a pKa of 5.19. It is present in the milk of many mammals, and along with C10 is particularly high in goat milk [69]. Studies on the mechanism of action of C8 as a PE have been mainly conducted with C10 as the MCFA [70–72], and C8 alone was dealt with in the study of the TPE™ technology applied to Mycapssa® [51]. In the 1980s, studies on the application of C8 were conducted for rectal suppositories and nasal applications. In these studies, the opening of TJs by Ca^{2+} chelation was suggested as a mechanism of C8 [63,71]. In the 1990s, studies on the effect of C8 and C10 on different molecular sizes and diffusion coefficients, from urea to PEG 900 and inulin in the colon of rats, were conducted to elucidate the mechanisms of C8 and C10 [70]. They argued that the permeability enhancement of C8 and C10 is mainly achieved through the paracellular pathway, which is divided into the shunt pathway (large pore pathway), that is not limited by the molecular size, and the small pore pathway that is limited by the molecular size.

However, these early studies lack evidence to support their asserted mechanism. A study on the permeation enhancement mechanism of TPE™ formulation was conducted in the TPE™ formulation study, which successfully led to the FDA-approval of oral octreotide with a formulation containing C8. This study suggested a paracellular pathway by TJ opening through the reorganization of ZO-1 and claudin proteins [51]. Contrary to the paracellular mechanism asserted in early C8 and TPE studies, recent studies have highlighted evidence for the transcellular pathway in the mechanism of MCFAs including C8 [72], thus classifying C8 as a transcellular PE with surfactant-like action [65,73].

Most studies on the PE effect of C8 have been conducted with C10. A common finding in many studies is that C8 is less potent than C10. In terms of surfactant PE, C8 has a higher CMC value than C10 and has faster membrane-inserting kinetics [72]. Nevertheless, C8 has a lower permeation-enhancing potency compared to C10, probably due to its insufficient chain length because it is composed of carbon numbers close to the threshold of MCFAs that have a PE effect [72,74]. According to a recent molecular dynamics simulation study, since C8 has a greater membrane expulsion tendency after being inserted into the membrane than C10, the ratio of the remaining C8 inserted into the membrane is small, and is thought to reduce the membrane disruption effect [75].

C8 is considered a key PE of the TPE™ technology that has led to the successful launch of Mycapssa®. Thus far, only TPE™ has entered clinical trials using C8 as a PE. When the TPE™ formulation was applied to a fluorescent marker (FITC-labeled dextran of 4.4 kDa, FD4) in the intrajejunal administration rat model, it was shown that the area under the curve (AUC, 0–90 min) value increased by over 10 times. In addition, in the absorption enhancing effect experiment, according to the increase in molecular weight of FITC-dextran (4.4–70 kDa) absorption enhancement was shown to be up to 40 kDa, and insignificant absorption enhancement was detected at 70 kDa. This is the result of absorption enhancement of the TPE™ formulation (oily suspension containing C8), which is easily overinterpreted as the permeation-enhancing effect of only C8. In effect, compared to the permeation enhancement of the combination of the FD4 and TPE™ formulation, FD4 and C8 in saline solution showed a relative value of one-fifth [51].

3.2. Sodium Caprate (C10)

C10, also called sodium decanoate, is a sodium salt of a saturated fatty acid composed of 10 carbons, with a molecular weight of 194.25 g/mol and a pKa value of 4.95. C10 is a representative MCFA PE and there have been active studies on its ability to enhance the permeability of various drugs, from low permeable chemical drugs [76–79] to antisense oligonucleotides and peptides (Table 2) [80,81].

Table 2. Studies on the permeation enhancement ability of sodium caprate (C10).

Peptide (MW)	Experimental Model	Dosing	Enhancement Ratio	Reference
In vitro assay				
D-decapeptide (~1.2 kDa)	Caco-2 cell monolayer	20–25 mM	~7	[82]
Ile-Pro-Pro (325 Da) Leu-Lys-Pro (389 Da)	Caco-2 cell monolayer	5 mM	~2.5 (Ile-Pro-Pro) ~2 (Leu-Lys-Pro)	[83]
Cyclopeptide, (EMD121974) (589 Da)	Caco-2 cell monolayer	10 mM	10.6	[84]
Vasopressin (1.2 kDa)	Caco-2 cell monolayer	13 mM	10	[85]
Recombinant human epidermal growth factor (6 kDa)	Caco-2 cell monolayer	1% (50 mM)	10.6	[86]
Ex vivo/in vivo assay				
D-decapeptide (~1.2 kDa)	Rat, ileal instillation	0.5 mmol/kg	~5	[82]
Ebiratide (996 Da)	Rat, Ussing chamber (jejunum and colon)	20 mM	1.50 (jejunum) 3.84 (colon)	[87]
Enalaprilat (349 Da)	Rat, single-pass intestinal perfusion	10 mg/mL	9	[88]
Hexarelin (887 Da)	Rat, single-pass intestinal perfusion	5~20 mg/mL	Not enhanced	[88]
Insulin (5.8 kDa)	Rat, Ussing chamber (jejunum and colon)	20 mM	0.97 (jejunum) 2.50 (Colon)	[89]
Horseradish peroxidase (45 kDa)	Human, Ussing chamber (Colon)	10 mM	~2	[90]
Insulin (5.8 kDa)	Rat, loop administration	1% (50 mM)	Duodenum: not enhanced * Jejunum: enhanced * Ileum: 1.67 * Colon: 9 *	[91]
Salmon calcitonin (3.4 kDa)	Rat, colonal instillation	0.1% (5 mM)	Enhanced *	[92]
Insulin (5.8 kDa)	Rat, rectal infusion	50 mM	24.31 *	[93]
DMP728 (657 Da)	Rat and dog, oral administration	Rat (8 mg/kg) Dog (2 mg/kg)	2.70 (Rat) 1.36 (Dog)	[94]
Insulin (5.8 kDa)	Rat, oral administration	0.5% (25 mM)	3.79*	[95]
Elcatonin (3.4 kDa)	Rabbit, rectal suppository	30 mg	1.61*	[96]

* Pharmacodynamic results.

Various methods and experimental models have explored the mechanism of C10 as an MCFA PE (Table 3). The mechanism suggested by the first study that utilized MCFAs as a PE was that MCFA opened TJs by chelating intercellular Ca^{2+} [63]. However, several subsequent studies on the mechanism of action of C10 have denied the Ca^{2+} chelating mechanism. According to Anderberg et al. [97], the presence or absence of Ca^{2+} in the apical (donor) part of the Caco-2 cell monolayer permeability assay did not affect the permeation-enhancing effect, and there was no change in cell integrity when Ca^{2+} was removed from the apical part. Rather, Ca^{2+} showed a negative effect by precipitating C10 in the buffer. In the study of Tomita et al. [98], the mechanism of action of C10 was explored through comparison with ethylenediaminetetraacetic acid (EDTA), a representative Ca^{2+} chelating agent. When EDTA was added to the basolateral (acceptor) part. rather than the apical part of Caco-2 cell monolayer permeability assay, the permeation effect was superior. Conversely, when C10 was applied to the apical and basolateral parts, there was no difference between the two. In this respect, the permeation-enhancing mechanism of C10 by Ca^{2+} chelation was denied.

Table 3. Studies on the permeation enhancement mechanism of sodium caprate (C10).

Experimental Model	Proposed Mechanism of Action (Rationale)	Evidence	Reference
Caco-2 cell monolayer	TJ modulation	*TEM* - TJ dilatation was observed after treatment with 13 mM C10. *Fluorescence microscopy* - It is observed that the peri-junctional F actin ring disbands over time, which corresponds to the permeation enhancement timeline of ^{14}C-Mannitol.	[97]
Caco-2 cell monolayer	TJ modulation	*TEM* - TJ dilatation was observed after treatment with 10 mM C10. - Frequency of dilatations after exposure to C10 was more than 40% (much higher than C8 and C12). *Fluorescence microscopy* - F actin rings were shown to be disbanded after exposure to C10.	[74]
Caco-2 cell monolayer	TJ modulation (PLC activation and CaM-dependent contraction of actin filament)	*Intracellular Ca^{2+} measurement (Fluorometric Ca^{2+} analyzer)* - C10 increased the intracellular Ca^{2+} regardless of the presence or absence of extracellular Ca^{2+} (0.05%–0.25% of C10, especially at 0.25%). *Inhibitor treatment for PLC-CaM signaling* - Treatment with KN-62 reduced the permeation-enhancing effect of C10 on FD-4K. - Treatment with KN-62 and W7 inhibited the C10-induced TEER reduction effect.	[38]
Ex vivo Ussing chamber (Rat ileum)	TJ modulation	*TEM* - C10 (10 mM) caused dilatations in 34% of the visualized TJ regions. *Comparison of patterns with Cytochalasin B* - Dose-response curve (C10: 2.5–10 mM, CytB: 60–300 µM) for transepithelial potential difference and [^{51}Cr]EDTA P_{app} are similar.	[99]

Table 3. Cont.

Experimental Model	Proposed Mechanism of Action (Rationale)	Evidence	Reference
Human airway epithelial cell	TJ modulation (Ca^{2+}-independent mechanism and direct effect on the TJ protein)	*Fluo-4 Ca^{2+} assay* - 30 mM C10 induced a rapid increase in Ca^{2+} from ER and returned to control levels by 300 s after exposure. *The effect of BAPTP-AM, La^{3+}, and thapsigargin* - The addition of BAPTP-AM (intracellular Ca^{2+} chelator) did not affect the decrease in the TEER value of C10. - The addition of La^{3+} (membrane Ca^{2+}-ATPase inhibitor) and thapsigargin (ER Ca^{2+}-ATPase inhibitor) that maintained an increase in intracellular Ca^{2+}, did not affect the decrease in the R_T value of C10. *The effect of signaling inhibitor* - Each treatment of U7, 48/80, H7, W7, and KN62 did not affect the reduction of the R_T value of C10. *Immunofluorescent Labeling and Confocal microscopy* - JAM and actin were clearly redistributed after exposure to C10 (ZO-1 did not change). - The redistribution was not blocked by BAPTA-AM. - Claudin-1 and -4 were redistributed immediately after C10 treatment.	[100]
- MDCK cell monolayer - Lipid raft isolation study	Membrane perturbation (Lipid raft disruption) TJ modulation (Displacement of specific TJ proteins)	*Western-blot analysis* - Claudin -4,-5, and occludin were displaced from the lipid raft.	[101]

Table 3. Cont.

Experimental Model	Proposed Mechanism of Action (Rationale)	Evidence	Reference
- HEK-293 Cell expressing claudin-5-YFP, MDCK-2-Cell expressing Flag-claudin-5 - Ex vivo mouse brain capillary	TJ modulation (by reducing the membranous claudin-5 amount and the F-actin content)	*Immunofluorescent Labeling and Confocal microscopy* - Claudin-5-YFP homophilic interaction was lost and fragmented by treatment with 5, 7.5, and 10 mM C10 for 20 min, and recovered after removal of C10. Treatment with C10 yielded no significant change in CellMask, a membrane-inserting dye. (Compared to MβCD, which is a membrane disruptor.) *Immunoblotting* - 7.5 mM C10 reduced membranous claudin-5 and intracellular F-actin in TJ-containing MDCK-2-Cells and in brain endothelial cells. (There was no change in ZO-1.) - Claudin-5 was found to be displaced from the triton-insoluble (lipids) fraction of MDCK cells after treatment with C10.	[102]
- HT-29/B6 Cell	TJ modulation (by reversible removal of tricellulin from the tricellular TJ)	*Two-path impedance spectroscopy* - A significant decrease in paracellular resistance was observed by C10, although transcellular resistance was not significantly changed. *Immunofluorescent Labeling and Confocal microscopy* - C10 specifically induced a decrease in tricellulin and claudin-5 signals, which was reversible after washout. *Localization of Sulfo-NHS-SS-biotin Permeation sites* - Biotin signal was detected only within or below tricellular cell contacts (not detected in bicellular cell contacts).	[103]

Table 3. *Cont.*

Experimental Model	Proposed Mechanism of Action (Rationale)	Evidence	Reference
- Caco-2 cell monolayer - Ex vivo Ussing chamber (Rat colon) - Rat intestinal instillation	Membrane perturbation	*Quantitative real-time PCR and gene expression microarrays* - After exposure to 8.5 mM C10 for 60 min, IL-8, an inflammatory signal, increased 11-fold and 26-fold at 1 and 4 h of recovery, respectively, and then decreased to the control level after 24 h. *Attenuation Effect of misoprostol* - Pre-exposure of monolayers to the misoprostol (10 and 100 nM) for 30 min prior to 8.5 mM C10 addition for 60 min significantly attenuated C10's capacity to reduce TEER and increase the [^{14}C]-mannitol and FD-4K P_{app}. - The protective effect of pre-incubation with misoprostol against C10 was detected by TEM. - In a rat colonic loop instillation experiment, misoprostol reduced the mean AUC and C_{max} of FD4K by 24% and 33%, respectively, compared with the results treatment with C10 alone. - SC51322 (EP$_1$ receptor antagonist) negated the effect of misoprostol in preventing the C10-induced changes in the intracellular Ca^{2+}, mitochondrial membrane potential, and plasma membrane permeability.	[104]
Caco-2 cell monolayer	Membrane perturbation (initial and fundamental mechanism) TJ modulation (by intracellular pathway arising from initial plasma membrane perturbation)	*Immunofluorescence of TJ proteins* - At 5 mM or higher C10, ZO-1 was internalized, and claudin-5 and occludin were also relocated and internalized. *Cytotoxicity assay* - LDH-Glo™, CellTox Green™, Neutral Red, and JC-1 assay results showed a decrease in the integrity of the plasma, nuclear, and mitochondrial membrane that was concentration-dependent (usually at 5 mM or higher) of C10. (This pattern was not observed in SNAC.)	[105]

Table 3. Cont.

Experimental Model	Proposed Mechanism of Action (Rationale)	Evidence	Reference
- CG-MD simulation - US simulation - TIRF microscopy (FRAP analysis)	Membrane perturbation (insertion of C10 into membrane and transmembrane perturbation)	*CG-MD simulation* - When 100 mM C10 in the fluid composition of the fasting state was applied to the POPC membrane, it was inserted into the membrane at a level of 70–80% in 6 μs. *US simulation (PMF profile)* - In a POPC bilayer with a thickness of 4.05 nm, C10 had an energy minima at a distance of 1.46 nm from the membrane center. (Energy minima represent the maximum probability of finding the molecule.) *TIRF Microscopy (FRAP analysis)* - In the POPC-C10 mixed membrane composed of various concentrations of C10, the membrane diffusivity increased in a C10 concentration-dependent manner. - When the pure POPC membrane was treated with 100 mM C10, diffusivity was increased, and it was observed that the generated bleached holes were recovered after 60 s when C10 was removed.	[72]

TEM, transmission electron microscope; TJ, tight junction; PLC, phospholipase C; CaM, calmodulin; FD, FITC-dextran; TEER, transepithelial electrical resistance; ER, endoplasmic reticulum; P_{app}, apparent permeability; JAM, junctional adhesion molecule; YFP, yellow fluorescence protein; ZO-1, zonula occludens-1; EP_1 receptor, prostaglandin E2 receptor 1; POPC, 1-Palmitoyl-2-oleoylphosphatidylcholine; CG-MD, coarse-grained molecular dynamics; US, umbrella sampling; TIRF, total internal reflection fluorescence; PMF, potential of mean force; FRAP, fluorescent recovery after photobleaching.

Subsequent mechanistic studies have mainly focused on TJ modulation by C10 treatment and its intracellular pathway. Tomita et al. [38] found that C10 increased intracellular Ca^{2+} and that the permeation enhancing effect of C10 was inhibited when treated with a phospholipase C (PLC)-calmodulin (CaM) signaling inhibitor. However, in a subsequent study of the impact of C10 on airway epithelial cells, Coyne et al. [100] suggested that C10 induces an increase in intracellular Ca^{2+}, albeit that the PE effect of C10 is Ca^{2+}-independent. They observed the effect of C10 when intracellular Ca^{2+} was removed with an intracellular Ca^{2+} chelator; increased intracellular Ca^{2+} was maintained by treatment with a Ca^{2+}-ATPase inhibitor and after treatment with the PLC-CaM signaling inhibitor. In all cases, there was no effect on the reduction of C10 transepithelial resistance, and the redistribution of the TJ protein by C10 was also not affected by the removal of intracellular Ca^{2+}.

While the initial study focused on the TJ observation through transmission electron microscopy [48] and the change in TJ proteins through immunofluorescence, active research on the effect of C10 on lipid membranes based on membrane perturbation or disruption is underway [101,104,105]. These studies focus more on the interaction with the lipid membrane, whereby C10 is a surfactant that successfully inserts into the membrane. Sugibayashi et al. [101] investigated the mechanism of C10 using a lipid raft model, which is relatively robust due to the enrichment of cholesterol and sphingomyelin and has resistance to nonionic surfactants such as Triton X-100. When comparing C10 and Methyl-β-Cyclodextrin (MβCD), which disrupts the lipid raft by depleting cholesterol, MβCD displaced claudin-1,-4,-5 and occludin, while C10 displaced claudin-4,-5 and occludin from the lipid raft. Brayden et al. [104] suggested that the underlying mechanism of C10 could be attributed to membrane perturbation via misoprostol pretreatment. Misoprostol is a synthetic PEG_1 methyl ester analog that protects gastric and duodenal mucosal perturbation-, NSAID-, aspirin-, and alcohol-induced ulcers [106]. Pretreatment with 10 nM misoprostol for 30 min significantly reduced the PE effect of C10 in both in vivo and ex vivo experiments, and this reduction effect was negated by SC51322, a prostaglandin EP-1 receptor antagonist. In addition to the permeability of the marker, the intracellular Ca^{2+} and mitochondrial membrane potential increase—indicators of the mechanism of action of C10—also showed the same trend with misoprostol and SC51322, respectively. More recently, there have been ongoing in silico studies to predict the molecular dynamic interaction between surfactant-based PEs such as C10 and the lipid membrane. This is an experimental technique that can further characterize C10 membrane perturbation by computing the insertion fraction of C10 into the membrane on the micro-second level [72] and predicting the behavior after membrane insertion, i.e., flip-flop or migration from the membrane to the aqueous phase [75]. However, since it is currently simulated in a simple virtual membrane composed of 1-palmitoyl-2-oleoyl-sn-glycero-3-phosphatidylcholine (POPC), evaluating the effect of the perturbation of such a membrane on TJ proteins or intracellular changes by C10, including an increase in intracellular Ca^{2+}, is challenging.

Research on the mechanism of C10 has yielded varying results and hypotheses for TJ modulation and membrane perturbation (Figure 3). However, there remains the possibility of a complex mechanism of C10 that is not among the two established categories, and the definitive mechanism remains unknown. Early research on the mechanism was focused on TJ modulation, but subsequent studies put weight on membrane perturbation according to the surfactant structure of C10. Paracellular routes by TJ modulation and transcellular routes by membrane perturbation are often regarded as two separate mechanisms. However, in a recent study by Brayden et al., a PE exhibiting a mild surfactant structure showed that membrane perturbation was its fundamental mechanism, suggesting the possibility of association with TJ modulation [47,105]. This means that TJ modulation and membrane perturbation may not be independent or completely dichotomous mechanisms, and a link between the two may exist. Through this new insight, a new direction was suggested for the study of the mechanism of C10, whose exact mechanism is unknown.

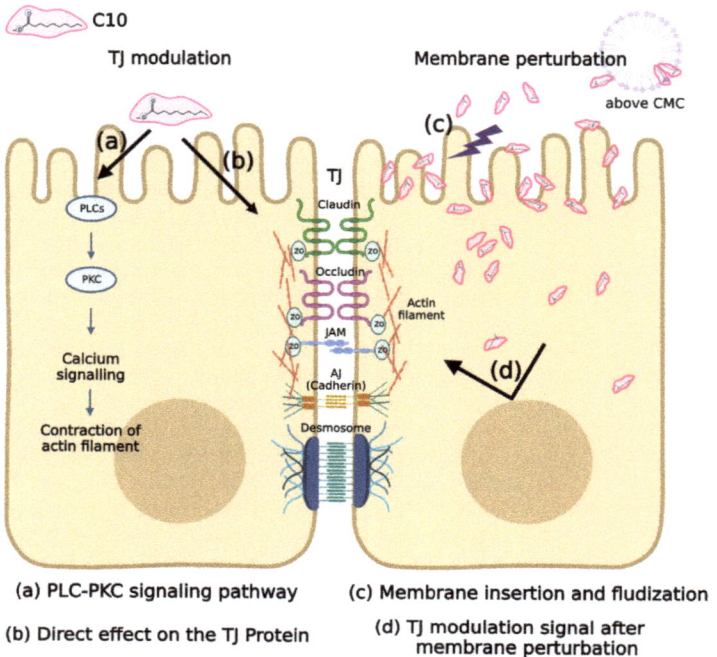

Figure 3. Hypotheses on the mechanism of C10. The diagram shows the simple classification of the mechanisms of C10 proposed to date. It is essentially divided into tight junction (TJ) modulation (left) and membrane perturbation mechanisms [68]. The TJ modulation hypothesis is divided into a Ca^{2+}-dependent PLC-PKC pathway mechanism (**a**) and a Ca2+-independent TJ protein modulation (**b**). As per the membrane perturbation hypothesis, the mechanism of action of C10 can be its insertion into the membrane to fluidize the membrane and enhance absorption into the transcellular pathway (**c**), and an unknown TJ modulation signal due to membrane perturbation (**d**).

C10 has been applied in in vitro and in vivo experiments to enhance the permeability of various peptides, ranging from small peptides with a molecular weight of 300 Da to peptides with a molecular weight of 7 kDa (Table 2). In an in vitro experiment (Caco-2 cell monolayer permeability assay), C10 was principally used at concentrations of 2.5–25 mM, which is a concentration range considered for cell viability and the CMC value of C10. The peptide permeability enhancement ratio of C10, which does not include the pharmacodynamic parameters of C10, was shown to be increased by up to 10 times.

The development of oral peptide drugs using C10 as a permeation enhancer started in earnest with the Gastro-Intestinal Permeation Enhancement Technology (GIPET™) of Merrion Pharmaceuticals [107]. It has consistently demonstrated the efficacy of solution-state peptides and C10 via in vitro and in vivo experiments. However, for the actual development of an oral peptide drug to which PEs are applied, a solid dosage form must be implemented. Moreover, in the final formulation, decomposition by gastric acid and simultaneous or optimized release of C10 and peptides at the absorption site should be considered. The relevance of GIPET™ lies in their performance in studies of the design of an actual solid formulation of C10 as a PE. GIPET™ has been developed and studied in three versions of the formulation so far, and the exact composition of the exact components and concentrations of the formulation has not been fully unveiled.

GIPET™ 1 formulation is a solid formulation in the form of an enteric-coated tablet containing C10. GIPET™ 2 contains C8 and C10 mono/diglycerides, and the solid formulation is in the form of an enteric-coated soft gel/hard capsule shell. Information on GIPET™ 3 has not been disclosed [108].

In a patent embodiment using fondaparinux as an active pharmaceutical ingredient (API), it is known that GIPET™ 1 (High) contains 550 mg of C10 and GIPET™ 1 (Low) contains 275 mg of C10 per 5 mg of fondaparinux [109]. GIPET™ 2 is a C8 and C10 microemulsion formulation esterified with glycerol, known as Capmul®. GIPET™ 2 Form 1 is a formulation based on Capmul® MCM (glyceryl caprylate caprate) and is composed of 41.9% Capmul® MCM, 23.3% PEG 400, 21.3% Tween® 80, 5% Captex® (glyceryl tricaprylate caprate), and 0.5% (5 mg) of fondaparinux. GIPET™ 2 Form 2 is a formulation based on Capmul® MCM C10 (Glyceryl caprate), and consists of 36.6% Capmul® MCM C10, 23.3% PEG400, 21.3% Tween® 80, 13.3% Captex® 300, and 0.5% (5 mg) of fondaparinux. The pharmacokinetic (PK) parameters of these four GIPET™ 1,2 formulations were measured using a dog's intra-duodenal instillation model, and compared with 1 mg subcutaneous formulation. Results of GIPET™ 1 (High) 16.94%, GIPET™ 1 (Low) 11.09%, GIPET™ 2 (Form 1) 18.48%, and GIPET™ 2 (Form 2) 9.61% were shown. Furthermore, compared to the unenhanced administration group to which permeation enhancer was not applied, GIPET™ 1 (High) increased by 3.2 times, GIPET™ 1 (Low) increased by 2.1 times, GIPET™ 2 (Form 1) increased by 3.4 times, and GIPET™ 2 (Form 2) increased by 1. 9 times.

Clinical trials have applied the GIPET™ technology to several peptides and proteins (Table S1). According to a comprehensive paper on the results of phase 1, GIPET™ 1 has an oral bioavailability of 8.4%, 9.0%, and 8.0% for alendronate, LMWH (MW 4400), and LMWH (MW 6010), respectively. Desmopressin, to which GIPET™ 2 was applied, showed an oral bioavailability of 2.4%. Alendronate and desmopressin showed 5-fold and 13-fold increased absorption compared to oral control, respectively [108,110]. In a clinical study of GIPET™ application to acyline, a GnRH antagonist peptide, 10 mg, 20 mg, and 40 mg of acyline were administered to subjects. All three concentrations of GIPET™-enhanced oral acyline decreased the serum follicle-stimulating hormone, luteinizing hormone, and testosterone for almost 12 h. Serum acyline concentration increased immediately after oral administration, but it was difficult to observe differences in pharmacokinetics parameters by dose due to large variability between subjects [111]. Merrion pharmaceutical's GIPET™ technology has entered into a license agreement for the development of Novo Nordisk's oral GLP-1 agonist and oral insulin. In particular, it has been applied to the development of oral insulin formulations and has entered clinical trials; however, it is known to have been discontinued [112]. Biocon's insulin tregopil project is currently developing oral insulin through C10. Insulin tregopil is a novel PEGylated insulin with a structure in which a short PEG is attached to the ε-amino group of Lysβ29 of human insulin [113]. According to the development paper of insulin tregopil, it is a simple, uncoated tablet formulation containing 5–15 mg of insulin tregopil, C10 as a PE, and mannitol, PVP, colloidal silica, and magnesium stearate as the remaining excipients. This tablet targets drug absorption in the stomach and is designed to elute more than 75% of the drug within 15 min [114].

C10, which has been extensively studied as a PE, has positioned itself as a representative MCFA PE. Recently, in addition to classic tablets or enteric capsules, there are ongoing studies on the application of next-generation formulation, such as 3D printed capsules that break under pressure in the antropyloric region and microcontainers that unidirectionally release drugs and PE [115,116].

4. Permeation Enhancer: Eligen™ Technology-Based PEs

Unlike naturally occurring MCFAs, Eligen™ technology-based PEs are a family of compounds developed for permeation enhancement. Eligen™ technology, based on PEs developed by Emisphere, has undergone a development process. They originally targeted the oral delivery of peptides through microspheres composed of thermally condensed α-amino acids [117]. In that process, it was necessary to develop a hydrophobic α-amino acid with a low molecular weight for microsphere preparation. They chose a method of derivatizing soy protein hydrolysate with phenylsulfonyl chloride, and through this, they successfully manufactured microspheres. In subsequent permeability experiments, empty microspheres were found to enhance the intestinal absorption of peptides loaded into microspheres. Through additional experiments, they discovered that (phenylsulfonyl)-α-amino acids themselves had the effect of a PE, and through this, they began screening for the PE activity of the modified α-amino acids themselves, and not through the microsphere strategy [53]. This initial study concluded that there is insufficient evidence that the increase in peptide absorption occurs by classical mechanisms such as protease/peptidase inhibition and penetration enhancement, and the research team focused on the possibility of enhancing permeation by specific interactions between peptides and Eligen™ technology-based PEs. Based on the flow of these studies, it can be observed that they were not limited to α-amino acids, but continuously screened for the difference in the permeability enhancing effect according to the changes in the substituents of N-acylated-non-α-amino acid, lipophilicity, etc. [118]. Subsequently, Emisphere's research team conducted a study on the mechanism of PE action with candidates obtained by screening (not including SNAC, the current leading compound). They argued that their PE acts as a "carrier" for protein/peptide delivery and that the passive/transcellular pathway is the main pathway (Figure 4). More specifically, their carriers stabilize the partially unfolded conformer of protein/peptide through non-covalent bonding, which exposes the hydrophobic side chain of protein/peptide and increases solubility in lipid membranes [119].

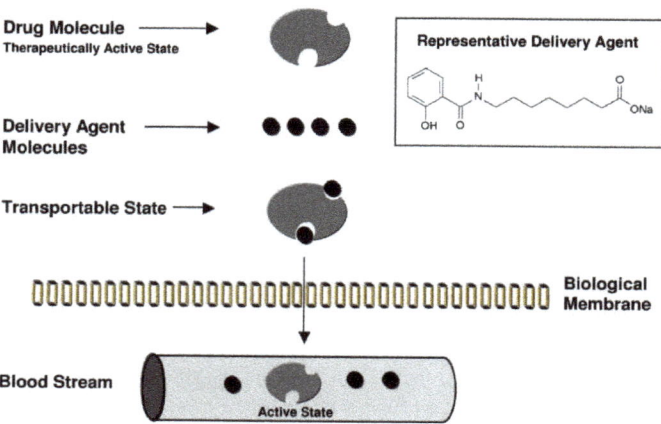

Figure 4. Schematic diagram of the mechanism of the Eligen™ technology (carrier mechanism). Emisphere researchers have argued that small carrier molecules with hydrophobic moieties increase lipophilicity through the formation of weak non-covalent bonds with drug molecules [120].

Through this journey, SNAC (N-[8-(2-hydroxybenzoyl)amino] caprylate) was developed, which also led to the development of oral semaglutide and other leading compounds such as 5-CNAC (8-(N-2-hydroxy-5-chloro-benzoyl)-amino-caprylate) and 4-CNAB (N-(4-chlorosalicyloyl)-4-aminobutyrate) (Figure 5). The most advanced of these is SNAC, which has been applied in clinical trials with insulin [121], heparin [122,123], ibandronate [124], and peptide YY3-36 (PYY3-36) [125], and led to the successful development of oral vitamin B12 and semaglutide products. The remaining leading compounds are 5-CNAC and 4-CNAB. The compound 5-CNAC has been applied to salmon calcitonin and has moved to phase 3 clinical trials [126]. The compound 4-CNAB, for its part, has been applied to insulin, and phase 1 clinical trials have been completed [127].

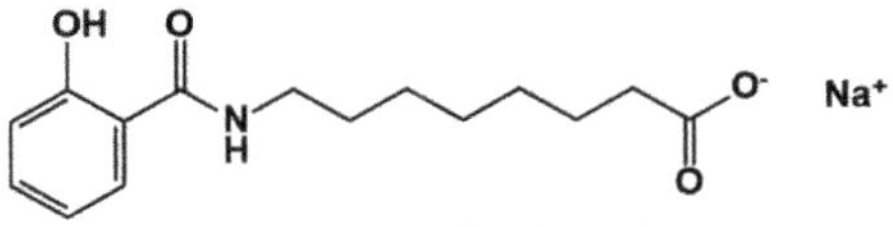

(a) salcaprozate sodium (SNAC)
MW 301.31 g/mol, pKa = 5.01

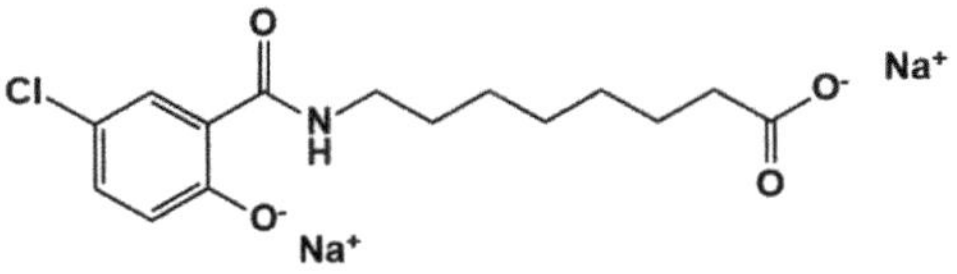

(b) 5-CNAC Disodium
MW 357.74

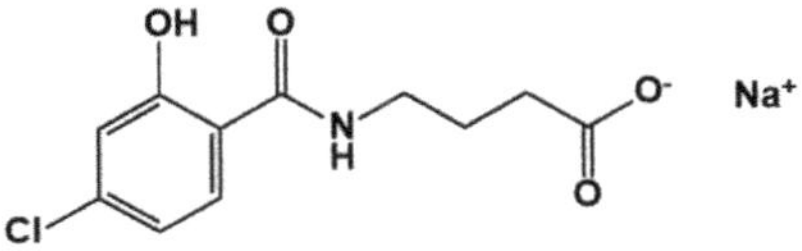

(c) salclobuzate sodium (4-CNAB)
MW 279.65

Figure 5. Structures of (**a**) SNAC, (**b**) 5-CNAC, and (**c**) 4-CNAB.

SNAC (N-[8-(2-hydroxybenzoyl)amino] caprylate), also called sodium salcaprozate, has a pKa value of 5.01 and a molecular weight of 301.31 Da [128]. It shares structural similarity with MCFA in that it has a fatty acid moiety, but unlike MCFA, it does not adequately demonstrate the tendency of surfactant-like action membrane insertion/perturbation. SNAC has a salicylamide structure at the molecular terminal, in addition to the carboxyl group of fatty acid shared with MCFA, and has a larger distribution of hydrophilic groups. In effect, the computed topological polar surface area of SNAC is more dispersed, with it being 40.1 Å for C10 and 89.5 Å for SNAC [129]. In a recent in silico-based research model, the tendency of SNAC to disrupt the membrane was calculated to be less than that of MCFA due to the presumed salicylamide structure. Moreover, the tendency of expulsion from the membrane leaflet after insertion into the membrane was also greater [75].

There have been studies on SNAC, a representative material of Eligen™ technology-based PEs, for the oral administration of insulin, octreotide, etc. (Table 4). This has led to the successful development of Rybelsus® (oral semaglutide). Most studies on the mechanism of SNAC have agreed that it acts as a transcellular PE (Table 5). Furthermore, many studies have concluded that SNAC does not exhibit surfactant-like action and membrane perturbation tendencies, as MCFA does. The representative mechanism of SNAC is the carrier mechanism. That is, SNAC forms a non-covalent complex with a drug to increase lipophilicity and membrane permeability, which is the mechanism claimed by Emisphere, who developed SNAC [54,130]. The PE mechanism of SNAC cannot be generalized to a single drug (a peptide) due to the nature of the mechanism of non-covalent binding to the drug. Albeit, SNAC exposed the hydrophobic region of insulin and there were no changes in TJ proteins or membrane integrity, represented by an LDH assay and a mannitol transport assay in an insulin-modeled study [54]. There are also studies that contradict the carrier mechanism. A study on the application of SNAC to cromolyn sodium, a low-molecular-weight molecule with low absorption in the GI tract due to its high hydrophilicity, presented results conflicting with the carrier mechanism. When observed through the partitioning solvent system, the lipophilicity change in cromolyn sodium by SNAC was not observed, and SNAC was observed to increase the membrane fluidity of the Caco-2 cell monolayer [131]. The change in membrane fluidity was observed by the treatment with 83 mM SNAC, with the difference existing at the concentration levels higher than that of 33–55 mM SNAC used in the existing carrier mechanism study.

Table 4. Studies on the permeation enhancement of SNAC.

Peptide (MW)	Model	Dosing	Enhancement Ratio	Reference
Insulin (5808 Da)	Caco-2 cell monolayer	5 mM	~10	[54]
Semaglutide (4114 Da)	NCI-N87 cell monolayer	80 mM	~7	[61]
Octreotide (1019 Da)	Ex vivo Ussing chamber of rat (colon, ileum, upper jejunum, duodenum, and stomach) and human (colon)	20 mM 40 mM	Rat (20 mM): 1.4~3.4 Human: 1.5 (20 mM), 2.1 (40 mM)	[128]
SHR-2042 (GLP-1RA) (~4.5 kDa)	Rat, duodenal perfusion	0.6 g/kg 1.2 g/kg	7.8 (0.6 g/kg) 69 (1.2 g.kg)	[132]

Table 5. Studies on the permeation enhancement mechanism of SNAC.

Experimental Method and Model Drugs	Proposed Mechanism of Action	Evidence	Reference
Fluorescence microscopy, Heparin	The transcellular pathway that does not involve membrane permeabilization and does not appear to be endocytosis.	*Fluorescence and confocal microscopy in the Caco-2 monolayer* - Uptake of ALEXA FLUOR™ 488 labeled heparin was observed in over 33 mM SNAC, which was present in the cytoplasm and nucleus (endocytic vesicles were not observed). - Permeation of ALEXA FLUOR™ 488 hydrazide, a fluorescent probe, and YOYO-1, a membrane-impermeable DNA dye, was not observed when treated with 33 mM SNAC. - During actin staining of the apical monolayer, no change was observed until treatment with 66 mM SNAC.	[130]
Voltage clamp method, 6-Carboxy-fluorescein (6-CF)	Transcellular pathway	*Voltage clamp experiment* - 10 mM EDTA increased the paracellular flux rate of 6-CF by 3.1-fold and the transcellular flux rate by 1.3-fold, whereas 33 mM SNAC caused a 1.6-fold and 7.2-fold increase, respectively. *TEER measurement and mannitol transport assay* - There were no significant changes in TEER and Mannitol P_{app} in 33–66 mM SNAC, showing an increase in the permeability of 6-CF.	[133]
Fluorescence microscopy, Insulin	Increased lipophilicity by non-covalent binding and the resulting transcellular pathway	*Fluorescence and confocal microscopy in Caco-2 monolayer* - Fluorescently labeled insulin was detected in the cytoplasm and along the plasma membrane. - Treatment with 55 mM SNAC/80 μM insulin did not change the distribution of the peri-junctional ring and occludin.	[54]
The standard shake-flask method and steady-state fluorescence emission anisotropy, Cromolyn sodium	Increased membrane fluidity, but not increased lipophilicity in cromolyn sodium	*The standard shake-flask method* - All three n-Octanol-, chloroform-, and PGDP-/water systems showed differences in cromolyn sodium concentration in the aqueous layer in the presence and absence of SNAC, albeit without statistical significance. *Steady-state fluorescence emission anisotropy* - 83 mM SNAC alone or mixed with 10 mM cromolyn sodium significantly increased the fluidity of the core hydrophobic region as well as the surface polar region of Caco-2 cell membranes (not observed in 10 mM and 63 mM SNAC).	[131]

Table 5. Cont.

Experimental Method and Model Drugs	Proposed Mechanism of Action	Evidence	Reference
Various in vitro, in vivo/ex vivo assays	Protection against enzymatic degradation via local buffering actions and semaglutide-specific transcellular absorption in the stomach	For transcellular mechanism - (In vitro) In the NCI-N87 cell monolayer, both SNAC and EDTA increased the P_{app} of semaglutide similarly, but SNAC-induced intracellular accumulation of semaglutide and EDTA did not. - (In vitro) SNAC yielded a gradual reduction in the main transition temperature (T_m) of DMPC membrane. - (Ex vivo) As a result of immunofluorescence and TEM imaging of semaglutide immunoreactivity, semaglutide was present in the intracellular region, especially in the cytoplasm, via SNAC. For semaglutide and SNAC specificity - (In vivo) SNAC did not enhance the absorption of liraglutide, and the *ortho*-isomer of SNAC did not enhance the absorption of semaglutide. For local buffering action - (In vitro) Semaglutide/SNAC tablets augmented the pH of SGF from acidic to neutral within 5 to 15 min, the semaglutide tablet without SNAC had no apparent effect on the pH. - (In vitro) In the stability test of semaglutide in solutions of various pH values, including pepsin, $t_{1/2}$ at pH 2.6 was 16 min, $t_{1/2}$ at pH 5.0 was 34 min, and at pH 7.4, almost no degradation was observed over 50 min. For absorption in the stomach - (In vivo) As a result of gamma scintigraphic imaging, it was confirmed that complete erosion of the semaglutide/SNAC tablet was achieved in the human stomach in an average of 57 min. - (In vivo) Plasma concentrations of semaglutide were comparable in pyloric ligated and non-ligated dogs.	[61]

Table 5. *Cont.*

Experimental Method and Model Drugs	Proposed Mechanism of Action	Evidence	Reference
- CG-MD simulation - US simulation - TIRF microscopy (FRAP analysis)	SNAC does not appear to exhibit a transcellular mechanism by membrane insertion and perturbation.	*CG-MD simulation* - When 100 mM SNAC in the fluid composition of the fasting state was applied to the POPC membrane, fewer molecules of SNAC than those of C10 and C8 were adsorbed onto and incorporated into the membrane surface. *US simulation (PMF profile)* - In a POPC bilayer with a thickness of 4.05 nm, SNAC had an energy minima at a distance of 1.93 nm from the membrane center (energy minima represent the maximum probability of finding the molecule). *TIRF Microscopy (FRAP analysis)* - In the POPC–SNAC mixed membrane composed of various concentrations of SNAC, the membrane diffusivity decreased in a SNAC concentration–dependent manner.	[72]

PGDP, propylene glycol dipelargonate; DMPC, 1,2-dimyristoyl-*sn*-glycero-3-phosphocholine; SGF, simulated gastric fluid.

Oral semaglutide studies have suggested another mechanism of SNAC. Novo Nordisk presented a mechanism by which SNAC enhances oral absorption of semaglutide using various in vitro, in vivo, ex vivo, and clinical studies [61]. They put forth that the PE mechanism of SNAC works specifically for semaglutide. They found that SNAC protects semaglutide from enzymatic degradation in the stomach during uptake by elevating the local pH, and equally increases the transcellular uptake of semaglutide by the mechanism of induction of monomerization of semaglutide and increase in membrane fluidity (Figure 6). One of the major hurdles to the oral administration of peptide/protein drugs is the degradation by the pH environment and enzymes in the stomach. Therefore, an enteric coating is used commonly in many strategies utilizing PEs, to prevent the breakdown of the payload in the stomach and mainly target absorption in the small intestine [48,108,134,135]. In contrast, Novo Nordisk's oral semaglutide, Rybelsus®, is a formulation designed to be absorbed after erosion of the entire tablet in the stomach, rather than applying an enteric coating technology. They conducted a study on the optimization of Rybelsus® formulations through ex vivo experiments using dogs and gamma scintigraphic imaging of healthy adults [61,136]. They mentioned that the small intestine, which has a large surface area, is the main absorption site for drugs, disregarding the stomach as the absorption site for peptide/protein drugs. Nevertheless, they suggested that it is appropriate to target absorption in the stomach, as is the case with semaglutide, which must be co-formulated with a PE such as SNAC. Their strategy was to devise a formulation in which complete tablet erosion (CTE) occurs in the stomach by local disintegration by sinking to the lower part of the stomach through optimization of the formulation. CTE was confirmed in the stomach when taken with 240 mL of water on an empty stomach, and the average time to reach CTE was predicted to be about 1 h. Furthermore, clinical trials analyzed the absorption pattern of semaglutide according to the amount of water consumed. Regardless of the water intake, the Rybelsus tablet reached CTE in the stomach; however, it was found that when ingested with a relatively small amount of water (50 mL), the erosion time of the tablet increased, resulting in higher plasma semaglutide exposure [61,136]. Consequently, the mechanism of SNAC has been studied as a carrier mechanism based on a non-covalent bond, and a semaglutide-specific mechanism studied during the development of oral semaglutide. Therefore, it seems difficult to specify and define the general mechanism of SNAC as a PE.

Emisphere, which developed SNAC, tested it for vitamin B12, heparin, and insulin. After this technology was transferred to Novo Nordisk, numerous clinical trials on semaglutide have been conducted (Table S2). In addition, SNAC was further applied to peptide drugs such as Novo Nordisk's new GLP-a agonist (NNC0113-2023) and PCSK9 inhibitor (NNC0385-0434).

Numerous clinical trials conducted with semaglutide and SNAC for the successful development of Rybelsus® can be broadly classified into three categories. First, the efficacy, safety, PK profiling, and dosage setting of semaglutide/SNAC. In terms of efficacy, a phase 3 trial targeting patients with T2DM managed only with diet and exercise (PIONEER 1) and patients with T2DM uncontrolled with metformin (PIONEER 2) demonstrated superiority. In PIONEER 1, oral administration of 3–14 mg of semaglutide caused a dose-dependent decrease in HbA_{1c} of 0.7–1.4%, and the highest dose of 14 mg also showed a significant weight loss in participants of 2.3 kg [137]. In PIONEER 2, semaglutide was compared with empagliflozin, an SGLT-2 inhibitor, which has a weight loss and hypoglycemic effect. When administered at 26 weeks, semaglutide showed superior HbA_{1c} reduction compared to empagliflozin, and at 52 weeks of administration, it showed superiority in both HbA_{1c} and weight loss [138]. For PK and safety, clinical trials were conducted not only on healthy subjects but also on renal [139] and hepatic [140] impaired subjects and patients with diseases in the upper gastrointestinal tract [141], which is the site of absorption of semaglutide. In all cases, there was no significant effect on the PK profile and safety concerns of semaglutide, and there was no specific safety concern due to the disease.

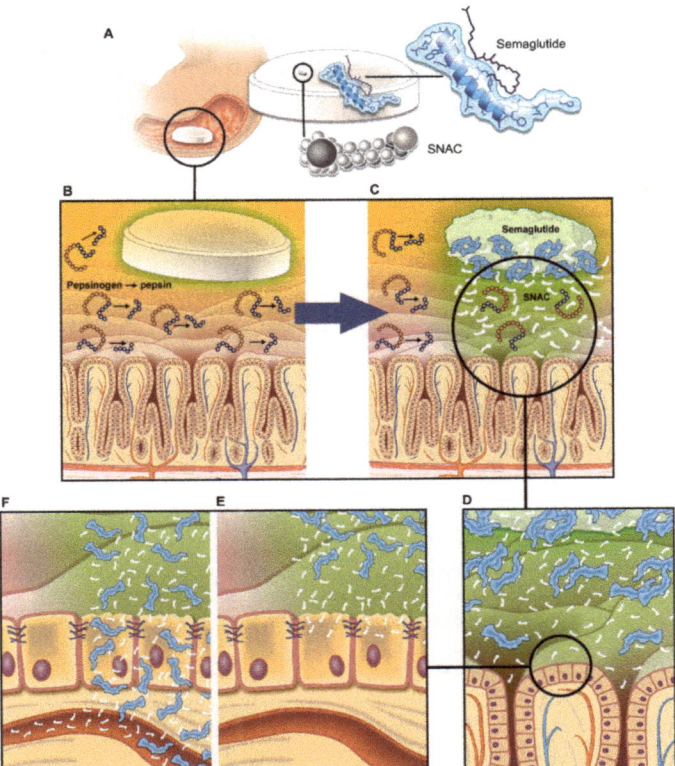

Figure 6. Formulation design of the Rybelsus® tablet and schematic diagram of the semaglutide absorption enhancement mechanism of SNAC (published by the Novo Nordisk research team) [61]. The Rybelsus® tablet (**A**) is completely eroded from the gastric mucosal surface (**B**,**C**) and SNAC increases the local pH to prevent the degradation of semaglutide from pepsin (**C**). Moreover, it indirectly weakens the self-association of semaglutide and helps to maintain the monomer state (**D**), and increases transcellular absorption by increasing membrane fluidity (**E**,**F**). Reprinted with permission from ref. [61]. Copyright 2018 *Science*.

The second category is the effect on reciprocal PK with concomitant drugs. In particular, due to the nature of the indications of semaglutide for chronic diseases such as diabetes and obesity, the patient is likely to be on multiple drugs in combination. In addition, since PE is used, it is also necessary to investigate the effect of the PE on the drug used in combination. Thus far, 11 concomitant drugs have been investigated at the clinical trial stage. Among them, the PK of four concomitant drugs: ethynylestradiol/levonorgestrel, digoxin, lisinopril, and warfarin, were not affected by semaglutide/SNAC [142,143]. Conversely, there was an increase in exposure to rosuvastatin, furosemide, levothyroxine, and metformin with the combination of semaglutide/SNAC [142–144].

The third category is the study of formulations. Beyond optimizing the basic semaglutide/SNAC dose, Novo Nordisk has conducted clinical trials on combinations of other excipients (otherwise called helping agents). Although the results of the clinical trial were not disclosed, they suggested that the study of excipients added together with the oral formulation to which PE is applied is more important than that of conventional oral formulations. In effect, the two clinical trials conducted by Novo Nordisk aimed to examine the effect of an additional helping agent on the dosage strength of semaglutide. That is, compared to the classical excipient, it functions as a more active type of excipient that can help the complex action of peptide API and PE.

Riley et al. extensively studied the safety of SNAC at the in vivo level and in the course of Rybelsus' clinical trials [145]. In vivo toxicity studies were conducted in a rat model for subchronic toxicity and peri- and post-natal developmental toxicity of SNAC. In Sprague Dawley rats (male (n = 20), female (n = 20)) given SNAC at 2 g/kg/day for 13 weeks, the mortality rate was 20% in males and 50% in females, showing a significant mortality rate, especially in females. Although the exact cause of death has not been elucidated, in comparison to the control group, changes in behavioral patterns (decreased activity, prostration, unkempt appearance, etc.) that persisted for several hours after SNAC administration; decreased globulin concentrations, especially in male rats; and a slight increase in liver and kidney weights were observed in the SNAC group. A sub-chronic toxicity study in Wistar rats was conducted with SNAC treatment at 0.1, 0.5, and 1 g/kg/day for 13 weeks. No death or clinical signs were observed at the highest dose of 1 g/kg/day, and they concluded that the no-adverse-effect level (NOAEL) for the Wistar rats was 1 g/kg/day. In the peri- and post-natal developmental toxicity study, oral administration of 1 g/kg/day from implantation to lactation of rats was conducted to evaluate the exposure and toxicity of SNAC in the uterus and breast milk of the offspring. There was no effect on the growth and development of surviving offspring exposed to SNAC, albeit that an increase in the number of stillbirths during pregnancy was observed [146]. Unlike MCFA, given that it does not exist in nature, SNAC may have more safety considerations. However, it has obtained FDA's GRAS status due to the accumulation of preclinical and clinical trial data that have been conducted so far, and has been established as key in the development of oral semaglutides without serious side effects.

5. Discussion

Oral administration of peptides using PEs is a simpler approach compared to strategies using nanoparticles and microneedle devices. However, there are still some limitations to be solved and issues to be considered. The first concern is the safety, efficacy, and reproducibility of PEs. MCFA and SNAC have independent safety status, and through this it has been possible to overcome regulatory hurdles. However, many PEs still need more research regarding their safety. As with MCFA and SNAC, most PEs have no established mechanism of action. Therefore, a more extensive toxicological investigation such as the off-target action in the intestine and the entire body is required in addition to the safety concerns directly related to the presumed mechanism. Damage to the intestinal tissue and related intestinal inflammation are the main safety concerns in transcellular PEs caused by membrane perturbation. Whereas the absorption of unwanted substances (enterotoxin, etc.), changes in the TJ integrity of other tissues after systemic absorption, and off-target action by sub-signaling are emerging as representative safety concerns for paracellular PEs based on TJ modulation. Additionally, as the development trend in peptide drugs for metabolic diseases increases, continuous dosing is required. Accordingly, the effect of long-term administration of PEs on the intestinal normal flora has been pointed out.

It seems that simply combining peptide drugs and PEs does not yet yield sufficient efficacy. The efficacy of a PE is directly related to the required amount of the peptide drug, an API. The first example of this is oral semaglutide (Rybelsys®). The bioavailability of Rybelsys® was 1% in a dog model [61]. In effect, the initial dose of injectable semaglutide (Wegovy®) administered once a week is 0.25 mg and the maintenance dose is 0.5–2 mg, whereas Rybelsus® is administered with an initial dose of 3 mg and a maintenance dose of 7 or 14 mg per day. That is, the amount of semaglutide consumed in the oral drug is about 80 or more times higher than that in the injectable formulation. An example of this can also be found in oral octreotide (Mycapssa®) [147]. In a phase 1 study of Mycapssa®, an oral octreotide does of 20 mg showed equivalent PK parameters to the 0.1 mg dose of the subcutaneous injectable octreotide. When comparing the actual dose of Mycapssa® with existing injectable products, 0.1 mg is administered 2–3 times a day for the subcutaneous injectable formulation, and 10–30 mg is injected once a month for the depot formulation. Conversely, Mycapssa® requires 20 mg of octreotide twice a day. In this way, the PE is as important as the API in terms of safety and efficacy.

In addition to safety and efficacy, reproducibility is an important concept. This is because if the effect of enhancing the absorption of peptides by a PE is vulnerable to differences between individuals and dosing conditions within individuals, a decrease in the therapeutic effect or side effects may be induced. In effect, there were cases where it was not possible to derive the difference in the PK parameter according to the administered dose due to the large variability between subjects in the clinical trials [111]. Another study equally mentions the need to lower the variability between subjects in future research, with an SD value of 4% and an average value of relative oral bioavailability of 7% [127].

The second point to be considered is the construction of an experimental model and the design of the formulation considering the action of PEs in the dynamic environment of the actual gastrointestinal tract. The in vitro experiment using the Caco-2 monolayer—the center of PE research—is a static experimental model and does not represent the actual dynamic environment of the gastrointestinal tract. This leads to a poor prediction of the effect of PEs in subsequent in vivo and clinical studies, implying that the effect of PEs is practically negligible and may lead to the failure of oral peptide development. The two main causes of the discrepancy between the static experimental model and the actual gastrointestinal tract are considered to be dilution and temporal synchronization of the PE and peptide in the gastrointestinal tract. First, in the case of dilution, as the PE and peptide are eluted into the bulk fluid of the gastrointestinal tract, PE is diluted to a concentration below the threshold that enhances absorption, and the peptide to be absorbed is moved away from the absorption site. In Rybelsus®, targeting absorption in the stomach, the Rybelsus® tablet is designed to localize and stay in the lower part of the stomach and CTE occurs. The design of the formulation appears to reduce the dilution of SNAC and semaglutide in the gastrointestinal tract. Novo Nordisk's research team investigated the difference in absorption of semaglutide according to the amount of water consumed along with the drug in a clinical trial, and found that the AUC of semaglutide increased when taking it with a small amount of water [136]. They mentioned the possibility that higher concentrations of SNAC and semaglutide in the stomach facilitate absorption, as well as slowing erosion and increasing gastric retention in the stomach. This is actually reflected in dosing regimens; patients are guided to take the tablets with less than 4 ounces of water. Recently, as a method to ensure proper synchronization of the PE and peptide, and to prevent dilution, the development of formulations capable of uni-directional release, i.e., gastrointestinal patches [148,149] and microcontainers [150,151], is emerging. Whatever its shape, it releases the PE and peptide only in the direction of the mucous membrane of the gastrointestinal tract, preventing dilution by elution into the bulk fluid, ensuring their synchronization by simultaneously or sequentially eluting the PE and peptide.

The third consideration is the properties of the peptide drug to be considered for establishing a PE strategy. Foremost, the natural properties of the peptide itself can be a determinant of the degree of its absorption in the gastrointestinal tract. The first of these properties is its susceptibility to enzymes in the gastrointestinal tract. In addition to overcoming the epithelial barrier expected from the PE, the other big task to be solved is overcoming the enzymatic barrier. A study on the stability of various peptides in gastrointestinal fluid confirmed that the enzymatic stability differs greatly depending on the sequence and structure of the peptide. GnRH analogues (-relin), including leuprolide and goserelin, have resistance to pepsin due to the amino acid substituted with the D-form at position 6, and show good stability in gastric fluid (GF). On the contrary, it does not have a protective effect on other intestinal enzymes including trypsin and chymotrypsin, and it has been confirmed that it is rapidly decomposed in intestinal fluid (IF). Moreover, the cyclic peptides cyclosporine, desmopressin, and octreotide showed excellent stability compared to other peptides in both GF and IF [152]. Furthermore, the stability of these three cyclic peptides in the gastrointestinal tract seems to have contributed to the development of some oral products: Sadimmun®, Minirin®, and Mycapssa®. Consequently, in overcoming the enzymatic barrier, the properties of the peptide itself are important, and to improve this, chemical modifications such as amino acid substitution and cyclization can be useful.

The subsequent consideration is the effect of peptide charge and modifications such as acylation. This is related to the migration of the peptide to the epithelial cell membrane in the gastrointestinal tract. This migratory behavior will also affect the establishment of the PE strategy. The charge of the peptide will affect the migration to and behavior near the membrane. Therefore, a PE strategy considering these characteristics should be established. A study on PIP640, a peptide PE and a TJ modulator, investigated the absorption enhancement effect for exenatide and calcitonin, which have similar hydrodynamic sizes but pI values of 4.9 and 9.3, respectively. It was observed that positively charged calcitonin had more improved bioavailability than negatively charged exenatide after treatment with PIP640 [153]. This suggests that the properties of the peptide, such as charge, can affect the absorption enhancement effect caused by the PE. Changes in properties due to peptide modification are also major factors to consider. A typical modification is acylation, which is intended to increase the half-life through albumin binding. A study comparing absorption enhancement patterns by transcellular PE (SDS) and paracellular PE (EGTA) for GLP-2 and its acylation derivatives observed varying absorption patterns dependent on acylation and the length of its carbon chain. The amount of GLP-2 bound to the cell membrane or uptaken into the cytoplasm increased according to the increase in the carbon chain length (C8–C12–C16), and for C8 to C12, the amount permeated into the increased acceptor compartment also increased. However, when acylated with C16, a lower absorption compared to the control was found. In addition, when comparing the absorption-enhancing effect of GLP-2 acylated with C16 by treatment with SDS and EGTA separately, the absorption enhancement by SDS was found to be superior. This was not observed in the control group and the group acylated with a shorter carbon chain. Furthermore, the research team observed an increase in self-association between peptides by acylation, and argued that this could cause a change in the permeability pattern [154]. These results indicate the need for a PE strategy that considers the increased interaction with the membrane by acylation. A PE strategy that reflects this can be seen in the examples of semaglutide and SNAC. For semaglutide, an acylated peptide, a strategy for the transcellular pathway was used via SNAC. Equally, another strategy was monomerization of semaglutide by SNAC.

The fourth issue concerns the regulatory approval of oral peptides to which the PE strategy has been applied. Considering the flow of changes in the biowaiver criteria of API belonging to BCS Classes 1 and 3 of immediate release solid formulations, it can be seen that regulatory agencies are taking a more restrictive standard for excipients. According to the 2017 FDA guidance, the excipient of the drug belonging to BCS Class 1 would not affect the absorption of the API [155]. Exceptionally, it was specified that surfactants such as polysorbate and excipients such as sorbitol and mannitol, which increase the GI fluid volume to decrease the residence time in the small intestine and affect drug absorption, should not differ qualitatively and must be quantitatively similar. Then, in 2020, the International Council for Harmonisation of Technical Requirements for Pharmaceuticals for Human Use (ICH) published "M9 guideline on biopharmaceutics classification system-based biowaivers (Step 5)", and the FDA published "M9 Biopharmaceutics Classification System-Based Biowaivers" reflecting this in the next year, which replaced the 2017 FDA guidance [156]. The difference from the 2017 guidance was the disappearance of the direct statement "The excipient has no effect on the absorption of APIs belonging to BCS Class 1", and even in the case of BCS Class 1, expression of concern that excipients may affect the absorption of APIs was emphasized. Of course, since peptide drugs belong to BCS Class 3, quantitative and qualitative differences from the excipients of the reference product were strict from the beginning of the introduction of the biowaiver concept. However, this regulatory flow is an example that reflects the stricter regulations being applied to excipients, more specifically, absorption-modifying excipients [157]. Unlike classical excipients, PE is a substance added 'intentionally' with the more active purpose of enhancing the absorption of APIs. Therefore, there is no doubt that there will be higher regulatory hurdles on the existing concepts of excipients. In particular, in the case of PEs which have obtained the safety status of food additives, such as MCFA, and GRAS, such as SNAC, or PEs that have not been approved as an excipient by regulatory agencies, the corresponding authorization for a new chemical entity may be applied. Similarly, due to the characteristics of a PE, it may not be appropriate to apply the concept of a biowaiver in the existing BCS Class 3 APIs at the time of approval of the generic product of oral peptide pharmaceuticals to which the PE is applied.

A final point to consider is the economics of oral peptide pharmaceuticals. As in the examples of Rybelsus® and Mycapssa® mentioned above, the oral formulation of the peptide developed with the PE strategy reaches almost 100 times the amount of peptide consumed compared to the conventional injectable dosage form. This increases the production cost of oral dosage forms which is unreasonably high and thus they have a very low economic feasibility. However, it is premature to judge the production cost and economic feasibility of oral peptide pharmaceuticals simply by the amount of peptide used as an active ingredient. Novo Nordisk argued that Rybelsus® had a higher API cost than Victoza® (liraglutide injectable product), but that the unit cost was not significantly different when considering the delivery cost of the injectable formulation [158]. The delivery cost of the injectable formulation includes the device for injection and the aseptic conditioning process involved in its production. This raises an opportunity to consider the increase in unit cost due to the production of injectable products and the direction of the development of oral peptide pharmaceuticals, given that this is the unit cost evaluated in Rybelsus® with oral bioavailability at approximately 1% level. If the oral bioavailability increases to a level greater than 1%, oral dosage forms can have a much lower unit cost compared to injectable dosage forms.

6. Conclusions

Oral macromolecule (peptides/proteins) delivery has been studied for decades, and a strategy using PE has recently yielded results at the peptide level. It was oral semaglutide that opened the door to oral peptide drug products. In particular, insulin, which has been a target of oral delivery since the beginning of the study of oral macromolecules, has not yet achieved clear results, despite numerous studies. Therefore, oral semaglutide by Novo Nordisk is evaluated to be more meaningful in the successful initiation of oral peptide drugs. The subsequent oral octreotide also became an example of a successful conversion to an oral dosage form because the existing dosage forms had obvious disadvantages, such as subcutaneous injectable formulations that required frequent administration and depot dosage forms that cause considerable pain during administration.

Despite the successful development history of Rybelsus® and Mycapssa®, the strategy of using PEs still has many limitations. Firstly, in terms of safety and regulation, the practically available PEs are not diverse. This means that a specific approval procedure for PEs should be established through a more extensive and systematic safety study on chemical entities that can be used as PEs and regulatory scientific research on PEs. Secondly, there is a need for research on more effective formulations. This includes research on the development of potent PEs that can further increase the bioavailability of macromolecules and research on next-generation formulations, such as unidirectional drug release considering the actual intestinal environment. These studies will reduce the required amount of peptide as an API in the process of converting from an injectable formulation to an oral formulation and will ensure the justification for the development of an oral peptide drug from an economic point of view.

Supplementary Materials: The following supporting information can be downloaded at: https://www.mdpi.com/article/10.3390/ph15121585/s1, Table S1: Clinical studies of oral drug formulations using sodium caprate (C10); Table S2: Clinical studies of oral drug formulations using SNAC.

Author Contributions: Conceptualization, J.C.K. and D.H.N.; methodology, J.C.K.; software, J.C.K.; investigation, J.C.K. and E.J.P.; data curation, J.C.K. and E.J.P.; writing—original draft preparation, J.C.K.; writing—review and editing, E.J.P. and D.H.N.; visualization, J.C.K. and E.J.P.; supervision, E.J.P. and D.H.N.; funding acquisition, D.H.N. All authors have read and agreed to the published version of the manuscript.

Funding: This work was supported by the National Research Foundation of Korea (NRF) grant funded by the Ministry of Science and ICT (NRF-2018R1A2B3004266) and by the Technology Innovation Program (20012631, Development of BiConTech based oral protein pharmaceutical product technology), funded by the Ministry of Trade, Industry & Energy (MOTIE, Korea). This research was supported by the Chung-Ang University Graduate Research Scholarship in 2021.

Institutional Review Board Statement: Not applicable.

Informed Consent Statement: Not applicable.

Data Availability Statement: Data is contained within the article and supplementary material.

Conflicts of Interest: The authors declare no conflict of interest.

References

1. Lau, J.L.; Dunn, M.K. Therapeutic peptides: Historical perspectives, current development trends, and future directions. *Bioorganic. Med. Chem.* **2018**, *26*, 2700–2707. [CrossRef] [PubMed]
2. Al Shaer, D.; Al Musaimi, O.; Albericio, F.; de la Torre, B.G. 2019 FDA TIDES (Peptides and Oligonucleotides) Harvest. *Pharmaceuticals* **2020**, *13*, 40. [CrossRef] [PubMed]
3. Wang, L.; Wang, N.; Zhang, W.; Cheng, X.; Yan, Z.; Shao, G.; Wang, X.; Wang, R.; Fu, C. Therapeutic peptides: Current applications and future directions. *Signal Transduct. Target. Ther.* **2022**, *7*, 48. [CrossRef] [PubMed]
4. Erak, M.; Bellmann-Sickert, K.; Els-Heindl, S.; Beck-Sickinger, A.G. Peptide chemistry toolbox—Transforming natural peptides into peptide therapeutics. *Bioorganic Med. Chem.* **2018**, *26*, 2759–2765. [CrossRef]
5. Tsomaia, N. Peptide therapeutics: Targeting the undruggable space. *Eur. J. Med. Chem.* **2015**, *94*, 459–470. [CrossRef] [PubMed]
6. Trier, S.; Linderoth, L.; Bjerregaard, S.; Strauss, H.M.; Rahbek, U.L.; Andresen, T.L. Acylation of salmon calcitonin modulates in vitro intestinal peptide flux through membrane permeability enhancement. *Eur. J. Pharm. Biopharm.* **2015**, *96*, 329–337. [CrossRef]
7. Na, D.H.; Youn, Y.S.; Park, E.J.; Lee, J.M.; Cho, O.R.; Lee, K.R.; Lee, S.D.; Yoo, S.D.; DeLuca, P.P.; Lee, K.C. Stability of PEGylated salmon calcitonin in nasal mucosa. *J. Pharm. Sci.* **2004**, *93*, 256–261. [CrossRef]
8. Na, D.H.; Faraj, J.; Capan, Y.; Leung, K.P.; DeLuca, P.P. Stability of Antimicrobial Decapeptide (KSL) and Its Analogues for Delivery in the Oral Cavity. *Pharm. Res.* **2007**, *24*, 1544–1550. [CrossRef]
9. Muttenthaler, M.; King, G.F.; Adams, D.J.; Alewood, P.F. Trends in peptide drug discovery. *Nat. Rev. Drug Discov.* **2021**, *20*, 309–325. [CrossRef]
10. Park, E.J.; Choi, J.; Lee, K.C.; Na, D.H. Emerging PEGylated non-biologic drugs. *Expert Opin. Emerg. Drugs* **2019**, *24*, 107–119. [CrossRef]
11. Park, E.J.; Lim, S.M.; Lee, K.C.; Na, D.H. Exendins and exendin analogs for diabetic therapy: A patent review (2012-2015). *Expert Opin. Ther. Pat.* **2016**, *26*, 833–842. [CrossRef] [PubMed]
12. Sheahan, K.H.; Wahlberg, E.A.; Gilbert, M.P. An overview of GLP-1 agonists and recent cardiovascular outcomes trials. *Postgrad. Med. J.* **2019**, *96*, 156–161. [CrossRef] [PubMed]
13. Lamberts, S.W.; van der Lely, A.-J.; de Herder, W.W.; Hofland, L.J. Octreotide. *N. Engl. J. Med.* **1996**, *334*, 246–254. [CrossRef]
14. McKeage, K.; Cheer, S.; Wagstaff, A.J. Octreotide Long-Acting Release (LAR): A review of its use in the management of acromegaly. *Drugs* **2003**, *63*, 2473–2499. [CrossRef] [PubMed]
15. Murty, S.B.; Na, D.H.; Thanoo, B.; DeLuca, P.P. Impurity formation studies with peptide-loaded polymeric microspheres: Part II. In vitro evaluation. *Int. J. Pharm.* **2005**, *297*, 62–72. [CrossRef]
16. Na, D.H.; DeLuca, P.P. PEGylation of Octreotide: I. Separation of Positional Isomers and Stability Against Acylation by Poly(D,L-lactide-co-glycolide). *Pharm. Res.* **2005**, *22*, 736–742. [CrossRef]
17. Ahn, J.H.; Park, E.J.; Lee, H.S.; Lee, K.C.; Na, D.H. Reversible Blocking of Amino Groups of Octreotide for the Inhibition of Formation of Acylated Peptide Impurities in Poly(Lactide-co-Glycolide) Delivery Systems. *AAPS PharmSciTech* **2011**, *12*, 1220–1226. [CrossRef]
18. Gadelha, M.R.; Wildemberg, L.E.; Kasuki, L. The Future of Somatostatin Receptor Ligands in Acromegaly. *J. Clin. Endocrinol. Metab.* **2021**, *107*, 297–308. [CrossRef]

19. Bornschein, J.; Drozdov, I.; Malfertheiner, P. Octreotide LAR: Safety and tolerability issues. *Expert Opin. Drug Saf.* **2009**, *8*, 755–768. [CrossRef]
20. Geho, W.B.; Rosenberg, L.N.; Schwartz, S.L.; Lau, J.R.; Gana, T.J. A Single-blind, Placebo-controlled, Dose-ranging Trial of Oral Hepatic-directed Vesicle Insulin Add-on to Oral Antidiabetic Treatment in Patients With Type 2 Diabetes Mellitus. *J. Diabetes Sci. Technol.* **2014**, *8*, 551–559. [CrossRef]
21. Rachmiel, M.; Barash, G.; Leshem, A.; Sagi, R.; Doenyas-Barak, K.; Koren, S. OR14-1 Pharmacodynamics, Safety, Tolerability, and Efficacy of Oral Insulin Formulation (Oshadi Icp) among Young Adults with Type 1 Diabetes: A Summary of Clinical Studies Phases I, Ib, and Ii. *J. Endocr. Soc.* **2019**, *3*. [CrossRef]
22. Tan, X.; Liu, X.; Zhang, Y.; Zhang, H.; Lin, X.; Pu, C.; Gou, J.; He, H.; Yin, T.; Zhang, Y.; et al. Silica nanoparticles on the oral delivery of insulin. *Expert Opin. Drug Deliv.* **2018**, *15*, 805–820. [CrossRef] [PubMed]
23. Pangeni, R.; Kang, S.; Jha, S.K.; Subedi, L.; Park, J.W. Intestinal membrane transporter-mediated approaches to improve oral drug delivery. *J. Pharm. Investig.* **2021**, *51*, 137–158. [CrossRef]
24. Leonaviciute, G.; Bernkop-Schnürch, A. Self-emulsifying drug delivery systems in oral (poly)peptide drug delivery. *Expert Opin. Drug Deliv.* **2015**, *12*, 1703–1716. [CrossRef] [PubMed]
25. Noh, G.; Keum, T.; Bashyal, S.; Seo, J.-E.; Shrawani, L.; Kim, J.H.; Lee, S. Recent progress in hydrophobic ion-pairing and lipid-based drug delivery systems for enhanced oral delivery of biopharmaceuticals. *J. Pharm. Investig.* **2021**, *52*, 75–93. [CrossRef]
26. Abramson, A.; Caffarel-Salvador, E.; Khang, M.; Dellal, D.; Silverstein, D.; Gao, Y.; Frederiksen, M.R.; Vegge, A.; Hubálek, F.; Water, J.J.; et al. An ingestible self-orienting system for oral delivery of macromolecules. *Science* **2019**, *363*, 611–615. [CrossRef]
27. Abramson, A.; Caffarel-Salvador, E.; Soares, V.; Minahan, D.; Tian, R.Y.; Lu, X.; Dellal, D.; Gao, Y.; Kim, S.; Wainer, J.; et al. A luminal unfolding microneedle injector for oral delivery of macromolecules. *Nat. Med.* **2019**, *25*, 1512–1518. [CrossRef]
28. Hashim, M.; Korupolu, R.; Syed, B.; Horlen, K.; Beraki, S.; Karamchedu, P.; Dhalla, A.K.; Ruffy, R.; Imran, M. Jejunal wall delivery of insulin via an ingestible capsule in anesthetized swine—A pharmacokinetic and pharmacodynamic study. *Pharmacol. Res. Perspect.* **2019**, *7*, e00522. [CrossRef]
29. Fricker, G.; Fahr, A.; Beglinger, C.; Kissel, T.; Reiter, G.; Drewe, J. Permeation enhancement of octreotide by specific bile salts in rats and human subjects: In vitro, in vivo correlations. *J. Cereb. Blood Flow Metab.* **1996**, *117*, 217–223. [CrossRef]
30. Lee, Y.-H.; Sinko, P.J. Oral delivery of salmon calcitonin. *Adv. Drug Deliv. Rev.* **2000**, *42*, 225–238. [CrossRef]
31. Stern, W. DRUG DELIVERY—Oral Delivery of Peptides by Peptelligence Technology. Available online: https://drug-dev.com/oral-delivery-of-peptides-by-peptelligence-technology/ (accessed on 28 September 2022).
32. Petersen, S.B.; Nielsen, L.G.; Rahbek, U.L.; Guldbrandt, M.; Brayden, D.J. Colonic absorption of salmon calcitonin using tetradecyl maltoside (TDM) as a permeation enhancer. *Eur. J. Pharm. Sci.* **2013**, *48*, 726–734. [CrossRef]
33. Kondoh, M.; Masuyama, A.; Takahashi, A.; Asano, N.; Mizuguchi, H.; Koizumi, N.; Fujii, M.; Hayakawa, T.; Horiguchi, Y.; Watanbe, Y. A Novel Strategy for the Enhancement of Drug Absorption Using a Claudin Modulator. *Mol. Pharmacol.* **2004**, *67*, 749–756. [CrossRef]
34. Gopalakrishnan, S.; Pandey, N.; Tamiz, A.P.; Vere, J.; Carrasco, R.; Somerville, R.; Tripathi, A.; Ginski, M.; Paterson, B.M.; Alkan, S.S. Mechanism of action of ZOT-derived peptide AT-1002, a tight junction regulator and absorption enhancer. *Int. J. Pharm.* **2009**, *365*, 121–130. [CrossRef] [PubMed]
35. Krug, S.M.; Hayaishi, T.; Iguchi, D.; Watari, A.; Takahashi, A.; Fromm, M.; Nagahama, M.; Takeda, H.; Okada, Y.; Sawasaki, T.; et al. Angubindin-1, a novel paracellular absorption enhancer acting at the tricellular tight junction. *J. Control. Release* **2017**, *260*, 1–11. [CrossRef] [PubMed]
36. Bocsik, A.; Gróf, I.; Kiss, L.; Ötvös, F.; Zsíros, O.; Daruka, L.; Fülöp, L.; Vastag, M.; Kittel, Á.; Imre, N.; et al. Dual Action of the PN159/KLAL/MAP Peptide: Increase of Drug Penetration across Caco-2 Intestinal Barrier Model by Modulation of Tight Junctions and Plasma Membrane Permeability. *Pharmaceutics* **2019**, *11*, 73. [CrossRef] [PubMed]
37. Artursson, P.; Magnusson, C. Epithelial Transport of Drugs in Cell Culture. II: Effect of Extracellular Calcium Concentration on the Paracellular Transport of Drugs of Different Lipophilicities across Monolayers of Intestinal Epithelial (Caco-2) Cells. *J. Pharm. Sci.* **1990**, *79*, 595–600. [CrossRef] [PubMed]
38. Tomita, M.; Hayashi, M.; Awazu, S. Absorption-Enhancing Mechanism of EDTA, Caprate, and Decanoylcarnitine in Caco-2 Cells. *J. Pharm. Sci.* **1996**, *85*, 608–611. [CrossRef]
39. Zhao, D.; Hirst, B.H. Comparison of Bile Salt Perturbation of Duodenal and Jejunal Isolated Brush-Border Membranes. *Digestion* **1990**, *47*, 200–207. [CrossRef]
40. Bonengel, S.; Jelkmann, M.; Abdulkarim, M.; Gumbleton, M.; Reinstadler, V.; Oberacher, H.; Prüfert, F.; Bernkop-Schnürch, A. Impact of different hydrophobic ion pairs of octreotide on its oral bioavailability in pigs. *J. Control. Release* **2018**, *273*, 21–29. [CrossRef]
41. Song, K.-H.; Chung, S.-J.; Shim, C.-K. Enhanced intestinal absorption of salmon calcitonin (sCT) from proliposomes containing bile salts. *J. Control. Release* **2005**, *106*, 298–308. [CrossRef]
42. LeCluyse, E.; Appel, L.E.; Sutton, S.C. Relationship Between Drug Absorption Enhancing Activity and Membrane Perturbing Effects of Acylcarnitines. *Pharm. Res.* **1991**, *8*, 84–87. [CrossRef] [PubMed]
43. Sutton, S.C.; Forbes, A.E.; Cargill, R.; Hochman, J.H.; LeCluyse, E.L. Simultaneous in Vitro Measurement of Intestinal Tissue Permeability and Transepithelial Electrical Resistance (TEER) Using Sweetana–Grass Diffusion Cells. *Pharm. Res.* **1992**, *09*, 316–319. [CrossRef] [PubMed]

44. LeCluyse, E.; Sutton, S.C.; Fix, J.A. In vitro effects of long-chain acylcarnitines on the permeability, transepithelial electrical resistance and morphology of rat colonic mucosa. *J. Pharmacol. Exp. Ther.* **1993**, *265*, 955–962. [PubMed]
45. Petersen, S.B.; Nolan, G.; Maher, S.; Rahbek, U.L.; Guldbrandt, M.; Brayden, D.J. Evaluation of alkylmaltosides as intestinal permeation enhancers: Comparison between rat intestinal mucosal sheets and Caco-2 monolayers. *Eur. J. Pharm. Sci.* **2012**, *47*, 701–712. [CrossRef]
46. Griesser, J.; Hetényi, G.; Moser, M.; Demarne, F.; Jannin, V.; Bernkop-Schnürch, A. Hydrophobic ion pairing: Key to highly payloaded self-emulsifying peptide drug delivery systems. *Int. J. Pharm.* **2017**, *520*, 267–274. [CrossRef]
47. McCartney, F.; Rosa, M.; Brayden, D.J. Evaluation of Sucrose Laurate as an Intestinal Permeation Enhancer for Macromolecules: Ex Vivo and In Vivo Studies. *Pharmaceutics* **2019**, *11*, 565. [CrossRef]
48. Banerjee, A.; Ibsen, K.; Brown, T.; Chen, R.; Agatemor, C.; Mitragotri, S. Ionic liquids for oral insulin delivery. *Proc. Natl. Acad. Sci. USA* **2018**, *115*, 7296–7301. [CrossRef]
49. Brayden, D.J.; Maher, S. Transient Permeation Enhancer®(TPE®) technology for oral delivery of octreotide: A technological evaluation. *Expert Opin. Drug Deliv.* **2021**, *18*, 1501–1512. [CrossRef]
50. Biermasz, N.R. New medical therapies on the horizon: Oral octreotide. *Pituitary* **2017**, *20*, 149–153. [CrossRef]
51. Tuvia, S.; Pelled, D.; Marom, K.; Salama, P.; Levin-Arama, M.; Karmeli, I.; Idelson, G.H.; Landau, I.; Mamluk, R. A Novel Suspension Formulation Enhances Intestinal Absorption of Macromolecules Via Transient and Reversible Transport Mechanisms. *Pharm. Res.* **2014**, *31*, 2010–2021. [CrossRef]
52. Salama, P.; Mamluk., R.; Marom., K.; Weinstein., I.; Tzabari., M. Pharmaceuical Compositions and Related Methods of Delivery. US20100105627A1, 2009.
53. Leone-Bay, A.; Santiago, N.; Achan, D.; Chaudhary, K.; DeMorin, F.; Falzarano, L.; Haas, S.; Kalbag, S.; Kaplan, D.; Leipold, H.; et al. N-Acylated.alpha.-Amino Acids as Novel Oral Delivery Agents for Proteins. *J. Med. Chem.* **1995**, *38*, 4263–4269. [CrossRef] [PubMed]
54. Malkov, D.; Angelo, R.; Wang, H.-Z.; Flanders, E.; Tang, H.; Gomez-Orellana, I. Oral Delivery of Insulin with the eligen(®) Technology: Mechanistic Studies. *Curr. Drug Deliv.* **2005**, *2*, 191–197. [CrossRef] [PubMed]
55. Lewis, A.L.; McEntee, N.; Holland, J.; Patel, A. Development and approval of rybelsus (oral semaglutide): Ushering in a new era in peptide delivery. *Drug Deliv. Transl. Res.* **2021**, *12*, 1–6. [CrossRef] [PubMed]
56. Lee, S.-H.; Lee, S.; Youn, Y.; Na, D.H.; Chae, S.Y.; Byun, A.Y.; Lee, K.C. Synthesis, Characterization, and Pharmacokinetic Studies of PEGylated Glucagon-like Peptide-1. *Bioconjugate Chem.* **2005**, *16*, 377–382. [CrossRef]
57. Son, S.; Lim, S.M.; Chae, S.Y.; Kim, K.; Park, E.J.; Lee, K.C.; Na, D.H. Mono-lithocholated exendin-4-loaded glycol chitosan nanoparticles with prolonged antidiabetic effects. *Int. J. Pharm.* **2015**, *495*, 81–86. [CrossRef]
58. Lee, W.; Park, E.J.; Kwak, S.; Lee, K.C.; Na, D.H.; Bae, J.-S. Trimeric PEG-Conjugated Exendin-4 for the Treatment of Sepsis. *Biomacromolecules* **2016**, *17*, 1160–1169. [CrossRef]
59. Husain, M.; Birkenfeld, A.L.; Donsmark, M.; Dungan, K.; Eliaschewitz, F.G.; Franco, D.R.; Jeppesen, O.K.; Lingvay, I.; Mosenzon, O.; Pedersen, S.D.; et al. Oral Semaglutide and Cardiovascular Outcomes in Patients with Type 2 Diabetes. *N. Engl. J. Med.* **2019**, *381*, 841–851. [CrossRef]
60. Knudsen, L.B.; Lau, J. The Discovery and Development of Liraglutide and Semaglutide. *Front. Endocrinol.* **2019**, *10*, 155. [CrossRef]
61. Buckley, S.T.; Baekdal, T.A.; Vegge, A.; Maarbjerg, S.J.; Pyke, C.; Ahnfelt-Ronne, J.; Madsen, K.G.; Scheele, S.G.; Alanentalo, T.; Kirk, R.K.; et al. Transcellular stomach absorption of aderivatized glucagon-like peptide-1 receptor agonist. *Sci. Transl. Med.* **2018**, *10*, eaar7047. [CrossRef]
62. Kitao, K.; Nishimura, K. Adsuvant for Promoting Absorption of Pharmacologically Active Substances through the Rectum. US4338306A, 6 July 1982.
63. Nishimura, K.; Nozaki, Y.; Yoshimi, A.; Nakamura, S.; Kitagawa, M.; Kakeya, N.; Kitao, K. Studies on the promoting effects of carboxylic acid derivatives on the rectal absorption of.BETA.-lactam antibiotics in rats. *Chem. Pharm. Bull.* **1985**, *33*, 282–291. [CrossRef]
64. Lindmark, T.; Söderholm, J.D.; Olaison, G.; Alván, G.; Ocklind, G.; Artursson, P. Mechanism of Absorption Enhancement in Humans After Rectal Administration of Ampicillin in Suppositories Containing Sodium Caprate. *Pharm. Res.* **1997**, *14*, 930–935. [CrossRef] [PubMed]
65. Maher, S.; Geoghegan, C.; Brayden, D.J. Intestinal permeation enhancers to improve oral bioavailability of macromolecules: Reasons for low efficacy in humans. *Expert Opin. Drug Deliv.* **2020**, *18*, 273–300. [CrossRef] [PubMed]
66. Hossain, S.; Berg, S.; Bergström, C.A.S.; Larsson, P. Aggregation Behavior of Medium Chain Fatty Acids Studied by Coarse-Grained Molecular Dynamics Simulation. *AAPS PharmSciTech* **2019**, *20*, 61. [CrossRef] [PubMed]
67. Food Additive Status List. Available online: https://www.fda.gov/food/food-additives-petitions/food-additive-status-list#abb (accessed on 30 September 2022).
68. Mortensen, A.; Aguilar, F.; Crebelli, R.; Di Domenico, A.; Dusemund, B.; Frutos, M.J.; Galtier, P.; Gott, D.; Gundert-Remy, U.; Leblanc, J.C.; et al. Re-evaluation of fatty acids (E 570) as a food additive. *EFSA J.* **2017**, *15*, e04785. [CrossRef] [PubMed]
69. Jia, W.; Dong, X.; Shi, L.; Chu, X. Discrimination of Milk from Different Animal Species by a Foodomics Approach Based on High-Resolution Mass Spectrometry. *J. Agric. Food Chem.* **2020**, *68*, 6638–6645. [CrossRef]
70. Sawada, T.; Ogawa, T.; Tomita, M.; Hayashi, M.; Awazu, S. Role of Paracellular Pathway in Nonelectrolyte Permeation Across Rat Colon Epithelium Enhanced by Sodium Caprate and Sodium Caprylate. *Pharm. Res.* **1991**, *08*, 1365–1371. [CrossRef]

71. Mishima, M.; Wakita, Y.; Nakano, M. Studies on the promoting effects of medium chain fatty acid salts on the nasal absorption of insulin in rats. *J. Pharmacobio-Dynamics* **1987**, *10*, 624–631. [CrossRef]
72. Hossain, S.; Joyce, P.; Parrow, A.; Jõemetsa, S.; Höök, F.; Larsson, P.; Bergström, C.A.S. Influence of Bile Composition on Membrane Incorporation of Transient Permeability Enhancers. *Mol. Pharm.* **2020**, *17*, 4226–4240. [CrossRef]
73. Maher, S.; Mrsny, R.J.; Brayden, D.J. Intestinal permeation enhancers for oral peptide delivery. *Adv. Drug Deliv. Rev.* **2016**, *106*, 277–319. [CrossRef]
74. Lindmark, T.; Nikkilä, T.; Artursson, P. Mechanisms of absorption enhancement by medium chain fatty acids in intestinal epithelial Caco-2 cell monolayers. *J. Pharmacol. Exp. Ther.* **1995**, *275*, 958–964.
75. Kneiszl, R.; Hossain, S.; Larsson, P. In Silico-Based Experiments on Mechanistic Interactions between Several Intestinal Permeation Enhancers with a Lipid Bilayer Model. *Mol. Pharm.* **2021**, *19*, 124–137. [CrossRef] [PubMed]
76. Ates, M.; Kaynak, M.S.; Sahin, S. Effect of permeability enhancers on paracellular permeability of acyclovir. *J. Pharm. Pharmacol.* **2016**, *68*, 781–790. [CrossRef] [PubMed]
77. Shanmugam, S.; Im, H.T.; Sohn, Y.T.; Kim, K.S.; Kim, Y.-I.; Yong, C.S.; Kim, J.O.; Choi, H.-G.; Woo, J.S. Zanamivir Oral Delivery: Enhanced Plasma and Lung Bioavailability in Rats. *Biomol. Ther.* **2013**, *21*, 161–169. [CrossRef] [PubMed]
78. Lo, Y.-L.; Huang, J.-D. Effects of sodium deoxycholate and sodium caprate on the transport of epirubicin in human intestinal epithelial Caco-2 cell layers and everted gut sacs of rats. *Biochem. Pharmacol.* **2000**, *59*, 665–672. [CrossRef]
79. Dos Santos, I.; Fawaz, F.; Lagueny, A.M.; Bonini, F. Improvement of norfloxacin oral bioavailability by EDTA and sodium caprate. *Int. J. Pharm.* **2003**, *260*, 1–4. [CrossRef]
80. Raoof, A.A.; Chiu, P.; Ramtoola, Z.; Cumming, I.K.; Teng, C.; Weinbach, S.P.; Hardee, G.E.; Levin, A.A.; Geary, R. Oral bioavailability and multiple dose tolerability of an antisense oligonucleotide tablet formulated with sodium caprate. *J. Pharm. Sci.* **2004**, *93*, 1431–1439. [CrossRef]
81. Raoof, A.A.; Ramtoola, Z.; McKenna, B.; Yu, R.Z.; Hardee, G.; Geary, R.S. Effect of sodium caprate on the intestinal absorption of two modified antisense oligonucleotides in pigs. *Eur. J. Pharm. Sci.* **2002**, *17*, 131–138. [CrossRef]
82. Chao, A.C.; Nguyen, J.V.; Broughall, M.; Griffin, A.; Fix, J.A.; Daddona, P.E. In vitro and in vivo evaluation of effects of sodium caprate on enteral peptide absorption and on mucosal morphology. *Int. J. Pharm.* **1999**, *191*, 15–24. [CrossRef]
83. Gleeson, J.; Frias, J.; Ryan, S.M.; Brayden, D.J. Sodium caprate enables the blood pressure-lowering effect of Ile-Pro-Pro and Leu-Lys-Pro in spontaneously hypertensive rats by indirectly overcoming PepT1 inhibition. *Eur. J. Pharm. Biopharm.* **2018**, *128*, 179–187. [CrossRef]
84. Kamm, W.; Jonczyk, A.; Jung, T.; Luckenbach, G.; Raddatz, P.; Kissel, T. Evaluation of absorption enhancement for a potent cyclopeptidic $\alpha v \beta 3$-antagonist in a human intestinal cell line (Caco-2). *Eur. J. Pharm. Sci.* **2000**, *10*, 205–214. [CrossRef]
85. Lindmark, T.; Schipper, N.; Lazorová, L.; De Boer, A.G.; Artursson, P. Absorption Enhancement in Intestinal Epithelial Caco-2 Monolayers by Sodium Caprate: Assessment of Molecular Weight Dependence and Demonstration of Transport Routes. *J. Drug Target.* **1998**, *5*, 215–223. [CrossRef]
86. Kim, I.-W.; Yoo, H.-J.; Song, I.-S.; Chung, Y.-B.; Moon, D.-C.; Chung, S.-J.; Shim, C.-K. Effect of excipients on the stability and transport of recombinant human epidermal growth factor (rhEGF) across Caco-2 cell monolayers. *Arch. Pharmacal Res.* **2003**, *26*, 330–337. [CrossRef]
87. Yamamoto, A.; Okagawa, T.; Kotani, A.; Uchiyama, T.; Shimura, T.; Tabata, S.; Kondo, S.; Muranishi, S. Effects of Different Absorption Enhancers on the Permeation of Ebiratide, an ACTH Analogue, across Intestinal Membranes. *J. Pharm. Pharmacol.* **1997**, *49*, 1057–1061. [CrossRef] [PubMed]
88. Dahlgren, D.; Sjöblom, M.; Hedeland, M.; Lennernäs, H. The In Vivo Effect of Transcellular Permeation Enhancers on the Intestinal Permeability of Two Peptide Drugs Enalaprilat and Hexarelin. *Pharmaceutics* **2020**, *12*, 99. [CrossRef] [PubMed]
89. Uchiyama, T.; Sugiyama, T.; Quan, Y.-S.; Kotani, A.; Okada, N.; Fujita, T.; Muranishi, S.; Yamamoto, A. Enhanced Permeability of Insulin across the Rat Intestinal Membrane by Various Absorption Enhancers: Their Intestinal Mucosal Toxicity and Absorption-enhancing Mechanism of n-Lauryl-β-D-maltopyranoside. *J. Pharm. Pharmacol.* **1999**, *51*, 1241–1250. [CrossRef]
90. Wallon, C.; Braaf, Y.; Wolving, M.; Olaison, G.; Söderholm, J.D. Endoscopic biopsies in Ussing chambers evaluated for studies of macromolecular permeability in the human colon. *Scand. J. Gastroenterol.* **2005**, *40*, 586–595. [CrossRef]
91. Morishita, M.; Morishita, I.; Takayama, K.; Machida, Y.; Nagai, T. Site-Dependent Effect of Aprotinin, Sodium Caprate, Na2EDTA and Sodium Glycocholate on Intestinal Absorption of Insulin. *Biol. Pharm. Bull.* **1993**, *16*, 68–72. [CrossRef]
92. Imai, T.; Sakai, M.; Ohtake, H.; Azuma, H.; Otagiri, M. Absorption-enhancing effect of glycyrrhizin induced in the presence of capric acid. *Int. J. Pharm.* **2005**, *294*, 11–21. [CrossRef]
93. Muranushi, N.; Mack, E.; Kim, S.W. The Effects of Fatty Acids and Their Derivatives on the Intestinal Absorption of insulin in Rat. *Drug Dev. Ind. Pharm.* **1993**, *19*, 929–941. [CrossRef]
94. Burcham, D.L.; Aungst, B.A.; Hussain, M.; Gorko, M.A.; Quon, C.Y.; Huang, S. The Effect of Absorption Enhancers on the Oral Absorption of the GP IIB/IIIA Receptor Antagonist, DMP 728, in Rats and Dogs. *Pharm. Res.* **1995**, *12*, 2065–2070. [CrossRef]
95. Radwan, M.A.; Aboul-Enein, H.Y. The effect of oral absorption enhancers on the in vivo performance of insulin-loaded poly(ethylcyanoacrylate) nanospheres in diabetic rats. *J. Microencapsul.* **2002**, *19*, 225–235. [CrossRef]
96. Watanabe, Y.; Mizufune, Y.; Kubomura, A.; Kiriyama, M.; Utoguchi, N.; Matsumoto, M. Studies of Drug Delivery Systems for a Therapeutic Agent Used in Osteoporosis. I. Pharmacodynamics (Hypocalcemic Effect) of Elcatonin in Rabbits Following Rectal Administration of Hollow-Type Suppositories Containing Elcatonin. *Biol. Pharm. Bull.* **1998**, *21*, 1187–1190. [CrossRef]

97. Anderberg, E.K.; Lindmark, T.; Artursson, P. Sodium Caprate Elicits Dilatations in Human Intestinal Tight Junctions and Enhances Drug Absorption by the Paracellular Route. *Pharm. Res.* **1993**, *10*, 857–864. [CrossRef]
98. Tomita, M.; Hayashi, M.; Awazu, S. Comparison of Absorption-Enhancing Effect between Sodium Caprate and Disodium Ethylenediaminetetraacetate in Caco-2 Cells. *Biol. Pharm. Bull.* **1994**, *17*, 753–755. [CrossRef]
99. Soderholm, J.D.; Oman, H.; Blomquist, L.; Veen, J.; Lindmark, T.; Olaison, G. Reversible increase in tight junction permeability to macromolecules in rat ileal mucosa in vitro by sodium caprate, a constituent of milk fat. *Dig. Dis. Sci.* **1998**, *43*, 1547–1552. [CrossRef] [PubMed]
100. Coyne, C.B.; Ribeiro, C.M.P.; Boucher, R.C.; Johnson, L.G. Acute Mechanism of Medium Chain Fatty Acid-Induced Enhancement of Airway Epithelial Permeability. *J. Pharmacol. Exp. Ther.* **2003**, *305*, 440–450. [CrossRef] [PubMed]
101. Sugibayashi, K.; Onuki, Y.; Takayama, K. Displacement of tight junction proteins from detergent-resistant membrane domains by treatment with sodium caprate. *Eur. J. Pharm. Sci.* **2009**, *36*, 246–253. [CrossRef] [PubMed]
102. Del Vecchio, G.; Tscheik, C.; Tenz, K.; Helms, H.C.; Winkler, L.; Blasig, R.; Blasig, I.E. Sodium Caprate Transiently Opens Claudin-5-Containing Barriers at Tight Junctions of Epithelial and Endothelial Cells. *Mol. Pharm.* **2012**, *9*, 2523–2533. [CrossRef]
103. Krug, S.M.; Amasheh, M.; Dittmann, I.; Christoffel, I.; Fromm, M.; Amasheh, S. Sodium caprate as an enhancer of macromolecule permeation across tricellular tight junctions of intestinal cells. *Biomaterials* **2012**, *34*, 275–282. [CrossRef]
104. Brayden, D.J.; Maher, S.; Bahar, B.; Walsh, E. Sodium caprate-induced increases in intestinal permeability and epithelial damage are prevented by misoprostol. *Eur. J. Pharm. Biopharm.* **2015**, *94*, 194–206. [CrossRef]
105. Twarog, C.; Liu, K.; O'Brien, P.J.; Dawson, K.A.; Fattal, E.; Illel, B.; Brayden, D.J. A head-to-head Caco-2 assay comparison of the mechanisms of action of the intestinal permeation enhancers: SNAC and sodium caprate (C10). *Eur. J. Pharm. Biopharm.* **2020**, *152*, 95–107. [CrossRef] [PubMed]
106. Jones, J.B.; Bailey, R.T., Jr. Misoprostol: A Prostaglandin E$_1$ Analog with Antisecretory and Cytoprotective Properties. *DICP* **1989**, *23*, 276–282. [CrossRef] [PubMed]
107. Maher, S.; Leonard, T.W.; Jacobsen, J.; Brayden, D.J. Safety and efficacy of sodium caprate in promoting oral drug absorption: From in vitro to the clinic. *Adv. Drug Deliv. Rev.* **2009**, *61*, 1427–1449. [CrossRef] [PubMed]
108. Leonard, T.W.; Lynch, J.; McKenna, M.J.; Brayden, D. Promoting absorption of drugs in humans using medium-chain fatty acid-based solid dosage forms: GIPET™. *Expert Opin. Drug Deliv.* **2006**, *3*, 685–692. [CrossRef]
109. Leonard, T.W.; Coughlan, D.C.; Cullen, A. Pharmaceutical Compositions of Selective Factor Xa Inhibitors for Oral Administration. WO2011120033A1, 29 September 2011.
110. Walsh, E.G.; Adamczyk, B.E.; Chalasani, K.B.; Maher, S.; O'Toole, E.B.; Fox, J.S.; Leonard, T.W.; Brayden, D.J. Oral delivery of macromolecules: Rationale underpinning Gastrointestinal Permeation Enhancement Technology (GIPET®). *Ther. Deliv.* **2011**, *2*, 1595–1610. [CrossRef]
111. Amory, J.K.; Leonard, T.W.; Page, S.T.; O'Toole, E.; McKenna, M.J.; Bremner, W.J. Oral administration of the GnRH antagonist acyline, in a GIPET®-enhanced tablet form, acutely suppresses serum testosterone in normal men: Single-dose pharmacokinetics and pharmacodynamics. *Cancer Chemother. Pharmacol.* **2009**, *64*, 641–645. [CrossRef]
112. Twarog, C.; Fattah, S.; Heade, J.; Maher, S.; Fattal, E.; Brayden, D.J. Intestinal Permeation Enhancers for Oral Delivery of Macromolecules: A Comparison between Salcaprozate Sodium (SNAC) and Sodium Caprate (C10). *Pharmaceutics* **2019**, *11*, 78. [CrossRef]
113. Ramaswamy, S.G.; Nayak, V.G.; Jha, S.K.; Hegde, V.; Waichale, V.S.; Melarkode, R.; Chirmule, N.; Rao, A.U.; Sengupta, N. Development and validation of an electrochemiluminescent ELISA for quantitation of oral insulin tregopil in diabetes mellitus serum. *Bioanalysis* **2017**, *9*, 975–986. [CrossRef]
114. Hazra, P.; Adhikary, L.; Dave, N.; Khedkar, A.; Manjunath, H.S.; Anantharaman, R.; Iyer, H. Development of a process to manufacture PEGylated orally bioavailable insulin. *Biotechnol. Prog.* **2010**, *26*, 1695–1704. [CrossRef]
115. Berg, S.; Krause, J.; Björkbom, A.; Walter, K.; Harun, S.; Granfeldt, A.; Janzén, D.; Nunes, S.F.; Antonsson, M.; Van Zuydam, N.; et al. In Vitro and In Vivo Evaluation of 3D Printed Capsules with Pressure Triggered Release Mechanism for Oral Peptide Delivery. *J. Pharm. Sci.* **2020**, *110*, 228–238. [CrossRef]
116. Jørgensen, J.R.; Jepsen, M.L.; Nielsen, L.H.; Dufva, M.; Nielsen, H.M.; Rades, T.; Boisen, A.; Müllertz, A. Microcontainers for oral insulin delivery—In vitro studies of permeation enhancement. *Eur. J. Pharm. Biopharm.* **2019**, *143*, 98–105. [CrossRef] [PubMed]
117. Steiner., S.; Rosen., R. Delivery Systems for Pharmacological Agents Encapsulated with Proteinoids. US4925673A, 15 May 1990.
118. Leone-Bay, A.; Ho, K.-K.; Agarwal, R.; Baughman, R.A.; Chaudhary, K.; DeMorin, F.; Genoble, L.; McInnes, C.; Lercara, C.; Milstein, S.; et al. 4-[4-[(2-Hydroxybenzoyl)amino]phenyl]butyric Acid as a Novel Oral Delivery Agent for Recombinant Human Growth Hormone. *J. Med. Chem.* **1996**, *39*, 2571–2578. [CrossRef]
119. Milstein, S.J.; Leipold, H.; Sarubbi, D.; Leone-Bay, A.; Mlynek, G.M.; Robinson, J.R.; Kasimova, M.; Freire, E. Partially unfolded proteins efficiently penetrate cell membranes—implications for oral drug delivery. *J. Control. Release* **1998**, *53*, 259–267. [CrossRef]
120. Arbit, E.; Goldberg, M.; Gomez-Orellana, I.; Majuru, S. Oral heparin: Status review. *Thromb. J.* **2006**, *4*, 6. [CrossRef]
121. Kidron, M.; Dinh, S.; Menachem, Y.; Abbas, R.; Variano, B.; Goldberg, M.; Arbit, E.; Bar-On, H. A novel per-oral insulin formulation: Proof of concept study in non-diabetic subjects. *Diabet. Med.* **2004**, *21*, 354–357. [CrossRef] [PubMed]
122. Mousa, S.A.; Zhang, F.; Aljada, A.; Chaturvedi, S.; Takieddin, M.; Zhang, H.; Chi, L.; Castelli, M.C.; Friedman, K.; Goldberg, M.M.; et al. Pharmacokinetics and Pharmacodynamics of Oral Heparin Solid Dosage Form in Healthy Human Subjects. *J. Clin. Pharmacol.* **2007**, *47*, 1508–1520. [CrossRef] [PubMed]

123. Berkowitz, S.D.; Marder, V.J.; Kosutic, G.; Baughman, R.A. Oral heparin administration with a novel drug delivery agent (SNAC) in healthy volunteers and patients undergoing elective total hip arthroplasty. *J. Thromb. Haemost.* **2003**, *1*, 1914–1919. [CrossRef]
124. Bittner, B.; McIntyre, C.; Tian, H.; Tang, K.; Shah, N.; Phuapradit, W.; Ahmed, H.; Chokshi, H.; Infeld, M.; Fotaki, N.; et al. Phase I clinical study to select a novel oral formulation for ibandronate containing the excipient sodium N-[8-(2-hydroxybenzoyl) amino] caprylate (SNAC). *Die Pharm.* **2012**, *67*, 233–241.
125. Steinert, R.E.; Poller, B.; Castelli, M.C.; Drewe, J.; Beglinger, C. Oral administration of glucagon-like peptide 1 or peptide YY 3-36 affects food intake in healthy male subjects. *Am. J. Clin. Nutr.* **2010**, *92*, 810–817. [CrossRef]
126. Karsdal, M.; Byrjalsen, I.; Alexandersen, P.; Bihlet, A.; Andersen, J.; Riis, B.; Bay-Jensen, A.; Christiansen, C. Treatment of symptomatic knee osteoarthritis with oral salmon calcitonin: Results from two phase 3 trials. *Osteoarthr. Cartil.* **2015**, *23*, 532–543. [CrossRef]
127. Kapitza, C.; Zijlstra, E.; Heinemann, L.; Castelli, M.C.; Riley, G.; Heise, T. Oral Insulin: A Comparison With Subcutaneous Regular Human Insulin in Patients With Type 2 Diabetes. *Diabetes Care* **2010**, *33*, 1288–1290. [CrossRef]
128. Fattah, S.; Ismaiel, M.; Murphy, B.; Rulikowska, A.; Frias, J.M.; Winter, D.C.; Brayden, D.J. Salcaprozate sodium (SNAC) enhances permeability of octreotide across isolated rat and human intestinal epithelial mucosae in Ussing chambers. *Eur. J. Pharm. Sci.* **2020**, *154*, 105509. [CrossRef]
129. Salcaprozate Sodium. Available online: https://pubchem.ncbi.nlm.nih.gov/compound/Salcaprozate-sodium (accessed on 5 October 2022).
130. Malkov, D.; Wang, H.; Dinh, S.; Gomez-Orellana, I. Pathway of oral absorption of heparin with sodium N-[8-(2-hydroxybenzoyl)amino] caprylate. *Pharm. Res.* **2002**, *19*, 1180–1184. [CrossRef]
131. Alani, A.W.G.; Robinson, J.R. Mechanistic Understanding of Oral Drug Absorption Enhancement of Cromolyn Sodium by an Amino Acid Derivative. *Pharm. Res.* **2007**, *25*, 48–54. [CrossRef] [PubMed]
132. Chen, H.; Lu, Y.; Shi, S.; Zhang, Q.; Cao, X.; Sun, L.; An, D.; Zhang, X.; Kong, X.; Liu, J. Design and Development of a New Glucagon-Like Peptide-1 Receptor Agonist to Obtain High Oral Bioavailability. *Pharm. Res.* **2022**, *39*, 1891–1906. [CrossRef] [PubMed]
133. Hess, S.; Rotshild, V.; Hoffman, A. Investigation of the enhancing mechanism of sodium N-[8-(2-hydroxybenzoyl)amino]caprylate effect on the intestinal permeability of polar molecules utilizing a voltage clamp method. *Eur. J. Pharm. Sci.* **2005**, *25*, 307–312. [CrossRef] [PubMed]
134. Zhang, Y.; Zhou, W.; Shen, L.; Lang, L.; Huang, X.; Sheng, H.; Ning, G.; Wang, W. Safety, Pharmacokinetics, and Pharmacodynamics of Oral Insulin Administration in Healthy Subjects: A Randomized, Double-Blind, Phase 1 Trial. *Clin. Pharmacol. Drug Dev.* **2022**, *11*, 606–614. [CrossRef] [PubMed]
135. Binkley, N.; Bolognese, M.; Sidorowicz-Bialynicka, A.; Vally, T.; Trout, R.; Miller, C.; Buben, C.E.; Gilligan, J.P.; Krause, D.S. A phase 3 trial of the efficacy and safety of oral recombinant calcitonin: The oral calcitonin in postmenopausal osteoporosis (ORACAL) trial. *J. Bone Miner. Res.* **2012**, *27*, 1821–1829. [CrossRef]
136. Bækdal, T.A.; Donsmark, M.; Hartoft-Nielsen, M.; Søndergaard, F.L.; Connor, A. Relationship Between Oral Semaglutide Tablet Erosion and Pharmacokinetics: A Pharmacoscintigraphic Study. *Clin. Pharmacol. Drug Dev.* **2021**, *10*, 453–462. [CrossRef]
137. Aroda, V.R.; Rosenstock, J.; Terauchi, Y.; Altuntas, Y.; Lalic, N.M.; Villegas, E.C.M.; Jeppesen, O.K.; Christiansen, E.; Hertz, C.L.; Haluzík, M.; et al. PIONEER 1: Randomized Clinical Trial of the Efficacy and Safety of Oral Semaglutide Monotherapy in Comparison With Placebo in Patients With Type 2 Diabetes. *Diabetes Care* **2019**, *42*, 1724–1732. [CrossRef]
138. Rodbard, H.W.; Rosenstock, J.; Canani, L.H.; Deerochanawong, C.; Gumprecht, J.; Lindberg, S.; Lingvay, I.; Søndergaard, A.L.; Treppendahl, M.B.; Montanya, E.; et al. Oral Semaglutide Versus Empagliflozin in Patients With Type 2 Diabetes Uncontrolled on Metformin: The PIONEER 2 Trial. *Diabetes Care* **2019**, *42*, 2272–2281. [CrossRef] [PubMed]
139. Granhall, C.; Søndergaard, F.L.; Thomsen, M.; Anderson, T.W. Pharmacokinetics, Safety and Tolerability of Oral Semaglutide in Subjects with Renal Impairment. *Clin. Pharmacokinet.* **2018**, *57*, 1571–1580. [CrossRef] [PubMed]
140. Baekdal, T.A.; Thomsen, M.; Kupčová, V.; Hansen, C.W.; Msc, T.W.A. Pharmacokinetics, Safety, and Tolerability of Oral Semaglutide in Subjects With Hepatic Impairment. *J. Clin. Pharmacol.* **2018**, *58*, 1314–1323. [CrossRef]
141. Overgaard, R.V.; Navarria, A.; Ingwersen, S.H.; Bækdal, T.A.; Kildemoes, R.J. Clinical Pharmacokinetics of Oral Semaglutide: Analyses of Data from Clinical Pharmacology Trials. *Clin. Pharmacokinet.* **2021**, *60*, 1335–1348. [CrossRef]
142. Jordy, A.B.; Albayaty, M.; Breitschaft, A.; Anderson, T.W.; Christiansen, E.; Houshmand-Øregaard, A.; Manigandan, E.; Bækdal, T.A. Effect of Oral Semaglutide on the Pharmacokinetics of Levonorgestrel and Ethinylestradiol in Healthy Postmenopausal Women and Furosemide and Rosuvastatin in Healthy Subjects. *Clin. Pharmacokinet.* **2021**, *60*, 1171–1185. [CrossRef]
143. Bækdal, T.A.; Borregaard, J.; Hansen, C.W.; Thomsen, M.; Anderson, T.W. Effect of Oral Semaglutide on the Pharmacokinetics of Lisinopril, Warfarin, Digoxin, and Metformin in Healthy Subjects. *Clin. Pharmacokinet.* **2019**, *58*, 1193–1203. [CrossRef]
144. Hauge, C.; Breitschaft, A.; Hartoft-Nielsen, M.-L.; Jensen, S.; Bækdal, T.A. Effect of oral semaglutide on the pharmacokinetics of thyroxine after dosing of levothyroxine and the influence of co-administered tablets on the pharmacokinetics of oral semaglutide in healthy subjects: An open-label, one-sequence crossover, single-center, multiple-dose, two-part trial. *Expert Opin. Drug Metab. Toxicol.* **2021**, *17*, 1139–1148. [CrossRef]
145. Riley, M.G.I.; Castelli, M.C.; Paehler, E.A. Subchronic Oral Toxicity of Salcaprozate Sodium (SNAC) in Sprague-Dawley and Wistar Rats. *Int. J. Toxicol.* **2009**, *28*, 278–293. [CrossRef] [PubMed]

146. Riley, M.G.I.; York, R.G. Peri- and Postnatal Developmental Toxicity of Salcaprozate Sodium (SNAC) in Sprague-Dawley Rats. *Int. J. Toxicol.* **2009**, *28*, 266–277. [CrossRef] [PubMed]
147. Tuvia, S.; Atsmon, J.; Teichman, S.L.; Katz, S.; Salama, P.; Pelled, D.; Landau, I.; Karmeli, I.; Bidlingmaier, M.; Strasburger, C.J.; et al. Oral Octreotide Absorption in Human Subjects: Comparable Pharmacokinetics to Parenteral Octreotide and Effective Growth Hormone Suppression. *J. Clin. Endocrinol. Metab.* **2012**, *97*, 2362–2369. [CrossRef]
148. Banerjee, A.; Wong, J.; Gogoi, R.; Brown, T.; Mitragotri, S. Intestinal micropatches for oral insulin delivery. *J. Drug Target.* **2017**, *25*, 608–615. [CrossRef]
149. Eiamtrakarn, S.; Itoh, Y.; Kishimoto, J.; Yoshikawa, Y.; Shibata, N.; Murakami, M.; Takada, K. Gastrointestinal mucoadhesive patch system (GI-MAPS) for oral administration of G-CSF, a model protein. *Biomaterials* **2002**, *23*, 145–152. [CrossRef]
150. Jørgensen, J.R.; Yu, F.; Venkatasubramanian, R.; Nielsen, L.H.; Nielsen, H.M.; Boisen, A.; Rades, T.; Müllertz, A. In Vitro, Ex Vivo and In Vivo Evaluation of Microcontainers for Oral Delivery of Insulin. *Pharmaceutics* **2020**, *12*, 48. [CrossRef]
151. Mazzoni, C.; Jacobsen, R.D.; Mortensen, J.; Jørgensen, J.R.; Vaut, L.; Jacobsen, J.; Gundlach, C.; Müllertz, A.; Nielsen, L.H.; Boisen, A. Polymeric Lids for Microcontainers for Oral Protein Delivery. *Macromol. Biosci.* **2019**, *19*, e1900004. [CrossRef]
152. Wang, J.; Yadav, V.; Smart, A.L.; Tajiri, S.; Basit, A.W. Toward Oral Delivery of Biopharmaceuticals: An Assessment of the Gastrointestinal Stability of 17 Peptide Drugs. *Mol. Pharm.* **2015**, *12*, 966–973. [CrossRef] [PubMed]
153. Almansour, K.; Taverner, A.; Turner, J.R.; Eggleston, I.M.; Mrsny, R.J. An intestinal paracellular pathway biased toward positively-charged macromolecules. *J. Control. Release* **2018**, *288*, 111–125. [CrossRef]
154. Trier, S.; Linderoth, L.; Bjerregaard, S.; Andresen, T.L.; Rahbek, U.L. Acylation of Glucagon-Like Peptide-2: Interaction with Lipid Membranes and In Vitro Intestinal Permeability. *PLoS ONE* **2014**, *9*, e109939. [CrossRef] [PubMed]
155. Hofsäss, M.A.; Dressman, J.B. The Discriminatory Power of the BCS-Based Biowaiver: A Retrospective With Focus on Essential Medicines. *J. Pharm. Sci.* **2019**, *108*, 2824–2837. [CrossRef]
156. Metry, M.; Polli, J.E. Evaluation of Excipient Risk in BCS Class I and III Biowaivers. *AAPS J.* **2022**, *24*, 20. [CrossRef] [PubMed]
157. Benson, K.; Cramer, S.; Galla, H.-J. Impedance-based cell monitoring: Barrier properties and beyond. *Fluids Barriers CNS* **2013**, *10*, 5. [CrossRef]
158. Capital Markets Day 2017. Available online: https://www.novonordisk.com/content/dam/nncorp/global/en/investors/irmaterial/cmd/2017/00_CMD%20Presentation%20combined.pdf (accessed on 5 October 2022).

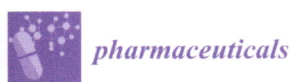

Review

KIF1A-Associated Neurological Disorder: An Overview of a Rare Mutational Disease

Ayushi Nair [1], Alosh Greeny [1], Rajalakshmi Rajendran [1], Mohamed A. Abdelgawad [2,3], Mohammed M. Ghoneim [4], Roshni Pushpa Raghavan [1,*], Sachithra Thazhathuveedu Sudevan [5], Bijo Mathew [5] and Hoon Kim [6,*]

1. Department of Pharmacy Practice, Amrita School of Pharmacy, Amrita Vishwa Vidyapeetham, Amrita Health Science Campus, Kochi 682041, India
2. Department of Pharmaceutical Chemistry, College of Pharmacy, Jouf University, Sakaka, Al Jouf 72341, Saudi Arabia
3. Department of Pharmaceutical Organic Chemistry, Faculty of Pharmacy, Beni-Suef University, Beni-Suef 62514, Egypt
4. Department of Pharmacy Practice, College of Pharmacy, AlMaarefa University, Ad Diriyah 13713, Saudi Arabia
5. Department of Pharmaceutical Chemistry, Amrita School of Pharmacy, Amrita Vishwa Vidyapeetham, AIMS Health Sciences Campus, Kochi 682 041, India
6. Department of Pharmacy, and Research Institute of Life Pharmaceutical Sciences, Sunchon National University, Suncheon 57922, Republic of Korea
* Correspondence: roshnipr@aims.amrita.edu (R.P.R.); hoon@sunchon.ac.kr (H.K.)

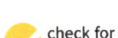

Citation: Nair, A.; Greeny, A.; Rajendran, R.; Abdelgawad, M.A.; Ghoneim, M.M.; Raghavan, R.P.; Sudevan, S.T.; Mathew, B.; Kim, H. KIF1A-Associated Neurological Disorder: An Overview of a Rare Mutational Disease. *Pharmaceuticals* 2023, 16, 147. https://doi.org/10.3390/ph16020147

Academic Editors: Silviya Petrova Zustiak and Era Jain

Received: 2 December 2022
Revised: 12 January 2023
Accepted: 17 January 2023
Published: 19 January 2023

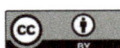

Copyright: © 2023 by the authors. Licensee MDPI, Basel, Switzerland. This article is an open access article distributed under the terms and conditions of the Creative Commons Attribution (CC BY) license (https://creativecommons.org/licenses/by/4.0/).

Abstract: KIF1A-associated neurological diseases (KANDs) are a group of inherited conditions caused by changes in the microtubule (MT) motor protein KIF1A as a result of *KIF1A* gene mutations. Anterograde transport of membrane organelles is facilitated by the kinesin family protein encoded by the MT-based motor gene *KIF1A*. Variations in the *KIF1A* gene, which primarily affect the motor domain, disrupt its ability to transport synaptic vesicles containing synaptophysin and synaptotagmin leading to various neurological pathologies such as hereditary sensory neuropathy, autosomal dominant and recessive forms of spastic paraplegia, and different neurological conditions. These mutations are frequently misdiagnosed because they result from spontaneous, non-inherited genomic alterations. Whole-exome sequencing (WES), a cutting-edge method, assists neurologists in diagnosing the illness and in planning and choosing the best course of action. These conditions are simple to be identified in pediatric and have a life expectancy of 5–7 years. There is presently no permanent treatment for these illnesses, and researchers have not yet discovered a medicine to treat them. Scientists have more hope in gene therapy since it can be used to cure diseases brought on by mutations. In this review article, we discussed some of the experimental gene therapy methods, including gene replacement, gene knockdown, symptomatic gene therapy, and cell suicide gene therapy. It also covered its clinical symptoms, pathogenesis, current diagnostics, therapy, and research advances currently occurring in the field of KAND-related disorders. This review also explained the impact that gene therapy can be designed in this direction and afford the remarkable benefits to the patients and society.

Keywords: KAND; *KIF1A* gene; microtubule; kinesin motor protein; neurological disorder

1. Introduction

KIF1A-associated neurological diseases (KAND) are a group of neurological illnesses caused by changes in the microtubule (MT) motor protein KIF1A as a consequence of a *KIF1A* gene mutation. These genetic changes might produce pathogenic mutations and lead to neurological disorders in patient [1]. Due to the limited availability of full gene sequencing and exome sequencing at the time, these illnesses were originally discovered in 2011, and many patients received the wrong diagnosis [2]. There are various KAND variations that can be passed down both dominantly and recessively. Researchers have noted various types of mutations in the same proteins in patients, and intriguingly, the majority of them exhibit private variants, opening up the possibility for further investigation and the discovery of further variants in these KIF1A-related disorders (KRD) [3]. This uncommon illness, which can also damage the vision, muscles, and nerves, primarily targets the neurons in the brain [4]. Studies on metabolic diseases, such as diabetes mellitus, have found that the *KIF1A* gene is more expressed and more immunoreactive [5]. Furthermore, this might eventually cause other neurological issues including encephalopathy and brain shrinkage [6].

The molecular motor KIF1A affects the survival and development of sensory neurons in our body as well as the movement of membrane-bound cargo [7]. If there are any disturbances in these neuronal trafficking pathways, which are strictly controlled due to the functional compartmentalization of neurons and connect the neuron's body, dendrites, and axons, neurodegenerative diseases would result [8]. The KIF1A protein's normal function can be altered by one mutation or numerous mutations in the gene that codes for it, resulting in this disorder [3]. Due to the serious life-threatening problems brought on by genetic abnormalities in this condition, patients' quality of life and life expectancy might be greatly affected [2]. The detailed work flow of current work is outlined in PRISMA diagram (Figure 1)

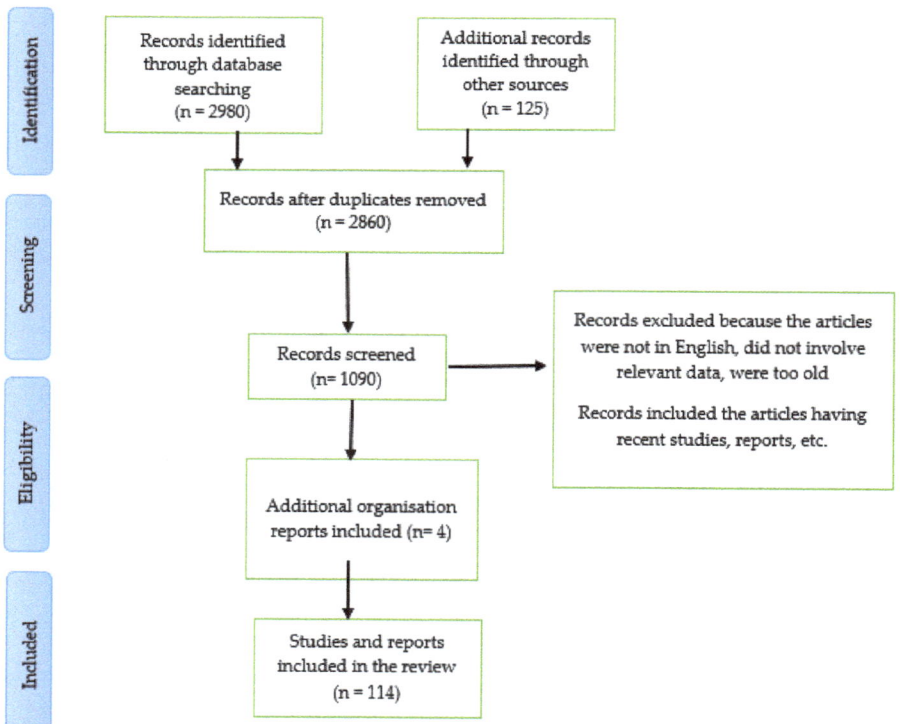

Figure 1. Work flow of this review and systematic review.

2. KIF1A Gene

Kinesin-like proteins, better known as axonal transporter of the synaptic vesicles, are MT-centered motors belonging to the kinesin family of proteins, and are involved in anterograde transport of some major membrane organelles, vesicles, macro-protein, and mRNA along the microtubular structures. This in itself explains that the *KIF1A* gene plays an important role in axonal transport as well as meiosis and mitosis processes [8]. The KIF1A is also required for neuronal dense core vesicles (DCV) transport to the dendritic spines and axons [9].

KIF1A protein comprises a neck region, a tail, and an N-terminal motor domain, as illustrated in Figure 2 [10]. The motor-domain has MT-dependent ATPase activity and MT-binding actions, whereas the tail consists of a stalk domain for protein binding, and a pleckstrin-homology [PH] domain is used for lipid binding. A small strand "neck linker" and the neck coil regions play an important role in the dimerization process of kinesin-3-motor and the processive motility [11–13]. The *KIF1A* gene initially exists as an inactive dimer and this stage is maintained by autoinhibitory mechanisms. It gets activated when bound to cargo, forming a homo-dimer enabling the transport of synaptic vesicle precursors along the MT [10,11,14].

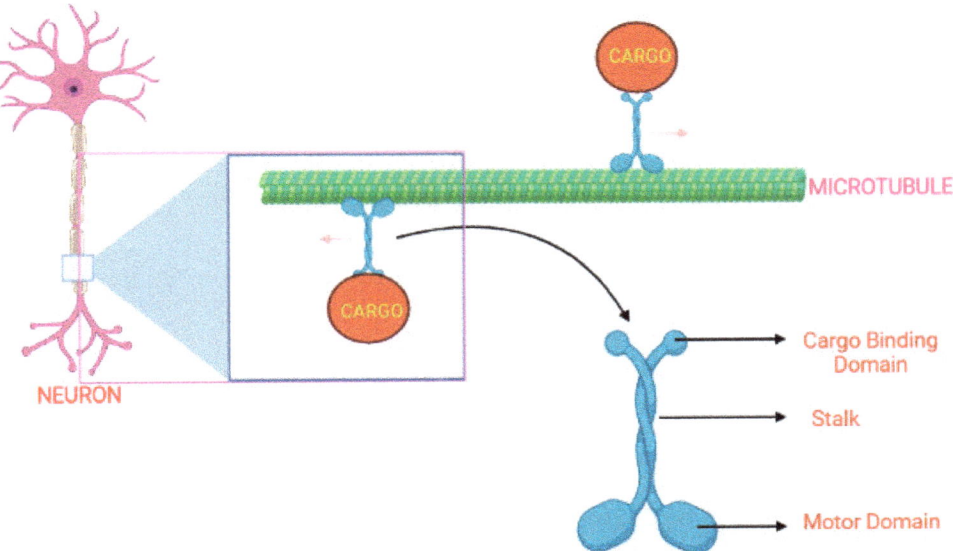

Figure 2. The KIF1A protein's typical shape and movement along the MT surface in a healthy neuronal cell [15]. (Created with Biorender.com).

Variations in the *KIF1A* gene have been associated with various clinical conditions and are described in a database known as Online Mendelian Inheritance in Man (OMIM). Variants in KIF1A were studied in various neurodegenerative diseases with dominant and recessive inheritance (Figure 3). In patients suffering from severe neurodegenerative disorders, homozygous recessive mutations in the *KIF1A* gene were first described as hereditary sensory and autonomic neuropathy type 2 and as three consanguineous families with an autosomal recessive form of hereditary spastic paraplegia (HSP) with an autosomal dominant form of SPG30 [16]. A particular mutation p.T99M was reported in patients having an intellectual disability (ID), spasticity and axial hypotonia [17]. A partially over-lapping phenotype-brain atrophy with progressive encephalopathy was recently found to be associated with *de-novo* KIF1A mutations [6]. Several *de-novo* variations and mutations in patients were classified as either pure or complicated. The complicated type is accompanied by axonal neuropathy and brain cerebellar atrophy [18,19].

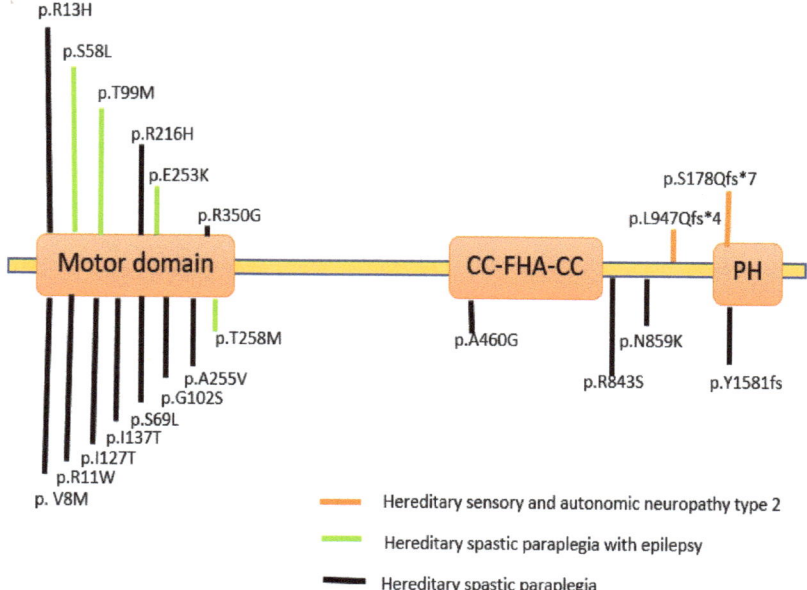

Figure 3. KIF1A protein depicted schematically, along with the locations of mutations in human KIF1A linked to several neurological diseases. The KIF1A subunit protein peptide contains these mutations in a variety of regions and domains [20–23]. (Created with Biorender.com).

3. KIF1A—As a Super Engaging Motor

KIF1A protein has the unique ability to be kinetically tuned to become a super engaging motor that ensures its proper functioning and integrity under hindering conditions when under loads [24]. The ability of these kinesin motor proteins under mechanical loads is very important for the proper intracellular transport of the cargo. The high loads on the kinesin motor will affect the motor speed as well as the MT attachment lifetime. As the KIF1A belongs to the kinesin-3 family, the super processive behavior under zero loads of these proteins will purely depend upon the loops and cores of this proteins [10,25,26]. Serapion et al. and Allison et al. found that the processive runs done by the KIF1A get terminated when under load and thus low average termination forces are required as compared to KIF5B, by comparing two different motors, i.e., KIF1A and KIF5B. Hence, therefore, it shows that KIF1A uses a different mechanism to work under loads to increase its efficiency and is not similar to other kinesin motors.

The distinct feature of KIF1A is its ability to form reengagement structures with the aid of different loops. Loop 12 plays a significant role in the motility of these proteins, and especially the positively charged K loop insert present in loop 12 has a crucial role [27–30]. In some studies, the scientists tried to replace the lysine (K) and remove the charge from loop 12 from the motor and this resulted in a lack of ability of the protein to work under load [24]. MT nucleotide and loop 12 influence the motor's ability to reengage under mechanical load. The degree of expansion of the MT lattice and the polymerization of the MT with different nucleotides affects the rate at which the reengagement takes place [31–33]. Thus, all these studies reveal that the proper functioning of loop 12 and the arrangement of MT nucleotides aids in the adaptive nature of KIF1A and its novel mechanism of transport of cargo by super engagement and reengagement methods.

4. Symptoms

KAND has a broad phenotypic spectrum of signs and symptoms. Intellectual disability, spasticity, inherited progressive spastic paraplegia, cerebral atrophy, optic nerve atrophy, and microcephaly are a few of these (Figure 4). But most frequently, most individuals show signs of seizures [3]. Cerebellar function impairment has also been reported in some clinical investigations, and some patients have also shown dysautonomic symptoms such as temperature instability and urine retention. Due to gastrointestinal dysfunction, people with severe diseases could need parenteral nourishment [2]. Several studies state that the mutation in the KIF1A gene directly affects the motility of hetero-dimeric motors [3,34,35].

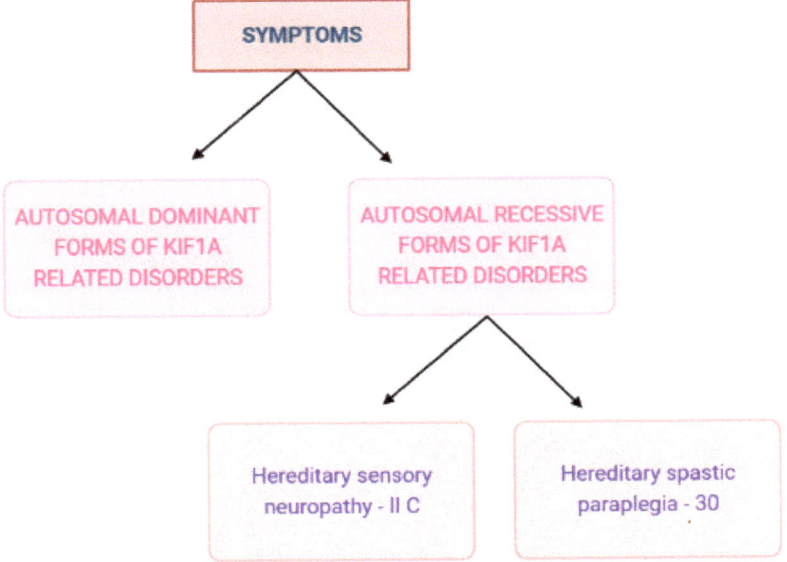

Figure 4. KAND symptoms on a clinical basis [36]. II C is a type of autosomal recessive disorder and can be represented as 2C also. (Created with BioRender.com.).

The following examples are the typical services that a KAND patient may require [36];

- Neurologist—neurological abnormality, seizures, and spasticity
- Ophthalmologist—impaired vision
- Pediatrician—developmental delay
- Specialized therapist—issues with speech and coordination
- A team of specialists—intellectual disability

4.1. Autosomal Dominant Variety of KRD [KIF1A-Related Disorders]

Developmental delays, cerebellar atrophy, peripheral neuropathy, ptosis, facial diplegia, intention tremors, strabismus, nystagmus, clumsiness, and ataxia are some of the typical symptoms. Other symptoms include hypertonia (increased muscle tone), hyperreflexia (exaggerated reflexes), spasticity (muscle tightness), and hyperreflexia [36,37].

4.2. Autosomal Recessive Forms of KIF1A-Related Disorders

4.2.1. Hereditary Sensory Neuropathy IIC (Also Represented as 2C)

The deterioration of the neurons that results in the loss of feeling is the cause of this neuropathy. Other signs, such as numbness and tingling, are also detected and eventually lead to the loss of sensation. As a result of this affecting sensory neurons, automatic or involuntary body movements are also directly impacted [36,38,39].

4.2.2. HSP

There are more than 80 genetically different types of HSP [40]. These types of spastic paraplegias are caused due to variations in the *KIF1A* gene and are referred to as an autosomal dominant type of Spastic Paraplegia (SPG30). The major symptoms include neurological difficulties, severe leg weakness, and spasticity [38,41,42]. The major sites of mutations in the human KAND protein are depicted in Figure 3.

5. Diagnosis

Traditional diagnostic methods such as multiplex probe amplification, karyotyping, genetic testing, and chromosomal microarray analysis were employed to screen out all forms of neurological disorders, including KAND [43–47]. The main drawback of these procedures was that different mutation types began exhibiting comparable clinical traits. A cutting-edge method called whole-exome sequencing (WES) is now becoming more widely used [48]. The WES aids in the diagnosis of the condition and the selection of the most effective treatment plan for the neurologist, particularly the pediatric neurologist [49]. Although WES is frequently used to diagnose KAND, it has several technical limitations that make it difficult to detect trinucleotide repeats, big indels, and epigenetic modifications that could impede the diagnosis of the illness [50,51]. Some of the newer fields such as the cytogenetics, chromosomal aberration, molecular diagnostic technique, carrier detection techniques are recently being explored by scientists to develop a novel method for the diagnosis of KAND.

6. Treatment

There is currently no effective therapy or cure for KAND. However, because gene therapies have the potential to treat many neurological disorders, researchers are working on them. Some of the fundamental experimental approaches for gene therapy are listed in Table 1. Even while there is no concrete evidence that gene therapy may entirely cure KAND, the preliminary findings from research trials enable the researchers to focus more on creating a treatment plan. These treatments will target the genes that cause the condition as well as the neurotrophic factors that support the healthy function and survival of the neuronal cell [52]. The use of nanoparticles, engineered microRNA, plasmid transfection, viral vector design, polymer-mediated gene delivery, clustered regularly interspaced short palindromic repeats (CRISPR)-based therapeutics, and other technologies has advanced this field [52]. Because surgical treatment cannot cure KAND and there is currently no approved standard pharmacological treatment, gene-based therapeutics are crucial [53]. By fully comprehending the pathophysiology of the disease and then treating it at the molecular level, these technologies also have the advantage of repairing genes and treating disorders that are not at all treatable by utilizing conventional medical procedures [54,55].

Table 1. The fundamental experimental approach for gene therapy used four theoretical modes of action [56].

Sl no.	Modes of Action	Specification
1.	Gene replacement [57]	This is done when the disease is caused due to the loss of functionality of the gene.
2.	Gene knockdown [58]	This is employed when a function has been toxically increased or when gene metabolites or gene products have accumulated.
3.	Pro-survival or symptomatic gene therapy [56]	Here the pathological condition is reversed by using a pro-survival gene that is non-specific in nature.
4.	Cell suicide gene therapy [59]	This is typically thought of as the last option. This is primarily used in cancer treatment, where it is necessary to eradicate malignant cells. In the case of KAND, this method's application is constrained.

The choice of a gene transfer vector is crucial because it directly affects how effective the treatment will be. The selection process takes into account a number of variables, including affinity and blood-brain barrier (BBB) crossing capability. Adenovirus (Ad), Herpes-Simplex virus (HSV), Lentivirus (LV), and recombinant Adeno-Associated virus (rAAV) are some of the most often employed viral vectors [56]. Even though all these methods exist to treat KAND, there is no conclusive clinical evidence that they can also be used to treat KRDs. The effectiveness percentage is still unknown.

7. *De Novo* Variations in the KIF1A Gene

De novo variants are primarily seen in patients who also have comorbid conditions like cognitive impairment, muscle stiffness, or optic nerve atrophy. These conditions co-occur with clinical symptoms caused by recessive mutations in the *KIF1A* gene, making them more harmful. The majority of mutations are found in the motor domain and are easily anticipated since they have an impact on the protein's ability to operate normally as a motor because of the change in the original structure [60]. Only a limited amount of information is known regarding *de novo* mutations because there haven't been many reports on these mutations published (Table 2). The missense mutations are observed at the c.296C > T/p.Thr99Met location of the KIF1A gene, which can affect the amino acid produced which will directly have an impact on the protein functions [17]. The prediction algorithms used are Scale Invariant Feature Transform (SIFT) [61], Polymorphism Phenotyping v2 (PolyPhen-2) [62], and PANTHER [63].

Table 2. Various parts of the KIF1A protein susceptible to mutation [26–29].

Sl no.	Domains	Proteins under Mutations.
1.	Motor domain	p.S58L p.G102D p.V144F p.R167C p.A202P p.S215R p.R216P p.L249Q p.E253K p.R316W
2.	Forkhead-associated domain	p.L947Rfs*4
3.	Pleckstrin homology	p.S1758Qfs*7

The following clinical manifestations are observed in people with *de novo* mutations in the motor domain:

- Intellectual disability—delay in cognitive development occurs in all cases
- Cerebellar atrophy—diagnosed using magnetic resonance imaging
- Optic nerve atrophy
- Spastic paraplegia—mainly affecting lower limbs
- Peripheral neuropathy [14]

8. Relation between KIF1A Variants and HSP

8.1. HSP

An uncommon neurological condition called HSP causes stiffness or wasting of the bladder or lower limbs [37]. It is caused by X chromosome-linked inheritance patterns, autosomal dominant and recessive mutations, as well as other factors that are categorized in OMIM [64]. Autosomal dominant paraplegia HSP subtype SPG30 is a result of homozygous missense variants, SPG7 and SPG11 in the *KIF1A* gene whereas the dominant form of HSP is observed due to variation in the 'SPAST' gene [38,65,66]. HSP can manifest basically in the form of spasticity and weakness in the patient. Although they may also experience hyperuricemia, these patients' life expectancies are unaffected. In more severe cases of HSP, peripheral and optic neuropathy as well as mental impairment may also be present. Currently, 79 specific and fixed positions are located in chromosomes with 61 corresponding genes that have a link to HSP condition [37].

The following types are the commonly recognized HSP disorders:
- Spastic paraplegia + Peripheral motor neuropathy + Distal wasting
- Spastic paraplegia + Cognitive impairment
- Spastic paraplegia + Ataxia
- Spastic paraplegia + Neuroimaging abnormality
- Spastic paraplegia + Additional neurologic + Systemic abnormalities [66].

8.2. KIF1A Variants and Spastic Paraplegia

KIF1A mutations are seen in three regions; the motor domain, regulatory region, and cargo binding region and these are mainly responsible for the development of SPG30. Specific mutations affect the gene function in a specific manner. These changes in the functions will ultimately result in the mislocalization of cellular cargoes, i.e., it will make the KIF1A protein unable to regulate its motility and subsequently, it fails to bind to the cargo. The severity of SPG30 depends on to what extent the *KIF1A* gene has undergone mutations [15]. The loss of functioning in the motor domain of KIF1A can affect the structural domain which is essential for various functions such as hydrolyzing ATP, providing mechanical force, and MT-binding (loop L8). Examples of these can be mutations residing in Switch I represented as R216C and Switch II which is represented as E253K and mutations that cause destabilization of loop L8 [66,67]. Switch II is better understood as E253K and ATP-binding cassette (ABC), that is the ATP-binding cassette mutant which drastically slows down the motility of this motor protein resulting in the inability to move to the distal portion of the neuronal axon.

The variants which result in the loss of functionality of the gene located outside the kinesin domain of the motor region lead to a defect in normal functioning that causes a problem known as functional intolerance [68,69]. Interestingly, a gain of function has also been observed in SPG30. Making use of a single-molecule assay procedure, Chiba et al. reported V8M, R350G, and A255V, the three KIF1A mutants casual in SPG30 had higher rates of settling on MTs and had higher velocity as compared to wild type (WT) KIF1A, indicating that excessive cargo accumulation can be harmful. In cohort studies done by Maartje Pennings et al., 20 heterozygous KIF1A variants were reported by clinical exome sequencing and the resulting SPG due to KIF1A was pure. It was observed that phenotypic differences in the KIF1A-related diseases may be due to different levels of impairment in transport. Parental testing done by the team revealed the deletion of chr2q37 in a few families. *KIF1A* gene is localized in the cytogenic 2q37.3 band and microdeletion of chromosome 2q37 is deleted in patients suffering from 2q37 microdeletion syndrome that can be observed by intellectual disability, brachydactyly, weight gain, hypotonia, characteristic facial features, autism, and epilepsy [37,67]. Eleven of the 20 variants reported in the studies done by Maartje Pennings et al. were found to be missense variants located at the motor domain that cause dominant SPG. The rest nine variants detected outside the motor domain included variants that showed loss of functionality of gene (some were *de novo* occurrences) and chr2q37 deletion which indicates that loss of function variants has the ability to cause autosomal dominant SPG [37].

In another study done by Stephan Klebe et al., using targeted NGS, p.R350G variant was identified, which has a direct effect on amino acid in the motor domain of kinesin 1A, and surprisingly this variant was found to be compatible with phenotype expressed by HSP patients. In the same studies, whole-genome genotyping done in a Palestinian family revealed that there is the presence of a unique homozygous c.756>T [p. Ala255Val] mutation that caused the phenotypic symptoms. Studies have shown that the nature of mutations could help scientists to foresee the phenotype expressed. Non-sense mutations which can lead to complete loss of functionality of the protein can cause significant clinical manifestations in the peripheral nervous system (PNS), as peripheral neuropathy is common in more than 60% of the SPG30 patients [22,70,71].

9. KIF1A and Brain Atrophy

Homozygous mutation in KIF1A is one of the main reasons for the rare hereditary sensory and autonomic neuropathy (HSAN) and HSP, but experiments that were done in vitro suggest that homozygous mutations influence the transport through synaptic vesicles and can lead to axon degeneration [22,66]. For example, in a child, a pathogenic variant, p.T99M *de novo* variation that causes cerebellar atrophy was reported, indicating these mutations may alter the neuronal function by disabling kinesin-mediated cargo transport. It has been observed that the homozygous inactivation KIF1A gene in mice can cause severe motor as well as sensory disturbances [72]. In studies done by Sahar Esmaeeli Nieh et al. [6] on 6 different patients, five *de novo* mutations were identified out of which two patients were observed who had *de novo* c.296C>T change that contained a substitution of threonine to methionine also represented as T99M [17]. Mutations like p.E253K also represented as c.757G>A and p.R316W were reported in the other two patients tested. The rest two patients had changes in the amino acid residues that were again getting mutated to form a third amino acid variant [19]. All these mutations were identified within a conserved region of the motor domain and they have the capacity to cause damage by using PolyPhen-2 [73,74].

In another study done by Chihiro Ohba et al., 5 missense mutations were found in five patients and were confirmed by Sanger sequencing to be *de novo* events. Magnetic resonance imaging done by the same team noticed that the patients had some difficulties in the gait along with exaggerated reflexes from locations such as deep tendons and in a few patients, cerebellar atrophy was observed. All *de novo* mutations observed during this study are located in the motor domain which mostly affects motor function. In this study, all the mutations observed were identified in the motor domain. The mutation p.Arg316Trp had been previously reported [72], at the same time Arg254, Arg307, and Arg307 were found on n loop L11. The α5 helix that helps to induce phosphate release during the hydrolysis of adenosine triphosphate molecule and facilitates KIF1A protein to bind onto MTs was also found to be mutated in some individuals [19,69,75]. The mutations can exhibit some unique actions on the structures present near them such as the p.Glu253Lys mutation adjacent to Arg254 can suppress γ-phosphate release [19], while p.Arg316Trp mutation disrupts the stability of loop 8 which forms a bond with the MT [69].

9.1. NESCAV Syndrome

NESCAV syndrome (NESCAVS), also referred to as autosomal dominant 9 or intellectual disability, is a neurodegenerative disorder characterized by global development delay with delayed walking or difficulty in walking due to spasticity in the lower limbs leading to loss of independent ambulation [2]. Some of the clinical features include optic nerve atrophy and varying degrees of brain atrophy, microcephaly, joint contractures, kyphosis, clubfoot, spasticity, and cerebellar atrophy [76]. It has been observed that NESCAVS is caused due to *de novo* heterozygous T99M mutation in the *KIF1A* gene. This study was done on an 8-year-old Japanese boy having axial hypotonia, peripheral spasticity, and global development delay with additional clinical manifestations like growth hormone deficiency, neurogenic bladder, and constipation [77]. In a few other studies involving unrelated patients, other manifestations like cortical visual impairment, optic neuropathy, movement disorders [6], hyperreflexia, hypermetrophic astigmatism, oculomotor apraxia, and distal muscle weakness [60]. Hamdan et al. (2011), identified a *de novo* missense mutation in the *KIF1A* gene in a patient with NESCAVS. In his study, he inserted a KIF1A MD-EGFP fusion construct into the hippocampal neurons present in rats and showed that the distal localization gets greatly reduced in neurites carrying the T99M mutation which leads to increased accumulation [17]. These mutations are found by whole-genome sequencing which can be later confirmed by sanger sequencing [60].

9.2. PEHO Syndrome [OMIM No. 260565]

PEHO syndrome characterized by progressive encephalopathy along with edema, and hypsarrhythmia is a rare neurodegenerative disease which leads to total loss of granules in the neurons resulting in an extreme condition of cerebellar atrophy [78]. This condition was first reported in 14 Finnish families in the year 1991. The basis for the diagnosis of PEHO syndrome has been put out by Somer et al. [79] who recognized the necessary features of this condition, i.e., jerking along with spasms, brain atrophy on neuroimaging studies, especially in the cerebellum and few regions of the brain stem with mild supratentorial atrophy [80]. In studies done by Sylvie Langlois et al., which involved the genomic study of patients with PEHO syndrome is being described; nine candidate genes were identified using trio WES out of which eight genes were heterozygous variants and a gene was *de novo* variant. The missense variant, p.(T99M) in KIF1A residing in chromosome number 2 is considered pathogenic [81]. Sanger sequencing was also carried out on the female patient and the unaffected parents and it was proved that the patient was heterozygous for the variant. Before this study was made, 24 patients had been reported with *de novo* heterozygous variants affecting the motor domain of KIF1A protein and the functional impact of these variants was demonstrated by Lee et al. The main clinical features reported were moderate to severe developmental delay, cerebellar atrophy, optic nerve atrophy, progressive spasticity affecting lower limbs, and peripheral neuropathy [19].

10. KIF1A and Autism Spectrum Disorder [ASD]

ASD also known as autism is a type of neurodevelopmental disorder in which the patients show a deficit in communication as well as the processing of language and expression of thoughts. This disorder directly or indirectly can influence the social life of the patient to a great extent. There are several genes implicated in ASD but approximately 10–15% of cases are due to mutations in a single gene [82]. Reports suggest that the patients exhibiting complex phenotypes are characterized by axonal neuropathy, spasticity, and majorly ASD. The genetic examination of these patients revealed about 21,683 variants in the coding regions [83]. Another study reports that there is a link between the KIF1A mutations and autism and is normally characterized by other neurological conditions like sensory disturbance, hyperactivity, spastic paraplegia, and epilepsy. Normally the c.38 g>A [R13H] mutation exhibits autism and hyperactivity, but in some special cases, all the neurological symptoms are exhibited by c.37C>T (p.R13C) which is a *de novo* mutation [84].

In the majority of the research studies done on KAND, the peripheral blood is used as the sample and the DNA is extracted and the gene sequencing is mainly done by WES technology. There are modern tools also available for predicting the structure such as the SWISS-MODEL and Mutation Tester that utilize a different strategy for reporting [85]. If a patient is found to have harmful variants such as c.664A>C (p. Asn222His), a type of *de novo* variant, it is suggested that the patient is at a higher risk of getting ASD [85]. Not only this, one interesting thing to be noted is that along with KIF1A mutations, the mutations on the HUWE1 gene have also led to the expression of ASD and other conditions like epilepsy. This is mainly due to the 22q11.2 duplication (a penetrant copy number variant) [86]. These studies suggest that ASD is having a close association with KAND.

11. Recent Studies in the Field of KAND

Transport of cargo is very much important as far as a cell is concerned. If proper translocation does not take place, the cargo can get accumulated and lead to cell necrosis. The transport of cargo is done by three major methods:

- Regulation of motor ATPase activity by the process of autoinduction.
- Regulation of cargo adaptors
- Modifications on the cytoskeletal tract.

There have been tremendous efforts done by a lot of scientists to discover the in vivo functioning of each part of the *KIF1A* gene and its protein. Recent advancements in technology have led to the discovery of newer models such as the DNA origami scaffold model which provides a much more precise picture of what is happening *in vivo*. We have included some of the latest discoveries in KAND in this paper. In a few studies done recently, it was proved that a more bound linker will allow the cargo motors to attach to the MT track. It was found that KIF1A, KIF13B, and KIF16 regulate the parts of the KIF1A protein, especially the coiled domain [30]. Another study shows that the kinesin-3 monomers can be multimerized which results in the transport of cargo [87]. Most of the studies done on the regulation of motor domains are normally carried out using the pure components of proteins, particularly in the motor domain but there are a few exemptions to be noted here such as the functioning of two opposite domains in the protein [88–92].

When transport of the cargo does not take place in a neuronal cell, the kinesin motors especially the kinesin-3 subfamily adopt the mechanism of autoinhibited conformation. In such a case, the UNC-104KIF1A gets activated automatically. To date, the mechanism of activation is not understood fully. This condition leads to the enhancement in cargo transport in the form of vesicles in the cell. This also explains to us the cause of motor hyperactivation associated with this disease [93]. In some cases, it is reported that there can be a disruption of motor domain/CC1 domain-mediated autoinhibition due to the actions of dominant suppressors. To be more specific, the mutations at C184 can disrupt the inter-domain packing, while if the mutation takes place at the G421 then there will be a sudden turn between the CC1a and CC1b that can indirectly lead to interference in packing [12,94–97].

12. Gene Therapy

In order for the transgene to integrate with the host DNA (retrovirus) and make up for the defective gene's lack of expression, the transgene must be introduced into the target cells through gene transfer therapy. Scientists have developed a wide range of carriers for the successful delivery of genes to their targets and the majority of them comprise of plasmid DNA and oligonucleotides [98]. Despite the fact that gene therapy overcomes the difficulties associated with conventional treatment, it is not without drawbacks. They include the high cost of gene therapy, which restricts its use, ethical concerns about changes made to the germline, immune rejection of the transferred gene, and the route of administration [96]. Due to their low pathogenicity, cellular tropism, replication incompetency, and simplicity of manipulation, LV and AAVs are being investigated as delivery modalities for the introduction of transgenes in clinical trials. A naturally occurring serotype of AAV called AAV9 has the capacity to penetrate the BBB and target neurons, astrocytes, and microglia in the brain. The capsid proteins of these serotypes distinguish them and help determine the corresponding cellular tropism [99].

Due to its cell-specific transduction abilities, rAAV9 is the most recommended CNS delivery technique for neurological diseases. Both dividing and non-dividing cells can be transduced by rAAVs [98]. The three most effective gene editing techniques used for modifying cellular DNA at the native locus are CRISPR and CRISPR-associated (Cas) proteins, transcription activator-like effector nucleases (TALENs), and zinc finger nucleotides (ZFN). ZFNs are the first programmable nucleases that can cleave particular regions of DNA using an altered *Fok*I endonuclease to change the way double-stranded breaks are repaired in DNA [100]. Target gene alterations can be carried out using TALENs, which can recognize random target sequences. TALENs merge *Fok*I endonuclease with transcription activator-like effectors (TALEs) modular DNA binding domain [101].

The foundation of gene editing techniques is the introduction of genomic breaks and the precise allocation of these breaks by nuclease enzymes. Genome editing depends on two biological pathways: non-homologous end joining (NHEJ) and homology-directed repair (HDR) [102]. While NHEJ is frequently observed in cells that are not dividing, such as neurons, HDR occurs across all cell cycle phases. The NHEJ repair process has been used by researchers to support gene editing techniques. Several unique gene editing techniques have been created thus far for non-dividing cells, including, HITI (homology independent targeted integration) [103], HITI-based SATI approach (Single homology Arm donor mediated Intron-Targeting Integration) [104], CRISPR Prime editing [105], HMEJ (homology mediated end joining) [106], vSLENDR (virus-mediated single-cell labelling of endogenous proteins via HDR) [107], PITCh (precise integration into targeted chromosome) [108].

A genomic technique known as whole exome sequencing (WES) is used to sequence the protein-coding sections of genomic DNA (exons) and find the causative mutations that lead to specific genetic disorders [109,110]. WES has been extensively utilized to diagnose KRDs [48,70]. The use of gene therapy to treat neurogenetic disorders has risen dramatically over the past several years, with KAND increasingly displacing more traditional approaches. As previously stated, there is no known treatment for KAND. The development of gene therapy offers hope for the existing therapeutic approaches. Gene editing tools now make it possible to change genes, and there is a chance that the conditions could be reversed. However, there are several drawbacks to gene therapy, such as inserted gene over- or under-expression, vector capacity to carry the gene, and mutant gene product attacking the wild-type allele. The constraints of gene therapy have been overcome by the emergence of gene editing tools like CRISPR Cas9.

13. Conclusions

In this paper, we addressed all the available information, recent studies, and newer advancements concerning the KAND. The main cause of this disease is the mutations that take place in the *KIF1A* gene which can result in loss of function or gain of mutated functions. These mutations directly result in the mis-delivery of essential cargo transported inside the neurons. These cargoes play a very important role in neuronal growth, differentiation, and survival. Another problem is that there can be different phenotypic expressions even for the same mutation in the gene making the diagnosis difficult even with the help of expensive testing. It was observed that there can be two different forms of KIF1A-related disorders which are the autosomal dominant forms as well as autosomal recessive forms. One such condition is spastic paraplegia, which has been discussed earlier in this paper. Spastic paraplegia can be pure when symptoms are confined to stiffness in the legs and bladder. When these symptoms are accompanied by other neurological disturbances, then it is termed as complicated. KIF1A mutations are also linked to brain atrophy, encephalopathy, PEHO syndrome and autism spectrum disorder and all the disorders were observed to occur due to *de novo* variations in the *KIF1A* gene. Very few reports were available regarding the *de novo* variation, which has been mentioned in the article.

There are various organizations and foundations that provide information and spread awareness about KAND. Some are governmental while others are privately funded organizations. These organizations consist of the patients, family members of the patient as well as the physicians, clinicians, research scholars, and other paramedical staff. Although this disorder is rare and there are still many research gaps in the field of KAND in neuroscience, the possibility of the development of a new drug or an active chemical moiety cannot be predicted as of now. To date, there is no existing cure that guarantees the recovery of the patient, but we expect that newer advancements in neuroscience can enhance the treatment and management of KAND. A better understanding of the in vivo functioning of the motor domain, the part where most of the mutations take place can give us a lead to improve the existing difficulties faced by the patients. Newer models like the DNA origami scaffold model are used by scientists to provide more information on what is happening *in vivo*. Newer technologies such as gene therapy have the potential to pave way for advanced therapies and thereby increasing the quality of life of the patients.

Author Contributions: R.P.R. provided the title and did the proofreading. A.N. and A.G. wrote the original draft. M.M.G. and S.T.S. wrote the revision parts. R.R., M.A.A., B.M. and H.K. read the drafts and did proofreading. All authors have read and agreed to the published version of the manuscript.

Funding: This research received no external funding.

Informed Consent Statement: Not applicable.

Data Availability Statement: The data sets used, analyzed, and reviewed were collected from the corresponding authors and online research databases.

Conflicts of Interest: The authors declare no conflict of interest.

Abbreviations

ABC	ATP binding cassette
ASD	autism spectrum disorder
CRISPR	Clustered regularly interspaced short palindromic repeats
DNA	Deoxyribonucleic acid
DRD1	Dopamine receptor D1
FHA	Forkhead associated domain
HSAN	Hereditary sensory and autonomic neuropathy
HSP	Hereditary spastic paraplegia
HSV	Herpes simplex virus
KAND	KIF1A associated neurological disorders
KRD	KIF1A related disorders
LV	Lenti virus
OMIM	Online Mendelian Inheritance in Man
PEHO	Progressive encephalopathy with oedema, Hypsarrhythmia and optic atrophy
PH	Pleckstrin homology
rAAV	recombinant Adenome associated virus
SIFT	Scale in variant feature transform
SPG30	Spastic paraplegia 30
WES	Whole exome sequencing

References

1. Roda, R.H.; Schindler, A.B.; Blackstone, C. Multigeneration family with dominant SPG30 hereditary spastic paraplegia. *Ann. Clin. Transl. Neurol.* **2017**, *4*, 821–824. [CrossRef]
2. Nemani, T.; Steel, D.; Kaliakatsos, M.; DeVile, C.; Ververi, A.; Scott, R.; Getov, S.; Sudhakar, S.; Male, A.; Mankad, K.; et al. KIF1A-related disorders in children: A wide spectrum of central and peripheral nervous system involvement. *J. Peripher. Nerv. Syst.* **2020**, *25*, 117–124. [CrossRef] [PubMed]
3. Boyle, L.; Rao, L.; Kaur, S.; Fan, X.; Mebane, C.; Hamm, L.; Thornton, A.; Ahrendsen, J.T.; Anderson, M.P.; Christodoulou, J.; et al. Genotype and defects in microtubule-based motility correlate with clinical severity in KIF1A-associated neurological disorder. *Hum. Genet. Genom. Adv.* **2021**, *2*, 100026. [CrossRef] [PubMed]
4. Di Fabio, R.; Comanducci, G.; Piccolo, F.; Santorelli, F.M.; DE Berardinis, T.; Tessa, A.; Sabatini, U.; Pierelli, F.; Casali, C. Cerebellar Atrophy in Congenital Fibrosis of the Extraocular Muscles Type 1. *Cerebellum* **2012**, *12*, 140–143. [CrossRef] [PubMed]
5. Baptista, F.; Pinto, M.J.; Elvas, F.; Almeida, R.; Ambrósio, A.F. Diabetes Alters KIF1A and KIF5B Motor Proteins in the Hippocampus. *PLoS ONE* **2013**, *8*, e65515. [CrossRef]
6. Nieh, S.E.; Madou, M.R.Z.; Sirajuddin, M.; Fregeau, B.; McKnight, D.; Lexa, K.; Strober, J.; Spaeth, C.; Hallinan, B.E.; Smaoui, N.; et al. De novo mutations in KIF1A cause progressive encephalopathy and brain atrophy. *Ann. Clin. Transl. Neurol.* **2015**, *2*, 623–635. [CrossRef]
7. Montenegro-Garreaud, X.; Hansen, A.W.; Khayat, M.M.; Chander, V.; Grochowski, C.M.; Jiang, Y.; Li, H.; Mitani, T.; Kessler, E.; Jayaseelan, J.; et al. Phenotypic expansion in KIF1A-related dominant disorders: A description of novel variants and review of published cases. *Hum. Mutat.* **2020**, *41*, 2094–2104. [CrossRef]
8. Aguilera, C.; Hümmer, S.; Masanas, M.; Gabau, E.; Guitart, M.; Jeyaprakash, A.A.; Segura, M.F.; Santamaria, A.; Ruiz, A. The Novel KIF1A Missense Variant (R169T) Strongly Reduces Microtubule Stimulated ATPase Activity and Is Associated with NESCAV Syndrome. *Front. Neurosci.* **2021**, *15*, 618098. [CrossRef]
9. Bharat, V.; Siebrecht, M.; Burk, K.; Ahmed, S.; Reissner, C.; Kohansal-Nodehi, M.; Steubler, V.; Zweckstetter, M.; Ting, J.T.; Dean, C. Capture of Dense Core Vesicles at Synapses by JNK-Dependent Phosphorylation of Synaptotagmin-4. *Cell Rep.* **2017**, *21*, 2118–2133. [CrossRef]

10. Okada, Y.; Yamazaki, H.; Sekine-Aizawa, Y.; Hirokawa, N. The neuron-specific kinesin superfamily protein KIF1A is a uniqye monomeric motor for anterograde axonal transport of synaptic vesicle precursors. *Cell* **1995**, *81*, 769–780. [CrossRef]
11. Hammond, J.; Cai, D.; Blasius, T.L.; Li, Z.; Jiang, Y.; Jih, G.T.; Meyhofer, E.; Verhey, K.J. Mammalian Kinesin-3 Motors Are Dimeric In Vivo and Move by Processive Motility upon Release of Autoinhibition. *PLOS Biol.* **2009**, *7*, e1000072. [CrossRef]
12. Klopfenstein, D.R.; Tomishige, M.; Stuurman, N.; Vale, R.D. Role of Phosphatidylinositol(4,5)bisphosphate Organization in Membrane Transport by the Unc104 Kinesin Motor. *Cell* **2002**, *109*, 347–358. [CrossRef] [PubMed]
13. Huo, L.; Yue, Y.; Ren, J.; Yu, J.; Liu, J.; Yu, Y.; Ye, F.; Xu, T.; Zhang, M.; Feng, W. The CC1-FHA Tandem as a Central Hub for Controlling the Dimerization and Activation of Kinesin-3 KIF1A. *Structure* **2012**, *20*, 1550–1561. [CrossRef] [PubMed]
14. Lee, J.-R.; Shin, H.; Ko, J.; Choi, J.; Lee, H.; Kim, E. Characterization of the Movement of the Kinesin Motor KIF1A in Living Cultured Neurons. *J. Biol. Chem.* **2003**, *278*, 2624–2629. [CrossRef] [PubMed]
15. Gabrych, D.R.; Lau, V.Z.; Niwa, S.; Silverman, M.A. Going Too Far Is the Same as Falling Short†: Kinesin-3 Family Members in Hereditary Spastic Paraplegia. *Front. Cell. Neurosci.* **2019**, *13*, 419. [CrossRef] [PubMed]
16. Citterio, A.; Arnoldi, A.; Panzeri, E.; Merlini, L.; D'Angelo, M.G.; Musumeci, O.; Toscano, A.; Bondi, A.; Martinuzzi, A.; Bresolin, N.; et al. Variants in KIF1A gene in dominant and sporadic forms of hereditary spastic paraparesis. *J. Neurol.* **2015**, *262*, 2684–2690. [CrossRef] [PubMed]
17. Hamdan, F.F.; Gauthier, J.; Araki, Y.; Lin, D.-T.; Yoshizawa, Y.; Higashi, K.; Park, A.-R.; Spiegelman, D.; Dobrzeniecka, S.; Piton, A.; et al. Excess of De Novo Deleterious Mutations in Genes Associated with Glutamatergic Systems in Nonsyndromic Intellectual Disability. *Am. J. Hum. Genet.* **2011**, *88*, 306–316. [CrossRef]
18. Ylikallio, E.; Kim, D.; Isohanni, P.; Auranen, M.; Kim, E.; Lönnqvist, T.; Tyynismaa, H. Dominant transmission of de novo KIF1A motor domain variant underlying pure spastic paraplegia. *Eur. J. Hum. Genet.* **2015**, *23*, 1427–1430. [CrossRef]
19. Lee, J.-R.; Srour, M.; Kim, D.; Hamdan, F.F.; Lim, S.-H.; Brunel-Guitton, C.; Décarie, J.-C.; Rossignol, E.; Mitchell, G.A.; Schreiber, A.; et al. De Novo Mutations in the Motor Domain of KIF1A Cause Cognitive Impairment, Spastic Paraparesis, Axonal Neuropathy, and Cerebellar Atrophy. *Hum. Mutat.* **2015**, *36*, 69–78. [CrossRef]
20. Niwa, S.; Lipton, D.M.; Morikawa, M.; Zhao, C.; Hirokawa, N.; Lu, H.; Shen, K. Autoinhibition of a Neuronal Kinesin UNC-104/KIF1A Regulates the Size and Density of Synapses. *Cell Rep.* **2016**, *16*, 2129–2141. [CrossRef]
21. Iqbal, Z.; Rydning, S.L.; Wedding, I.M.; Koht, J.; Pihlstrøm, L.; Rengmark, A.H.; Henriksen, S.P.; Tallaksen, C.M.E.; Toft, M. Targeted high throughput sequencing in hereditary ataxia and spastic paraplegia. *PLoS ONE* **2017**, *12*, e0174667. [CrossRef]
22. Rivière, J.-B.; Ramalingam, S.; Lavastre, V.; Shekarabi, M.; Holbert, S.; Lafontaine, J.; Srour, M.; Merner, N.; Rochefort, D.; Hince, P.; et al. KIF1A, an Axonal Transporter of Synaptic Vesicles, Is Mutated in Hereditary Sensory and Autonomic Neuropathy Type 2. *Am. J. Hum. Genet.* **2011**, *89*, 219–230. [CrossRef]
23. Chiba, K.; Takahashi, H.; Chen, M.; Obinata, H.; Arai, S.; Hashimoto, K.; Oda, T.; McKenney, R.J.; Niwa, S. Disease-associated mutations hyperactivate KIF1A motility and anterograde axonal transport of synaptic vesicle precursors. *Proc. Natl. Acad. Sci. USA* **2019**, *116*, 18429–18434. [CrossRef]
24. Pyrpassopoulos, S.; Gicking, A.M.; Zaniewski, T.M.; Hancock, W.O.; Ostap, E.M. KIF1A is kinetically tuned to be a super-engaging motor under hindering loads. *Biophys. Comput. Biol.* **2023**, *120*, e2216903120. [CrossRef]
25. Hirokawa, N.; Noda, Y.; Tanaka, Y.; Niwa, S. Kinesin superfamily motor proteins and intracellular transport. *Nat. Rev. Mol. Cell Biol.* **2009**, *10*, 682–696. [CrossRef]
26. Budaitis, B.G.; Jariwala, S.; Rao, L.; Yue, Y.; Sept, D.; Verhey, K.J.; Gennerich, A. Pathogenic mutations in the kinesin-3 motor KIF1A diminish force generation and movement through allosteric mechanisms. *J. Cell Biol.* **2021**, *220*, e202004227. [CrossRef]
27. Okada, Y.; Hirokawa, N. A Processive Single-Headed Motor: Kinesin Superfamily Protein KIF1A. *Science* **1999**, *283*, 1152–1157. [CrossRef]
28. Soppina, V.; Verhey, K.J. The family-specific K-loop influences the microtubule on-rate but not the superprocessivity of kinesin-3 motors. *Mol. Biol. Cell* **2014**, *25*, 2161–2170. [CrossRef]
29. Okada, Y.; Hirokawa, N. Mechanism of the single-headed processivity: Diffusional anchoring between the K-loop of kinesin and the C terminus of tubulin. *Proc. Natl. Acad. Sci. USA* **2000**, *97*, 640–645. [CrossRef]
30. Soppina, V.; Norris, S.R.; Dizaji, A.S.; Kortus, M.; Veatch, S.; Peckham, M.; Verhey, K.J. Dimerization of mammalian kinesin-3 motors results in superprocessive motion. *Proc. Natl. Acad. Sci. USA* **2014**, *111*, 5562–5567. [CrossRef]
31. Alushin, G.M.; Lander, G.C.; Kellogg, E.H.; Zhang, R.; Baker, D.; Nogales, E. High-Resolution Microtubule Structures Reveal the Structural Transitions in αβ-Tubulin upon GTP Hydrolysis. *Cell* **2014**, *157*, 1117–1129. [CrossRef] [PubMed]
32. Zhang, R.; LaFrance, B.; Nogales, E. Separating the effects of nucleotide and EB binding on microtubule structure. *Proc. Natl. Acad. Sci. USA* **2018**, *115*, E6191–E6200. [CrossRef] [PubMed]
33. Zhang, R.; Alushin, G.M.; Brown, A.; Nogales, E. Mechanistic Origin of Microtubule Dynamic Instability and Its Modulation by EB Proteins. *Cell* **2015**, *162*, 849–859. [CrossRef] [PubMed]
34. Montemurro, N.; Ricciardi, L.; Scerrati, A.; Ippolito, G.; Lofrese, G.; Trungu, S.; Stoccoro, A. The Potential Role of Dysregulated miRNAs in Adolescent Idiopathic Scoliosis and 22q11.2 Deletion Syndrome. *J. Pers. Med.* **2022**, *12*, 1925. [CrossRef] [PubMed]
35. Anazawa, Y.; Kita, T.; Iguchi, R.; Hayashi, K.; Niwa, S. De novo mutations in KIF1A-associated neuronal disorder (KAND) dominant-negatively inhibit motor activity and axonal transport of synaptic vesicle precursors. *Proc. Natl. Acad. Sci.* **2022**, *119*, e2113795119. [CrossRef]

36. Lumpkins, C. KIF1A-Related Disorder. NORD (National Organization for Rare Disorders). Available online: https://rarediseases.org/rare-diseases/kif1a-related-disorder/ (accessed on 21 July 2022).
37. Pennings, M.; Schouten, M.I.; van Gaalen, J.; Meijer, R.P.P.; de Bot, S.T.; Kriek, M.; Saris, C.G.J.; Berg, L.H.V.D.; van Es, M.A.; Zuidgeest, D.M.H.; et al. KIF1A variants are a frequent cause of autosomal dominant hereditary spastic paraplegia. *Eur. J. Hum. Genet.* **2019**, *28*, 40–49. [CrossRef]
38. Klebe, S.; Lossos, A.; Azzedine, H.; Mundwiller, E.; Sheffer, R.; Gaussen, M.; Marelli, C.; Nawara, M.; Carpentier, W.; Meyer, V.; et al. KIF1A missense mutations in SPG30, an autosomal recessive spastic paraplegia: Distinct phenotypes according to the nature of the mutations. *Eur. J. Hum. Genet.* **2012**, *20*, 645–649. [CrossRef]
39. McEntagart, M.E.; Reid, S.L.; Irtthum, A.; Douglas, J.B.; Eyre, K.E.D.; Donaghy, M.J.; Anderson, N.E.; Rahman, N. Confirmation of a hereditary motor and sensory neuropathy IIC locus at chromosome 12q23-q24. *Ann. Neurol.* **2005**, *57*, 293–297. [CrossRef]
40. Hedera, P. Hereditary Spastic Paraplegia Overview. In *GeneReviews®*; Adam, M., Everman, D., Mirzaa, G., Pagon, R., Wallace, S., Bean, L.J., Gripp, K., Amemiya, A., Eds.; University of Washington: Seattle, WA, USA, 1993. Available online: http://www.ncbi.nlm.nih.gov/books/NBK1509/ (accessed on 20 July 2022).
41. Hebbar, M.; Shukla, A.; Nampoothiri, S.; Bielas, S.; Girisha, K.M. Locus and allelic heterogeneity in five families with hereditary spastic paraplegia. *J. Hum. Genet.* **2018**, *64*, 17–21. [CrossRef]
42. Fink, J.K. Chapter 77—Hereditary Spastic Paraplegia. In *Rosenberg's Molecular and Genetic Basis of Neurological and Psychiatric Disease*, 5th ed.; Rosenberg, R.N., Pascual, J.M., Eds.; Academic Press: Cambridge, MA, USA, 2015; pp. 891–906. [CrossRef]
43. Rauch, A.; Hoyer, J.; Guth, S.; Zweier, C.; Kraus, C.; Becker, M.; Zenker, M.; Hüffmeier, U.; Thiel, C.; Rüschendorf, F.; et al. Diagnostic yield of various genetic approaches in patients with unexplained developmental delay or mental retardation. *Am. J. Med. Genet. Part A* **2006**, *140A*, 2063–2074. [CrossRef]
44. Miller, D.T.; Adam, M.P.; Aradhya, S.; Biesecker, L.G.; Brothman, A.R.; Carter, N.P.; Church, D.M.; Crolla, J.A.; Eichler, E.E.; Epstein, C.J.; et al. Consensus Statement: Chromosomal Microarray Is a First-Tier Clinical Diagnostic Test for Individuals with Developmental Disabilities or Congenital Anomalies. *Am. J. Hum. Genet.* **2010**, *86*, 749–764. [CrossRef]
45. Costain, G.; Cordeiro, D.; Matviychuk, D.; Mercimek-Andrews, S. Clinical Application of Targeted Next-Generation Sequencing Panels and Whole Exome Sequencing in Childhood Epilepsy. *Neuroscience* **2019**, *418*, 291–310. [CrossRef]
46. Demos, M.; Guella, I.; DeGuzman, C.; McKenzie, M.B.; Buerki, S.E.; Evans, D.M.; Toyota, E.B.; Boelman, C.; Huh, L.L.; Datta, A.; et al. Diagnostic Yield and Treatment Impact of Targeted Exome Sequencing in Early-Onset Epilepsy. *Front. Neurol.* **2019**, *10*, 434. [CrossRef]
47. Watson, E.; Davis, R.; Sue, C.M. New diagnostic pathways for mitochondrial disease. *J. Transl. Genet. Genom.* **2020**, *4*, 188–202. [CrossRef]
48. Lee, H.; Chi, C.; Tsai, C. Diagnostic yield and treatment impact of whole-genome sequencing in paediatric neurological disorders. *Dev. Med. Child Neurol.* **2020**, *63*, 934–938. [CrossRef]
49. KIF1A. Wikipedia. 2022. Available online: https://en.wikipedia.org/w/index.php?title=KIF1A&oldid=1077108149 (accessed on 22 July 2022).
50. Barbitoff, Y.A.; Polev, D.E.; Glotov, A.S.; Serebryakova, E.A.; Shcherbakova, I.V.; Kiselev, A.M.; Kostareva, A.A.; Glotov, O.S.; Predeus, A.V. Systematic dissection of biases in whole-exome and whole-genome sequencing reveals major determinants of coding sequence coverage. *Sci. Rep.* **2020**, *10*, 2057. [CrossRef]
51. Clark, M.M.; Stark, Z.; Farnaes, L.; Tan, T.Y.; White, S.M.; Dimmock, D.; Kingsmore, S.F. Meta-analysis of the diagnostic and clinical utility of genome and exome sequencing and chromosomal microarray in children with suspected genetic diseases. *npj Genom. Med.* **2018**, *3*, 16. [CrossRef]
52. Pena, S.A.; Iyengar, R.; Eshraghi, R.S.; Bencie, N.; Mittal, J.; Aljohani, A.; Mittal, R.; Eshraghi, A.A. Gene therapy for neurological disorders: Challenges and recent advancements. *J. Drug Target.* **2019**, *28*, 111–128. [CrossRef]
53. Simonato, M.; Bennett, J.; Boulis, N.M.; Castro, M.; Fink, D.J.; Goins, W.F.; Gray, S.J.; Lowenstein, P.R.; Vandenberghe, L.H.; Wilson, T.J.; et al. Progress in gene therapy for neurological disorders. *Nat. Rev. Neurol.* **2013**, *9*, 277–291. [CrossRef]
54. Puranik, N.; Yadav, D.; Chauhan, P.S.; Kwak, M.; Jin, J.-O. Exploring the Role of Gene Therapy for Neurological Disorders. *Curr. Gene Ther.* **2021**, *21*, 11–22. [CrossRef]
55. Choong, C.-J.; Baba, K.; Mochizuki, H. Gene therapy for neurological disorders. *Expert Opin. Biol. Ther.* **2015**, *16*, 143–159. [CrossRef] [PubMed]
56. Manfredsson, F.P.; Mandel, R.J. Development of gene therapy for neurological disorders. *Discov. Med.* **2010**, *9*, 204–211. [PubMed]
57. Khan, S.M.; Bennett, J.P. Development of Mitochondrial Gene Replacement Therapy. *J. Bioenerg. Biomembr.* **2004**, *36*, 387–393. [CrossRef] [PubMed]
58. Shan, G. RNA interference as a gene knockdown technique. *Int. J. Biochem. Cell Biol.* **2010**, *42*, 1243–1251. [CrossRef] [PubMed]
59. Bonini, C.; Bondanza, A.; Perna, S.K.; Kaneko, S.; Traversari, C.; Ciceri, F.; Bordignon, C. The Suicide Gene Therapy Challenge: How to Improve a Successful Gene Therapy Approach. *Mol. Ther.* **2007**, *15*, 1248–1252. [CrossRef]
60. Ohba, C.; Haginoya, K.; Osaka, H.; Kubota, K.; Ishiyama, A.; Hiraide, T.; Komaki, H.; Sasaki, M.; Miyatake, S.; Nakashima, M.; et al. De novo KIF1A mutations cause intellectual deficit, cerebellar atrophy, lower limb spasticity and visual disturbance. *J. Hum. Genet.* **2015**, *60*, 739–742. [CrossRef]
61. Ng, P.C.; Henikoff, S. SIFT: Predicting amino acid changes that affect protein function. *Nucleic Acids Res.* **2003**, *31*, 3812–3814. [CrossRef]

62. Sunyaev, S. Prediction of deleterious human alleles. *Hum. Mol. Genet.* **2001**, *10*, 591–597. [CrossRef]
63. Thomas, P.D.; Kejariwal, A.; Guo, N.; Mi, H.; Campbell, M.J.; Muruganujan, A.; Lazareva-Ulitsky, B. Applications for protein sequence-function evolution data: mRNA/protein expression analysis and coding SNP scoring tools. *Nucleic Acids Res.* **2006**, *34*, W645–W650. [CrossRef]
64. Giudice, T.L.; Lombardi, F.; Santorelli, F.M.; Kawarai, T.; Orlacchio, A. Hereditary spastic paraplegia: Clinical-genetic characteristics and evolving molecular mechanisms. *Exp. Neurol.* **2014**, *261*, 518–539. [CrossRef]
65. Klebe, S.; Azzedine, H.; Durr, A.; Bastien, P.; Bouslam, N.; Elleuch, N.; Forlani, S.; Charon, C.; Koenig, M.; Melki, J.; et al. Autosomal recessive spastic paraplegia (SPG30) with mild ataxia and sensory neuropathy maps to chromosome 2q37.3. *Brain* **2006**, *129*, 1456–1462. [CrossRef]
66. Fink, J. Hereditary Spastic Paraplegia: Clinical Principles and Genetic Advances. *Semin. Neurol.* **2014**, *34*, 293–305. [CrossRef]
67. Doherty, E.S.; Lacbawan, F.L. 2q37 Microdeletion Syndrome—Retired Chapter, For Historical Reference Only. In *GeneReviews®*; Adam, M., Everman, D., Mirzaa, G., Pagon, R., Wallace, S., Bean, L.J., Gripp, K., Amemiya, A., Eds.; University of Washington: Seattle, WA, USA, 1993.
68. Cheon, C.K.; Lim, S.-H.; Kim, Y.-M.; Kim, D.; Lee, N.-Y.; Yoon, T.-S.; Kim, N.-S.; Kim, E.; Lee, J.-R. Autosomal dominant transmission of complicated hereditary spastic paraplegia due to a dominant negative mutation of KIF1A, SPG30 gene. *Sci. Rep.* **2017**, *7*, 12527. [CrossRef]
69. Nitta, R.; Kikkawa, M.; Okada, Y.; Hirokawa, N. KIF1A Alternately Uses Two Loops to Bind Microtubules. *Science* **2004**, *305*, 678–683. [CrossRef]
70. Erlich, Y.; Edvardson, S.; Hodges, E.; Zenvirt, S.; Thekkat, P.; Shaag, A.; Dor, T.; Hannon, G.J.; Elpeleg, O. Exome sequencing and disease-network analysis of a single family implicate a mutation in *KIF1A* in hereditary spastic paraparesis. *Genome Res.* **2011**, *21*, 658–664. [CrossRef]
71. Schule, R.; Kremer, B.P.H.; Kassubek, J.; Auer-Grumbach, M.; Kostic, V.; Klopstock, T.; Klimpe, S.; Otto, S.; Boesch, S.; van de Warrenburg, B.P.; et al. SPG10 is a rare cause of spastic paraplegia in European families. *J. Neurol. Neurosurg. Psychiatry* **2008**, *79*, 584–587. [CrossRef]
72. Yonekawa, Y.; Harada, A.; Okada, Y.; Funakoshi, T.; Kanai, Y.; Takei, Y.; Terada, S.; Noda, T.; Hirokawa, N. Defect in Synaptic Vesicle Precursor Transport and Neuronal Cell Death in KIF1A Motor Protein–deficient Mice. *J. Cell Biol.* **1998**, *141*, 431–441. [CrossRef]
73. Adzhubei, I.A.; Schmidt, S.; Peshkin, L.; Ramensky, V.E.; Gerasimova, A.; Bork, P.; Kondrashov, A.S.; Sunyaev, S.R. A method and server for predicting damaging missense mutations. *Nat. Methods* **2010**, *7*, 248–249. [CrossRef]
74. Altschul, S.F.; Gish, W.; Miller, W.; Myers, E.W.; Lipman, D.J. Basic local alignment search tool. *J. Mol. Biol.* **1990**, *215*, 403–410. [CrossRef]
75. Kikkawa, M.; Sablin, E.P.; Okada, Y.; Yajima, H.; Fletterick, R.J.; Hirokawa, N. Switch-based mechanism of kinesin motors. *Nature* **2001**, *411*, 439–445. [CrossRef]
76. Nescav Syndrome Disease: Malacards—Research Articles, Drugs, Genes, Clinical Trials. Available online: https://www.malacards.org/card/nescav_syndrome (accessed on 6 August 2022).
77. Okamoto, N.; Miya, F.; Tsunoda, T.; Yanagihara, K.; Kato, M.; Saitoh, S.; Yamasaki, M.; Kanemura, Y.; Kosaki, K. KIF1A mutation in a patient with progressive neurodegeneration. *J. Hum. Genet.* **2014**, *59*, 639–641. [CrossRef] [PubMed]
78. Chitty, L.S.; Robb, S.; Berry, C.; Silver, D.; Baraitser, M. PEHO or PEHO-like syndrome? *Clin. Dysmorphol.* **1996**, *5*, 143–152. [CrossRef] [PubMed]
79. Somer, M. Diagnostic criteria and genetics of the PEHO syndrome. *J. Med. Genet.* **1993**, *30*, 932–936. [CrossRef] [PubMed]
80. Yiş, U.; Hız, S.; Anal, O.; Dirik, E. Progressive encephalopathy with edema, hypsarrhythmia, and optic atrophy and PEHO-like syndrome: Report of two cases. *J. Pediatr. Neurosci.* **2011**, *6*, 165–168. [CrossRef] [PubMed]
81. Richards, S.; Aziz, N.; Bale, S.; Bick, D.; Das, S.; Gastier-Foster, J.; Grody, W.W.; Hegde, M.; Lyon, E.; Spector, E.; et al. Standards and guidelines for the interpretation of sequence variants: A joint consensus recommendation of the American College of Medical Genetics and Genomics and the Association for Molecular Pathology. *Anesthesia Analg.* **2015**, *17*, 405–424. [CrossRef]
82. Levy, S.E.; Mandell, D.S.; Schultz, R.T. Autism. *Lancet* **2009**, *374*, 1627–1638. [CrossRef]
83. Tomaselli, P.J.; Rossor, A.M.; Horga, A.; Laura, M.; Blake, J.C.; Houlden, H.; Reilly, M.M. A de novo dominant mutation in *KIF1A* associated with axonal neuropathy, spasticity and autism spectrum disorder. *J. Peripher. Nerv. Syst.* **2017**, *22*, 460–463. [CrossRef]
84. Kurihara, M.; Ishiura, H.; Bannai, T.; Mitsui, J.; Yoshimura, J.; Morishita, S.; Hayashi, T.; Shimizu, J.; Toda, T.; Tsuji, S. A Novel de novo KIF1A Mutation in a Patient with Autism, Hyperactivity, Epilepsy, Sensory Disturbance, and Spastic Paraplegia. *Intern. Med.* **2020**, *59*, 839–842. [CrossRef]
85. Huang, Y.; Jiao, J.; Zhang, M.; Situ, M.; Yuan, D.; Lyu, P.; Li, S.; Wang, Z.; Yang, Y.; Huang, Y. A study on KIF1A gene missense variant analysis and its protein expression and structure profiles of an autism spectrum disorder family trio. *Zhonghua Yi Xue Yi Chuan Xue Za Zhi* **2021**, *38*, 620–625. [CrossRef]
86. Demily, C.; Lesca, G.; Poisson, A.; Till, M.; Barcia, G.; Chatron, N.; Sanlaville, D.; Munnich, A. Additive Effect of Variably Penetrant 22q11.2 Duplication and Pathogenic Mutations in Autism Spectrum Disorder: To Which Extent Does the Tree Hide the Forest? *J. Autism Dev. Disord.* **2018**, *48*, 2886–2889. [CrossRef]
87. Schimert, K.I.; Budaitis, B.G.; Reinemann, D.N.; Lang, M.J.; Verhey, K.J. Intracellular cargo transport by single-headed kinesin motors. *Proc. Natl. Acad. Sci. USA* **2019**, *116*, 6152–6161. [CrossRef]

88. Derr, N.D.; Goodman, B.S.; Jungmann, R.; Leschziner, A.E.; Shih, W.M.; Reck-Peterson, S.L. Tug-of-War in Motor Protein Ensembles Revealed with a Programmable DNA Origami Scaffold. *Science* **2012**, *338*, 662–665. [CrossRef]
89. Hariadi, R.F.; Sommese, R.F.; Sivaramakrishnan, S. Tuning myosin-driven sorting on cellular actin networks. *Elife* **2015**, *4*, e05472. [CrossRef]
90. Toropova, K.; Mladenov, M.; Roberts, A.J. Intraflagellar transport dynein is autoinhibited by trapping of its mechanical and track-binding elements. *Nat. Struct. Mol. Biol.* **2017**, *24*, 461–468. [CrossRef]
91. Driller-Colangelo, A.R.; Chau, K.W.; Morgan, J.M.; Derr, N.D. Cargo rigidity affects the sensitivity of dynein ensembles to individual motor pausing. *Cytoskeleton* **2016**, *73*, 693–702. [CrossRef]
92. Furuta, K.; Furuta, A.; Toyoshima, Y.Y.; Amino, M.; Oiwa, K.; Kojima, H. Measuring collective transport by defined numbers of processive and nonprocessive kinesin motors. *Proc. Natl. Acad. Sci. USA* **2012**, *110*, 501–506. [CrossRef]
93. Cong, D.; Ren, J.; Zhou, Y.; Wang, S.; Liang, J.; Ding, M.; Feng, W. Motor domain-mediated autoinhibition dictates axonal transport by the kinesin UNC-104/KIF1A. *PLOS Genet.* **2021**, *17*, e1009940. [CrossRef]
94. Ren, J.; Wang, S.; Chen, H.; Wang, W.; Huo, L.; Feng, W. Coiled-coil 1-mediated fastening of the neck and motor domains for kinesin-3 autoinhibition. *Proc. Natl. Acad. Sci. USA* **2018**, *115*, E11209–E11942. [CrossRef]
95. Kanai, Y.; Wang, D.; Hirokawa, N. KIF13B enhances the endocytosis of LRP1 by recruiting LRP1 to caveolae. *J. Cell Biol.* **2014**, *204*, 395–408. [CrossRef]
96. Hanada, T.; Lin, L.; Tibaldi, E.V.; Reinherz, E.L.; Chishti, A.H. GAKIN, a Novel Kinesin-like Protein Associates with the Human Homologue of the Drosophila Discs Large Tumor Suppressor in T Lymphocytes. *J. Biol. Chem.* **2000**, *275*, 28774–28784. [CrossRef]
97. Miki, H.; Setou, M.; Kaneshiro, K.; Hirokawa, N. All kinesin superfamily protein, KIF, genes in mouse and human. *Proc. Natl. Acad. Sci. USA* **2001**, *98*, 7004–7011. [CrossRef] [PubMed]
98. Frontiers | Breaking Boundaries in the Brain—Advances in Editing Tools for Neurogenetic Disorders. Available online: https://www.frontiersin.org/articles/10.3389/fgeed.2021.623519/full (accessed on 8 January 2023).
99. Westhaus, A.; Cabanes-Creus, M.; Rybicki, A.; Baltazar, G.; Navarro, R.G.; Zhu, E.; Drouyer, M.; Knight, M.; Albu, R.F.; Ng, B.H.; et al. High-Throughput In Vitro, Ex Vivo, and In Vivo Screen of Adeno-Associated Virus Vectors Based on Physical and Functional Transduction. *Hum. Gene Ther.* **2020**, *31*, 575–589. [CrossRef] [PubMed]
100. Kim, Y.G.; Chandrasegaran, S. Chimeric restriction endonuclease. *Proc. Natl. Acad. Sci. USA* **1994**, *91*, 883–887. [CrossRef] [PubMed]
101. Carlson, D.F.; Tan, W.; Lillico, S.G.; Stverakova, D.; Proudfoot, C.; Christian, M.; Voytas, D.F.; Long, C.R.; Whitelaw, C.B.A.; Fahrenkrug, S.C. Efficient TALEN-mediated gene knockout in livestock. *Proc. Natl. Acad. Sci. USA* **2012**, *109*, 17382–17387. [CrossRef]
102. Iyama, T.; Wilson, D.M., III. DNA repair mechanisms in dividing and non-dividing cells. *DNA Repair* **2013**, *12*, 620–636. [CrossRef]
103. Suzuki, K.; Tsunekawa, Y.; Hernandez-Benitez, R.; Wu, J.; Zhu, J.; Kim, E.J.; Hatanaka, F.; Yamamoto, M.; Araoka, T.; Li, Z.; et al. In vivo genome editing via CRISPR/Cas9 mediated homology-independent targeted integration. *Nature* **2016**, *540*, 144–149. [CrossRef]
104. Suzuki, K.; Yamamoto, M.; Hernandez-Benitez, R.; Li, Z.; Wei, C.; Soligalla, R.D.; Aizawa, E.; Hatanaka, F.; Kurita, M.; Reddy, P.; et al. Precise in vivo genome editing via single homology arm donor mediated intron-targeting gene integration for genetic disease correction. *Cell Res.* **2019**, *29*, 804–819. [CrossRef]
105. Anzalone, A.V.; Randolph, P.B.; Davis, J.R.; Sousa, A.A.; Koblan, L.W.; Levy, J.M.; Chen, P.J.; Wilson, C.; Newby, G.A.; Raguram, A.; et al. Search-and-replace genome editing without double-strand breaks or donor DNA. *Nature* **2019**, *576*, 149–157. [CrossRef]
106. Homology-Mediated End Joining-Based Targeted Integration Using CRISPR/Cas9 | Cell Research. Available online: https://www.nature.com/articles/cr201776 (accessed on 10 January 2023).
107. Nishiyama, J.; Mikuni, T.; Yasuda, R. Virus-Mediated Genome Editing via Homology-Directed Repair in Mitotic and Postmitotic Cells in Mammalian Brain. *Neuron* **2017**, *96*, 755–768.e5. [CrossRef]
108. Microhomology-Mediated End-Joining-Dependent Integration of Donor DNA in Cells and Animals Using TALENs and CRISPR/Cas9 | Nature Communications. Available online: https://www.nature.com/articles/ncomms6560 (accessed on 10 January 2023).
109. Płoski, R. Next Generation Sequencing—General Information about the Technology, Possibilities, and Limitations. In *Clinical Applications for Next-Generation Sequencing*; Academic Press: Cambridge, MA, USA, 2016; pp. 1–18. [CrossRef]
110. Cheng, E.Y. 18—Prenatal Diagnosis. In *Avery's Diseases of the Newborn*, 10th ed.; Gleason, C.A., Juul, S.E., Eds.; Elsevier: Amsterdam, The Netherlands, 2018; pp. 190–200. [CrossRef]

Disclaimer/Publisher's Note: The statements, opinions and data contained in all publications are solely those of the individual author(s) and contributor(s) and not of MDPI and/or the editor(s). MDPI and/or the editor(s) disclaim responsibility for any injury to people or property resulting from any ideas, methods, instructions or products referred to in the content.

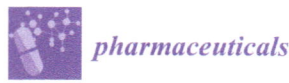

Review

Renal Proximal Tubular Cells: A New Site for Targeted Delivery Therapy of Diabetic Kidney Disease

Hao Li, Wenni Dai, Zhiwen Liu and Liyu He *

Department of Nephrology, The Second Xiangya Hospital of Central South University, Hunan Key Laboratory of Kidney Disease and Blood Purification, Changsha 410011, Hunan, China
* Correspondence: heliyu1124@csu.edu.cn; Tel.: +86-731-8529-2064

Abstract: Diabetic kidney disease (DKD) is a major complication of diabetes mellitus (DM) and the leading cause of end-stage kidney disease (ESKD) worldwide. A significant number of drugs have been clinically investigated for the treatment of DKD. However, a large proportion of patients still develop end-stage kidney disease unstoppably. As a result, new effective therapies are urgently needed to slow down the progression of DKD. Recently, there is increasing evidence that targeted drug delivery strategies such as large molecule carriers, small molecule prodrugs, and nanoparticles can improve drug efficacy and reduce adverse side effects. There is no doubt that targeted drug delivery strategies have epoch-making significance and great application prospects for the treatment of DKD. In addition, the proximal tubule plays a very critical role in the progression of DKD. Consequently, the purpose of this paper is to summarize the current understanding of proximal tubule cell-targeted therapy, screen for optimal targeting strategies, and find new therapeutic approaches for the treatment of DKD.

Keywords: diabetic nephropathies; drug delivery systems; kidney tubules; proximal; molecular targeted therapy; diabetes mellitus

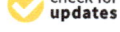

Citation: Li, H.; Dai, W.; Liu, Z.; He, L. Renal Proximal Tubular Cells: A New Site for Targeted Delivery Therapy of Diabetic Kidney Disease. *Pharmaceuticals* **2022**, *15*, 1494. https://doi.org/10.3390/ph15121494

Academic Editors: Silviya Petrova Zustiak and Era Jain

Received: 6 November 2022
Accepted: 29 November 2022
Published: 30 November 2022

Publisher's Note: MDPI stays neutral with regard to jurisdictional claims in published maps and institutional affiliations.

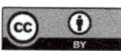

Copyright: © 2022 by the authors. Licensee MDPI, Basel, Switzerland. This article is an open access article distributed under the terms and conditions of the Creative Commons Attribution (CC BY) license (https://creativecommons.org/licenses/by/4.0/).

1. Introduction

Diabetic kidney disease (DKD) is one of the main complications of diabetes mellitus (DM) and is also the main cause of end-stage kidney disease (ESKD). The prevalence of ESKD in the general adult population in mainland China is 10.8%. With the rapid development of the world economy and the increasingly serious aging of the population, the incidence of ESKD is increasing year by year [1,2]. At present, there are approximately 100 million DKD patients in the world, resulting in huge medical costs and a huge economic burden [3]. The main treatment methods for DKD are blood pressure control and blood glucose control, and commonly used drugs include angiotensin-converting enzyme inhibitors (ACEI), angiotensin II receptor blockers (ARB), mineralocorticoid receptor antagonists (MRAs), dipeptidyl peptidase 4(DPP-4) inhibitor glucagon-like peptide-1 (GLP-1) receptor agonist, and sodium glucose cotransporter 2(SGLT2) inhibition [4–9]. In addition, in recent years, papers have reported new drugs for the treatment of DKD, such as: luteolin attenuates, protein arginine methyltranferase-1, stanniocalcin-1 (STC-1), adiponectin, and microRNA-122-5p [10–14]. However, these drugs make it difficult for them to control the progression of DKD due to their side effects or difficulties in achieving effective accumulation in the kidney. In such cases, many patients inevitably develop ESKD. Therefore, new therapeutic methods are urgently needed to be developed and applied to DKD.

Targeted drug delivery therapy refers to the use of the specific carrier to wrap active pharmaceutical ingredients [15] that can be transported to designated organs or cells via the carrier. In this way, its local drug concentration can be greatly increased and its side effects can be deeply reduced. Targeted drug delivery therapy is a new treatment method that has been widely used in various tumors, such as urothelial carcinoma, breast cancer, non-small cell lung cancer, and so on [16–18]. The study of kidney-targeted drug delivery began in 1990, and the concept was comprehensively proposed by Haas in 2002 [19]. During these two decades, various studies on kidney-targeted drug delivery have been published. It is well known that the kidney consists of basic renal units, which are composed of glomeruli and tubules, and the main pathological changes in DKD are glomerulosclerosis, tubular dysfunction, and tubulointerstitial fibrosis [20–22]. Therefore, the targeted treatment of DKD to glomeruli and tubules is of great significance. In current studies, the main focus is on glomerular podocytes, glomerular mesangial cells, and proximal tubular cells [23]. The purpose of this paper is to provide a comprehensive and important update on the development of drug delivery strategies for this target in proximal tubular epithelial cells, to summarize the rationale of its targeting and the associated drug carriers, in order to find new methods for the treatment of DKD.

2. Renal Proximal Tubular Cells

Targeted drug delivery to proximal tubular cells not only significantly enhances the efficiency of drug effects but also extremely reduces the negative side effects caused by drug action to other sites. This provides a new idea for the treatment of pathological changes such as tubulointerstitial fibrosis caused by DKD. In order to understand the targeted drug delivery to proximal tubular cells, we must first understand the physiological characteristics of the proximal tubule, its relationship with DKD, and its mechanism of drug uptake.

2.1. Physiological Characteristics of Proximal Tubule Cells

The kidney consists of basic renal units, which are composed of glomeruli and tubules. The renal tubule consists of a single layer of epithelial cells arranged on the proximal tubule, distal tubule, and collecting duct, which undertakes the exchange of substances between blood and urine. Therefore, the main physiological functions of renal tubules are reabsorption and secretion [24]. The proximal tubule plays a primary role in reabsorption, participating in the reabsorption of approximately two-thirds of the filtrate and recovering many compounds from the urine [25]. In addition, proximal tubules also have a potent secretory role, especially activated proximal tubular epithelial cells, which can promote the formation and development of tubulointerstitial lesions, reduced renal function, interstitial inflammation, and fibrosis through chemotaxis, antigen presentation, and cytokine autocrine and paracrine patterns [26,27]. This is very closely related to the development of DKD.

2.2. Relationship with DKD Progression

Currently, the most significant research on diabetes kidney disease has been focused on the glomerulus-centered research model. The pathological changes of the glomerulus, such as glomerular basement membrane thickening, mesangial expansion, increased resistance of endothelial cell fenestrations and podocyte injury [28–31], are the main pathological changes of DKD and are closely related to proteinuria, which is the signature of DKD. However, it has been shown that some patients with advanced disease show neither substantial glomerulopathy nor proteinuria but demonstrate a decline in traditional indicators of renal function (such as the presence of microalbuminuria or a decrease in glomerular filtration rate) [32]. Thus, structural and functional alterations of the renal tubules have an irreplaceable role in the progression of DKD. Renal tubular injury, mostly in the proximal tubule, is associated with abnormal activation of the AGEs-RAGE signaling pathway and is closely related to tubulointerstitial fibrosis, interstitial inflammation, and decreased renal function [33]. The mechanism that causes its injury is that due to the dependence of the proximal tubule itself on high energy and aerobic metabolism, when ischemic injury occurs in diabetic patients, increased consumption, impaired utilization, and reduced delivery of oxygen lead to apoptosis and fibrosis in the renal unit of the proximal tubule [34].

2.3. Mechanism of Proximal Tubule Uptake of Drugs

Although the renal tubules consist of proximal tubules, distal tubules, and collecting ducts, most tubule-targeting systems are aimed at the proximal tubules [35]. According to the anatomy of the kidney, drugs have to travel from the blood circulation to the proximal tubular cells, and there are two anatomical barriers between them, glomerular filtration barriers and basolateral barriers [36]. The glomerular filtration barrier is a highly specialized capillary wall that consists of three parts, including endothelial cells, podocytes, and basement membrane [37]. First, glomerular endothelial cells have the function of window opening, and the diameter of their window opening is approximately 70–100 nm [38]. There is an endothelial surface layer consisting of a membrane-bound layer of proteoglycans, glycosaminoglycans, and salivary proteins, a glycocalyx, and a loosely attached endothelial cell shell. Since salivary proteins, sulfated glycosaminoglycans, and hyaluronic acid in the endothelial surface layer are negatively charged, positively charged carriers pass through more easily [39]. Second, the glomerular basement membrane is composed of laminins, collagen IV, nidogens, and the heparan sulfate proteoglycans agrin, perlecan, and collagen XVIII. GBM is negatively charged due to the presence of negatively charged heparan sulfate proteoglycans agrin, which facilitates the passage of positively charged carriers [40]. Third, the podocyte is the terminally differentiated epithelial cell of the glomerulus, and its structure is traditionally divided into three distinct subcellular compartments: the cell body, the microtubule-driven membrane-extended primary process, and the actin-driven membrane-extended peduncle [41,42]. Adjacent podocyte cross each other at their foot processes, which are also called the slit diaphragm. The size of these slit diaphragms determines the size of the carrier that can pass through, with a passable carrier diameter of approximately 5–7 nm [43]. The basolateral barrier consists of the periportal capillary endothelium and the tubular mesenchyme between the capillaries and the proximal tubular cells. In order to cross this barrier, it first depends on the windowing of the peritubular capillary endothelium, which has a diameter of approximately 60–70 nm [44]. These opening windows are covered by a septum of approximately 3–5 nm thickness, which is composed of radial fibrils. The pore size to pass through these fibers is approximately 5.0–5.5 nm [45–47]. The surface layer of peritubular capillary endothelial cells contains negatively charged heparan sulfate so that positively charged drug carriers pass through more easily than negatively charged ones [48,49].

As the above description shows, it is easy to know that positively charged drugs with sizes smaller than 5–7 nm can reach proximal tubule cells from the bloodstream relatively easily and smoothly through the anatomical barrier. However, there are two ways that the drugs are taken up by the proximal tubule, one is the transporter protein, and the other is the receptor-mediated endocytosis [50]. The SLC subgroup is the uptake of drugs following chemical gradient-mediated passive transport. The ABC family is the uptake of drugs relying on ATP-depleted active transport [51,52]. Although there are so many transporter proteins, the feasibility of choosing them as transporters for targeted drug uptake is not high. First, as they are mainly involved in the uptake of small endogenous molecules and small molecules, targeted drugs with carriers may be too large for them. Second, the drug that is transported in by a transporter protein on one side of the proximal tubule may be quickly transported out again by the same or a different transporter protein on the other side. This may make it difficult to achieve effective drug concentrations in the proximal tubule. Finally, these transport proteins are widely distributed not only in the kidney but also in other organs [53,54]. This is the most limiting point for its application, because the most important thing for our targeted therapy is to increase the concentration of the drug in the kidney and reduce its side effects in other sites.

Consequently, we have to focus on receptor-mediated endocytosis (Figure 1). There are four receptors associated with targeted therapy, namely: megalin, cubilin, amnionless(AMN), and folate receptors [35]. Megalin and cubilin are present in the parietal membrane of proximal tubule epithelial cells, and it was shown that megalin cooperates with cubilin to facilitate the reabsorption of almost all filtered plasma proteins [55,56].

Megalin, as a multispecific clearance receptor, has a large extracellular structural domain, a single transmembrane structural domain, and a small cytoplasmic structural domain. In contrast, cubilin has only one extracellular structural domain and lacks the transmembrane and cytoplasmic structural domains, and it must interact with other membrane proteins for endocytosis. AMN has an extracellular structural domain, transmembrane structural domain, and cytoplasmic structural domain, and its main role is to assist the endocytosis of cubilin [57,58]. Based on differences in cellular ultrastructure, the proximal tubule is anatomically divided into three distinct segments S1 to S3, and it was shown that the s1 segment is highly specialized for receptor-mediated endocytosis [59,60]. Therefore, it is not difficult to conclude that the s1 fragment is the primary location where our targeted therapeutic drug is taken up by the proximal tubule. Megalin and cubilin combine and mediate endocytosis of a large and highly diverse set of ligands, including plasma proteins, peptides, enzymes, vitamin-binding proteins, hormones, and hormone-binding proteins, as well as drugs and toxins. Even though these two receptors have a wide range of ligands, their interaction with the ligands is specific [61]. As for the folate receptor (FR), its main role is to reabsorb folate from the renal tubular lumen. Among the four folate receptor subtypes identified in humans, the membrane-associated folate receptors FRα and FRβ were detected only in proximal renal tubule cells, which have a high specificity. In addition, folate receptors are overexpressed in a variety of malignant tissues and have been used for tumor-targeted delivery of anticancer drugs [62,63]. In summary, receptor-mediated endocytosis will be an important mechanism for our proximal tubule-targeted therapy.

(A) Ligand–receptor binding: Cubilin, due to its lack of transmembrane and cytoplasmic structural domains, must form a dual receptor complex with megelin or amnionless (AMN) for endocytosis to occur. Different ligands bind to the corresponding receptors with different affinities.

(B) Vesicle transport: After receptor–ligand binding, lattice proteins wrap the vesicles and transport them to the corresponding organelles (e.g., lysosomes) for further processing.

(C) Receptor recycling: After vesicle release of ligand, the receptor is recycled to the cell membrane by the apical tubules (DATs).

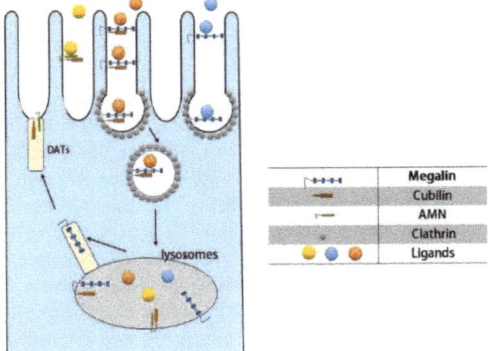

Figure 1. Receptor-mediated endocytosis of proximal tubules.

3. Targeted Drug Delivery Strategy

As previously discussed, the glomerular filtration barrier requires drugs smaller than 5–7 nm in diameter and positively charged to cross the barrier and reach the proximal tubule. Carriers that can be used as proximal tubule cell-targeted therapeutics include common proteins and peptides, polymers, small molecule prodrugs, and nanoparticles. I will summarize and discuss the applications and feasibility of these carriers in detail in the following sections.

3.1. Protein-Based and Peptide-Based Carriers

Low molecular weight proteins are the most widely researched carriers, which reach renal tubular cells via receptor-mediated endocytosis. The most popular of the low-molecular-weight proteins is lysozyme, with a molecular weight of approximately 14 kDa, which freely passes through the glomerular basement membrane and is endocytosed into proximal tubular cells expressing the giant protein receptor. Haas et al. [64] used lysozyme as a carrier to wrap naproxen targeted to the proximal tubule, resulting in a significant increase in naproxen accumulation in the kidney of approximately 70-fold. Dolman et al. [65] linked sunitinib analogs to lysozyme via a platinum-based linker to target them to the proximal tubule. The area of subcurvilinear renal drug levels was increased by 28-fold compared to equimolar doses of sunitinib malate, and its toxicity was substantially reduced. In spite of the fact that lysozyme is widely studied, the carrier itself can cause adverse effects such as systemic blood pressure and adverse effects on renal function [66]. In addition to lysozyme, another low molecular weight protein is the human serum protein fragment. Vegt et al. [67] first suggested in 2008 that the serum albumin fragment could be targeted to the kidney. Z.-x. Yuan et al. [68] used human serum albumin as the starting material, cleaved it into albumin fragments, and separated and purified the degradation products using Superdex 75 and CM-Sepharose FF to obtain three peptide fragments with specific sequences (PF-A_{1-123}, PF-$A_{124-298}$, and PF-$A_{299-585}$). By studying their nephrotoxicity and cellular uptake, it was concluded that the human serum protein fragments not only showed good targeting (with PF-$A_{299-585}$ being the best) but also no nephrotoxicity despite concentrations up to 5.00 mg/mL. Furthermore, in their next study [69], they applied PF-A299–585 as a vector to carry the Chinese herbal medicine rehmannia methylestradiol, which successfully targeted the kidney and alleviated the symptoms in a rodent model of membranous nephropathy. This certainly indicates that human serum protein fragment is an effective targeting carrier. Moreover, other proteins that can be reabsorbed by renal tubules, such as streptavidin [70] and somatostatin [71], also have some potential to become proximal tubule carriers. Thus, low molecular weight proteins have a bright and wide application prospect as targeting carriers for proximal tubule cells.

3.2. Polymeric Carriers

A number of studies have demonstrated that polymers can be used as carriers for proximal tubule targeting. The ability of polymers to accumulate in the renal tubules depends primarily on the type of anionic group, the copolymer monomer content, and the molecular weight of the final polymer. For example, low molecular weight polyvinylpyrrolidone (PVP) is excreted in the urine and does not accumulate in the kidney. However, anionized polyvinylpyrrolidones can remain in the kidney and carboxylated PVP exhibits higher renal accumulation than sulfonated PVPs. Kodeira et al. [72] found that carboxylated PVP accumulated in the kidney at 30% of the injected dose 3 h after administration, and most carboxylated PVP accumulated in the proximal tubule. On the basis of PVP, another PVP copolymer, poly (vinylpyrrolidone-co-dimethyl maleic anhydride) co-polymer (PVD), which has a higher renal accumulation, was investigated. Kamada et al. [73] found that approximately 80% of the 10-kDa PVD selectively accumulated in the kidney 4 h after intravenous administration of PVD to mice. Moreover, approximately 40% remained in the kidney 96 h after treatment. Yamamoto et al. [74], who used PVD as a carrier for the protein drug superoxide dismutase (SOD), showed that approximately six times more L-PVD-SOD than natural SOD was distributed to the kidney 3 h after intravenous injection.

Another targeting carrier that has been extensively studied is acetylated low molecular weight chitosan (LMWC). Using fluorescence imaging, Z.-X. Yuan et al. [75] found that random 50% N-acetylated low molecular weight chitosan (LMWC) selectively accumulated in the kidney, especially in the proximal tubule, and used LMWC as a carrier to piggyback on prednisolone and showed that the binding with a molecular weight of 19 kD had the highest accumulation rate in the kidney, and the total amount in the kidney was 13 times higher than that in the control prednisolone group D.-W. Wang et al. [76] constructed stepwise targeted chitosan triphenylphosphine-low molecular weight chitosan-curcumin (TPP-LMWC-CUR, TLC) and TLC in kidney tissue, causing rapid preferential distribution followed by specific internalization by renal tubular epithelial cells via interaction of the megalin with LMWC. LMWC is now well established for the targeted treatment of AKI and hyperuricemic kidney stones [76,77]; therefore, LMWC should have great potential as a vehicle for the treatment of DKD.

A recently emerging research trend is the use of various amino-acid-modified polyamide amine dendrimers as targeting carriers, which have been extensively investigated in tumors as well as osteoporosis [78,79]. Matsuura et al. [80] used L-serine (Ser)-modified polyamide amine dendrimers (PAMAM) as effective kidney-targeting drug carriers and showed that 3 h after intravenous injection, approximately in contrast, unmodified PAMAM, L-threonine-modified PAMAM, and L-tyrosine-modified PAMAM resulted in 28%, 35%, and 31% renal accumulation, respectively. The results suggest that Ser modification is a promising approach for renal targeting using macromolecular drug carriers.

Other carriers with proximal tubule targeting potential have been reported in the literature. For example, poly(N-(2-hydroxypropyl) methacrylamide) (pHPMA), which was applied for targeted tumor therapy, is currently being used [81,82]. In a study of the distribution of pHPMA in tumor-bearing mice, Kissel et al. [83] found a 33-fold higher concentration of biotin-pHPMA than HPMA in proximal tubular cells of both kidneys by day 7 after intravenous injection. This suggests that biotinylated pHPMA has the potential to target the kidney. However, its application is limited by the non-degradable nature of its backbone [84].

Similarly, poly-l-glutamic acid (PG) is widely used as a carrier for the delivery of anti-cancer chemotherapeutic drugs [85,86]. H.-J. Chai et al. [87] administered 3H-deoxycytidine-labeled PG and 3H-deoxycytidine intravenously to normal and streptozotocin-induced diabetic rats. The results showed that in normal rats, the renal accumulation was 7- or 15-fold higher in the group injected with PG carrier conjugates than in the non-injected group at 24 h after injection. In the kidneys of diabetic rats, the PG conjugate injected group was 8-fold higher than the control group. Additionally, after 24 h of injection, PG can be selectively deposited in the renal tubular epithelium. This study demonstrates the favorable accumulation properties of PG in normal and oxidative stress-induced kidneys with the potential for proximal tubule-targeted drug carriers. With the advancement of technology, more and more polymers are being invented, and polymer carriers have strong application prospects.

3.3. Small-Molecule Prodrugs

Prodrugs are simple chemical derivatives that require one or two enzymatic or chemical transformations to produce an active drug [88]. Large molecule drugs such as proteins often encounter significant barriers to penetration, so small molecule prodrugs are urgently needed. Folic acid, a carrier that has long been widely used in tumor-targeted therapy [89–91], works on the principle that tumor cells express folate receptors. Normal renal proximal tubules also express several folate receptors, so folic acid can be used to target drugs to proximal renal tubular cells [92]. When Trump et al. [93] labeled folic acid conjugates with radionuclides to observe their distribution at the tumor site, they unexpectedly found a high initial uptake of radionuclides in the proximal tubules of the kidney (17% ID/g at five minutes), which increased to 48% ID/g after 4 h. A noteworthy point is that folate receptors are expressed not only in proximal tubules but also in activated macrophages/monocytes and in organs other than the kidney (e.g., liver) [94]. Therefore, folic acid is controversial as a carrier for proximal-tubule-targeted therapy. Hyaluronic acid (HA) is also a small molecule prodrug, and Hu et al. [95] developed an HA-curcumin (HA-CUR) polymeric prodrug targeting proximal tubular epithelial cells. The biodistribution results showed a 13.9-fold increase in the accumulation of HA-CUR in the kidney compared to free CUR. This indicates that HA has a high prospect for proximal tubule targeting applications. There is also a small molecule prodrug called glycosylated small molecule prodrug. Lin et al. [96] designed carbamate-glucosamine conjugate (PCG), a combination of 2-aminoglucose and prednisolone, to ascertain the renal targeting ability of 2-aminoglucose. The results were poor tissue-specific localization of prednisolone and selective accumulation of PCG in the kidney with an 8.1-fold increase in drug concentration in the kidney 60 min after intravenous administration. The specific structural modification of the parent drug is key to the development of renal-targeted prodrugs [97].

3.4. Nanoparticles

Nanoparticles are a popular research topic nowadays. Nanoparticles are defined as particles less than 100 nm in diameter. Nanoparticles include: nanoliposomes, solid lipid nanoparticles, inorganic nanoparticles, organic nanoparticles, and micelles [98,99]. Because of their distinctive physical properties, such as surface effect and volume, in the past few years, nanoparticles have been successfully applied in many fields of medicine, such as cancer, diabetes, osteoarthritis, etc. [100–102]. The kidney has always been an important area for nanoparticle applications as well, not only because of the important role of the kidney in physiology but also because of the important role of the kidney in the filtration and excretion of nanoparticles [103]. Therefore, targeting nanoparticles to the renal tubules for the treatment of diabetic nephropathy is also very prospective. Whether the nanoparticles can reach the specified cellular destination depends on the size, homogeneity, surface potential, and drug loading of nanoparticles [104]. In the following, we detail the studies concerning these nanoparticles targeting the renal tubules.

First, nanoliposomes are an ideal and safe form of drug delivery with a characteristic lipid bilayer similar to the cytoplasmic membrane. They can incorporate a wide range of drug candidates in their hydrophilic and hydrophobic compartments [105]. Nanoliposomes can be administered by a variety of routes, including intravenous, transdermal, subcutaneous, or inhalation [106]. Nanoliposomes already have applications in Alzheimer's disease, osteoporosis, and cancer, as well as promising applications in the treatment of kidney disease [107–109]. In a study by C. Huang et al. [110] they have prepared calycosin-loaded nanoliposomes for the treatment of diabetic nephropathy. The particle size, zeta potential, drug loading, and entrapment efficiency of this microparticle were 80 nm, -20.53 ± 3.57, $7.48 \pm 1.19\%$, and $88.37 \pm 2.28\%$, respectively. They used calycosin, an antioxidant, that plays a key role in reducing oxidative stress damage in kidney cells. As we mentioned before, oxidative stress is a key mechanism for tubular damage in diabetic nephropathy. They found that calycosin-loaded nanoliposomes not only reduced the first-pass effect of calycosin to improve its oral absorption but also prolonged its mean bioavailability to provide a slow release.

Second, the concept of solid lipid nanoparticles was first introduced in the early 1990s and has developed rapidly during the last three decades [111]. Solid lipid nanoparticles were investigated intensively as drug delivery systems for a number of delivery pathways, such as oral, parenteral, dermal, and topical delivery [112,113]. In contrast to nanoliposomes, solid lipid nanoparticles are devoid of cavities made up of bilayers. Ahangarpour et al. [114–116] utilized solid lipid nanoparticles of myricitrin, which has poor bioavailability, to successfully improve oxidative stress in proximal tubules induced by hyperglycemia. The microparticles they designed were spherical in shape with an average particle size, zeta potential, encapsulation efficiency, and encapsulation capacity of 76.1 nm, -5.51 mV, 56.2%, and 5.62% respectively. It is definitely exciting news for us to target proximal tubule cells for the treatment of DKD. In addition, in a work by M. H. Asfour et al. [117], they ingeniously designed all-trans retinoic acid loaded chitosan/tripolyphosphate lipid hybrid nanoparticles to treat DKD. This is a chitosan-coated solid lipid nanoparticle encapsulated with all-trans retinoic acid, which can greatly increase the oral availability of the drug. All-trans retinoic acid can protect renal tubules in the progression of DKD by inhibiting fibrosis [118]. They have produced spherical microparticles with a size of 338.26 nm and an encapsulation efficiency of 94.19%. Furthermore, when designing the solid nanoparticles, they have applied the characteristic surface effect of nanoparticles to increase the surface area and solubility of the drug.

Third, as for organic nanoparticles, Liu et al. [119] wrapped Chinese medicine monomer Gypenoside (Gyp) XLIX with polymeric nanoparticles to form polylactic acid-co-glycoside (PLGA)-Gyp XLIX nanoparticles. Particle size, zeta potential, encapsulation rate, and drug loading capacity of the microparticles, which they prepared by applying nanoprecipitation and nano-self-assembly methods, were 128 ± 5.89 nm, -35.6 ± 3.18 mV, $82.4 \pm 5.36\%$, and $9.04 \pm 0.76\%$, respectively. The microparticles they prepared targeted the kidney and effectively inhibited tubular fibrosis and tubular necrosis, which are pathological changes found in DKD. Oroojalian et al. [120] used polymyxin-polyetherimide/DNA nanoparticles formulated with polymyxin B to successfully target proximal tubule cells expressing the megalin and demonstrated that it has higher transfection efficiency and lower cytotoxicity than unmodified PEIs/DNA nanoparticles. The microparticles sizes and zeta potentials prepared were 143–180 nm and 16.4 ± 1.87 to 23.43 ± 1.25 mV, correspondingly.

Fourth, inorganic nanoparticles, such as Fe_3O_4 magnetic nanoparticles, attenuated renal tubular injury and effectively inhibited tubular fibrosis with Fe_3O_4 magnetic albumin nanoparticles in a study by Liu et al. [121]. The hydrodynamic size and zeta potential of these microparticles were 102 nm and -18.6 mV, respectively. The intelligent use of albumin-coated iron particles effectively prolonged the in vivo circulation time of the particles and reduced off-target side effects [122].

Finally, Micelles are nanoparticles in the size range of 10–100 nm formed by the polymerization of monomers consisting of a hydrophilic head group and a hydrophobic tail group. J. Wang et al. [123] used micelles linked to kidney-targeting peptide (Lys-Lys-Glu-Glu-Glu)3-Lys) to successfully target the megalin on renal tubular epithelial cells. The average diameter of these particles was 15.0 ± 0.0 nm with the zeta potential of -7.8 ± 0.5 mV.

On the other hand, mesoscale nanoparticles refer to the larger gamut of nanoparticles above 100 nm in diameter. In the study by Williams et al. [124,125], they prepared a type of mesoscale nanoparticles with a diameter of approximately 400 nm that were formed from poly (lactic-co-glycolic acid) conjugated to polyethylene glycol, and observed that the nanoparticles could selectively and stably localize to the renal proximal tubular epithelial cells in experimental animals by the fluorescent tracer method. This microparticle size and surface charge were 347.6 ± 21.0 nm and -19.0 ± 0.3 mV, respectively. Their studies found that surface PEGylation facilitated particle localization to the kidney, long-term degradation, and controlled payload release. Moreover, they found that their localization efficiency in the kidney was 26–94 times higher than that in other organs, and they specifically targeted the renal tubules, and they had no inhibitory effect on renal function and no systemic toxicity. This carrier particle has already been successfully applied to encapsulate the selective TLR9 antagonist ODN2088 renal tubular targeting to treat tubular necrosis, inflammation, and apoptosis. This certainly encourages its application for therapeutic studies in DKD [126].

In addition, nanomaterials are not only nanoparticles but also nanotubes, nanocapsules, nanofibers and nanofilms. The tunneling nanotube is a channel that connects cells over long distances and has a diameter of 20–500 nm. The tunneling nanotube-TNFAIP2/M-sec system is used to treat autophagy of podocytes in DKD [127]. From this, we can look forward to future studies to discover whether new proteins present in the renal tubules are involved in the formation of tunneling nanotubes for the targeted treatment of DKD. Nanocapsules are also a common nanomaterial that has great potential in the therapy of DKD. In a study by M. Yu et al. [128], they used reactive-oxygen-species-responsive nanocapsules wrapped around adropin to effectively control blood glucose and lipid levels in DKD mice, inhibit the production of reactive oxygen species, and alleviate oxidative stress in DKD.

4. Conclusions and Future Perspectives

Drug targeting to proximal renal tubular cells is an increasingly sophisticated technique with great potential for development. The proximal tubular cell is a very promising targeting cell because it can transport and accumulate carriers into proximal tubular cells via receptor-mediated endocytosis to achieve appropriate drug concentrations and reduce drug side effects. We summarize four types of carriers that can target proximal tubule cells, including protein- and peptide-based carriers, polymeric carriers, small-molecule prodrugs, and nanoparticles. (Table 1) Among them, nanoparticles may be the most promising carriers for future clinical practice. Compared with the other three carriers, it has lower nephrotoxicity than protein and peptide carriers, better properties than polymer carriers with almost no renal excretion, and better targeting efficiency and retention than small molecule pre-drugs. Nanoparticles have their own unique nano-effects, such as surface effects that can greatly increase the surface area of the encapsulated drug to increase its absorbability. At present, the point that needs to be overcome for nanoparticle carriers is whether mass production and more precise targeting can be achieved. Nanotechnology is developing rapidly today, with technologies such as nanoenzymes, atomic force microscopes, and nanochips making a splash in various fields. We believe that with the future expansion of the field of nanotechnology, it is hopeful that nanoparticles with the ability to mass-produce and precisely target proximal renal tubular cells will be developed to slow down the progression of DKD and cur more and more patients with DKD.

Table 1. Drug carriers targeting proximal tubule cells.

Carriers	Applications	Limitations
Protein-based and peptide-based carriers	Lysozyme Albumin fragment Streptavidin Somatostatin	Systemic hypotension and nephrotoxicity
Polymeric carriers	PVP PVD LMWC PAMAM pHPMA PG	Inferior biodegradability
Small-molecule prodrugs	Folic acid Hyaluronic acid PCG	Low targeting efficiency, retentiveness, and poor cell permeability
Nanoparticles	Nanoliposomes Solid lipid nanoparticles Organic nanoparticles Inorganic nanoparticles Micelles	Difficulty in mass production and lack of technology

Author Contributions: Writing—original draft preparation: H.L.; writing—review and editing, H.L.; W.D.; Z.L.; L.H. All authors have read and agreed to the published version of the manuscript.

Funding: This research was funded by [Hunan Provincial Natural Science Foundation for Outstanding Youth] grant number [No. 2022JJ10093], [the Scientific Research Fund of Hunan Provincial Health Commission] grant number [B202303056777], [Natural Science Foundation of China] grant number [81870500]. And The APC was funded by [The Second Xiangya Hospital of Central South University].

Institutional Review Board Statement: Not applicable.

Informed Consent Statement: Not applicable.

Data Availability Statement: Not applicable.

Conflicts of Interest: The authors declare no conflict of interest.

References

1. Chen, Z.; Zhang, W.; Chen, X.; Hsu, C.-Y. Trends in end-stage kidney disease in Shanghai, China. *Kidney Int.* **2019**, *95*, 232. [CrossRef] [PubMed]
2. Wang, J.; Zhang, L.; Tang, S.C.-W.; Kashihara, N.; Kim, Y.-S.; Togtokh, A.; Yang, C.-W.; Zhao, M.-H. Disease burden and challenges of chronic kidney disease in North and East Asia. *Kidney Int.* **2018**, *94*, 22–25. [CrossRef] [PubMed]
3. Deng, Y.; Li, N.; Wu, Y.; Wang, M.; Yang, S.; Zheng, Y.; Deng, X.; Xiang, D.; Zhu, Y.; Xu, P.; et al. Global, Regional, and National Burden of Diabetes-Related Chronic Kidney Disease From 1990 to 2019. *Front. Endocrinol.* **2021**, *12*, 672350. [CrossRef] [PubMed]
4. Pollock, C.; Stefánsson, B.; Reyner, D.; Rossing, P.; Sjöström, C.D.; Wheeler, D.C.; Langkilde, A.M.; Heerspink, H.J.L. Albuminuria-lowering effect of dapagliflozin alone and in combination with saxagliptin and effect of dapagliflozin and saxagliptin on glycaemic control in patients with type 2 diabetes and chronic kidney disease (DELIGHT): A randomised, double-blind, placebo-controlled trial. *Lancet Diabetes Endocrinol.* **2019**, *7*, 429–441.
5. Barrera-Chimal, J.; Lima-Posada, I.; Bakris, G.L.; Jaisser, F. Mineralocorticoid receptor antagonists in diabetic kidney disease—Mechanistic and therapeutic effects. *Nat. Rev. Nephrol.* **2022**, *18*, 56–70.
6. Mann, J.F.E.; Ørsted, D.D.; Brown-Frandsen, K.; Marso, S.P.; Poulter, N.R.; Rasmussen, S.; Tornøe, K.; Zinman, B.; Buse, J.B. Liraglutide and Renal Outcomes in Type 2 Diabetes. *N. Engl. J. Med.* **2017**, *377*, 839–848. [CrossRef]
7. Cherney, D.; Perkins, B.A.; Lytvyn, Y.; Heerspink, H.; Rodríguez-Ortiz, M.E.; Mischak, H. The effect of sodium/glucose cotransporter 2 (SGLT2) inhibition on the urinary proteome. *PLoS ONE* **2017**, *12*, e0186910. [CrossRef]
8. Lytvyn, Y.; Bjornstad, P.; Van Raalte, D.H.; Heerspink, H.L.; Cherney, D.Z.I. The New Biology of Diabetic Kidney Disease-Mechanisms and Therapeutic Implications. *Endocr. Rev.* **2020**, *41*, 202–231.
9. Ravindran, S.; Munusamy, S. Renoprotective mechanisms of sodium-glucose co-transporter 2 (SGLT2) inhibitors against the progression of diabetic kidney disease. *J. Cell. Physiol.* **2022**, *237*, 1182–1205. [CrossRef]
10. Zhang, M.; He, L.; Zhou, L. Luteolin Attenuates Diabetic Nephropathy through Suppressing Inflammatory Response and Oxidative Stress by Inhibiting STAT3 Pathway. *Exp. Clin. Endocrinol. Diabetes* **2021**, *129*, 729–739. [CrossRef]
11. Chen, Y.; Yang, Y.; Liu, Z.; He, L. Adiponectin promotes repair of renal tubular epithelial cells by regulating mitochondrial biogenesis and function. *Metabolism* **2022**, *128*, 154959. [CrossRef] [PubMed]
12. Liu, Z.; Liu, H.; Xiao, L.; Liu, G.; Sun, L.; He, L. STC-1 ameliorates renal injury in diabetic nephropathy by inhibiting the expression of BNIP3 through the AMPK/SIRT3 pathway. *Lab. Invest.* **2019**, *99*, 684–697. [CrossRef] [PubMed]
13. Chen, Y.-Y.; Peng, X.-F.; Liu, G.-Y.; Liu, J.-S.; Sun, L.; Liu, H.; Xiao, L.; He, L.-Y. Protein arginine methyltranferase-1 induces ER stress and epithelial-mesenchymal transition in renal tubular epithelial cells and contributes to diabetic nephropathy. *Biochim. Biophys. Acta Mol. Basis Dis.* **2019**, *1865*, 2563–2575. [CrossRef] [PubMed]
14. Cheng, L.; Qiu, X.; He, L.; Liu, L. MicroRNA-122-5p ameliorates tubular injury in diabetic nephropathy via FIH-1/HIF-1α pathway. *Ren. Fail.* **2022**, *44*, 293–303. [CrossRef]
15. Bae, Y.H.; Park, K. Advanced drug delivery 2020 and beyond: Perspectives on the future. *Adv. Drug. Deliv. Rev.* **2020**, *158*, 4–16. [CrossRef]
16. Arbour, K.C.; Riely, G.J. Systemic Therapy for Locally Advanced and Metastatic Non-Small Cell Lung Cancer: A Review. *JAMA* **2019**, *322*, 764–774. [CrossRef] [PubMed]
17. Li, Y.; Wu, J.; Qiu, X.; Dong, S.; He, J.; Liu, J.; Xu, W.; Huang, S.; Hu, X.; Xiang, D.-X. Bacterial outer membrane vesicles-based therapeutic platform eradicates triple-negative breast tumor by combinational photodynamic/chemo-/immunotherapy. *Bioact. Mater.* **2023**, *20*, 548–560. [CrossRef]
18. Kleinmann, N.; Matin, S.F.; Pierorazio, P.M.; Gore, J.L.; Shabsigh, A.; Hu, B.; Chamie, K.; Godoy, G.; Hubosky, S.; Rivera, M.; et al. Primary chemoablation of low-grade upper tract urothelial carcinoma using UGN-101, a mitomycin-containing reverse thermal gel (OLYMPUS): An open-label, single-arm, phase 3 trial. *Lancet Oncol.* **2020**, *21*, 776–785. [CrossRef]
19. Haas, M.; Moolenaar, F.; Meijer, D.K.F.; de Zeeuw, D. Specific drug delivery to the kidney. *Cardiovasc. Drugs Ther.* **2002**, *16*, 489–496. [CrossRef]
20. Vallon, V.; Thomson, S.C. Renal function in diabetic disease models: The tubular system in the pathophysiology of the diabetic kidney. *Annu. Rev. Physiol.* **2012**, *74*, 351–375. [CrossRef]
21. Qian, Y.; Feldman, E.; Pennathur, S.; Kretzler, M.; Brosius, F.C. From fibrosis to sclerosis: Mechanisms of glomerulosclerosis in diabetic nephropathy. *Diabetes* **2008**, *57*, 1439–1445. [CrossRef] [PubMed]
22. Ponchiardi, C.; Mauer, M.; Najafian, B. Temporal profile of diabetic nephropathy pathologic changes. *Curr. Diab. Rep.* **2013**, *13*, 592–599. [CrossRef] [PubMed]
23. Liu, C.-P.; Hu, Y.; Lin, J.-C.; Fu, H.-L.; Lim, L.Y.; Yuan, Z.-X. Targeting strategies for drug delivery to the kidney: From renal glomeruli to tubules. *Med. Res. Rev.* **2019**, *39*, 561–578. [CrossRef] [PubMed]
24. Geng, H.; Lan, R.; Liu, Y.; Chen, W.; Wu, M.; Saikumar, P.; Weinberg, J.M.; Venkatachalam, M.A. Proximal tubule LPA1 and LPA2 receptors use divergent signaling pathways to additively increase profibrotic cytokine secretion. *Am. J. Physiol. Renal. Physiol.* **2021**, *320*, F359–F374. [CrossRef] [PubMed]
25. Stormark, T.A.; Strømmen, K.; Iversen, B.M.; Matre, K. Three-dimensional ultrasonography can detect the modulation of kidney volume in two-kidney, one-clip hypertensive rats. *Ultrasound. Med. Biol.* **2007**, *33*, 1882–1888. [CrossRef]

26. Zou, Z.; Chung, B.; Nguyen, T.; Mentone, S.; Thomson, B.; Biemesderfer, D. Linking receptor-mediated endocytosis and cell signaling: Evidence for regulated intramembrane proteolysis of megalin in proximal tubule. *J. Biol. Chem.* **2004**, *279*, 34302–34310. [CrossRef]
27. Christensen, E.I.; Gburek, J. Protein reabsorption in renal proximal tubule-function and dysfunction in kidney pathophysiology. *Pediatr. Nephrol.* **2004**, *19*, 714–721. [CrossRef]
28. Dai, H.; Liu, Q.; Liu, B. Research Progress on Mechanism of Podocyte Depletion in Diabetic Nephropathy. *J. Diabetes Res.* **2017**, *2017*, 2615286. [CrossRef]
29. Finch, N.C.; Fawaz, S.S.; Neal, C.R.; Butler, M.J.; Lee, V.K.; Salmon, A.J.; Lay, A.C.; Stevens, M.; Dayalan, L.; Band, H.; et al. Reduced Glomerular Filtration in Diabetes Is Attributable to Loss of Density and Increased Resistance of Glomerular Endothelial Cell Fenestrations. *J. Am. Soc. Nephrol.* **2022**, *33*, 1120–1136. [CrossRef]
30. Kim, D.; Li, H.Y.; Lee, J.H.; Oh, Y.S.; Jun, H.-S. Lysophosphatidic acid increases mesangial cell proliferation in models of diabetic nephropathy via Rac1/MAPK/KLF5 signaling. *Exp. Mol. Med.* **2019**, *51*, 1–10. [CrossRef]
31. Zhang, J.; Wang, Y.; Gurung, P.; Wang, T.; Li, L.; Zhang, R.; Li, H.; Guo, R.; Han, Q.; Zhang, J.; et al. The relationship between the thickness of glomerular basement membrane and renal outcomes in patients with diabetic nephropathy. *Acta Diabetol.* **2018**, *55*, 669–679. [CrossRef] [PubMed]
32. Krolewski, A.S. Progressive renal decline: The new paradigm of diabetic nephropathy in type 1 diabetes. *Diabetes Care* **2015**, *38*, 954–962. [CrossRef] [PubMed]
33. Haraguchi, R.; Kohara, Y.; Matsubayashi, K.; Kitazawa, R.; Kitazawa, S. New Insights into the Pathogenesis of Diabetic Nephropathy: Proximal Renal Tubules Are Primary Target of Oxidative Stress in Diabetic Kidney. *Acta Histochem. Cytochem.* **2020**, *53*, 21–31. [CrossRef] [PubMed]
34. Gilbert, R.E. Proximal Tubulopathy: Prime Mover and Key Therapeutic Target in Diabetic Kidney Disease. *Diabetes* **2017**, *66*, 791–800. [CrossRef] [PubMed]
35. Christensen, E.I.; Birn, H.; Storm, T.; Weyer, K.; Nielsen, R. Endocytic receptors in the renal proximal tubule. *Physiology (Bethesda)* **2012**, *27*, 223–236. [CrossRef]
36. Kaissling, B.; Hegyi, I.; Loffing, J.; Le Hir, M. Morphology of interstitial cells in the healthy kidney. *Anat. Embryol.* **1996**, *193*, 303–318. [CrossRef]
37. Li, A.S.; Ingham, J.F.; Lennon, R. Genetic Disorders of the Glomerular Filtration Barrier. *Clin. J. Am. Soc. Nephrol.* **2020**, *15*, 1818–1828. [CrossRef]
38. Akilesh, S.; Huber, T.B.; Wu, H.; Wang, G.; Hartleben, B.; Kopp, J.B.; Miner, J.H.; Roopenian, D.C.; Unanue, E.R.; Shaw, A.S. Podocytes use FcRn to clear IgG from the glomerular basement membrane. *Proc. Natl. Acad. Sci. USA* **2008**, *105*, 967–972. [CrossRef]
39. Sverrisson, K.; Axelsson, J.; Rippe, A.; Asgeirsson, D.; Rippe, B. Dynamic, size-selective effects of protamine sulfate and hyaluronidase on the rat glomerular filtration barrier in Vivo. *Am. J. Physiol. Renal. Physiol.* **2014**, *307*, F1136–F1143. [CrossRef]
40. Naylor, R.W.; Morais MR, P.T.; Lennon, R. Complexities of the glomerular basement membrane. *Nat. Rev. Nephrol.* **2021**, *17*, 112–127.
41. Sever, S. Role of actin cytoskeleton in podocytes. *Pediatr. Nephrol.* **2021**, *36*, 2607–2614. [CrossRef] [PubMed]
42. Pavenstädt, H.; Kriz, W.; Kretzler, M. Cell biology of the glomerular podocyte. *Physiol. Rev.* **2003**, *83*, 253–307. [CrossRef] [PubMed]
43. Schipper, M.L.; Iyer, G.; Koh, A.L.; Cheng, Z.; Ebenstein, Y.; Aharoni, A.; Keren, S.; Bentolila, L.A.; Li, J.; Rao, J.; et al. Particle size, surface coating, and PEGylation influence the biodistribution of quantum dots in living mice. *Small* **2009**, *5*, 126–134. [CrossRef] [PubMed]
44. Satchell, S.C.; Braet, F. Glomerular endothelial cell fenestrations: An integral component of the glomerular filtration barrier. *Am. J. Physiol. Renal. Physiol.* **2009**, *296*, F947–F956. [CrossRef]
45. Rabelink, T.J.; Wijewickrama, D.C.; De Koning, E.J. Peritubular endothelium: The Achilles heel of the kidney? *Kidney Int.* **2007**, *72*, 926–930. [CrossRef]
46. Shaw, I.; Rider, S.; Mullins, J.; Hughes, J.; Péault, B. Pericytes in the renal vasculature: Roles in health and disease. *Nat. Rev. Nephrol.* **2018**, *14*, 521–534. [CrossRef]
47. Stan, R.V.; Kubitza, M.; Palade, G.E. PV-1 is a component of the fenestral and stomatal diaphragms in fenestrated endothelia. *Proc. Natl. Acad. Sci. USA* **1999**, *96*, 13203–13207. [CrossRef]
48. Alcorn, D.; Maric, C.; Mccausland, J. Development of the renal interstitium. *Pediatr. Nephrol.* **1999**, *13*, 347–354. [CrossRef]
49. Bearer, E.L.; Orci, L. Endothelial fenestral diaphragms: A quick-freeze, deep-etch study. *J. Cell Biol.* **1985**, *100*, 418–428. [CrossRef]
50. Ivanyuk, A.; Livio, F.; Biollaz, J.; Buclin, T. Renal Drug Transporters and Drug Interactions. *Clin. Pharmacokinet.* **2017**, *56*, 825–892.
51. Nigam, S.K. The SLC22 Transporter Family: A Paradigm for the Impact of Drug Transporters on Metabolic Pathways, Signaling, and Disease. *Annu. Rev. Pharmacol. Toxicol.* **2018**, *58*, 663–687. [CrossRef] [PubMed]
52. Yaneff, A.; Sahores, A.; Gómez, N.; Carozzo, A.; Shayo, C.; Davio, C. MRP4/ABCC4 As a New Therapeutic Target: Meta-Analysis to Determine cAMP Binding Sites as a Tool for Drug Design. *Curr. Med. Chem.* **2019**, *26*, 1270–1307. [PubMed]
53. Koepsell, H.; Lips, K.; Volk, C. Polyspecific organic cation transporters: Structure, function, physiological roles, and biopharmaceutical implications. *Pharm. Res.* **2007**, *24*, 1227–1251. [PubMed]

54. El-Sheikh, A.A.K.; Masereeuw, R.; Russel, F.G.M. Mechanisms of renal anionic drug transport. *Eur. J. Pharmacol.* **2008**, *585*, 245–255. [CrossRef] [PubMed]
55. Christensen, E.I.; Verroust, P.J.; Nielsen, R. Receptor-mediated endocytosis in renal proximal tubule. *Pflug. Arch.* **2009**, *458*, 1039–1048. [CrossRef]
56. Christensen, E.I.; Birn, H. Megalin and cubilin: Multifunctional endocytic receptors. *Nat. Rev. Mol. Cell Biol.* **2002**, *3*, 256–266. [PubMed]
57. Coudroy, G.; Gburek, J.; Kozyraki, R.; Madsen, M.; Trugnan, G.; Moestrup, S.K.; Verroust, P.J.; Maurice, M. Contribution of cubilin and amnionless to processing and membrane targeting of cubilin-amnionless complex. *J. Am. Soc. Nephrol.* **2005**, *16*, 2330–2337. [CrossRef]
58. Fyfe, J.C.; Madsen, M.; Højrup, P.; Christensen, E.I.; Tanner, S.M.; de la Chapelle, A.; He, Q.; Moestrup, S.K. The functional cobalamin (vitamin B12)-intrinsic factor receptor is a novel complex of cubilin and amnionless. *Blood* **2004**, *103*, 1573–1579. [CrossRef]
59. Carney, E.F. Endocytosis in the proximal tubule. *Nat. Rev. Nephrol.* **2019**, *15*, 2. [CrossRef]
60. Hall, A.M.; Polesel, M.; Berquez, M. The proximal tubule, protein uptake, and the riddle of the segments. *Kidney Int.* **2021**, *99*, 803–805. [CrossRef]
61. Leheste, J.R.; Rolinski, B.; Vorum, H.; Hilpert, J.; Nykjaer, A.; Jacobsen, C.; Aucouturier, P.; Moskaug, J.O.; Otto, A.; Christensen, E.I.; et al. Megalin knockout mice as an animal model of low molecular weight proteinuria. *Am. J. Pathol.* **1999**, *155*, 1361–1370. [CrossRef] [PubMed]
62. Qu, Y.; Hao, C.; Zhai, R.; Yao, W. Folate and macrophage folate receptor-β in idiopathic pulmonary fibrosis disease: The potential therapeutic target? *Biomed. Pharmacother.* **2020**, *131*, 110711. [PubMed]
63. Liu, J.; Chen, H.; Liu, Y.; Shen, Y.; Meng, F.; Kaniskan, H.Ü.; Jin, J.; Wei, W. Cancer Selective Target Degradation by Folate-Caged PROTACs. *J. Am. Chem. Soc.* **2021**, *143*, 7380–7387. [CrossRef] [PubMed]
64. Haas, M.; Kluppel, A.C.; Wartna, E.S.; Moolenaar, F.; Meijer, D.K.; de Jong, P.E.; de Zeeuw, D. Drug-targeting to the kidney: Renal delivery and degradation of a naproxen-lysozyme conjugate In Vivo. *Kidney Int.* **1997**, *52*, 1693–1699. [CrossRef] [PubMed]
65. Dolman, M.E.M.; Harmsen, S.; Pieters, E.H.E.; Sparidans, R.W.; Lacombe, M.; Szokol, B.; Orfi, L.; Kéri, G.; Storm, G.; Hennink, W.E.; et al. Targeting of a platinum-bound sunitinib analog to renal proximal tubular cells. *Int. J. Nanomed.* **2012**, *7*, 417–433.
66. Haverdings, R.F.; Haas, M.; Greupink, A.R.; de Vries, P.A.; Moolenaar, F.; de Zeeuw, D.; Meijer, D.K. Potentials and limitations of the low-molecular-weight protein lysozyme as a carrier for renal drug targeting. *Ren. Fail.* **2001**, *23*, 397–409. [CrossRef]
67. Vegt, E.; Van Eerd, J.E.M.; Eek, A.; Oyen, W.J.G.; Wetzels, J.F.M.; de Jong, M.; Russel, F.G.M.; Masereeuw, R.; Gotthardt, M.; Boerman, O.C. Reducing renal uptake of radiolabeled peptides using albumin fragments. *J. Nucl. Med.* **2008**, *49*, 1506–1511. [CrossRef]
68. Yuan, Z.-X.; He, X.-K.; Wu, X.-J.; Gao, Y.; Fan, M.; Song, L.-Q.; Xu, C.-Q. Peptide fragments of human serum albumin as novel renal targeting carriers. *Int. J. Pharm.* **2014**, *460*, 196–204. [CrossRef]
69. Yuan, Z.-X.; Wu, X.-J.; Mo, J.; Wang, Y.-l.; Xu, C.-q.; Lim, L.Y. Renal targeted delivery of triptolide by conjugation to the fragment peptide of human serum albumin. *Eur. J. Pharm. Biopharm.* **2015**, *94*, 363–371. [CrossRef]
70. Schechter, B.; Arnon, R.; Colas, C.; Burakova, T.; Wilchek, M. Renal accumulation of streptavidin: Potential use for targeted therapy to the kidney. *Kidney Int.* **1995**, *47*, 1327–1335. [CrossRef]
71. Reubi, J.C.; Horisberger, U.; Studer, U.E.; Waser, B.; Laissue, J.A. Human kidney as target for somatostatin: High affinity receptors in tubules and vasa recta. *J. Clin. Endocrinol. Metab.* **1993**, *77*, 1323–1328. [PubMed]
72. Kodaira, H.; Tsutsumi, Y.; Yoshioka, Y.; Kamada, H.; Kaneda, Y.; Yamamoto, Y.; Tsunoda, S.-i.; Okamoto, T.; Mukai, Y.; Shibata, H.; et al. The targeting of anionized polyvinylpyrrolidone to the renal system. *Biomaterials* **2004**, *25*, 4309–4315. [CrossRef] [PubMed]
73. Kamada, H.; Tsutsumi, Y.; Sato-Kamada, K.; Yamamoto, Y.; Yoshioka, Y.; Okamoto, T.; Nakagawa, S.; Nagata, S.; Mayumi, T. Synthesis of a poly(vinylpyrrolidone-co-dimethyl maleic anhydride) co-polymer and its application for renal drug targeting. *Nat. Biotechnol.* **2003**, *21*, 399–404. [CrossRef] [PubMed]
74. Yamamoto, Y.; Tsutsumi, Y.; Yoshioka, Y.; Kamada, H.; Sato-Kamada, K.; Okamoto, T.; Mukai, Y.; Shibata, H.; Nakagawa, S.; Mayumi, T. Poly(vinylpyrrolidone-co-dimethyl maleic acid) as a novel renal targeting carrier. *J. Control. Release* **2004**, *95*, 229–237. [CrossRef] [PubMed]
75. Yuan, Z.-X.; Sun, X.; Gong, T.; Ding, H.; Fu, Y.; Zhang, Z.-R. Randomly 50% N-acetylated low molecular weight chitosan as a novel renal targeting carrier. *J. Drug. Target* **2007**, *15*, 269–278. [CrossRef] [PubMed]
76. Wang, D.-W.; Li, S.-J.; Tan, X.-Y.; Wang, J.-H.; Hu, Y.; Tan, Z.; Liang, J.; Hu, J.-B.; Li, Y.-G.; Zhao, Y.-F. Engineering of stepwise-targeting chitosan oligosaccharide conjugate for the treatment of acute kidney injury. *Carbohydr. Polym.* **2021**, *256*, 117556. [CrossRef] [PubMed]
77. Kandav, G.; Bhatt, D.C.; Singh, S.K. Effect of Different Molecular Weights of Chitosan on Formulation and Evaluation of Allopurinol-Loaded Nanoparticles for Kidney Targeting and in Management of Hyperuricemic Nephrolithiasis. *AAPS PharmSciTech* **2022**, *23*, 144. [CrossRef]
78. Ren, M.; Li, Y.; Zhang, H.; Li, L.; He, P.; Ji, P.; Yang, S. An oligopeptide/aptamer-conjugated dendrimer-based nanocarrier for dual-targeting delivery to bone. *J. Mater. Chem. B* **2021**, *9*, 2831–2844. [CrossRef]
79. Hu, Q.; Wang, Y.; Xu, L.; Chen, D.; Cheng, L. Transferrin Conjugated pH- and Redox-Responsive Poly(Amidoamine) Dendrimer Conjugate as an Efficient Drug Delivery Carrier for Cancer Therapy. *Int. J. Nanomed.* **2020**, *15*, 2751–2764. [CrossRef]

80. Matsuura, S.; Katsumi, H.; Suzuki, H.; Hirai, N.; Hayashi, H.; Koshino, K.; Higuchi, T.; Yagi, Y.; Kimura, H.; Sakane, T.; et al. l-Serine-modified polyamidoamine dendrimer as a highly potent renal targeting drug carrier. *Proc. Natl. Acad. Sci. USA* **2018**, *115*, 10511–10516. [CrossRef]
81. Wang, Y.; Xia, H.; Chen, B.; Wang, Y. Rethinking nanoparticulate polymer-drug conjugates for cancer theranostics. *Wiley Interdiscip. Rev. Nanomed. Nanobiotechnol.* **2022**, e1828. [CrossRef]
82. Duan, Z.; Luo, Q.; Dai, X.; Li, X.; Gu, L.; Zhu, H.; Tian, X.; Zhang, H.; Gong, Q.; Gu, Z.; et al. Synergistic Therapy of a Naturally Inspired Glycopolymer-Based Biomimetic Nanomedicine Harnessing Tumor Genomic Instability. *Adv. Mater.* **2021**, *33*, e2104594. [CrossRef] [PubMed]
83. Kissel, M.; Peschke, P.; Subr, V.; Ulbrich, K.; Strunz, A.M.; Kühnlein, R.; Debus, J.; Friedrich, E. Detection and cellular localisation of the synthetic soluble macromolecular drug carrier pHPMA. *Eur. J. Nucl. Med. Mol. Imaging* **2002**, *29*, 1055–1062. [CrossRef]
84. Kukowska-Latallo, J.F.; Candido, K.A.; Cao, Z.; Nigavekar, S.S.; Majoros, I.J.; Thomas, T.P.; Balogh, L.P.; Khan, M.K.; Baker, J.R. Nanoparticle targeting of anticancer drug improves therapeutic response in animal model of human epithelial cancer. *Cancer Res.* **2005**, *65*, 5317–5324. [CrossRef]
85. Wang, Y.; Shen, N.; Wang, Y.; Li, M.; Zhang, W.; Fan, L.; Liu, L.; Tang, Z.; Chen, X. Cisplatin nanoparticles boost abscopal effect of radiation plus anti-PD1 therapy. *Biomater. Sci.* **2021**, *9*, 3019–3027. [CrossRef] [PubMed]
86. Cheah, H.Y.; Gallon, E.; Dumoulin, F.; Hoe, S.Z.; Japundžić-Žigon, N.; Glumac, S.; Lee, H.B.; Anand, P.; Chung, L.Y.; Vicent, M.J.; et al. Near-Infrared Activatable Phthalocyanine-Poly-L-Glutamic Acid Conjugate: Enhanced In Vivo Safety and Antitumor Efficacy toward an Effective Photodynamic Cancer Therapy. *Mol. Pharm.* **2018**, *15*, 2594–2605. [CrossRef]
87. Chai, H.-J.; Kiew, L.-V.; Chin, Y.; Norazit, A.; Mohd Noor, S.; Lo, Y.-L.; Looi, C.-Y.; Lau, Y.-S.; Lim, T.-M.; Wong, W.-F.; et al. Renal targeting potential of a polymeric drug carrier, poly-l-glutamic acid, in normal and diabetic rats. *Int. J. Nanomed.* **2017**, *12*, 577–591. [CrossRef] [PubMed]
88. Mishra, A.P.; Chandra, S.; Tiwari, R.; Srivastava, A.; Tiwari, G. Therapeutic Potential of Prodrugs Towards Targeted Drug Delivery. *Open Med. Chem. J.* **2018**, *12*, 111–123. [CrossRef] [PubMed]
89. Chen, Z.; Wang, W.; Li, Y.; Wei, C.; Zhong, P.; He, D.; Liu, H.; Wang, P.; Huang, Z.; Zhu, W.; et al. Folic Acid-Modified Erythrocyte Membrane Loading Dual Drug for Targeted and Chemo-Photothermal Synergistic Cancer Therapy. *Mol. Pharm.* **2021**, *18*, 386–402. [CrossRef]
90. Qiu, L.; Dong, C.; Kan, X. Lymphoma-targeted treatment using a folic acid-decorated vincristine-loaded drug delivery system. *Drug Des. Dev. Ther.* **2018**, *12*, 863–872. [CrossRef]
91. Lu, Y.; Low, P.S. Folate-mediated delivery of macromolecular anticancer therapeutic agents. *Adv. Drug Deliv. Rev.* **2002**, *54*, 675–693. [CrossRef] [PubMed]
92. Low, P.S.; Kularatne, S.A. Folate-targeted therapeutic and imaging agents for cancer. *Curr. Opin. Chem. Biol.* **2009**, *13*, 256–262. [CrossRef] [PubMed]
93. Trump, D.P.; Mathias, C.J.; Yang, Z.; Low, P.S.; Marmion, M.; Green, M.A. Synthesis and evaluation of 99mTc(CO)(3)-DTPA-folate as a folate-receptor-targeted radiopharmaceutical. *Nucl. Med. Biol.* **2002**, *29*, 569–573. [CrossRef] [PubMed]
94. Yang, Y.; Guo, L.; Wang, Z.; Liu, P.; Liu, X.; Ding, J.; Zhou, W. Targeted silver nanoparticles for rheumatoid arthritis therapy via macrophage apoptosis and Re-polarization. *Biomaterials* **2021**, *264*, 120390. [CrossRef]
95. Hu, J.-B.; Li, S.-J.; Kang, X.-Q.; Qi, J.; Wu, J.-H.; Wang, X.-J.; Xu, X.-L.; Ying, X.-Y.; Jiang, S.-P.; You, J.; et al. CD44-targeted hyaluronic acid-curcumin prodrug protects renal tubular epithelial cell survival from oxidative stress damage. *Carbohydr. Polym.* **2018**, *193*, 268–280. [CrossRef]
96. Lin, Y.; Li, Y.; Wang, X.; Gong, T.; Zhang, L.; Sun, X. Targeted drug delivery to renal proximal tubule epithelial cells mediated by 2-glucosamine. *J. Control. Release* **2013**, *167*, 148–156. [CrossRef]
97. Yuan, Z.-X.; Shang, Z.; Gu, J.; He, L. Renal targeting delivery systems. *Future Med. Chem.* **2019**, *11*, 2237–2240. [CrossRef]
98. Mukherjee, A.; Waters, A.K.; Kalyan, P.; Achrol, A.S.; Kesari, S.; Yenugonda, V.M. Lipid-polymer hybrid nanoparticles as a next-generation drug delivery platform: State of the art, emerging technologies, and perspectives. *Int. J. Nanomed.* **2019**, *14*, 1937–1952. [CrossRef]
99. Mu, H.; Holm, R. Solid lipid nanocarriers in drug delivery: Characterization and design. *Expert Opin. Drug Deliv.* **2018**, *15*, 771–785.
100. Xu, S.; Chang, L.; Zhao, X.; Hu, Y.; Lin, Y.; Chen, Z.; Ren, X.; Mei, X. Preparation of epigallocatechin gallate decorated Au-Ag nano-heterostructures as NIR-sensitive nano-enzymes for the treatment of osteoarthritis through mitochondrial repair and cartilage protection. *Acta Biomater.* **2022**, *144*, 168–182. [CrossRef]
101. Mei, X.; Hu, T.; Wang, H.; Liang, R.; Bu, W.; Wei, M. Highly dispersed nano-enzyme triggered intracellular catalytic reaction toward cancer specific therapy. *Biomaterials* **2020**, *258*, 120257. [CrossRef] [PubMed]
102. Luo, X.-M.; Yan, C.; Feng, Y.-M. Nanomedicine for the treatment of diabetes-associated cardiovascular diseases and fibrosis. *Adv. Drug Deliv. Rev.* **2021**, *172*, 234–248. [CrossRef] [PubMed]
103. Hauser, P.V.; Chang, H.M.; Yanagawa, N.; Hamon, M. Nanotechnology, Nanomedicine, and the Kidney. *Appl. Sci.* **2021**, *11*, 7187. [CrossRef]
104. Albanese, A.; Tang, P.S.; Chan, W.C.W. The effect of nanoparticle size, shape, and surface chemistry on biological systems. *Annu. Rev. Biomed. Eng.* **2012**, *14*, 1–16. [CrossRef] [PubMed]

105. Filipczak, N.; Pan, J.; Yalamarty, S.S.K.; Torchilin, V.P. Recent advancements in liposome technology. *Adv. Drug Deliv. Rev.* **2020**, *156*, 4–22. [PubMed]
106. Paluszkiewicz, P.; Martuszewski, A.; Zaręba, N.; Wala, K.; Banasik, M.; Kepinska, M. The Application of Nanoparticles in Diagnosis and Treatment of Kidney Diseases. *Int. J. Mol. Sci.* **2021**, *23*, 131. [CrossRef] [PubMed]
107. Chen, C.-H.; Weng, T.-H.; Chuang, C.-H.; Huang, K.-Y.; Huang, S.-C.; Chen, P.-R.; Huang, H.-H.; Huang, L.-Y.; Shen, P.-C.; Chuang, P.-Y.; et al. Transdermal nanolipoplex simultaneously inhibits subcutaneous melanoma growth and suppresses systemically metastatic melanoma by activating host immunity. *Nanomedicine* **2022**, *47*, 102628. [CrossRef]
108. Salave, S.; Rana, D.; Kumar, H.; Kommineni, N.; Benival, D. Anabolic Peptide-Enriched Stealth Nanoliposomes for Effective Anti-Osteoporotic Therapy. *Pharmaceutics* **2022**, *14*, 2417. [CrossRef]
109. Passeri, E.; Elkhoury, K.; Morsink, M.; Broersen, K.; Linder, M.; Tamayol, A.; Malaplate, C.; Yen, F.T.; Arab-Tehrany, E. Alzheimer's Disease: Treatment Strategies and Their Limitations. *Int. J. Mol. Sci.* **2022**, *23*, 13954.
110. Huang, C.; Xue, L.-F.; Hu, B.; Liu, H.-H.; Huang, S.-B.; Khan, S.; Meng, Y. Calycosin-loaded nanoliposomes as potential nanoplatforms for treatment of diabetic nephropathy through regulation of mitochondrial respiratory function. *J. Nanobiotechnol.* **2021**, *19*, 178. [CrossRef]
111. Müller, R.H.; Shegokar, R.; Keck, C.M. 20 years of lipid nanoparticles (SLN and NLC): Present state of development and industrial applications. *Curr. Drug Discov. Technol.* **2011**, *8*, 207–227. [CrossRef] [PubMed]
112. Subroto, E.; Andoyo, R.; Indiarto, R.; Wulandari, E.; Wadhiah, E.F.N. Preparation of Solid Lipid Nanoparticle-Ferrous Sulfate by Double Emulsion Method Based on Fat Rich in Monolaurin and Stearic Acid. *Nanomaterials* **2022**, *12*, 3054. [CrossRef] [PubMed]
113. Iqbal, M.A.; Md, S.; Sahni, J.K.; Baboota, S.; Dang, S.; Ali, J. Nanostructured lipid carriers system: Recent advances in drug delivery. *J. Drug Target.* **2012**, *20*, 813–830. [CrossRef]
114. Ahangarpour, A.; Oroojan, A.A.; Khorsandi, L.; Kouchak, M.; Badavi, M. Solid Lipid Nanoparticles of Myricitrin Have Antioxidant and Antidiabetic Effects on Streptozotocin-Nicotinamide-Induced Diabetic Model and Myotube Cell of Male Mouse. *Oxid. Med. Cell. Longev.* **2018**, *2018*, 7496936. [CrossRef] [PubMed]
115. Ahangarpour, A.; Oroojan, A.A.; Khorsandi, L.; Kouchak, M.; Badavi, M. Antioxidant, anti-apoptotic, and protective effects of myricitrin and its solid lipid nanoparticle on streptozotocin-nicotinamide-induced diabetic nephropathy in type 2 diabetic male mice. *Iran. J. Basic Med. Sci.* **2019**, *22*, 1424–1431.
116. Ahangarpour, A.; Oroojan, A.A.; Khorsandi, L.; Kouchak, M.; Badavi, M. Hyperglycemia-induced oxidative stress in isolated proximal tubules of mouse: The in vitro effects of myricitrin and its solid lipid nanoparticle. *Arch. Physiol. Biochem.* **2021**, *127*, 422–428. [CrossRef]
117. Asfour, M.H.; Salama, A.A.A.; Mohsen, A.M. Fabrication of All-Trans Retinoic Acid loaded Chitosan/Tripolyphosphate Lipid Hybrid Nanoparticles as a Novel Oral Delivery Approach for Management of Diabetic Nephropathy in Rats. *J. Pharm. Sci.* **2021**, *110*, 3208–3220. [CrossRef]
118. Sierra-Mondragon, E.; Rodríguez-Muñoz, R.; Namorado-Tonix, C.; Molina-Jijon, E.; Romero-Trejo, D.; Pedraza-Chaverri, J.; Reyes, J.L. All-Trans Retinoic Acid Attenuates Fibrotic Processes by Downregulating TGF-β1/Smad3 in Early Diabetic Nephropathy. *Biomolecules* **2019**, *9*, 525. [CrossRef]
119. Liu, Q.; Chen, X.; Kan, M.; Yang, J.; Gong, Q.; Jin, R.; Dai, Y.; Jin, J.; Zang, H. Gypenoside XLIX loaded nanoparticles targeting therapy for renal fibrosis and its mechanism. *Eur. J. Pharmacol.* **2021**, *910*, 174501. [CrossRef]
120. Oroojalian, F.; Rezayan, A.H.; Mehrnejad, F.; Nia, A.H.; Shier, W.T.; Abnous, K.; Ramezani, M. Efficient megalin targeted delivery to renal proximal tubular cells mediated by modified-polymyxin B-polyethylenimine based nano-gene-carriers. *Mater. Sci. Eng. C Mater. Biol. Appl.* **2017**, *79*, 770–782. [CrossRef]
121. Liu, L.; Xu, Q.; Zhang, L.; Sun, H.; Ding, F.; Li, Y.; Chen, P. FeO magnetic nanoparticles ameliorate albumin-induced tubulointerstitial fibrosis by autophagy related to Rab7. *Colloids Surf. B Biointerfaces* **2021**, *198*, 111470. [CrossRef] [PubMed]
122. Guo, L.; Luo, S.; Du, Z.; Zhou, M.; Li, P.; Fu, Y.; Sun, X.; Huang, Y.; Zhang, Z. Targeted delivery of celastrol to mesangial cells is effective against mesangioproliferative glomerulonephritis. *Nat. Commun.* **2017**, *8*, 878. [CrossRef] [PubMed]
123. Wang, J.; Poon, C.; Chin, D.; Milkowski, S.; Lu, V.; Hallows, K.R.; Chung, E.J. Design and in vivo characterization of kidney-targeting multimodal micelles for renal drug delivery. *Nano Res.* **2018**, *11*, 5584–5595. [CrossRef]
124. Williams, R.M.; Shah, J.; Ng, B.D.; Minton, D.R.; Gudas, L.J.; Park, C.Y.; Heller, D.A. Mesoscale nanoparticles selectively target the renal proximal tubule epithelium. *Nano Lett.* **2015**, *15*, 2358–2364. [CrossRef]
125. Williams, R.M.; Shah, J.; Tian, H.S.; Chen, X.; Geissmann, F.; Jaimes, E.A.; Heller, D.A. Selective Nanoparticle Targeting of the Renal Tubules. *Hypertension* **2018**, *71*, 87–94. [CrossRef] [PubMed]
126. Han, S.J.; Williams, R.M.; D'agati, V.; Jaimes, E.A.; Heller, D.A.; Lee, H.T. Selective nanoparticle-mediated targeting of renal tubular Toll-like receptor 9 attenuates ischemic acute kidney injury. *Kidney Int.* **2020**, *98*, 76–87. [CrossRef] [PubMed]
127. Barutta, F.; Bellini, S.; Kimura, S.; Hase, K.; Corbetta, B.; Corbelli, A.; Fiordaliso, F.; Bruno, S.; Biancone, L.; Barreca, A.; et al. Protective effect of the tunneling nanotube-TNFAIP2/M-sec system on podocyte autophagy in diabetic nephropathy. *Autophagy* **2022**, 1–20. [CrossRef]
128. Yu, M.; Wang, D.; Zhong, D.; Xie, W.; Luo, J. Adropin Carried by Reactive Oxygen Species-Responsive Nanocapsules Ameliorates Renal Lipid Toxicity in Diabetic Mice. *ACS Appl. Mater. Interfaces* **2022**, *14*, 37330–37344. [CrossRef]

Recent Advances in Doxorubicin Formulation to Enhance Pharmacokinetics and Tumor Targeting

Jihoon Lee [1], Min-Koo Choi [2] and Im-Sook Song [1,*]

1. BK21 FOUR Community-Based Intelligent Novel Drug Discovery Education Unit, Vessel-Organ Interaction Research Center (VOICE), Research Institute of Pharmaceutical Sciences, College of Pharmacy, Kyungpook National University, Daegu 41566, Republic of Korea; legadema0905@knu.ac.kr
2. College of Pharmacy, Dankook University, Cheon-an 31116, Republic of Korea; minkoochoi@dankook.ac.kr
* Correspondence: isssong@knu.ac.kr; Tel.: +82-53-950-8575; Fax: +82-53-950-8557

Abstract: Doxorubicin (DOX), a widely used drug in cancer chemotherapy, induces cell death via multiple intracellular interactions, generating reactive oxygen species and DNA-adducted configurations that induce apoptosis, topoisomerase II inhibition, and histone eviction. Despite its wide therapeutic efficacy in solid tumors, DOX often induces drug resistance and cardiotoxicity. It shows limited intestinal absorption because of low paracellular permeability and P-glycoprotein (P-gp)-mediated efflux. We reviewed various parenteral DOX formulations, such as liposomes, polymeric micelles, polymeric nanoparticles, and polymer-drug conjugates, under clinical use or trials to increase its therapeutic efficacy. To improve the bioavailability of DOX in intravenous and oral cancer treatment, studies have proposed a pH- or redox-sensitive and receptor-targeted system for overcoming DOX resistance and increasing therapeutic efficacy without causing DOX-induced toxicity. Multifunctional formulations of DOX with mucoadhesiveness and increased intestinal permeability through tight-junction modulation and P-gp inhibition have also been used as orally bioavailable DOX in the preclinical stage. The increasing trends of developing oral formulations from intravenous formulations, the application of mucoadhesive technology, permeation-enhancing technology, and pharmacokinetic modulation with functional excipients might facilitate the further development of oral DOX.

Keywords: doxorubicin (DOX); formulation strategy; drug resistance; oral formulation

1. Introduction

Although various options such as immunotherapy and targeted therapy have been developed for cancer treatment, chemotherapy remains an important treatment option for most cancers, especially metastatic cancer [1]. The goal of palliative chemotherapy is to help patients live longer comfortably without the influence of factors that harm their quality of life. This goal can be achieved through the development of oral administration therapy from intravenous chemotherapy. Advantages of oral therapy include noninvasiveness, convenience, and cost-effectiveness; moreover, it may reduce the need for hospital care [2,3].

In addition to providing better quality of life, switching to oral formulations of intravenous drugs may produce beneficial pharmacokinetic profiles. Intravenous injection or infusion contributes to toxicity, which is associated with the high peak plasma concentration of anticancer drugs [4]. In the U.S. pharmaceutical market, approximately 70% of anticancer drugs are oral formulations. However, 40% of drugs in the pipeline and 70% of developing candidate drugs exhibit poor water solubility or low oral bioavailability (BA) [5]. Thus, the development of oral dosage formulations and BA enhancement technology for candidate drugs seems to be at a critical stage [6]. However, there are many obstacles that may impede the development of oral dosage formulations, such as low intestinal solubility and permeability and the high intestinal first-pass effect [7–9].

Doxorubicin (DOX) (Figure 1), an anthracycline drug, is one of the most widely used chemotherapeutic drugs. It is indicated for hematopoietic malignancies and solid tumors and is prescribed to patients with breast and lung cancers, leukemia, and malignant lymphoma [10]. In general, DOX is known to exhibit two mechanisms of action: classical topoisomerase II inhibition and chromatin damage [11]. Topoisomerase II is an enzyme that prevents DNA from excessive or insufficient coiling by creating temporary double-stranded breaks and regenerating DNA via religation [12–14]. DOX intercalates into the DNA–topoisomerase II complex through its cyclohexane and sugar moieties and causes DNA damage, followed by p53 pathway-mediated cell cycle arrest [15] (Figure 1). Regarding chromatin damage, the sugar moiety of DOX migrates into DNA, occupying the histone space and causing collapse of the nucleosome [16,17], which leads to cell death [18].

Structure	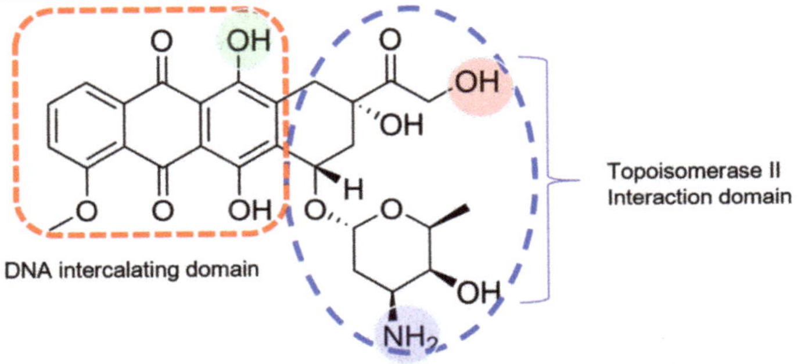 DNA intercalating domain / Topoisomerase II Interaction domain
Molecular weight	543.52 g/mol
pKa	pKa1 = 7.34 (green color); pKa2 = 8.46 (purple color); PKa3 = 9.46 (pink color)
Aqueous solubility	1.15 mg/mL
Permeability (P_{app})	A to B P_{app}: 1.02 ± 0.14 × 10^{-7} cm/s B to A P_{app}: 6.72 ± 1.49 × 10^{-7} cm/s Efflux ratio (B to A P_{app}/A to B P_{app}): 6.6
BCS type	Class 3 (high solubility, low permeability)
Metabolic enzyme	Carbonyl reductase, oxidoreductase, CYP3A4, CYP2D6

Figure 1. Chemical structure and physicochemical properties of DOX. Data are available at website (https://pubchem.ncbi.nlm.nih.gov/compound/Doxorubicin accessed on 19 May 2023) and reference [19]. P_{app}: permeability; A to B: apical to basal; B to A: basal to apical; BCS: biopharmaceutical classification system; CYP: cytochrome P450. Red and blue dotted line indicated DNA intercalating and Topoisomerase II interaction domain.

DOX toxicity and therapeutic resistance remain major problems, and resistance to chemotherapeutic drugs can cause treatment failure in >90% of patients with metastatic cancer [20]. DOX resistance may be associated with various mechanisms, including enhanced expression of multidrug resistance (MDR) transporters (such as P-glycoprotein [P-gp], breast cancer resistance protein [BCRP], and MDR-associated proteins [MRPs]), elevated xenobiotic metabolism, increased DNA repair capacity, and increased expression of growth and genetic factors [20,21]. Another obstacle that impedes the development of DOX formulation is its low BA. Limited intestinal permeability as well as the first-pass effect caused by P-gp- and MRP1-mediated efflux of DOX and drug-metabolizing enzymes result in low BA (<5%) [21,22]. DOX is a weakly basic drug and is classified in the biopharmaceutical classification system (BCS) as type 3 because of its high solubility (1.15 mg/mL) and low permeability (6.72×10^{-7} cm/s), with an efflux ratio of 6.6 (Figure 1). Therefore, research on oral DOX has mainly focused on enhancing permeability and maintaining the basic pH environment [23].

In this review, we discussed the research on the development of DOX formulations. First, we focused on DOX formulations that have undergone clinical trials and discussed whether they were successful. In addition to the clinical results, we reviewed the obstacles to DOX reformulation with regard to the gastrointestinal environment, drug resistance, and DOX-induced toxicity. Then, we examined the pharmaceutical trials and recent DOX formulations to overcome these obstacles.

2. DOX Formulations under Clinical Use or Trials

Remarkable progress has been made in the development of DOX formulations. However, only a few intravenous formulations have been applied as intravenous infusions in the clinical setting. The currently available nanotechnology platforms under clinical use or trials include liposomes, polymeric micelles (PMs), polymeric nanoparticles (PNPs), and polymer–drug conjugates (Table 1).

2.1. Liposomes

Liposomes have been used as a drug delivery system for many years since their discovery in 1965 [24]. Their biodegradable characteristics and ability to incorporate hydrophilic, hydrophobic, and amphiphilic drugs allow researchers to encapsulate several drug candidates within liposomes [25,26]. However, in the reticuloendothelial system, high liposome clearance and less effective targeting of liposomes to cancer cells are major obstacles. One of the most well-known modifications involves coating liposome surfaces with polyethylene glycol (PEG), a process known as PEGylation [27]. PEG is a US Food and Drug Administration (FDA)-approved molecule for human administration, which is characterized by nontoxic and nonimmunogenic properties. PEGylation can lead to the formation of a protective hydrophilic layer, can prevent self-aggregation, and can avoid interaction with blood components [28]. Thus, PEGylation reduces complement-mediated lysis by the immune system and prolongs blood circulation times [26,28]. Circulating PEGylated liposomes (PLs) of a size of 100–200 nm are mainly deposited in tumor cells that a have large, leaky spaces in pericytes but not in normal tissue with tight capillary junctions, in what is known as the enhanced permeation and retention (EPR) effect [29,30]. However, PLs block the surface zeta potential, which prevents protein adsorption and may decrease tumor targeting [31]. Decreasing the duration of PEGylation causes liposomes to diffuse out of the lipid membrane system, which are then delivered to the tumor site [32]. Moreover, a specific tumor enzyme that cleaves PEG from liposomes contributes to the detachment of PEG from the liposome system after reaching the target site [33].

In 1995, the first PEGylated liposomal DOX formulation, named Doxil (Janssen Biotech Inc., Horsham, PA, USA), was approved by the US FDA for treating ovarian cancer, Kaposi's sarcoma, metastatic breast cancer, and multiple myeloma [34]. A similar PEGylated liposomal DOX formulation known as Lipo-dox was approved as a generic version of Doxil by the US FDA in 2012. However, the therapeutic efficacy of Lipo-dox for ovarian cancer was not equivalent to that of Doxil [34]. Caelyx and Zolsketil, two PEGlylated liposomal formulations similar to Doxil, received marketing authorization in 2005 and 2022, respectively, by the European Medicine Agency (EMA) for treating breast and ovarian cancers, multiple myeloma, and Kaposi's sarcoma [26]. JNS002, a PEGylated liposomal DOX formulation, is under evaluation in a clinical phase III trial involving patients with ovarian cancer, primary fallopian tube cancer, and peritoneal cancer [35]. These formulations are expected to exert EPR effects with reduced cardiotoxicity based on the long circulation time in the blood and reduced distribution to the heart [34] (Table 1).

Phosphatidylcholine/cholesterol liposomes containing citrate (300 mM, pH 4.5) with a size of approximately 150 nm were successfully loaded with DOX with an encapsulation efficiency of over 95%. This formulation, known as Myocet, combined with cyclophosphamide was approved in 2000 by the EMA as a first-line treatment for metastatic breast cancer in adult women [36]. Myocet, a non-PEGylated liposomal DOX formulation, exhibited distinctive pharmacokinetics compared with free DOX and PLs (Doxil and Caelyx). It displayed higher area under the curve (AUC) values than free DOX but lower AUC values than PLs. However, Caelyx, which is characterized by low clearance and long circulating time, could penetrate into skin tissues (e.g., in cases of Kaposi's sarcoma), which could explain the increased potential to cause hand–foot syndrome, characterized by swelling, pain, and redness on the hands and feet [36]. Hand–foot syndrome is the main effect of the dose-limiting toxicity of PLs, such as Doxil and Caelyx. However, Myocet showed a low incidence of hand–foot syndrome [37].

During the development of active targeting liposomes, a glutathione-conjugated PEGylated liposomal DOX formulation (GSH–PL–DOX) was developed for the delivery of liposomal DOX to the brain through a GSH transporter across the blood–brain barrier. This was confirmed by the 5-fold increase in the delivery of DOX to mice brains compared with that of Doxil [38]. In the phase I/IIa clinical trials, the GSH–PL–DOX formulation was proven to be safe and well tolerated and showed intracranial and extracranial antitumor activity [39]. Human epidermal growth factor receptor 2 (HER2)-targeted antibody anchoring PL–DOX (HER2–PL–DOX) was designed to enhance targeting to HER2-positive advanced breast cancer cells. However, in the phase I clinical trial involving 47 patients with cancer, HER2–PL–DOX failed to show superior beneficial effects [34]. Similarly, epidermal growth factor receptor (EGFR)-targeted antibody (cetuximab) anchoring PL–DOX (EGFR–PL–DOX) targets EGFR-positive breast cancer cells. Patients who received EGFR–PL–DOX did not show hand–foot syndrome, cardiotoxicity, or cumulative toxicity even at the maximum tolerated dose (50 mg/m^2) [40,41] (Table 1).

2.2. PMs

PMs have the advantage of an extremely small particle size (10–100 nm), which makes them efficient for delivering drugs to solid or poorly vascularized tumors. The amphiphilic property allows them to self-assemble in a fluid in vivo after reaching the critical micellar concentration [42]. The structure of a PM entraps a hydrophobic drug in the core, while the hydrophilic shell prevents the removal of the PM via the reticuloendothelial effect, leading to a longer circulation time. This provides PMs an opportunity to accumulate in the tumor site via the EPR effect or actively target the tumor site using a specific ligand [43].

SP1049C is a DOX-loaded PM formulation composed of Pluronic L61 and Pluronic F127 as carrier materials that exert a P-gp inhibitory effect [44,45]. However, its pharmacokinetics and toxic characteristics are similar to those of DOX, and the response ratio of SP1049C in the clinical phase II study was 47% in cases of advanced adenocarcinoma of the esophagus and gastroesophageal junction [46–48]. NK911 is a DOX-loaded PEG–polyaspartic acid nanomicelle [49]. In phase II trials in patients with metastatic pancreatic cancer, NK911 was well tolerated and showed a partial response at a dosage of 50 mg/m^2 every 3 weeks. NK911 showed low plasma concentrations of DOX, suggesting that NK911 is less stable than Doxil [49] (Table 1).

2.3. Polymeric Nanoparticles (PNPs)

PNPs are composed of natural ingredients, such as chitosan, dextran, polylactic acid (PLA), polylactide-co-glycolide (PLGA), or polycaprolactone (PCL), with a particle size of 10–1000 nm. PNPs are manufactured as nanocapsules and nanospheres that can entrap drugs within or are associated with a polymer core. They have the advantages of biocompatibility, biodegradability, and design flexibility [50].

Livatag consists of DOX-loaded PNPs formed using alkyl cyanoacrylate (PACA) and covalently linked to squalene. It was developed using Onxeo's proprietary Transdrug™

technology. Livatag aims to promote the penetration of DOX into tumor cells and enhance the contact between target DNA and DOX, thus bypassing the P-gp-mediated resistance mechanism in tumor cells [51]. It is suitable for the clinical treatment of hepatocellular carcinoma (HCC), and early clinical trials have shown good results. The overall safety and tolerability of Livatag was favorable, with a fully manageable toxicity profile in patients with HCC who had long treatment periods of >1 year. In a clinical phase III trial, although the experimental group did not show the desired effects compared with the high survival rate of the control group that received other anticancer treatments, Livatag as a single agent tended to exhibit a similar level of efficacy as regorafenib [52]. Therefore, the US FDA recently placed Livatag for the treatment of primary liver cancer on a fast-track designation [34] (Table 1).

2.4. Polymer-Drug Conjugates

Polymer–drug conjugates can be manufactured by covalently binding a drug to a polymeric carrier. This conjugation confers numerous benefits, including enhanced solubility, controlled drug release, and improved pharmacokinetic drug properties [53]. Clinical evaluation is under way for FCE28068/PK1, N-(2-hydroxypropyl) methacrylamide (HPMA) conjugated to DOX using a Gly–Phe–Leu–Gly peptide spacer [54]. FCE28068/PK1 showed a prolonged plasma circulation time and was mainly cleared by the kidneys without accumulating in the liver [55]. FCE28068/PK1 had no significant cardiotoxicity up to an intravenous dose of 1680 mg/m^2. It was active against refractory tumors, and the maximum tolerable dose was 320 mg/m^2, which was 4–5 times higher than the clinical dose of DOX (60–80 mg/m^2) [55]. In the phase II clinical trial, FCE28068/PK1 showed a considerable response in some patients with breast cancer and non-small cell lung cancer but not in those with colon cancer [56] (Table 1). However, the lack of tissue-targeting ability and biodegradability led to the development of the second formulation.

FCE28069/PK2 is an HPMA polymer–DOX conjugate linked to a galactosamine structure, which binds to the hepatic asialoglycoprotein receptor. It was designed for treating primary liver cancer. When FCE28069/PK2 was intravenously administered to patients with primary or metastatic liver cancer, liver-specific DOX delivery could be achieved, and some patients showed a partial response. However, a patient who received FCE28069/PK2 at a dose of 160 mg/m^2 had grade 4 neutropenia and grade 3 mucositis, and DOX targeted to the liver was generally distributed to normal liver cells rather than to cancer cells. In other words, 16% of the dose was distributed to the liver but only 3% was distributed to tumor cells [57] (Table 1).

Table 1. DOX formulations under clinical use or trials.

Carrier Type	Formulation and Route of Administration	Name	Clinical Results	References
Liposomes	PEGylated liposome (PL), IV	Doxil, approved by the FDA	EPR Treatment of ovarian cancer, Kaposi's sarcoma, metastatic breast cancer, and multiple myeloma	[34]
	PL, IV	Lipo-dox, approved by the FDA	EPR Therapeutic efficacy was not equivalent to that of Doxil in patients with ovarian cancer	[34]
	PL, IV	Caelyx, approved by the EMA	EPR Treatment of ovarian cancer, Kaposi's sarcoma, metastatic breast cancer, and multiple myeloma	[26]
	PL, IV	Zolsketil, approved by the EMA	EPR Treatment of ovarian cancer, Kaposi's sarcoma, metastatic breast cancer, and multiple myeloma	[26]

Table 1. Cont.

Carrier Type	Formulation and Route of Administration	Name	Clinical Results	References
Liposomes	PL, IV	JNS002 Phase III	EPR Treatment of ovarian cancer, primary fallopian tube cancer, and peritoneal cancer	[35]
	Non-PEGylated liposome, IV	Myocet, approved by the EMA	EPR A first-line treatment for metastatic breast cancer in adult women, in combination with cyclophosphamide	[36]
	Glutathione-conjugated PL, IV	GSH–PL–DOX Phase I/IIa	Brain targeting through a GSH transporter across the blood–brain barrier Safe and well tolerated with intracranial and extracranial antitumor activity	[39]
	HER2-targeted antibody anchoring PL, IV	HER2–PL–DOX Phase I	HER2-targeting Failed to provide beneficial effect superior to Doxil in patients with breast cancer	[34]
	EGFR-targeted antibody anchoring PL, IV	EGFR–PL–DOX Phase I	EGFR-targeting At 50 mg/m^2, hand–foot syndrome, cardiotoxicity, or cumulative toxicity did not occur in any patient with glioblastoma and breast cancer	[40,41]
PMs	PM with two nonionic pluronic block copolymers, IV	SP1049C Phase III	Inhibition of P-gp-mediated DOX efflux In a phase II trial involving 21 patients, 9 patients had a partial response and 8 patients had a minor response. The overall response rate was 47%	[46,47]
	PEG–polyaspartic acid nanomicelle, IV	NK911 Phase II	EPR Well tolerated at 50 mg/m^2 in 23 metastatic pancreatic cancer patients, and a partial response was achieved	[49]
PNPs	Polyalkyl cyanoacrylate (PACA) nanoparticle, IV	Livatag Phase III	The phase III clinical trial did not achieve the desired effects in patients with advanced hepatocellular carcinoma	[51,52]
Polymer–drug conjugates	HPMA copolymer–GFLG–DOX, IV	FCE28069/PK1 Phase II	EPR and pinocytosis The maximum tolerable dose was 320 mg/m^2, and no polymer-related toxicities were observed A considerable response occurred in some patients with breast and non-small cell lung cancer, but no response was noted in colorectal cancer patients Lack of biodegradability of the polymer main chain	[54–56]
	HPMA copolymer–GFLG–DOX–galactosamine, IV	FCE28069/PK2 Phase II	Galactosamine-mediated uptake Liver-specific delivery using galactosamine-modified polymers, and a partial response was achieved in patients with liver cancer Grade 4 neutropenia and grade 3 mucositis	[57]

PL: PEGylated liposome; PM: polymeric micelle; PNP: polymeric nanoparticle; IV: intravenous injection; EPR: enhanced permeation and retention; FDA: Food and Drug Administration; EMA: European Medicine Agency; HPMA: N-(2-hydroxypropyl) methacrylamide; GFLG: glycyl-phenylalanyl-leucyl-glycine.

3. Obstacles in and Strategies for Formulating DOX to Enhance Oral BA and Tumor Targeting

As mentioned previously, all DOX formulations in clinical applications are currently administered intravenously. Therefore, many studies on anticancer drugs have focused on the development of oral formulations. Pharmaceutical and chemical strategies have been employed to increase chemical stability in gastrointestinal fluids, increase aqueous solubility, and reduce the first-pass effect. An oral formulation of trifluridine in combination with tipiracil, an inhibitor of thymidine phosphorylase, increased the oral BA of trifluridine by 38-fold and has been approved by the US FDA, the EMA, and the Ministry of Health, Labour and Welfare of Japan (MHLW) [58]. Successful oral formulations of Tegafur from intravenous 5-fluorouracil have been approved by the EMA and MHLW using a prodrug approach in combination with uracil, which acts as a metabolic inhibitor of dihydropyrimidine dehydrogenase [58].

Oral anticancer drugs are effective and convenient for patients. Knowledge regarding the pharmacokinetics-altering strategies of other drugs will guide DOX oral formulation. Therefore, we reviewed these challenges for oral DOX formulations in terms of pharmacokinetic obstacles as well as the occurrence of DOX resistance and the effort to overcome these limitations using a DOX formulation strategy (Figure 2).

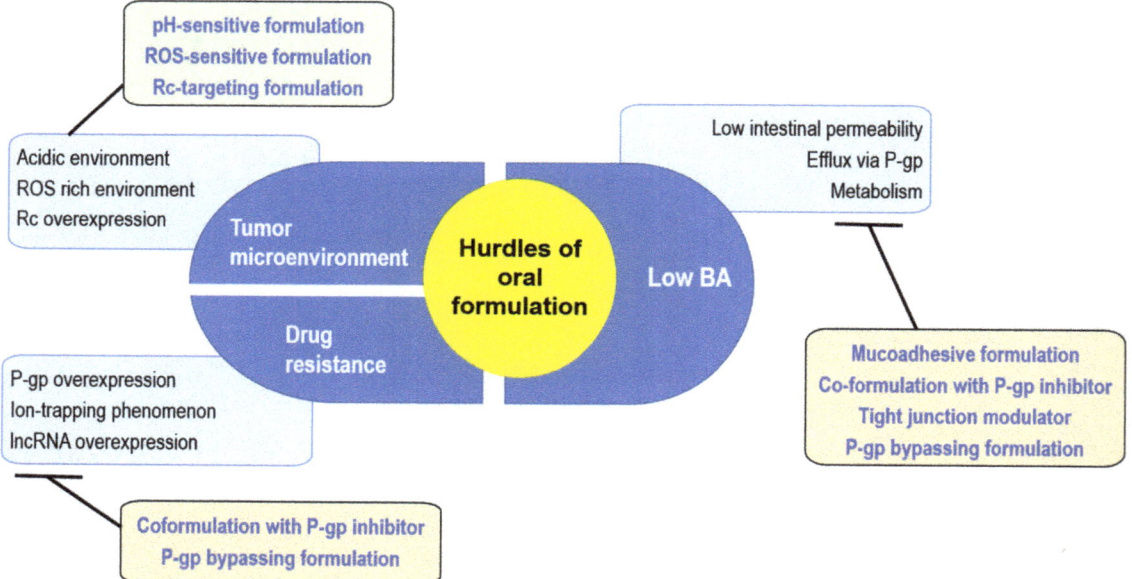

Figure 2. Challenges in the development of DOX oral formulations and the corresponding formulation strategies. ROS: reactive oxygen species; Rc: Receptor; P-gp: P-glycoprotein; lncRNA: long noncoding RNA; BA: bioavailability.

3.1. Formulation Strategy Based on Tumor Microenvironments for the Targetability of DOX in the Preclinical Stage

3.1.1. pH-Sensitive Formulation

Deregulated energy metabolism, insufficient perfusion, and uncontrolled proliferation collectively confer particular characteristics to the tumor microenvironment, including acidity, hypoxia, increased lactate concentrations, and reduced glucose concentrations [59]. Although the pH of the interstitial space of solid tumors ranges from slightly acidic to neutral (pH 6.4–7.0), the central regions of solid tumors are intensely acidic because of reduced O_2 and glucose concentrations and, correspondingly, increased H^+ and lactate concentrations that are observed with increasing distance from the vascular system [59].

To enhance drug release into tumor tissues, pH-sensitive liposomes are currently being researched. The most popular base lipid for fabricating pH-sensitive liposomes is phosphatidylethanolamine (PE). However, PE cannot form a stable liposome on its own; therefore, additional amphiphilic molecules are added as stabilizers. At physiological pH, these stabilizers are inserted between PE molecules in an ionized form, leading to the production of stable liposomes. In an acidic environment, however, protonated stabilizers cause the reversion of PE molecules and disrupt liposomes, leading to a burst release of inner contents, including DOX [60–62].

De Oliveira Silva et al. [63] synthesized a formulation of cholesteryl hemisuccinate (CHEMS) and distearoyl PE polyethyleneglycol2000 (DSPE-PEG2000) in a dioleoyl-phosphatidyl-ethanolamine (DOPE)-based pH-sensitive liposome (DOPE:CHEMS:DOPE-PEG2000 = 5.8:3.7:0.5) with a size distribution of 125–135 nm. This formulation showed higher uptake by tumors than by control tissue and higher specificity for tumors in 4T1 tumor-bearing mice. Moreover, the researchers continued the study in healthy mice to monitor acute cardiotoxicity and other side effects. Compared with normal DOX, this pH-sensitive liposome seemed to be more effective and safe, as indicated by the 2-fold reduction in QT interval prolongation on an electrocardiogram in the pH-sensitive liposome treatment group [64] (Table 2).

Bobde et al. [65] conjugated DOX and poly N-(2 hydroxypropyl) methacrylamide via hydrazone bonding and developed pH-sensitive PNP, i.e., HPMA–NH-DOX, which releases DOX 5 times faster in an acidic intratumor environment (pH 6.5). Further, a faster release is observed in a more acidic tumor environment (pH 5.5) in MCF-7 and 4T1 cell lines (Table 2).

pH-sensitive micelles composed of DSPE-PEG2000 and oleic acid at a ratio of 10:6 with a size of 12.8 nm and a zeta potential of −2.7 mV were prepared, and DOX was incorporated with a loading efficiency of 92% [66]. A mixture of DSPE-PEG2000 and oleic acid was self-assembled, wherein the hydrophobic DSPE constituted the inner core with DOX, and PEG2000, as a nontoxic hydrophilic polymer, produced a hydrophilic shell to provide steric stability and protection from opsonization. Oleic acid acts as a pH-sensitive indicator, and DOX incorporated into this micelle was released faster at pH 5.0 than at pH 7.4. As a result, pH-sensitive micelles showed a 7-fold tumor shrinkage in 4T1 tumor-bearing mice compared with free DOX when administered intravenously (5 mg/kg/day, every other day, four times) [66] (Table 2).

3.1.2. Reactive Oxygen Species (ROS)-Sensitive Formulation

Cancer initiation and progression can slightly increase ROS levels. Therefore, cancer cells thrive on moderately higher ROS levels than normal cells because they have developed stronger antioxidant systems. This feature renders cancer cells more sensitive to external stimuli that further increase ROS production [67]. An increasing number of therapeutic strategies are currently being developed to elevate ROS levels and overwhelm the redox adaptation of the same cells as well as ROS-responsive formulations containing anticancer therapeutics. Here, we summarized several DOX formulations that initiate burst release in response to elevated ROS levels in tumor cells.

ROS-sensitive liposomes using 10,10′-diselanediylbis decanoic acid (DDA) as a fundamental building block of various ratios of egg l-α-phosphatidylcholine (egg PC), DOPE, and 1,2-dioleoyl-sn-glycero-3-phosphocholine were prepared and characterized. The optimum formulation of DOPE/egg PC/DDA at a molar ratio of 37.5/60/2.5% showed a 30% burst release in 0.1% H_2O_2 at pH 6.5 through diselenide bond cleavage induced by the ROS signal. Intravenous injection of this redox-sensitive formulation containing DOX into C26-tumor-bearing mice showed a 40-fold higher AUC than that of free DOX, efficiently suppressed C26 tumor growth, and improved the distribution of DOX in tumor cells [68] (Table 2).

pH- and ROS-sensitive mesoporous silica nanoparticles (MSNs) with surface modifications using chitosan–folate conjugate (DOX–MSN-SS-CH-FA) have been developed for breast cancer therapy [69]. DOX release significantly increased in the presence of 10 mM GSH and at pH 5.5, suggesting a dual responsive (pH and ROS) formulation. DOX–MSN-SS-CH-FA was activated by ROS and acidic pH and was engulfed by the tumor via the folate receptor to release DOX into tumor cells following its intravenous injection in Ehrlich ascites carcinoma (EAC)-bearing BALB/c mice. DOX–MSN-CH-FA prolonged survival in EAC tumor-bearing mice with a decrease in tumor volume; however, the cardiotoxicity markers remained unchanged [69] (Table 2).

As mentioned previously, ROS-responsive formulations resulted in a positive therapeutic response by enhancing the targetability of the DOX formulation. Therefore, decreasing the ROS level might suppress the DOX response (Figure 2). Nuclear factor erythroid 2-related factor 2 (Nrf2) is a regulator gene that protects cells from oxidative stress and is known to play a key role in cancer progression [70,71]. Ryoo et al. [72] reported the upregulation of Nrf2 expression in DOX-resistant cancer cells, which resulted in reduced ROS levels in cancer cells, leading to decreased DOX efficacy. Moreover, cancer cells with low ROS levels have a tendency to express more P-gp in the cell membrane, as demonstrated by the positive association between Nrf2 and P-gp expression; accordingly, most DOX-resistant cancer cells showed Nrf2 overexpression [70,72]. To interfere with Nrf2 action using short hairpin RNA (shRNA) or small interfering RNA (siRNA) as a strategy to overcome drug resistance, Gu et al. [73] developed hyaluronidase-responsive multilayer liposomes (HLCNs) with cisplatin and Nrf2 siRNA. In vivo results revealed a 4-fold increase in cytotoxicity. Additionally, in mice with xenograft osteosarcoma, HLCN showed a 2-fold decrease in tumor volume with a low cytotoxic effect. This formulation showed favorable and sustained biodistribution of cisplatin in tumor tissues along with its rapid elimination in other organs.

3.1.3. Receptor (Rc)-Targeted Formulation

Prolonged blood circulating formulations are likely to accumulate in tumor tissue with an EPR effect due to the leakiness of tumor vasculature and poor lymphatic drainage [74]. Some receptors are overexpressed on the surface of tumor cells, which could guide targeted drug therapy. For example, formulations modified with tumor-targeting molecules such as folate and transferrin can be easily recognized and internalized by tumor cells due to their overexpression of folate or transferrin receptors [75]. Hyaluronic acid (HA) is an important linear polysaccharide component that exists in the extra-cellular matrix and has been reported with high specific affinity to CD44 receptors on cell surfaces [76], which broadened its application as a tumor targeting delivery system.

Wang et al. [77] prepared folate conjugated PEG-PLGA micelles containing DOX with or without SIS3, a potent P-gp and BCRP inhibitor (i.e., FA/DOX and FA/DOX/SIS3, respectively). Sustained release of DOX from both FA/DOX and FA/DOX/SIS3 micelles could be maintained for more than 48 h and both formulations significantly increased AUC and decreased the elimination half-life of DOX following IV injection compared with free DOX but showed comparable pharmacokinetic behavior between FA/DOX and FA/DOX/SIS3 micelles. In addition, FA/DOX showed a significantly higher intratumor DOX concentration and increased cytotoxicity in MCF-7 cells. By co-encapsulation of SIS3 (FA/DOX/SIS3), DOX concentration in tumor tissue significantly increased compared with FA/DOX in MCF-7/ADR cells. In addition, FA/DOX/SIS3 reduced tumor size more effectively and prolonged survival rate in MCF-7/ADR bearing BALB/c nude mice compared with FA/DOX treatment. Collectively, the results suggested the contribution of the folate targeted formulation and the co-delivery of the efflux pump inhibitor SIS3 to the better therapeutic efficacy and the reversal of DOX resistance [77] (Table 2).

Table 2. Formulation strategy using tumor microenvironments for tumor targetability of DOX in preclinical stage.

Carrier–Type	Formulation & Route of Administration	Experimental Research	Findings	References
pH-sensitive PLs	DOX-loaded PL (DOPE: CHEMS: DOPE-PEG2000 = 5.8:3.7:0.5), IV	4T1 tumor-bearing mice	Long circulating pH-sensitive liposome. Higher tumor uptake in 4T1 tumor-bearing mice	[63]
		Healthy mice	Less QT interval prolongation on an electrocardiogram (reduced cardiotoxicity)	[64]
pH-sensitive PNPs	DOX and pHPMA conjugates via hydrazone bond (HPMA-NH-DOX), IV	4T1, MCF-7 cell	A 5-fold faster DOX release in acidic intratumor (pH 6.5) and intratumor cellular (pH 5.5) environments than at pH 7.4	[65]
pH-sensitive PMs	DOX-loaded micelle (DSPE-PEG2000/OA = 10:6), IV	4T1 tumor-bearing mouse	pH-sensitive DOX release, 7-fold tumor shrinkage	[66]
ROS-sensitive liposomes	DOPE/Egg PC/DDA = 37.5/60/2.5%, IV	Walker 256 carcinosarcoma-bearing rat	A 3-fold faster DOX release at pH 5.0 than at pH 7.4 A 3-fold higher apoptosis rate	[68]
pH- and ROS-sensitive MSNs	Chitosan-folate conjugated MSN (DOX-MSN-SS-CH-FA), IV	C26-tumor-bearing mice	A 30% burst release in 0.1% H_2O_2 at pH 6.5 through the diselenide bond cleavage induced by the ROS signal The DOX-loaded liposome showed a 40-fold higher AUC than free DOX, efficient suppression of C26 tumor growth, and improved DOX distribution in tumors	[69]
Rc-targeted PMs	Folate targeted PM co-delivery of DOX and SIS3 (FA/DOX/SIS3), IV	SD rat	EPR and folate Rc-mediated endocytosis P-gp and BCRP inhibition by SIS3 6.1-fold increased AUC and 3.9-fold decreased clearance of DOX compared with free DOX	[77]
	FA/DOX/SIS3, unilateral axillary injection	MCF-7/ADR bearing nude mice	EPR and folate Rc-mediated endocytosis P-gp and BCRP inhibition by SIS3 Increased DOX accumulation in tumor tissue Inhibited tumor growth and prolonged the lifetime in DOX resistant tumor mice	
Rc-targeted and pH-sensitive PMs	HOD PM enclosed DOX-NN-VES, IV	MCF-7/ADR bearing nude mice	EPR and CD44-mediated endocytosis pH-sensitive DOX release at acidic intratumor organelles by hydrazone bond cleavage Increased DOX accumulation in tumor tissue Increased apoptosis and 2.28-fold decreased tumor weight compared with free DOX	[78]
Rc-targeted and pH-sensitive PNPs	Transferrin (Tf)- and poloxamer-integrated pH-sensitive PLGA NPs (Tf–DOX–PLGA), IV	NCI/ADR ovarian tumor cells	P-gp inhibition in tumor cells Significant decrease in cell viability from 80% to 20% compared with free DOX Arrested cell cycle in the G1 phase and increased apoptotic cell death by 2-fold	[79]

PL: PEGylated liposome; PNP: polymeric nanoparticles; PM: Polymeric micelles; MSN: mesoporous silicate nanoparticles; IV: intravenous injection; Rc: Receptor; CHEMS: cholesteryl hemi succinate; DSPE-PEG2000: distearoyl phosphatidyl ethanolamine polyethyleneglycol2000; DOPE: dioleoyl phosphatidyl ethanolamine; pHPMA: Poly N-(2 hydroxypropyl) methacrylamide; OA: oleic acid; ROS: reactive oxygen species; AUC: area under the curve; HOD PM enclosed DOX-NN-VES: HA-2-(octadecyloxy)-1,3-dioxan-5-amine (HOD) PM incorporating a conjugate of DOX and vitamin E succinate using a hydrazone bond (DOX-NN-VES).

Qiu et al. [78] prepared pH-sensitive and tumor targeting HA-2-(octadecyloxy)-1,3-dioxan-5-amine (HOD) PM and incorporated an acid-sensitive DOX-NN-VES prodrug (i.e., a conjugate of DOX and vitamin E succinate (VES) using a hydrazone bond (NN)). The pH-sensitive HOD PMs are internalized by CD44-mediated endocytosis via HA conjugates. Inside the tumor cells, HOD polymers are depolymerized to release the prodrug DOX-NN-VES. The hydrazone bond of DOX-NN-VES is also rapidly broken in the acidic environment to release the free DOX and VES. VES can inhibit the P-gp efflux pump to increase the accumulation of DOX in MCF-7/ADR cells. Therefore, this formulation can display higher efficiency in overcoming DOX resistance. In MCF-7/ADR tumor bearing mice, the HOD PM enclosed DOX-NN-VES prodrug reduced tumor weight by 2.28-fold, accompanied by reduced cardiotoxic side effect [78].

Scheeren et al. [79] proposed transferrin (Tf) and poloxamer-integrated pH-sensitive PLGA nanoparticles (Tf–DOX–PLGA) to bypass the P-gp-mediated DOX efflux. During the cell cycle, dividing cells show high expression of the transferrin receptor (TfR) for iron intake. TfR has the ability to uptake molecules via TF-mediated endocytosis, and the Tf-incorporated formulation could be uptaken by TfR. The engulfed Tf–DOX–PLGA nanoparticles release DOX and poloxamer into the cells. Poloxamer has been reported to have multiple functions in P-gp overexpressed cells, such as inhibiting P-gp and depleting ATP in mitochondria, resulting in ROS generation and cytochrome c release, which lead to apoptosis [80]. Tf–DOX–PLGA treatment in DOX-resistant NCI/ADR ovarian tumor cells showed a significant decrease in cell viability, from 80% to 20%, compared with free DOX treatment. In addition, the results of a cell cycle arrest study showed that most cells affected by Tf–DOX–PLGA treatment were arrested in the G1 phase, with a 2-fold increase in apoptotic cell death [79] (Table 2).

3.2. Formulation Strategy for Overcoming DOX Resistance in the Preclinical Stage

3.2.1. Overexpression of P-gp in Tumor Cells

P-gp is found not only in the gastrointestinal tract but also in tissues associated with various other cancers, especially melanoma and central nervous system cancer, with extremely high expression in renal and colon cancers [81]. Unexpectedly, DOX could induce P-gp expression in cancer cell membranes; it shows significant correlation with increased P-gp expression in cancer cells and enhanced resistance to DOX [20]. DOX activates the phosphatidylinositol 3-kinase/AKT/mammalian target of the rapamycin signaling cascade and subsequently enhances P-gp expression and promotes the proliferation of cancer cells [82]. DOX also activates the mitogen-activated protein kinase (MAPK)/extracellular signal-regulated kinase pathway, which promotes the proliferation of tumor cells and protects them from oxidative stress [83].

Glucose-regulated protein 78 (GRP78), a chaperone heat shock protein, activates this signaling pathway [84]. Under DOX stress, GRP78 is overexpressed in the cell membrane and induces disordered protein status on membranes, including P-gp. Gemcitabine resistance in breast cancer is associated with overexpressed GRP78 and consecutive AKT elevation, leading to the overexpression of P-gp. It can be interpreted that DOX induces stress in cancer cells, which then overexpress GRP78 and consequently lead to P-gp overexpression, which increases DOX resistance [85]. Colon and prostate cancer cells have shown high GRP78 expression during treatment with celecoxib [86,87]. Collectively, to develop an oral DOX formulation and reduce the occurrence of DOX resistance, the modulation of P-gp function and expression remains a major challenge. Therefore, we also reviewed many DOX formulation studies focusing on the inhibition of P-gp.

3.2.2. P-gp Inhibition in a Cellular Environment to Overcome Drug Resistance

To increase DOX sensitivity, studies have focused on DOX coupled with small molecules or excipients that exert a P-gp inhibitory effect. Grabarnick et al. synthesized PEGylated liposomes incorporating DOX, indocyanine green (ICG), and P-gp inhibitor quinine (ICG + PEGylated liposomes with DOX and quinine [PLDQ]) [88]. ICG is an FDA-approved photosensitizer and is known to be superior to other photosensitizers in terms of tissue penetration and safety [89]. When ICG was exposed to near-infrared light, it generated excessive levels of ROS and caused oxidative stress, leading to ROS-induced cell death [90,91]. When quinine was used as a P-gp inhibitor, PLDQ increased the cellular accumulation of DOX and reduced tumor volume by 25% in mice with xenografted HT29-MDR1 positive cells (i.e., P-gp overexpressed HT29 colon cancer cells) compared with PLD (without quinine) [88]. Additionally, with the incorporation of ICG into PLDQ, the tumor volume of mice with xenografted HT29-MDR1 reduced by 75% following exposure to near-infrared light. The survival rate also showed a 2-fold increase with treatment with ICG + PLDQ. The results could be attributed to the P-gp inhibitory effect of quinine on ICG and DOX as both are substrates for P-gp [88] (Table 3).

An et al. [92] designed DOX-loaded apolipoprotein A1 (ApoA1)-modified cationic liposomes (ApoA1-LipDOX). Previously, ApoA1-modified liposomes increased the intake of the substrate drug by inhibiting the P-gp-mediated efflux [93]. In other words, the DOX concentration in the tumor tissues of 4T1 tumor-bearing mice treated with ApoA1-LipDOX was three times higher than the concentration of free DOX in the same region. Consequently, these mice also had a three times smaller tumor volume [92] (Table 3).

In DOX-resistant H69AR cancer cells, triphenylphosphonium (TPP)-conjugated DOX (TPP–DOX) efficiently accumulates in mitochondria and disrupts the membrane potential and ATP gradient. Consequently, P-gp is inactivated, and mitochondria-induced apoptosis causes cell death [94]. To achieve the targeting of TPP–DOX to tumor mitochondria, Zhou et al. designed a near-infrared (NIR) light- and acidity-activated micellar nanoplatform, known as PEGylated iPUTDN. Then, PEGylated iPUTDN was maintained in circulation. Upon NIR irradiation of the tumor region, PEG was cleaved from the light-sensitive cleavage polymer and 9-amino acid cyclic peptide (cCRGDKGPDC) could facilitate the intratumor penetration and tumor cell uptake of nanoparticles. The acidic condition in tumor cells disrupted the core shell via rapid protonation of poly(β-aminoester)-based nanoparticles and released TPP–DOX from the core. This disrupted the membrane potential and ATP gradient; consequently, P-gp was inactivated, and mitochondria-induced apoptosis caused cell death in the tumor region of H69AR lung cancer-bearing mice. In the tumor region, treatment with PEG-iPUTDN showed a 20-fold greater DOX accumulation than that with free DOX. Compared with TPP–DOX alone, tumor volume decreased by 10-fold following treatment with PEG-iPUTDN and NIR exposure [95] (Table 3).

Suppressing P-gp expression is another strategy to overcome P-gp-mediated DOX resistance. Tomentodione M (TTM), a novel natural syncarpic acid-conjugated monoterpene, increases the intracellular concentration of rhodamine 123 and DOX in K562/MDR human leukemia MDR cells and MCF-7/MDR breast cancer cells [96]. Further, high DOX sensitivity results in cell death when DOX and TTM are used in combination. TTM inhibits the p38 MAPK signaling pathway. P-gp expression stimulated by MAPK is inhibited by TTM, resulting in an increased uptake of DOX in tumor cells [96]. Tanshinone IIA (Tan IIA) is a lipophilic component derived from *Salvia miltiorrhiza*. Tan IIA is a potential candidate for combination with DOX because it not only inhibits DOX efflux but also reduces cardiotoxicity with a cardiovascular protective effect [97,98]. This effect could be explained by the Tan IIA-induced suppression of the PTEN/AKT signaling pathway that downregulates the expression of P-gp as well as BCRP and MRP1 in MCF-7 human breast cancer cells [99]. Collectively, the coadministration of DOX with Tan IIA is a promising candidate for increasing DOX sensitivity and reducing its cardiotoxicity [100].

Ascorbate not only reduces DOX efflux by inhibiting P-gp expression but also sensitizes DOX-resistant MCF-7 breast cancer cells (MCF-7/DOX) to DOX by inhibiting the ATP level [101]. In another attempt to use a combination of DOX and ascorbate, DOX and palmitoyl ascorbate (PA)-loaded liposomes (DOX–PA–liposomes) showed a 2.5-fold higher DOX uptake in MCF-7 cells compared with DOX-loaded liposomes (DOX–liposomes) [102]. Pharmacokinetics and efficacy studies using DOX–PA–liposomes were conducted in SD rats and MCF-7-bearing female BALB/c nude mice for comparison with DOX–liposomes.

Intravenous injection of DOX–PA–liposomes in rats showed a 10-fold elevation in DOX AUC compared with that of DOX–liposomes. DOX–PA–liposomes showed a 10-fold lower clearance compared with DOX–liposomes. This indicates that ascorbate reduces extracellular ROS generation and consequently downregulates P-gp expression, resulting in reduced clearance and increased DOX AUC. In addition, the administration of DOX–PA–liposomes in MCF-7-bearing female BALB/c nude mice resulted in a decrease in tumor size by 2-fold compared with that of DOX–liposomes [102].

As the tumor microenvironment is characterized by a low interstitial pH, overexpressed enzymes, and high GSH levels, two silicate nanoparticles (namely glucose oxidase-loaded silica nanoparticles with disulfide bonds in the shell and arginine on the surface [GOD@SiO$_2$-Arg] and DOX-loaded MSN [DOX–MSN]) were linked via methacrylated hyaluronic acid (HA–MA) to form hydrogels. Once this formulation was administered to the tumor tissue, hyaluronic acidase, which is overexpressed in tumor tissue, cleaved the crosslink between HA–MA and released GOD@SiO$_2$-Arg and DOX–MSN. In tumor cells, Arg generates NO in the presence of H$_2$O$_2$ and decreases P-gp expression, and the low pH environment facilitates DOX release from DOX–MSN. By combining these tumor microenvironment-responsive formulations, GOD@SiO$_2$-Arg and DOX–MSN hydrogel decreased P-gp expression and increased DOX therapeutic efficacy in DOX-resistant MCF-7/ADR cells [103]. In addition, in a nude mouse model of a subcutaneous xenograft tumor, GOD@SiO$_2$-Arg and DOX–MSN significantly reduced the tumor volume by 8-fold without causing significant histological abnormalities. The survival rate of tumor-bearing mice in GOD@SiO$_2$-Arg and DOX–MSN hydrogel treatment group increased from 15 to 30 days compared with that of DOX treatment group [103] (Table 3).

Pluronic F127 micelles with pH-sensitive polyacrylic acid at two terminals of the micelle carrier (PAA-PF127-PAA-PM) loaded with DOX had a spherical shape with a size of 100 nm. They showed a pH-sensitive DOX release profile, with a faster release at pH 5.0 and a slower release at pH 7.4. PAA-PF127-PAA-PM showed >80% viability at concentrations of <300 µg/mL; moreover, it showed a 3-fold higher apoptosis rate than free DOX in a Walker 256 carcinosarcoma-bearing rat [104]. Pluronic F127 micelles also exhibited a P-gp inhibitory effect [45]. Although the pharmacokinetics and in vivo anticancer efficacy of PAA-PF127-PAA-PM have not been investigated, the pH-sensitive drug release and P-gp reversal effect may have contributed to the therapeutic and pharmacokinetic benefits (Table 3).

3.2.3. Ion-Trapping Phenomenon

Another factor affecting DOX efficacy is the acidic pH of the tumor environment. When ionizable weak base anticancer drugs, such as anthraquinones, anthracyclines, and vinca alkaloids, come into contact with this acidic environment, they become charged, leading to decreased cellular uptake and low therapeutic efficacy. This phenomenon is known as ion-trapping [105,106]. As mentioned previously, the acidity of the central region of solid tumors increases compared with their overall acidity (pH 6.4–7.0). Under this condition, DOX is sequestered into acidic vesicles, reducing the resultant therapeutic efficacy. Treatment with imidazole and tamoxifen, which inhibit vesicle acidification, can increase DOX release into the cytoplasm and enhance its cytotoxicity [105,107,108].

Abumanhal-Masarweh et al. injected NaHCO$_3$-loaded HSPC-m2000PEG DSPE–liposomes along with DOX into 4T1 breast cancer-bearing mice. Results showed a 2–3-fold elevation in DOX concentration with NaHCO$_3$ coadministration, followed by a decrease in cell viability by 3-fold [109]. The average extracellular pH in tumor tissue increased to 7.38 compared with the acidic extracellular pH of 5.0–6.0 in tumor cells [110].

Ando et al. [111] analyzed per oral NaHCO$_3$-loaded liposomes with intravenous Doxil in colon 26 tumor-bearing mice. Both intravenous and orally administered NaHCO$_3$ showed clear DOX accumulation in the tumor tissue as well as a 9- and 2-fold decrease in tumor size compared with free DOX and Doxil alone, respectively. A previously reported diffusion model with MDA-MB-231 showed that orally administered bicarbonate had no influence on acidic tumor environment [112]. However, Ando et al. suggested that NaHCO$_3$ is a promising candidate for combination with DOX as long as it is released at a local tumor site [111] (Table 3).

3.2.4. Long Noncoding RNA (lncRNA) Overexpression

Recently, lncRNA has been reported to be associated with DOX resistance in osteosarcoma. The expression of LINC00426, a newly found lncRNA, was upregulated in DOX-resistant osteosarcoma [113]. Moreover, following siRNA-mediated LINC00426 knockdown in osteosarcoma cells, the IC$_{50}$ value of DOX decreased by 2-fold, and caspase-3 activity increased by 4-fold [113]. However, the role of lncRNA in DOX resistance is controversial, depending on the cancer type. AX747207, a lncRNA knockdown RUX3 tumor suppressor gene, induces DOX resistance in MCF-7 breast cancer cells [114]. BMP/OP-responsive gene, another lncRNA, induces DOX resistance by activating RPA1 and NF-kB in triple-negative breast cancer [115]. DOX stress induces prosurvival autophagy via lncRNA SOX2OT variant 7, which also results in DOX resistance in osteosarcoma cells. Epigallocatechin gallate in combination with DOX reduces the expression of lncRNA human SOX2 overlapping transcript (SOX2OT) variant 7 in osteosarcoma U20s and SaoS2 cells and reverses the DOX resistance [116].

Additionally, lncRNA SOX2OT variant 7 stimulates upstream Notch3/DLL3 signaling, leading to differentiation of osteosarcoma stem cells as well as breast, lung, and ovarian cancer cells [117]. Consequently, the use of lncRNA inhibitor as a DOX resistance target warrants further research.

3.2.5. Hypoglycemic Environment

Glucose is an important factor in DOX resistance at the cellular level. A hyperglycemic environment activates the mitochondrial function responsible for ROS generation, contributing to the downregulation of P-gp expression and thus increasing DOX sensitivity [118]. Dickkopf protein 4 (DKK4) is an important regulator of glucose uptake; it regulates ROS levels that further regulate P-gp expression [119]. DKK4 mRNA expression was downregulated in hepatoma and colorectal cancer cells (67.5% and 57.1%, respectively) compared with that in normal epithelium [120,121]. Downregulated DKK4 levels are associated with low glucose levels and can contribute to high P-gp expression, which facilitates DOX resistance. In contrast, a study reported the association of DKK4-mediated positive regulation of glucose and ROS and resultant P-gp upregulation; however, the types of cancer cells that upregulate DKK4 levels remain controversial [122].

3.3. Challenges in the Development of Oral Formulations
3.3.1. Low Intestinal Permeability

Orally administered DOX encounters a harsh gastrointestinal environment. Among factors inhibiting the BA of DOX, limited intestinal absorption is the most critical factor, with 82–99% of orally administered DOX remaining unabsorbed [19]. Nanoparticles are trapped in the mucus and epithelial barriers. Mucus is mostly composed of glycosylated proteins and is present throughout the gastrointestinal tract [123]. It acts as a first barrier, limiting diffusion and trapping drugs before they interact with the intestinal epithelium [124]. In addition, the epithelium acts as a barrier to drug absorption. DOX also has limited intestinal absorption and P-gp- and MRP1-mediated efflux are the main factors responsible for its low intestinal absorption and BA (Figure 3).

Table 3. Formulations for overcoming DOX resistance in the preclinical stage.

Carrier–Type	Formulation and Route of Administration	Experimental Model	Findings	References
PLs	PL incorporating DOX, ICG, and P-gp inhibitor quinine (ICG + PLDQ), IV	HT-29 MDR1 positive xenograft mice	P-gp inhibition in tumor cells Increased cellular uptake of DOX and reduction in tumor volume by 25% Increase in survival rate by 2-fold	[88]
Liposomes	DOX-loaded apolipoprotein A1-modified cationic liposome (ApoA1-LipDOX), IV	4T1 tumor-bearing mice	P-gp inhibition in tumor cells with 3-fold higher DOX concentration in tumor tissue Decrease in tumor volume by 3-fold	[92]
	DOX and palmitoyl ascorbate (PA)-loaded liposome (DOX-PA-liposome), IV	MCF-7 cells	P-gp inhibition in tumor cells Increased DOX uptake in MCF-7 cells by 2.5-fold	[102]
		SD rats	Elevation in DOX AUC by 10-fold compared with DOX–liposome AUC	
		MCF-7 breast cancer bearing mice	Tumor size decreased by 2-fold compared with DOX–liposome	
	DOX and NaHCO$_3$-loaded HSPC-m2000PEG DSPE–liposome, IV	4T1 breast cancer-bearing mouse	Increase in DOX concentration by 2–3-fold The average extracellular pH in tumor tissue increased to 7.38	[109]
	NaHCO$_3$-loaded liposome and Doxil combination, IV	colon26 tumor-bearing mouse	Decrease in tumor size by 9- and 2-fold compared with free DOX and Doxil, respectively	[111]
PMs	DOX-loaded Pluronic F127 micelles with pH-sensitive poly(acrylic acid) at two terminals (PAA-PF127-PAA-PM), IV	Walker 256 carcinosarcoma-bearing mice	A 3-fold faster DOX release at pH 5.0 than at pH 7.4 A 3-fold higher apoptosis rate compared with free DOX	[104]
PNPs	PEG-iPUTDN + NIR exposure, IP	H69AR lung cancer-bearing mice	Bypassed the P-gp-mediated efflux TPP-conjugated DOX was efficiently accumulated in mitochondria Tumor volume and weight decreased by 10-fold	[95]
MSNs	GOD@SiO$_2$-Arg and DOX-MSN hydrogels, SC	MCF-7/ADR cells	Arg generated NO in the presence of H$_2$O$_2$ and decreased P-gp expression. Low pH facilitated DOX release from DOX–MSN and increased its therapeutic efficacy	[103]
		MCF-7/ADR xenograft mice	Tumor volume reduced significantly by 8-fold without causing significant histological abnormalities Survival rate increased by 2-fold	

PL: PEGylated liposome; PMs: polymeric micelles; PNPs: Polymeric nanoparticles; IV: intravenous injection; IP: intraperitoneal injection; SC: subcutaneous injection; ICG: indocyanine green; GOD@SiO$_2$-Arg: glucose oxidase loaded silica nanoparticle with disulfide bonds in the shell and arginine on the surface; DOX-MSN: DOX loaded mesoporous nanosilicate; TPP: triphenylphosphonium; AUC: area under the curve.

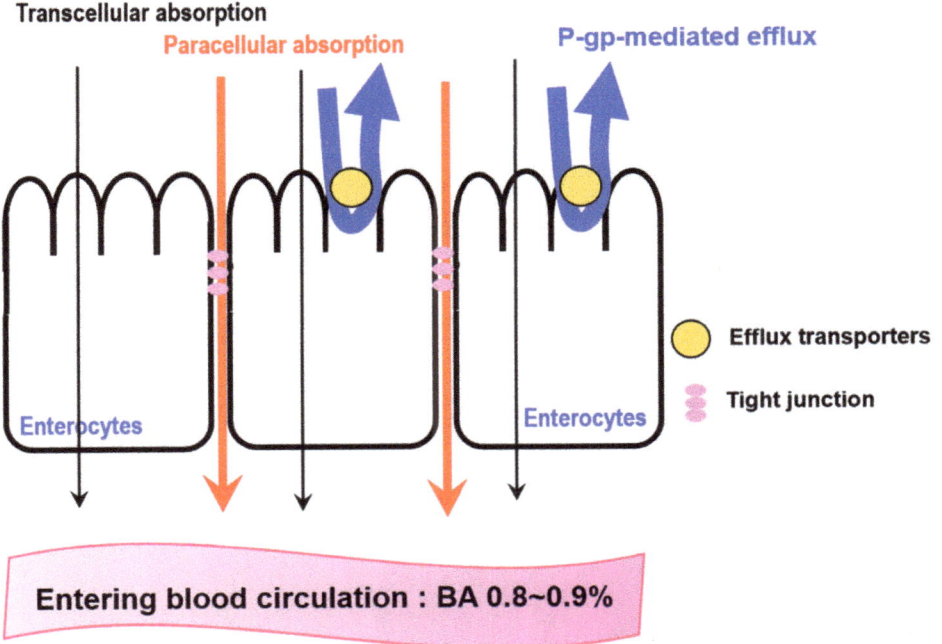

Figure 3. Intestinal absorption of DOX. P-gp: P-glycoprotein. BA: bioavailability, which was accessed in rats [19]. Black, red, and blue arrows represent transcellular absorption, paracellular absorption, and P-gp-mediated efflux, respectively.

Based on an analysis of bidirectional transport, DOX in Caco-2 cells cultured in a Ca^{2+}/Mg^{2+}-free medium showed a 20-fold increase in absorptive permeability ($P_{app,AB}$) compared with that in Caco-2 cells cultured in a Ca^{2+}/Mg^{2+}-positive medium, indicating that DOX is primarily absorbed from the intestinal epithelium through a paracellular route [125]. However, the secretory permeability ($P_{app,BA}$) of DOX was 6.6 times higher than that of $P_{app,AB}$, and the intestinal extraction of DOX via P-gp-mediated efflux accounts for 0.39–0.44 in rats. In the presence of an existing P-gp inhibitor, the $P_{app,BA}$ of DOX reduced significantly, whereas its $P_{app,AB}$ was rarely affected in Caco-2 cells. Collectively, as shown in Figure 3, DOX mainly penetrates the intestinal epithelium via the paracellular pathway, and P-gp-mediated efflux limits DOX absorption. This might be the reason for the low absorption of DOX. Therefore, the oral BA of DOX was 0.8–0.9% [19].

3.3.2. High First-Pass Metabolism of DOX

In addition to limited intestinal absorption, a previous study revealed that the hepatic first-pass extraction ratio of DOX in rats was 0.49–0.56 [19]. In another study, 45–50% DOX was eliminated via bilirubin excretion in the parent form, and the remaining DOX underwent metabolism [126] (Figure 4). Doxorubicinol (Figure 4B), a major metabolite of DOX-mediated toxicity by carbonyl reductase (CBR), is known to be an essential cardiotoxicity factor that disturbs the homeostasis of iron and calcium balances and induces mitochondrial dysfunction [127,128]. The quinone moiety in DOX is transformed into semiquinone (Figure 4C), another metabolite of DOX, by the cytochrome p450 oxidoreductase (POR) and NADPH dehydrogenase of the mitochondrial electron transport chain complex I [129]. This semiquinone regenerates into quinone and produces ROS. ROS production and cytochrome C, released via mitochondrial dysfunction together, activate caspase-3 and cause cell apoptosis, thus explaining DOX-induced cardiotoxicity [130].

Cardiomyocytes require high levels of ATP; therefore, the density of mitochondria is considerably higher than that of other tissues. Consequently, the heart sustains more damage by DOX than other tissues [131,132].

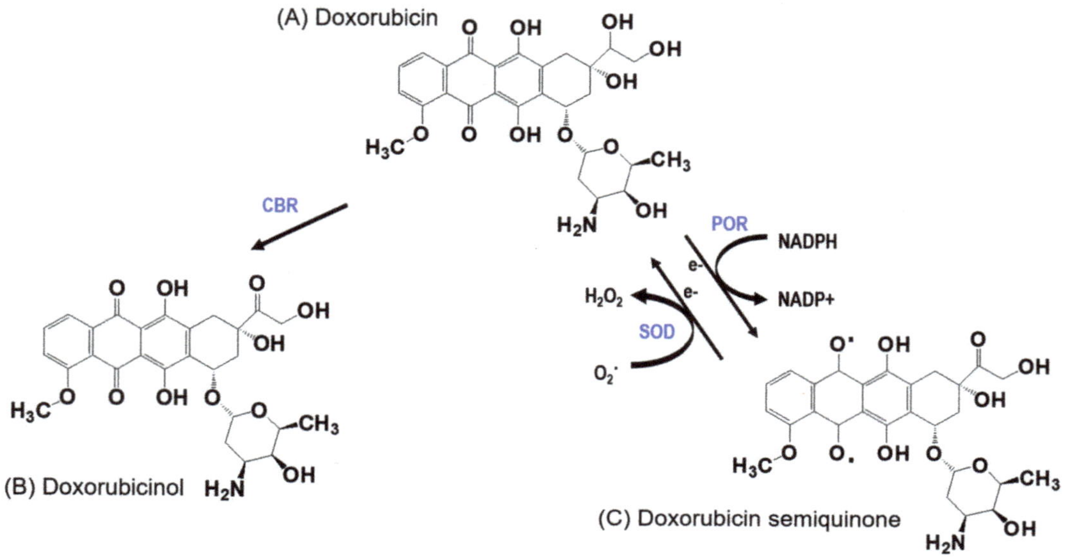

Figure 4. Metabolic pathway and related metabolic enzymes for the transformation of (**A**) DOX to (**B**) doxorubicinol and (**C**) doxorubicin semiquinone, major metabolites of DOX. CBR: carbonyl reductase; POR: cytochrome P450 oxidoreductase; SOD: superoxide dismutase. Arrows represent the metabolic conversion.

3.4. Formulation Strategy for Overcoming Low Oral BA in the Preclinical Stage

3.4.1. Coadministration with a P-gp Inhibitor to Increase Oral Absorption

Two cytosolic ATP-binding cassette (ABC) domains of a P-gp inhibitor and ATP hydrolysis alter the conformation of P-gp and allow the excretion of substrate drugs into the extracellular environment. Because the ABC domains and substrate binding sites are available for targeting with small molecules, to date, various P-gp inhibitors have been developed to downregulate the expression and activity of P-gp [133]. As described previously, the use of P-gp inhibitors is critical for achieving acceptable oral BA and preventing DOX resistance at the cellular level. Many research studies have focused on this issue.

The concomitant administration of a P-gp inhibitor with anticancer drugs as a strategy for BA enhancement has been studied in clinical trials. Elacridar (GF120918) is one of the third-generation P-gp and BCRP inhibitors that more specifically inhibits P-gp and BCRP while having no interaction with CYP enzymes [134]. Elacridar is a noncompetitive P-gp inhibitor and modulates ATPase activity by inhibiting ATP hydrolysis [135]. With the coadministration of elacridar, the oral BA of paclitaxel increased from 4% to 30–50% in humans [136,137]. Topotecan also showed a marked BA enhancement. With the coadministration of elacridar, the oral BA of topotecan increased from 42% to 97% in cancer patients. In other studies, interindividual variability decreased from 17% to 11% [138–140]. Similar clinical trials using potent P-gp inhibitors such as encequidar (HM30181A) with paclitaxel and docetaxel are underway [141]. Coadministration of the P-gp inhibitor ONT-093 with docetaxel resulted in BA enhancement from >10% to 26% and lowered interindividual variability from 90% to 44–70% [142].

A clinical trial explored DOX administration in combination with elacridar via IV injection in 46 patients. The DOX AUC tended to increase with increasing plasma elacridar concentrations, but only a small difference in AUC was observed between treatment with DOX alone and the combination of DOX and elacridar [126]. However, the plasma concentrations of doxorubicinol increased in some patients, which may be attributed to the decreased metabolism of doxorubicinol owing to the presence of elacridar. Similar results were reported in combination treatment with DOX and cyclosporin A or PSC-833 [143,144]. Therefore, unlike paclitaxel, the coadministration of elacridar with DOX may not provide the therapeutic benefit of DOX.

Zosuquidar (LY335979) is the most selective third-generation P-gp inhibitor and has no interaction with efflux transporters, such as BCRP and MRP transporters, or CYP. In UKFNB-3 neuroblastoma cells, DOX treatment with zosuquidar showed a 2-fold lower IC_{50} value than DOX alone [145]. With the coadministration of zosuquidar, Nielsen et al. reported a 2.5–35% increase in the oral BA of etoposide in rats [146]. However, currently, clinical trials based on the combination of zosuquidar and the CHOP regimen, which includes the intravenous infusion of vincristine (1.4 mg/m^2), DOX (50 mg/m^2) and cyclophosphamide (750 mg/m^2) and the oral administration of prednisolone (100 mg), have not revealed positive interactions between zosuquidar and P-gp substrates in the CHOP regimen (i.e., vincristine or DOX) [147].

As studies have reported a substantial contribution of P-gp to intestinal absorption, it is necessary to conduct clinical studies to investigate the effect of P-gp inhibitors on the oral BA of DOX. In addition, the effect of P-gp inhibitors on the oral BA of anticancer drugs is likely to benefit only certain drugs, especially those with highly variable drug concentrations, low oral BA, and anticancer activity primarily mediated by the parent drug with a demonstrated exposure–response relationship [58]. Some drugs such as etoposide did not significantly improve their oral BA despite promising preclinical evidence [38,148]. Therefore, additional functional inhibitors that can increase intestinal penetration as parent drugs are required for formulating DOX with P-gp inhibitors.

3.4.2. Mucoadhesive Formulation

Adhesion to and penetration across the thick mucosa in the gastrointestinal tract is an important aspect of oral administration, which has been a continuing concern in the development of oral therapies. In this regard, chitosan is a cationic polysaccharide derived from chitin that has been widely used because of its mucoadhesive property and ability to loosen the epithelial tight junction in the gastrointestinal tract, making it an important conjugate candidate for oral formulation [149,150]. Chitosan and stearic acid copolymer (CSO–SA) were used to form mixed micelles with a diameter of 32.7 nm in the aqueous phase, which were subsequently uptaken by cancer cells. DOX-conjugated CSO–SA PMs (DOX–CSO–SA) enhanced DOX uptake in MCF-7/ADR cells and human hepatocellular carcinoma-bearing nude mice. This formulation showed favorable drug release at an acidic pH (pH 5.0) compared with that at pH 7.0. DOX–CSO–SA micelles were sensitive in both DOX-sensitive MCF cells and DOX-resistant MCF-7/ADR cells. The reversal power, which was calculated based on the IC_{50} difference, against MCF-7/ADR cells was 10.5 [151]. Similar approaches have been applied to oral administration. Compared with free DOX, chitosan and linoleic acid-based PMs incorporating DOX (DOX–CS–LA) improved the oral BA of DOX by 166% in Sprague-Dawley (SD) rats by targeting the intestinal fatty acid transporter [152].

With the increasing development of multifunctional formulations, the addition of P-gp inhibitors and chitosan into the DOX formulation could increase its oral BA. Therefore, we examined DOX formulation studies that aimed to increase the oral BA of DOX.

3.4.3. Formulations to Increase the Oral BA of DOX

In addition to the DOX formulation in the clinical stage, many DOX formulations, such as PMs, PNPs, etc., that are mainly studied for increasing oral BA, targeting the tumor cells, and reducing adverse effects have been studied.

(1) PMs

In a previous study, DOX-loaded lysine-linked ditocopherol polyethylene glycol 2000 succinate micelle formulation (PLV2K–DOX) increased the intestinal absorption rate of DOX by 1.61–3.19-fold compared with free DOX in the duodenum, jejunum, and ileum [104]. In the presence of cyclosporine, a P-gp inhibitor, the cellular uptake of DOX was even higher than that with free DOX, suggesting that the increased intestinal permeability of DOX incorporated in PLV2K–DOX is attributed to P-gp inhibition by the ditocopherol polyethylene glycol 2000 succinate linkage. In addition, caveolin-mediated and caveolin-/clathrin-independent endocytosis facilitated the intestinal absorption of DOX. The pharmacokinetics of DOX in rats following oral administration of PLV2K–DOX revealed a 3.7- and 5.6-fold higher maximum plasma concentration (C_{max}) and plasma exposure (AUC), respectively, than those of free DOX [153,154] (Table 4).

Oleanolic acid (OA) is a naturally occurring pentacyclic triterpenoid saponin present in >1600 plant species [155]. It exerts hepatoprotective, anticancer, anti-inflammatory, and antioxidative effects. OA also induces ROS generation, apoptosis, and cell cycle arrest and attenuates DOX-mediated toxicity in patients with hepatocellular carcinoma [156]. Based on this effect, Kumbham et al. [155] developed a biodegradable micelle formulation encapsulating DOX and OA. The OA-conjugated methoxy-poly (ethylene glycol) (mPEG)-polylactide (PLA) micelle formulation loaded with DOX (mPEG–PLA–OA–DOX) enhanced DOX accumulation, increased cell cytotoxicity, and induced apoptotic signals. This formulation also increased DOX accumulation and antitumor activity in FaDu-HTB-43 spheroids isolated from a hypopharyngeal tumor of a patient with squamous cell carcinoma. The formulation showed a 30-fold enhancement in circulation time and a 30-fold reduction in the clearance time of DOX compared with free DOX following their oral administration in rats (Table 4).

(2) PNPs

Among the PNPs presented in Section 2, PLGA has been approved by the US FDA for encapsulating various drugs to achieve ease of administration, biocompatibility, and biodegradability [157,158]. Moreover, PLGA can be uptaken by M cells distributed in the Peyer's patches of the small intestinal epithelium for distribution in the lymphatic circulation. This route is crucial, as it can bypass the first-pass mechanism and P-gp-mediated efflux in the intestinal epithelium [159–161]. Biodegradable nanoparticles containing DOX–PLGA have been developed for treating glioblastoma and breast cancer in animal models, but they have not yet undergone clinical studies [162–164].

Several DOX formulation studies in experimental animals showing enhanced oral BA and therapeutic efficacy have been reported. The preparation of freeze–dried DOX-loaded PLGA nanoparticles resulted in a 3.63-fold BA enhancement, while its absorption time (T_{max}) was delayed from 6 to 36 h. The sustained release of DOX from freeze–dried DOX-loaded PLGA NPs also has the advantage of not causing cardiotoxicity [157]. Treatment with DOX-loaded PLGA NPs showed considerably greater cellular accumulation than that with free DOX and even greater cellular accumulation than that with free DOX and cyclosporine A. Orally administered DOX-loaded PLGA NPs showed a similar reduction in tumor size and burden to that of IV administered DOX, whereas oral free DOX was shown to be ineffective. This formulation increased the survival rate of breast tumor-bearing female rats compared with free DOX. Moreover, the increased levels of well-known cardiotoxicity markers—malondialdehyde, lactate dehydrogenase, and creatine phosphokinase—reduced with the decreasing levels of GSH [157,165]. Compared with elevated or reduced levels of markers in IV DOX, superoxide dismutase levels remained unchanged in DOX-loaded PLGA nanoparticles. Surface modification of PLGA NPs using Pluronic F127, zwitter ionic polydopamine, and PEGylation increased the mucus and epithelial permeability of DOX and showed a great improvement in its oral BA [166]. These three surfaced-modified PLGA NPs showed significantly increased mucus and epithelial penetration, cellular uptake, and transepithelial transport in HT29-MTX and TR146 cells. The in vivo effect of these surface-modified PLGA NPs has been evaluated (Table 4).

PEGylated DOX-loaded PLGA NPs were prepared to circumvent the effect of intestinal efflux transporters. This formulation had a size of approximately 200 nm and a zeta potential of -13.1 mV. It showed sustained release for 24 h. The plasma AUC of DOX was 13.8 times higher than that of free DOX, with a 2.1-fold delayed elimination rate. It also showed enhanced intestinal adhesion and penetration compared with non-PEGylated particles [167]. Another surface modification of PLGA NPs has been reported. Chitosan-coated daunorubicin–PLGA (Cs–DAU–PLGA) nanoparticles had the following characteristics: (1) biodegradability and biocompatibility owing to PLGA and (2) a mucoadhesive property and ability to open a tight junction owing to chitosan. The properties of controlled release were attributed to the formulated nanoparticles. These properties were demonstrated by the 3.5-fold increase in Caco-2 permeability and endocytotic intestinal uptake of the Cs–DAU–PLGA nanoparticle formulation, which were not observed with free dauonorubicin. Compared with free daunorubicin, the administration of Cs–DAU–PLGA nanoparticle formulation to rats revealed an 11.3-fold higher AUC with a 2.8-fold delay in elimination half-life. The enhanced absorption and delayed disposition could be due to encapsulation with daunorubicin, escape from P-gp-mediated efflux and CYP-mediated metabolism, and enterocytic endocytosis of the nanoparticle formulation [168] (Table 4).

As acidic conditions (pH < 6.0) are required to dissolve chitosan in an aqueous solution [169], acidic modification of chitosan has been attempted. Chitosan was modified to chitosan diacetate and chitosan triacetate, and DOX-loaded nanoparticles were prepared using modified chitosan diacetate (DOX–CDA) or modified chitosan triacetate (DOX–CTA) with loading efficacy of 58% and 80%, respectively. Both modified chitosan–DOX-loaded NPs showed a 2.1- and 1.8-fold increase in permeability in MCF-7 tumor cells compared with free DOX. DOX–CTA NPs showed a relatively sustained release of DOX over 24 h, and the oral administration of DOX–CTA NPs in rats showed a 3-fold AUC enhancement compared with that of free DOX [169] (Table 4).

Intestine-penetrating, pH-sensitive, and double-layered NPs with a mean size of 350 nm were developed. Hydrophobic polyortho-ester urethane, composed of PCL and polyoxyethylene (POE) blocks, constituted the core shell, and DOX was loaded into the core shell. Carboxymethyl chitosan and glutaraldehyde were crosslinked to the outer membranes. The outer coating of carboxymethyl chitosan loosened the tight junction of the intestinal epithelium, and glutaraldehyde stabilized the liposome in the harsh gastric environment (pH 0.9–1.5) without releasing DOX; therefore, it could bypass the first-pass effect of DOX [170]. The core POE block induced DOX accumulation at the tumor site and DOX release in the acidic tumor environment (pH 5–6). PO administration of these formulations in H22 tumor-bearing mice showed a relative BA of 75.4%, which effectively inhibited tumor growth. Importantly, orally administered intestine-penetrating, pH-sensitive, and double-layered DOX NPs showed reduced cardiac distribution compared with free DOX, and the DOX concentrations in the major tissues did not exceed the maximum tolerated concentration; approximately 40% of absorbed DOX was accumulated in tumor tissues [170] (Table 4).

The natural substance casein has become a candidate for anticancer formulations because of its advantages, such as low cost, biodegradability, nontoxicity, and ability to form nanomicelles and nanoparticles [171]. Sodium caseinate NPs incorporating DOX (DOX–NaCN), with a size of 271 nm, spherical shape, and zeta potential of -0.054 mV, have been prepared and characterized. They showed sustained DOX release over 24 h and a significantly higher cellular uptake. Orally administered DOX–NaCN decreased the tumor size by 8-fold compared with free DOX in 4T1-breast cancer-bearing mice. In addition, the oral administration of DOX–NaCN showed 8.34-fold higher DOX accumulation in tumor tissues than that of intravenous free DOX but was comparable to that of intravenous DOX–NaCN. However, the cardiac concentration of DOX following the oral administration of DOX–NaCN was the lowest among the four different treatment groups (i.e., free DOX administered orally or intravenously, DOX–NaCN administered orally or intravenously). These results suggest that nontoxic controlled release of DOX from NaCN has beneficial antitumor effects after PO administration [172] (Table 4).

(3) Multilayer micro-dispersing system (MMS)

Feng et al. [173] constructed MMS to enhance the oral BA of DOX. First, nanogels (NGs) incorporating DOX were constructed with chitosan to obtain a carboxymethyl chitosan complex (DOX:CS/CMCS-NGs), which was then crosslinked with Ca and carboxylate ions in the core of multilayer alginate beads. These beads were composed of a layer-by-layer structure with a porous core, along with quercetin (DOX:CS/CMCS-NGs/Qu-M-ALG-beads). At low pH of 7.0, DOX:CS/CMCS-NGs/Qu-M-ALG-beads resisted the swallowing test, but DOX:CS/CMCS-NGs and quercetin were gradually released at pH > 7.0. Chitosan induced mucoadhesion and, more importantly, the ability to open the tight junction in the intestinal epithelium, which promoted DOX paracellular permeation [149,150]. Quercetin, a P-gp inhibitor, enhanced DOX absorption by inhibiting the P-gp-mediated efflux of DOX. In addition, the M-cell-mediated endocytosis of DOX:CS/CMCS-NGs could increase the BA of DOX. As a result, orally administered DOX:CS/CMCS-NGs/Qu-M-ALG-beads had a 18.65-fold higher AUC compared with free oral DOX, and its absolute BA was calculated as 55.8% [173] (Table 4).

(4) MSNs

MSNs have been approved by the US FDA for clinical trials of cancer formulations because of their adjustable porous structure, ability to induce surface modification, high loading efficiency, excellent biocompatibility, and biodegradability [174]. The pharmacokinetics of DOX-loaded MSNs of three different sizes or shapes were evaluated in rats. The particle size of MSNs ranged from 100 to 200 nm with a stable negative zeta potential. The viability test in Caco-2 cells revealed that 80% of MSNs were nontoxic. DOX–MSN with a rod shape and size of 200 nm had higher C_{max} and greater AUC than orally administered free DOX. The relative BA enhancement of DOX–MSN with a rod shape was 5.9-fold compared with free DOX [175] (Table 4).

With the ease of surface modification in MSNs, DOX loading and surface functionalization of MSNs to modify their release profile and therapeutic efficacy have also been investigated. DOX-loaded MSNs modified with (3-aminopropyl)triethoxysilane (DOX–MSN–APTES) possess a negative charge under normal cell conditions (pH 7.4), which becomes positive after exposure to the acidic tumor environment (pH 5.0). The benefit of charge-reversible MSNs is long-term drug stability in the serum (pH 7.4), which permits the sustained release of DOX for 7 days in KB cells; in surface unmodified MSNs, DOX release was completed within 8 h [176].

Furthermore, DOX–MSN coated with soybean lecithin and DSPE-PEG2000 (DOX–MSN–phospholipids) have been formulated. DOX–MSN coated with phospholipids increased the zeta potential from −25 to −1.0 mV and enhanced the affinity toward the cell membrane lipid bilayer. Consequently, DOX–MSN–phospholipids showed a pH-sensitive release profile (i.e., 3.5–5-fold higher DOX release at pH 5.0 than at pH 7.4) and enhanced internalization of DOX–MSN–phospholipids. Despite the relatively low loading efficiency of 16%, DOX–MSN–phospholipids showed a 2-fold increase in cytotoxicity and 10-fold reduction in hemolysis percentage [177].

Dual-stimuli-responsive HA conjugated with MSN via a disulfide link was prepared. CD44 receptors were responsive to HA and actively uptook HA-modified MSNs encapsulating DOX, which resulted in 3-fold higher DOX uptake in CD44-positive HCT-116 cells than that in CD44-negative NIH-3T3 cells. Another study used GSH as a stimulant. High levels of GSH facilitated enhanced DOX release at low pH (pH 5.0) compared with that at pH 7.4 [178]. This surface modified MSN could be a strategy for stimuli-responsive targeted cancer therapy.

(5) Clay mineral formulation

Clay minerals are biocompatible and low-cost materials that have been shown to modify the release and increase the solubility of drugs [179]. Recently, hematite NPs were added to DOX loaded chitosan-poly vinyl pyrrolidone hydrogels to deliver DOX to MCF-7 cancer cells, based on its pH-responsiveness. This formulation enabled pH-sensitive delivery to cancer cells and sustained DOX release [180]. Montmorillonite (MMT) clay mineral has been frequently used as a drug carrier due to its excellent cation exchange capacity and biocompatibility. Rahmani et al. [181] prepared a pH—sensitive chitosan—MMT—nitrogen—doped carbon quantum dots (NCQDs) nanocomposite and loaded DOX. This formulation showed pH-sensitive sustained release of DOX at pH 5.4 over a 96-h period, but no diffusion was observed at pH 7.4. It also showed significantly higher cytotoxicity toward MCF-7 cells compared with free DOX [181]. In addition, MMT nanosheets effectively intercalated and stabilized DOX. MMT also showed pH-sensitive sustained release at pH 6.0 and increased cytotoxicity in MCF-7 cells. pH-sensitive release profiles of DOX from MMT nanosheets are related to the protonation of negatively charged nanoclays in weakly acidic solutions, which make it easier to dissociate with positively charged DOX [179,182].

Similarly, Huang et al. prepared four layers of MMT nanosheets that stably intercalated PEGylated chitosan (PEG-CS/MMT). The multilayered PEG-CS/MMT showed superior DOX loading efficiency, was located within acid organelles, and elicited cell apoptosis [183], which can give a rationale to MMT nanosheets as a cancer chemotherapeutic drug delivery system. Further investigations regarding the beneficial effects on the pharmacokinetics and therapeutic effects of DOX in in vivo preclinical and clinical studies need to be performed.

Table 4. DOX formulations to increase oral BA.

Carrier–Type	Formulation & Route of Administration	Experimental Model	Findings	References
PMs	Linolenic acid–chitosan-based PMs (DOX-CS-LA), PO	SD rat	Mucoadhesive formulation Targeting the intestinal fatty acid transporter Increase in relative BA by 166% compared with that of free DOX	[152]
	Lysine-linked ditocopherol polyethylene glycol 2000 succinate (PLV2K-DOX), PO	SD rat	Intestinal permeability of PLV2K–DOX was 3.19-, 1.61-, and 1.80-fold higher than that of free DOX in the duodenum, jejunum, and ileum Orally administered PLV2K–DOX showed 5.6-fold higher AUC than free DOX in rats	[153,154]
	Oleanolic acid conjugated methoxy-poly (ethylene glycol)-poly (D, L-lactide) (mPEG-PLA-OA), PO	Wistar rats	A 30-fold increased DOX circulation time and 30-fold reduced clearance time	[155]

Table 4. Cont.

Carrier–Type	Formulation & Route of Administration	Experimental Model	Findings	References
PNPs	DOX-loaded poly (lactic-co-glycolic acid) (PLGA) NPs, PO	SD rats	BA enhancement by 363% and reduced cardiotoxicity	[165]
		Breast cancer bearing rats	Reduced tumor size, increased survival rate, and reduced cardiotoxicity	
	Chitosan coated–daunorubicin PLGA–NPs, PO	Wistar rats	Compared with free daunorubicin, a 11.3-fold higher AUC and 2.8-fold delay in the elimination of daunorubicin from the plasma	[168]
	PEGylated-DOX-loaded-PLGA–NPs, PO	Wistar rats	Compared with free DOX, a 11.8-fold higher AUC and 2.1-fold delay in the elimination of DOX from the plasma	[167]
	Chitosan modified chitosan diacetate (CDA) and chitosan triacetate (CTA)-NPs, PO	MCF-7 cells	Approximately 2-fold increased permeability of DOX in MCF-7 cells	[169]
		SD rats	Compared with free DOX, sustained release for 24 h, and 3-fold increase in the AUC of DOX–CTA NPs	
	Intestine-penetrating, pH-sensitive and double layered NPs, PO	H22-tumor bearing mice	Relative BA of 75.4% with effective inhibition of tumor growth. DOX concentrations in major tissues did not exceed the maximum tolerated concentration. Approximately 40% of the absorbed DOX accumulated in the tumor tissue	[170]
	Sodium caseinate (NaCN) NPs, PO	4T1-breast cancer bearing mice	A 8-fold tumor shrinkage compared with that of free DOX. Following the oral administration of DOX–NaCN NPs, DOX in tumor tissues showed 8.34-fold higher accumulation than IV DOX and 1.27-fold higher accumulation than IV DOX–NaCN NPs	[172]
MMS	Mutilayer alginate beads with codelivery of chitosan-DOX nanogel and quercetin (DOX:CS/CMCS-NGs /Qu-M-ALG-Beads), PO	SD rats	pH-sensitive release at pH > 7.0. Chitosan increased DOX absorption via mucoadhesion and tight-junction opening. Quercetin increased DOX absorption by inhibiting P-gp. BA of DOX:CS/CMCS-NGs/Qu-M-ALG-beads was 55.8%	[173]
MSNs	DOX loaded MSN (DOX-MSN), PO	SD rats	DOX–MSN with a rod shape and size of 200 nm showed 5.9-fold enhancement in relative BA compared with free DOX	[175]

PM: Polymeric micelle; PNP: Polymeric nanoparticles; MMS: Multilayer micro-dispersing system; MSN: Mesoporous silica nanoparticles; DOX:CS/CMCS-NGs/Qu-M-ALG-Beads: DOX-chitosan complex incorporating carboxymethyl chitosan nanogels in the core of MMS and querctin modified alginate beads; AUC: Area under the curve; PO: per os.; BA: Bioavailability; SD rats: Sprague-Dawley rats.

4. Future Perspectives

IV administrations of liposomal DOX formulations have shown great improvement in terms of prolonged DOX circulation and reduced cardiotoxicity. Future DOX formulation strategies can be developed via three approaches: (1) increasing tumor targetability using the tumor microenvironment, (2) increasing therapeutic efficacy by achieving more favorable pharmacokinetic properties and reducing DOX resistance, and (3) enhancing the oral BA by switching from IV to PO formulation. DOX formulations that inhibit the P-gp function have been evaluated for developing more effective formulations that can reduce the occurrence of drug resistance and enhance oral absorption. However, the use of a simple P-gp inhibitor in DOX formulations seemed to be ineffective. In addition, pH- or ROS-sensitive DOX formulations (e.g., pH-sensitive PLs, PNPs, and PMs and ROS-sensitive liposomes and MSNs; Table 2) effectively increased DOX concentrations in tumor cells following parenteral administration. In particular, the use of ROS- or pH-sensitive excipients along with Rc-targeted ligands in the outer shell and DOX and P-gp inhibitor inside of core formulation have been reported to increase the targetability of the formulation and sequential release of DOX and P-gp inhibitors in tumor cells. Consequently, these DOX formulations reduced the tumor size (Table 3); however, they were also administered parenterally.

Regarding the oral formulation of DOX, multifunctional and sequential release of functional excipients may show promising BA enhancement and more effective anticancer activity. DOX undergoes limited intestinal absorption because of low paracellular permeability and P-gp-mediated efflux. To increase the intestinal absorption of DOX, a mucoadhesive agent, tight-junction modulator, and/or P-gp inhibitor must be used as the outer shell of the formulation. After absorption, DOX formulations with a pH- or ROS-sensitive core can show better tumor targetability and provide therapeutic benefits. Among the tested formulations, chitosan-modified or intestine-penetrating, pH-sensitive, and double-layered nanoparticles (PNP and MMS; Table 4) significantly increased oral BA, showed enhanced antitumor activity, and reduced cardiotoxicity [170]. Nevertheless, these oral DOX formulations have not yet been tested on humans.

These multifunctional and sequential-release DOX formulations warrant further validation in patients with cancer, and the success of these formulations will depend not only on improved efficacy, reduced toxicity, and enhanced oral BA in humans but also on improved manufacturing processes and market competition. We hope that this strategy of creating multifunctional and sequential-release DOX formulations using a mucoadhesive agent, tight-junction modulator, and P-gp inhibitor in the outer shell and a pH- or ROS-sensitive core will expand the oral administration of DOX.

Author Contributions: Conceptualization, J.L. and I.-S.S.; data curation, J.L. and I.-S.S.; writing—original draft preparation, J.L.; writing—review and editing, M.-K.C. and I.-S.S.; visualization, M.-K.C. and I.-S.S.; supervision, M.-K.C. and I.-S.S.; project administration, I.-S.S.; funding acquisition, I.-S.S. All authors have read and agreed to the published version of the manuscript.

Funding: This work was supported, in part, by a National Research Foundation of Korea (NRF) grant funded by the Korean government (MSIT) (No. NRF-2020R1I1A3074384 and NRF-2020R1A5A2017323).

Institutional Review Board Statement: Not applicable.

Informed Consent Statement: Not applicable.

Data Availability Statement: Not applicable.

Conflicts of Interest: The authors declare no conflict of interest.

References

1. Gotwals, P.; Cameron, S.; Cipolletta, D.; Cremasco, V.; Crystal, A.; Hewes, B.; Mueller, B.; Quaratino, S.; Sabatos-Peyton, C.; Petruzzelli, L.; et al. Prospects for combining targeted and conventional cancer therapy with immunotherapy. *Nat. Rev. Cancer* **2017**, *17*, 286–301. [CrossRef] [PubMed]
2. Le Lay, K.; Myon, E.; Hill, S.; Riou-Franca, L.; Scott, D.; Sidhu, M.; Dunlop, D.; Launois, R. Comparative cost-minimisation of oral and intravenous chemotherapy for first-line treatment of non-small cell lung cancer in the UK NHS system. *Eur. J. Health Econ.* **2007**, *8*, 145–151. [CrossRef] [PubMed]
3. Cassidy, J.; Douillard, J.Y.; Twelves, C.; McKendrick, J.J.; Scheithauer, W.; Bustová, I.; Johnston, P.G.; Lesniewski-Kmak, K.; Jelic, S.; Fountzilas, G.; et al. Pharmacoeconomic analysis of adjuvant oral capecitabine vs intravenous 5-FU/LV in Dukes' C colon cancer: The X-ACT trial. *Br. J. Cancer* **2006**, *94*, 1122–1129. [CrossRef] [PubMed]
4. Terwogt, J.M.; Schellens, J.H.; Huinink, W.W.; Beijnen, J.H. Clinical pharmacology of anticancer agents in relation to formulations and administration routes. *Cancer Treat. Rev.* **1999**, *25*, 83–101. [CrossRef]
5. Tu, L.; Cheng, M.; Sun, Y.; Fang, Y.; Liu, J.; Liu, W.; Feng, J.; Jin, Y. Fabrication of ultra-small nanocrystals by formation of hydrogen bonds: In vitro and in vivo evaluation. *Int. J. Pharm.* **2020**, *573*, 118730. [CrossRef]

6. Mohammad, I.S.; Hu, H.; Yin, L.; He, W. Drug nanocrystals: Fabrication methods and promising therapeutic applications. *Int. J. Pharm.* **2019**, *562*, 187–202. [CrossRef]
7. Lozoya-Agullo, I.; González-Álvarez, I.; González-Álvarez, M.; Merino-Sanjuán, M.; Bermejo, M. Development of an ion-pair to improve the colon permeability of a low permeability drug: Atenolol. *Eur. J. Pharm. Sci.* **2016**, *93*, 334–340. [CrossRef]
8. Zhao, J.; Yang, J.; Xie, Y. Improvement strategies for the oral bioavailability of poorly water-soluble flavonoids: An overview. *Int. J. Pharm.* **2019**, *570*, 118642. [CrossRef]
9. Yang, S.H.; Lee, M.G. Dose-independent pharmacokinetics of ondansetron in rats: Contribution of hepatic and intestinal first-pass effects to low bioavailability. *Biopharm. Drug Dispos.* **2008**, *29*, 414–426. [CrossRef]
10. Rivankar, S. An overview of doxorubicin formulations in cancer therapy. *J. Cancer Res. Ther.* **2014**, *10*, 853–858. [CrossRef]
11. Tewey, K.M.; Rowe, T.C.; Yang, L.; Halligan, B.D.; Liu, L.F. Adriamycin-induced DNA damage mediated by mammalian DNA topoisomerase II. *Science* **1984**, *226*, 466–468. [CrossRef] [PubMed]
12. Dong, K.C.; Berger, J.M. Structural basis for gate-DNA recognition and bending by type IIA topoisomerases. *Nature* **2007**, *450*, 1201–1205. [CrossRef] [PubMed]
13. Nitiss, J.L. DNA topoisomerase II and its growing repertoire of biological functions. *Nat. Rev. Cancer* **2009**, *9*, 327–337. [CrossRef] [PubMed]
14. Nitiss, J.L. Targeting DNA topoisomerase II in cancer chemotherapy. *Nat. Rev. Cancer* **2009**, *9*, 338–350. [CrossRef]
15. Perego, P.; Corna, E.; De Cesare, M.; Gatti, L.; Polizzi, D.; Pratesi, G.; Supino, R.; Zunino, F. Role of apoptosis and apoptosis-related genes in cellular response and antitumor efficacy of anthracyclines. *Curr. Med. Chem.* **2001**, *8*, 31–37. [CrossRef]
16. Pang, B.; Qiao, X.; Janssen, L.; Velds, A.; Groothuis, T.; Kerkhoven, R.; Nieuwland, M.; Ovaa, H.; Rottenberg, S.; van Tellingen, O.; et al. Drug-induced histone eviction from open chromatin contributes to the chemotherapeutic effects of doxorubicin. *Nat. Commun.* **2013**, *4*, 1908. [CrossRef]
17. Yang, F.; Kemp, C.J.; Henikoff, S. Doxorubicin enhances nucleosome turnover around promoters. *Curr. Biol.* **2013**, *23*, 782–787. [CrossRef]
18. Gorovsky, M.A.; Keevert, J.B. Absence of histone F1 in a mitotically dividing, genetically inactive nucleus. *Proc. Natl. Acad. Sci. USA* **1975**, *72*, 2672–2676. [CrossRef]
19. Kim, J.-E.; Cho, H.-J.; Kim, J.S.; Shim, C.-K.; Chung, S.-J.; Oak, M.-H.; Yoon, I.-S.; Kim, D.-D. The limited intestinal absorption via paracellular pathway is responsible for the low oral bioavailability of doxorubicin. *Xenobiotica* **2013**, *43*, 579–591. [CrossRef]
20. Bukowski, K.; Kciuk, M.; Kontek, R. Mechanisms of Multidrug Resistance in Cancer Chemotherapy. *Int. J. Mol. Sci.* **2020**, *21*, 3233. [CrossRef]
21. Lage, H. ABC-transporters: Implications on drug resistance from microorganisms to human cancers. *Int. J. Antimicrob. Agents* **2003**, *22*, 188–199. [CrossRef] [PubMed]
22. Hershman, D.L.; McBride, R.B.; Eisenberger, A.; Tsai, W.Y.; Grann, V.R.; Jacobson, J.S. Doxorubicin, cardiac risk factors, and cardiac toxicity in elderly patients with diffuse B-cell non-Hodgkin's lymphoma. *J. Clin. Oncol.* **2008**, *26*, 3159–3165. [CrossRef] [PubMed]
23. Gou, M.; Shi, H.; Guo, G.; Men, K.; Zhang, J.; Zheng, L.; Li, Z.; Luo, F.; Qian, Z.; Zhao, X.; et al. Improving anticancer activity and reducing systemic toxicity of doxorubicin by self-assembled polymeric micelles. *Nanotechnology* **2011**, *22*, 095102. [CrossRef] [PubMed]
24. Bangham, A.D.; Standish, M.M.; Watkins, J.C. Diffusion of univalent ions across the lamellae of swollen phospholipids. *J. Mol. Biol.* **1965**, *13*, 238–252. [CrossRef]
25. Choi, M.K.; Nam, S.J.; Ji, H.Y.; Park, M.J.; Choi, J.S.; Song, I.S. Comparative pharmacokinetics and pharmacodynamics of a novel sodium-glucose cotransporter 2 Inhibitor, DWP16001, with dapagliflozin and ipragliflozin. *Pharmaceutics* **2020**, *12*, 268. [CrossRef]
26. Taléns-Visconti, R.; Díez-Sales, O.; de Julián-Ortiz, J.V.; Nácher, A. Nanoliposomes in Cancer Therapy: Marketed Products and Current Clinical Trials. *Int. J. Mol. Sci.* **2022**, *23*, 4249. [CrossRef] [PubMed]
27. Green, A.E.; Rose, P.G. Pegylated liposomal doxorubicin in ovarian cancer. *Int. J. Nanomedicine* **2006**, *1*, 229–239.
28. Gheibi Hayat, S.M.; Jaafari, M.R.; Hatamipour, M.; Jamialahmadi, T.; Sahebkar, A. Harnessing CD47 mimicry to inhibit phagocytic clearance and enhance anti-tumor efficacy of nanoliposomal doxorubicin. *Expert. Opin. Drug Deliv.* **2020**, *17*, 1049–1058. [CrossRef]
29. Waterhouse, D.N.; Tardi, P.G.; Mayer, L.D.; Bally, M.B. A comparison of liposomal formulations of doxorubicin with drug administered in free form: Changing toxicity profiles. *Drug Saf.* **2001**, *24*, 903–920. [CrossRef]
30. Jain, R.K. Normalization of tumor vasculature: An emerging concept in antiangiogenic therapy. *Science* **2005**, *307*, 58–62. [CrossRef]
31. Fang, C.; Shi, B.; Pei, Y.Y.; Hong, M.H.; Wu, J.; Chen, H.Z. In vivo tumor targeting of tumor necrosis factor-alpha-loaded stealth nanoparticles: Effect of MePEG molecular weight and particle size. *Eur. J. Pharm. Sci.* **2006**, *27*, 27–36. [CrossRef] [PubMed]
32. Ambegia, E.; Ansell, S.; Cullis, P.; Heyes, J.; Palmer, L.; MacLachlan, I. Stabilized plasmid-lipid particles containing PEG-diacylglycerols exhibit extended circulation lifetimes and tumor selective gene expression. *Biochim. Biophys. Acta* **2005**, *1669*, 155–163. [CrossRef]

33. Hatakeyama, H.; Akita, H.; Kogure, K.; Oishi, M.; Nagasaki, Y.; Kihira, Y.; Ueno, M.; Kobayashi, H.; Kikuchi, H.; Harashima, H. Development of a novel systemic gene delivery system for cancer therapy with a tumor-specific cleavable PEG-lipid. *Gene Ther.* **2007**, *14*, 68–77. [CrossRef] [PubMed]
34. Zhu, L.; Lin, M. The Synthesis of Nano-Doxorubicin and its Anticancer Effect. *Anticancer Agents Med. Chem.* **2021**, *21*, 2466–2477. [CrossRef] [PubMed]
35. Motohashi, T.; Yabuno, A.; Michimae, H.; Ohishi, T.; Nonaka, M.; Takano, M.; Nishio, S.; Fujiwara, H.; Fujiwara, K.; Kondo, E.; et al. Randomized phase III trial comparing pegylated liposomal doxorubicin (PLD) at 50 mg/m^2 versus 40 mg/m^2 in patients with platinum-refractory and -resistant ovarian carcinoma: The JGOG 3018 Trial. *J. Gynecol. Oncol.* **2021**, *32*, e9. [CrossRef]
36. Swenson, C.E.; Perkins, W.R.; Roberts, P.; Janoff, A.S. Liposome technology and the development of Myocet™ (liposomal doxorubicin citrate). *Breast* **2001**, *10*, 1–7. [CrossRef]
37. Rafiyath, S.M.; Rasul, M.; Lee, B.; Wei, G.; Lamba, G.; Liu, D. Comparison of safety and toxicity of liposomal doxorubicin vs. conventional anthracyclines: A meta-analysis. *Exp. Hematol. Oncol.* **2012**, *1*, 10. [CrossRef]
38. Hudes, G. Boosting bioavailability of topotecan: What do we gain? *J. Clin. Oncol.* **2002**, *20*, 2918–2919. [CrossRef]
39. Kerklaan, B.M.; Jager, A.; Aftimos, P.; Dieras, V.; Altintas, S.; Anders, C.; Arnedos, M.; Gelderblom, H.; Soetekouw, P.; Gladdines, W.; et al. NT-23 phase 1/2a study of gluthathione PEGylated liposomal doxorubicin (2B3-101) in breast cancer patients with brain metastasis (BCMB) or recurrent high grade gliomas (HGC). *Neuro-Oncol.* **2014**, *16*, v163. [CrossRef]
40. Wicki, A.; Ritschard, R.; Loesch, U.; Deuster, S.; Rochlitz, C.; Mamot, C. Large-scale manufacturing of GMP-compliant anti-EGFR targeted nanocarriers: Production of doxorubicin-loaded anti-EGFR-immunoliposomes for a first-in-man clinical trial. *Int. J. Pharm.* **2015**, *484*, 8–15. [CrossRef]
41. Mamot, C.; Ritschard, R.; Wicki, A.; Stehle, G.; Dieterle, T.; Bubendorf, L.; Hilker, C.; Deuster, S.; Herrmann, R.; Rochlitz, C. Tolerability, safety, pharmacokinetics, and efficacy of doxorubicin-loaded anti-EGFR immunoliposomes in advanced solid tumours: A phase 1 dose-escalation study. *Lancet Oncol.* **2012**, *13*, 1234–1241. [CrossRef] [PubMed]
42. Kumari, P.; Ghosh, B.; Biswas, S. Nanocarriers for cancer-targeted drug delivery. *J. Drug Target.* **2016**, *24*, 179–191. [CrossRef]
43. Oerlemans, C.; Bult, W.; Bos, M.; Storm, G.; Nijsen, J.F.; Hennink, W.E. Polymeric micelles in anticancer therapy: Targeting, imaging and triggered release. *Pharm. Res.* **2010**, *27*, 2569–2589. [CrossRef]
44. Kwon, M.; Lim, D.Y.; Lee, C.H.; Jeon, J.H.; Choi, M.K.; Song, I.S. Enhanced intestinal absorption and pharmacokinetic modulation of berberine and its metabolites through the inhibition of P-glycoprotein and intestinal metabolism in rats using a berberine mixed micelle formulation. *Pharmaceutics* **2020**, *12*, 882. [CrossRef] [PubMed]
45. Choi, Y.A.; Yoon, Y.H.; Choi, K.; Kwon, M.; Goo, S.H.; Cha, J.S.; Choi, M.K.; Lee, H.S.; Song, I.S. Enhanced oral bioavailability of morin administered in mixed micelle formulation with PluronicF127 and Tween80 in rats. *Biol. Pharm. Bull.* **2015**, *38*, 208–217. [CrossRef] [PubMed]
46. Danson, S.; Ferry, D.; Alakhov, V.; Margison, J.; Kerr, D.; Jowle, D.; Brampton, M.; Halbert, G.; Ranson, M. Phase I dose escalation and pharmacokinetic study of pluronic polymer-bound doxorubicin (SP1049C) in patients with advanced cancer. *Br. J. Cancer* **2004**, *90*, 2085–2091. [CrossRef]
47. Valle, J.W.; Armstrong, A.; Newman, C.; Alakhov, V.; Pietrzynski, G.; Brewer, J.; Campbell, S.; Corrie, P.; Rowinsky, E.K.; Ranson, M. A phase 2 study of SP1049C, doxorubicin in P-glycoprotein-targeting pluronics, in patients with advanced adenocarcinoma of the esophagus and gastroesophageal junction. *Investig. New Drugs* **2011**, *29*, 1029–1037. [CrossRef]
48. Varela-Moreira, A.; Shi, Y.; Fens, M.H.A.M.; Lammers, T.; Hennink, W.E.; Schiffelers, R.M. Clinical application of polymeric micelles for the treatment of cancer. *Mater. Chem. Front.* **2017**, *1*, 1485–1501. [CrossRef]
49. Matsumura, Y.; Hamaguchi, T.; Ura, T.; Muro, K.; Yamada, Y.; Shimada, Y.; Shirao, K.; Okusaka, T.; Ueno, H.; Ikeda, M.; et al. Phase I clinical trial and pharmacokinetic evaluation of NK911, a micelle-encapsulated doxorubicin. *Br. J. Cancer* **2004**, *91*, 1775–1781. [CrossRef]
50. Razak, S.A.; Mohd Gazzali, A.; Fisol, F.A.; Abdulbaqi, I.M.; Parumasivam, T.; Mohtar, N.; Wahab, H.A. Advances in Nanocarriers for Effective Delivery of Docetaxel in the Treatment of Lung Cancer: An Overview. *Cancers* **2021**, *13*, 400. [CrossRef]
51. Mura, S.; Fattal, E.; Nicolas, J. From poly(alkyl cyanoacrylate) to squalene as core material for the design of nanomedicines. *J. Drug Target.* **2019**, *27*, 470–501. [CrossRef] [PubMed]
52. Graur, F.; Puia, A.; Mois, E.I.; Moldovan, S.; Pusta, A.; Cristea, C.; Cavalu, S.; Puia, C.; Al Hajjar, N. Nanotechnology in the Diagnostic and Therapy of Hepatocellular Carcinoma. *Materials* **2022**, *15*, 3893. [CrossRef] [PubMed]
53. Ekladious, I.; Colson, Y.L.; Grinstaff, M.W. Polymer-drug conjugate therapeutics: Advances, insights and prospects. *Nat. Rev. Drug Discov.* **2019**, *18*, 273–294. [CrossRef] [PubMed]
54. Duncan, R. Development of HPMA copolymer-anticancer conjugates: Clinical experience and lessons learnt. *Adv. Drug Deliv. Rev.* **2009**, *61*, 1131–1148. [CrossRef] [PubMed]
55. Vasey, P.A.; Kaye, S.B.; Morrison, R.; Twelves, C.; Wilson, P.; Duncan, R.; Thomson, A.H.; Murray, L.S.; Hilditch, T.E.; Murray, T.; et al. Phase I clinical and pharmacokinetic study of PK1 [N-(2-hydroxypropyl)methacrylamide copolymer doxorubicin]: First member of a new class of chemotherapeutic agents-drug-polymer conjugates. Cancer Research Campaign Phase I/II Committee. *Clin. Cancer Res.* **1999**, *5*, 83–94. [PubMed]

56. Seymour, L.W.; Ferry, D.R.; Kerr, D.J.; Rea, D.; Whitlock, M.; Poyner, R.; Boivin, C.; Hesslewood, S.; Twelves, C.; Blackie, R.; et al. Phase II studies of polymer-doxorubicin (PK1, FCE28068) in the treatment of breast, lung and colorectal cancer. *Int. J. Oncol.* **2009**, *34*, 1629–1636. [CrossRef]
57. Seymour, L.W.; Ferry, D.R.; Anderson, D.; Hesslewood, S.; Julyan, P.J.; Poyner, R.; Doran, J.; Young, A.M.; Burtles, S.; Kerr, D.J. Hepatic drug targeting: Phase I evaluation of polymer-bound doxorubicin. *J. Clin. Oncol.* **2002**, *20*, 1668–1676. [CrossRef]
58. Eisenmann, E.D.; Talebi, Z.; Sparreboom, A.; Baker, S.D. Boosting the oral bioavailability of anticancer drugs through intentional drug-drug interactions. *Basic Clin. Pharmacol. Toxicol.* **2022**, *130* (Suppl. 1), 23–35. [CrossRef]
59. Boedtkjer, E.; Pedersen, S.F. The Acidic Tumor Microenvironment as a Driver of Cancer. *Annu. Rev. Physiol.* **2020**, *82*, 103–126. [CrossRef] [PubMed]
60. Simões, S.; Moreira, J.N.; Fonseca, C.; Düzgüneş, N.; de Lima, M.C. On the formulation of pH-sensitive liposomes with long circulation times. *Adv. Drug Deliv. Rev.* **2004**, *56*, 947–965. [CrossRef]
61. Karanth, H.; Murthy, R.S. pH-sensitive liposomes–principle and application in cancer therapy. *J. Pharm. Pharmacol.* **2007**, *59*, 469–483. [CrossRef]
62. Koudelka, S.; Turanek Knotigova, P.; Masek, J.; Prochazka, L.; Lukac, R.; Miller, A.D.; Neuzil, J.; Turanek, J. Liposomal delivery systems for anti-cancer analogues of vitamin E. *J. Control. Release* **2015**, *207*, 59–69. [CrossRef] [PubMed]
63. de Oliveira Silva, J.; Miranda, S.E.M.; Leite, E.A.; de Paula Sabino, A.; Borges, K.B.G.; Cardoso, V.N.; Cassali, G.D.; Guimarães, A.G.; Oliveira, M.C.; de Barros, A.L.B. Toxicological study of a new doxorubicin-loaded pH-sensitive liposome: A preclinical approach. *Toxicol. Appl. Pharmacol.* **2018**, *352*, 162–169. [CrossRef] [PubMed]
64. de Oliveira Silva, J.; Fernandes, R.S.; Ramos Oda, C.M.; Ferreira, T.H.; Machado Botelho, A.F.; Martins Melo, M.; de Miranda, M.C.; Assis Gomes, D.; Dantas Cassali, G.; Townsend, D.M.; et al. Folate-coated, long-circulating and pH-sensitive liposomes enhance doxorubicin antitumor effect in a breast cancer animal model. *Biomed. Pharmacother.* **2019**, *118*, 109323. [CrossRef] [PubMed]
65. Bobde, Y.; Biswas, S.; Ghosh, B. PEGylated N-(2 hydroxypropyl) methacrylamide-doxorubicin conjugate as pH-responsive polymeric nanoparticles for cancer therapy. *React. Funct. Polym.* **2020**, *151*, 104561. [CrossRef]
66. Cavalcante, C.H.; Fernandes, R.S.; de Oliveira Silva, J.; Oda, C.M.R.; Leite, E.A.; Cassali, G.D.; Charlie-Silva, I.; Fernandes, B.H.V.; Ferreira, L.A.M.; de Barros, A.L.B. Doxorubicin-loaded pH-sensitive micelles: A promising alternative to enhance antitumor activity and reduce toxicity. *Biomed. Pharmacother.* **2021**, *134*, 111076. [CrossRef]
67. Perillo, B.; Di Donato, M.; Pezone, A.; Di Zazzo, E.; Giovannelli, P.; Galasso, G.; Castoria, G.; Migliaccio, A. ROS in cancer therapy: The bright side of the moon. *Exp. Mol. Med.* **2020**, *52*, 192–203. [CrossRef]
68. Mirhadi, E.; Mashreghi, M.; Askarizadeh, A.; Mehrabian, A.; Alavizadeh, S.H.; Arabi, L.; Badiee, A.; Jaafari, M.R. Redox-sensitive doxorubicin liposome: A formulation approach for targeted tumor therapy. *Sci. Rep.* **2022**, *12*, 11310. [CrossRef]
69. Bhavsar, D.B.; Patel, V.; Sawant, K.K. Design and characterization of dual responsive mesoporous silica nanoparticles for breast cancer targeted therapy. *Eur. J. Pharm. Sci.* **2020**, *152*, 105428. [CrossRef]
70. Mirzaei, S.; Zarrabi, A.; Hashemi, F.; Zabolian, A.; Saleki, H.; Azami, N.; Hamzehlou, S.; Farahani, M.V.; Hushmandi, K.; Ashrafizadeh, M. Nrf2 signaling pathway in chemoprotection and doxorubicin resistance: Potential application in drug discovery. *Antioxidants* **2021**, *10*, 349. [CrossRef]
71. Calcabrini, C.; Maffei, F.; Turrini, E.; Fimognari, C. Sulforaphane potentiates anticancer effects of doxorubicin and cisplatin and mitigates their toxic effects. *Front. Pharmacol.* **2020**, *11*, 567. [CrossRef]
72. Ryoo, I.-g.; Kim, G.; Choi, B.-h.; Lee, S.-h.; Kwak, M.-K. Involvement of NRF2 signaling in doxorubicin resistance of cancer stem cell-enriched colonospheres. *Biomol. Ther.* **2016**, *24*, 482. [CrossRef] [PubMed]
73. Gu, T.-T.; Li, C.; Xu, Y.; Zhang, L.; Shan, X.; Huang, X.; Guo, L.; Chen, K.; Wang, X.; Ge, H. Stimuli-responsive combination therapy of cisplatin and Nrf2 siRNA for improving antitumor treatment of osteosarcoma. *Nano Res.* **2020**, *13*, 630–637. [CrossRef]
74. Ojha, T.; Pathak, V.; Shi, Y.; Hennink, W.E.; Moonen, C.T.W.; Storm, G.; Kiessling, F.; Lammers, T. Pharmacological and physical vessel modulation strategies to improve EPR-mediated drug targeting to tumors. *Adv. Drug Deliv. Rev.* **2017**, *119*, 44–60. [CrossRef]
75. Xu, W.; Cui, Y.; Ling, P.; Li, L.B. Preparation and evaluation of folate-modified cationic pluronic micelles for poorly soluble anticancer drug. *Drug Deliv.* **2012**, *19*, 208–219. [CrossRef] [PubMed]
76. Jia, Y.; Chen, S.; Wang, C.; Sun, T.; Yang, L. Hyaluronic acid-based nano drug delivery systems for breast cancer treatment: Recent advances. *Front. Bioeng. Biotechnol.* **2022**, *10*, 990145. [CrossRef]
77. Wang, Y.; Tan, X.; Zhou, Q.; Geng, P.; Wang, J.; Zou, P.; Deng, A.; Hu, J. Co-delivery of doxorubicin and SIS3 by folate-targeted polymeric micelles for overcoming tumor multidrug resistance. *Drug Deliv. Transl. Res.* **2022**, *12*, 167–179. [CrossRef]
78. Qiu, L.; Xu, J.; Ahmed, K.S.; Zhu, M.; Zhang, Y.; Long, M.; Chen, W.; Fang, W.; Zhang, H.; Chen, J. Stimuli-responsive, dual-function prodrug encapsulated in hyaluronic acid micelles to overcome doxorubicin resistance. *Acta Biomater.* **2022**, *140*, 686–699. [CrossRef]
79. Scheeren, L.E.; Nogueira-Librelotto, D.R.; Macedo, L.B.; de Vargas, J.M.; Mitjans, M.; Vinardell, M.P.; Rolim, C.M. Transferrin-conjugated doxorubicin-loaded PLGA nanoparticles with pH-responsive behavior: A synergistic approach for cancer therapy. *J. Nanopart. Res.* **2020**, *22*, 1–18. [CrossRef]

80. Swider, E.; Koshkina, O.; Tel, J.; Cruz, L.J.; de Vries, I.J.M.; Srinivas, M. Customizing poly (lactic-co-glycolic acid) particles for biomedical applications. *Acta Biomater.* **2018**, *73*, 38–51. [CrossRef]
81. Waghray, D.; Zhang, Q. Inhibit or Evade Multidrug Resistance P-Glycoprotein in Cancer Treatment. *J. Med. Chem.* **2018**, *61*, 5108–5121. [CrossRef] [PubMed]
82. Lee, K.Y.; Shueng, P.W.; Chou, C.M.; Lin, B.X.; Lin, M.H.; Kuo, D.Y.; Tsai, I.L.; Wu, S.M.; Lin, C.W. Elevation of CD109 promotes metastasis and drug resistance in lung cancer via activation of EGFR-AKT-mTOR signaling. *Cancer Sci.* **2020**, *111*, 1652–1662. [CrossRef] [PubMed]
83. Christowitz, C.; Davis, T.; Isaacs, A.; Van Niekerk, G.; Hattingh, S.; Engelbrecht, A.-M. Mechanisms of doxorubicin-induced drug resistance and drug resistant tumour growth in a murine breast tumour model. *BMC Cancer* **2019**, *19*, 757. [CrossRef]
84. Ibrahim, I.M.; Abdelmalek, D.H.; Elfiky, A.A. GRP78: A cell's response to stress. *Life Sci.* **2019**, *226*, 156–163. [CrossRef] [PubMed]
85. Xie, J.; Tao, Z.-H.; Zhao, J.; Li, T.; Wu, Z.-H.; Zhang, J.-F.; Zhang, J.; Hu, X.-C. Glucose regulated protein 78 (GRP78) inhibits apoptosis and attentinutes chemosensitivity of gemcitabine in breast cancer cell via AKT/mitochondrial apoptotic pathway. *Biochem. Biophys. Res. Commun.* **2016**, *474*, 612–619. [CrossRef] [PubMed]
86. Tian, S.; Chang, W.; Du, H.; Bai, J.; Sun, Z.; Zhang, Q.; Wang, H.; Zhu, G.; Tao, K.; Long, Y. The interplay between GRP78 expression and Akt activation in human colon cancer cells under celecoxib treatment. *Anti-Cancer Drugs* **2015**, *26*, 964–973. [CrossRef]
87. Fu, Y.; Wey, S.; Wang, M.; Ye, R.; Liao, C.-P.; Roy-Burman, P.; Lee, A.S. Pten null prostate tumorigenesis and AKT activation are blocked by targeted knockout of ER chaperone GRP78/BiP in prostate epithelium. *Proc. Natl. Acad. Sci. USA* **2008**, *105*, 19444–19449. [CrossRef]
88. Grabarnick, E.; Andriyanov, A.V.; Han, H.; Eyal, S.; Barenholz, Y. PEGylated liposomes remotely loaded with the combination of doxorubicin, quinine, and indocyanine green enable successful treatment of multidrug-resistant tumors. *Pharmaceutics* **2021**, *13*, 2181. [CrossRef]
89. Treger, J.S.; Priest, M.F.; Iezzi, R.; Bezanilla, F. Real-time imaging of electrical signals with an infrared FDA-approved dye. *Biophys. J.* **2014**, *107*, L09–L12. [CrossRef]
90. Tamai, K.; Mizushima, T.; Wu, X.; Inoue, A.; Ota, M.; Yokoyama, Y.; Miyoshi, N.; Haraguchi, N.; Takahashi, H.; Nishimura, J. Photodynamic therapy using indocyanine green loaded on super carbonate apatite as minimally invasive cancer treatment. *Mol. Cancer Ther.* **2018**, *17*, 1613–1622. [CrossRef]
91. Master, A.; Livingston, M.; Gupta, A.S. Photodynamic nanomedicine in the treatment of solid tumors: Perspectives and challenges. *J. Control. Release* **2013**, *168*, 88–102. [CrossRef] [PubMed]
92. An, D.; Yu, X.; Jiang, L.; Wang, R.; He, P.; Chen, N.; Guo, X.; Li, X.; Feng, M. Reversal of multidrug resistance by apolipoprotein A1-modified doxorubicin liposome for breast cancer treatment. *Molecules* **2021**, *26*, 1280. [CrossRef] [PubMed]
93. Yuan, Y.; Wang, W.; Wang, B.; Zhu, H.; Zhang, B.; Feng, M. Delivery of hydrophilic drug doxorubicin hydrochloride-targeted liver using apoAI as carrier. *J. Drug Target.* **2013**, *21*, 367–374. [CrossRef] [PubMed]
94. Cui, H.; Huan, M.-l.; Ye, W.-l.; Liu, D.-z.; Teng, Z.-h.; Mei, Q.-B.; Zhou, S.-y. Mitochondria and nucleus dual delivery system to overcome DOX resistance. *Mol. Pharm.* **2017**, *14*, 746–756. [CrossRef]
95. Zhou, M.-X.; Zhang, J.-Y.; Cai, X.-M.; Dou, R.; Ruan, L.-F.; Yang, W.-J.; Lin, W.-C.; Chen, J.; Hu, Y. Tumor-penetrating and mitochondria-targeted drug delivery overcomes doxorubicin resistance in lung cancer. *Chin. J. Polym. Sci.* **2023**, *41*, 525–537. [CrossRef]
96. Zhou, X.-W.; Xia, Y.-Z.; Zhang, Y.-L.; Luo, J.-G.; Han, C.; Zhang, H.; Zhang, C.; Yang, L.; Kong, L.-Y. Tomentodione M sensitizes multidrug resistant cancer cells by decreasing P-glycoprotein via inhibition of p38 MAPK signaling. *Oncotarget* **2017**, *8*, 101965–101983. [CrossRef] [PubMed]
97. Liao, X.; Gao, Y.; Liu, J.; Tao, L.; Xie, J.; Gu, Y.; Liu, T.; Wang, D.; Xie, D.; Mo, S. Combination of Tanshinone IIA and Cisplatin Inhibits Esophageal Cancer by Downregulating NF-κB/COX-2/VEGF Pathway. *Front. Oncol.* **2020**, *10*, 1756. [CrossRef]
98. Wang, R.; Luo, Z.; Zhang, H.; Wang, T. Tanshinone IIA reverses gefitinib-resistance in human non-small-cell lung cancer via regulation of VEGFR/Akt pathway. *Onco. Targets Ther.* **2019**, 9355–9365. [CrossRef]
99. Ye, Y.T.; Zhong, W.; Sun, P.; Wang, D.; Wang, C.; Hu, L.M.; Qian, J.Q. Apoptosis induced by the methanol extract of Salvia miltiorrhiza Bunge in non-small cell lung cancer through PTEN-mediated inhibition of PI3K/Akt pathway. *J. Ethnopharmacol.* **2017**, *200*, 107–116. [CrossRef]
100. Jiang, Q.; Chen, X.; Tian, X.; Zhang, J.; Xue, S.; Jiang, Y.; Liu, T.; Wang, X.; Sun, Q.; Hong, Y.; et al. Tanshinone I inhibits doxorubicin-induced cardiotoxicity by regulating Nrf2 signaling pathway. *Phytomedicine* **2022**, *106*, 154439. [CrossRef] [PubMed]
101. Liu, Y.; Zhang, L.; Ma, Z.; Tian, L.; Liu, Y.; Liu, Y.; Chen, Q.; Li, Y.; Ma, E. Ascorbate promotes the cellular accumulation of doxorubicin and reverses the multidrug resistance in breast cancer cells by inducing ROS-dependent ATP depletion. *Free Radic. Res.* **2019**, *53*, 758–767. [CrossRef] [PubMed]
102. Yang, Y.; Lu, X.; Liu, Q.; Dai, Y.; Zhu, X.; Wen, Y.; Xu, J.; Lu, Y.; Zhao, D.; Chen, X.; et al. Palmitoyl ascorbate and doxorubicin co-encapsulated liposome for synergistic anticancer therapy. *Eur. J. Pharm. Sci.* **2017**, *105*, 219–229. [CrossRef] [PubMed]

103. Liu, Y.; Zhu, M.; Meng, M.; Wang, Q.; Wang, Y.; Lei, Y.; Zhang, Y.; Weng, L.; Chen, X. A dual-responsive hyaluronic acid nanocomposite hydrogel drug delivery system for overcoming multiple drug resistance. *Chin. Chem. Lett.* **2023**, *34*, 107583. [CrossRef]
104. Zhao, H.; Sun, S.; Wang, Z.; Hong, Y.; Shi, L.; Lan, M. pH-sensitive DOX-loaded PAA-PF127-PAA micelles combined with cryotherapy for treating walker 256 carcinosarcoma in a rat model. *J. Nanosci. Nanotechnol.* **2018**, *18*, 8070–8077. [CrossRef]
105. Mahoney, B.P.; Raghunand, N.; Baggett, B.; Gillies, R.J. Tumor acidity, ion trapping and chemotherapeutics: I. Acid pH affects the distribution of chemotherapeutic agents in vitro. *Biochem. Pharmacol.* **2003**, *66*, 1207–1218. [CrossRef] [PubMed]
106. Yoneda, T.; Hiasa, M.; Nagata, Y.; Okui, T.; White, F. Contribution of acidic extracellular microenvironment of cancer-colonized bone to bone pain. *Biochim. Biophys. Acta* **2015**, *1848*, 2677–2684. [CrossRef]
107. Dubowchik, G.M.; Padilla, L.; Edinger, K.; Firestone, R.A. Reversal of doxorubicin resistance and catalytic neutralization of lysosomes by a lipophilic imidazole. *Biochim. Biophys. Acta* **1994**, *1191*, 103–108. [CrossRef]
108. Altan, N.; Chen, Y.; Schindler, M.; Simon, S.M. Tamoxifen inhibits acidification in cells independent of the estrogen receptor. *Proc. Natl. Acad. Sci. USA* **1999**, *96*, 4432–4437. [CrossRef]
109. Abumanhal-Masarweh, H.; Koren, L.; Zinger, A.; Yaari, Z.; Krinsky, N.; Kaneti, G.; Dahan, N.; Lupu-Haber, Y.; Suss-Toby, E.; Weiss-Messer, E. Sodium bicarbonate nanoparticles modulate the tumor pH and enhance the cellular uptake of doxorubicin. *J. Control. Release* **2019**, *296*, 1–13. [CrossRef]
110. Kato, Y.; Ozawa, S.; Miyamoto, C.; Maehata, Y.; Suzuki, A.; Maeda, T.; Baba, Y. Acidic extracellular microenvironment and cancer. *Cancer Cell Int.* **2013**, *13*, 89. [CrossRef]
111. Ando, H.; Ikeda, A.; Tagami, M.; Matsuo, N.C.A.; Shimizu, T.; Ishima, Y.; Eshima, K.; Ishida, T. Oral administration of sodium bicarbonate can enhance the therapeutic outcome of Doxil®via neutralizing the acidic tumor microenvironment. *J. Control. Release* **2022**, *350*, 414–420. [CrossRef] [PubMed]
112. Robey, I.F.; Baggett, B.K.; Kirkpatrick, N.D.; Roe, D.J.; Dosescu, J.; Sloane, B.F.; Hashim, A.I.; Morse, D.L.; Raghunand, N.; Gatenby, R.A. Bicarbonate increases tumor pH and inhibits spontaneous metastases. *Cancer Res.* **2009**, *69*, 2260–2268. [CrossRef] [PubMed]
113. Wang, L.; Luo, Y.; Zheng, Y.; Zheng, L.; Lin, W.; Chen, Z.; Wu, S.; Chen, J.; Xie, Y. Long non-coding RNA LINC00426 contributes to doxorubicin resistance by sponging miR-4319 in osteosarcoma. *Biol. Direct.* **2020**, *15*, 1–11. [CrossRef]
114. Huang, L.; Zeng, L.; Chu, J.; Xu, P.; Lv, M.; Xu, J.; Wen, J.; Li, W.; Wang, L.; Wu, X. Chemoresistance-related long non-coding RNA expression profiles in human breast cancer cells Erratum in/10.3892/mmr. 2019.10003. *Mol. Med. Rep.* **2018**, *18*, 243–253. [CrossRef]
115. Gooding, A.J.; Zhang, B.; Gunawardane, L.; Beard, A.; Valadkhan, S.; Schiemann, W.P. The lncRNA BORG facilitates the survival and chemoresistance of triple-negative breast cancers. *Oncogene* **2019**, *38*, 2020–2041. [CrossRef]
116. Wang, W.; Chen, D.; Zhu, K. SOX2OT variant 7 contributes to the synergistic interaction between EGCG and Doxorubicin to kill osteosarcoma via autophagy and stemness inhibition. *J. Exp. Clin. Cancer Res.* **2018**, *37*, 1–16. [CrossRef]
117. Zhang, Y.; Chen, B.; Wang, Y.; Zhao, Q.; Wu, W.; Zhang, P.; Miao, L.; Sun, S. NOTCH3 Overexpression and Posttranscriptional Regulation by miR-150 Were Associated with EGFR-TKI Resistance in Lung Adenocarcinoma. *Oncol. Res.* **2019**, *27*, 751–761. [CrossRef] [PubMed]
118. Pandey, V.; Chaube, B.; Bhat, M.K. Hyperglycemia regulates MDR-1, drug accumulation and ROS levels causing increased toxicity of carboplatin and 5-fluorouracil in MCF-7 cells. *J. Cell Biochem.* **2011**, *112*, 2942–2952. [CrossRef] [PubMed]
119. Chouhan, S.; Singh, S.; Athavale, D.; Ramteke, P.; Vanuopadath, M.; Nair, B.G.; Nair, S.S.; Bhat, M.K. Sensitization of hepatocellular carcinoma cells towards doxorubicin and sorafenib is facilitated by glucose-dependent alterations in reactive oxygen species, P-glycoprotein and DKK4. *J. Biosci.* **2020**, *45*, 1–23. [CrossRef]
120. Liao, C.H.; Yeh, C.T.; Huang, Y.H.; Wu, S.M.; Chi, H.C.; Tsai, M.M.; Tsai, C.Y.; Liao, C.J.; Tseng, Y.H.; Lin, Y.H. Dickkopf 4 positively regulated by the thyroid hormone receptor suppresses cell invasion in human hepatoma cells. *Hepatology* **2012**, *55*, 910–920. [CrossRef]
121. Baehs, S.; Herbst, A.; Thieme, S.E.; Perschl, C.; Behrens, A.; Scheel, S.; Jung, A.; Brabletz, T.; Göke, B.; Blum, H. Dickkopf-4 is frequently down-regulated and inhibits growth of colorectal cancer cells. *Cancer Lett.* **2009**, *276*, 152–159. [CrossRef]
122. Xi, Y.; Formentini, A.; Nakajima, G.; Kornmann, M.; Ju, J. Validation of biomarkers associated with 5-fluorouracil and thymidylate synthase in colorectal cancer. *Oncol. Rep.* **2008**, *19*, 257–262. [CrossRef] [PubMed]
123. Ensign, L.M.; Cone, R.; Hanes, J. Oral drug delivery with polymeric nanoparticles: The gastrointestinal mucus barriers. *Adv. Drug Deliv. Rev.* **2012**, *64*, 557–570. [CrossRef] [PubMed]
124. Cone, R.A. Barrier properties of mucus. *Adv. Drug Deliv Rev.* **2009**, *61*, 75–85. [CrossRef]
125. Ma, T.Y.; Tran, D.; Hoa, N.; Nguyen, D.; Merryfield, M.; Tarnawski, A. Mechanism of extracellular calcium regulation of intestinal epithelial tight junction permeability: Role of cytoskeletal involvement. *Microsc. Res. Tech.* **2000**, *51*, 156–168. [CrossRef]
126. Speth, P.; Van Hoesel, Q.; Haanen, C. Clinical pharmacokinetics of doxorubicin. *Clin. Pharmacokine* **1988**, *15*, 15–31. [CrossRef] [PubMed]
127. Rawat, P.S.; Jaiswal, A.; Khurana, A.; Bhatti, J.S.; Navik, U. Doxorubicin-induced cardiotoxicity: An update on the molecular mechanism and novel therapeutic strategies for effective management. *Biomed. Pharmacother.* **2021**, *139*, 111708. [CrossRef]

128. Reis-Mendes, A.; Carvalho, F.; Remião, F.; Sousa, E.; Bastos, M.d.L.; Costa, V.M. The main metabolites of fluorouracil+ adriamycin+ cyclophosphamide (FAC) are not major contributors to FAC toxicity in H9c2 cardiac differentiated cells. *Biomolecules* **2019**, *9*, 98. [CrossRef]
129. Mordente, A.; Meucci, E.; Silvestrini, A.; Martorana, G.E.; Giardina, B. New developments in anthracycline-induced cardiotoxicity. *Curr. Med. Chem.* **2009**, *16*, 1656–1672. [CrossRef]
130. Green, P.S.; Leeuwenburgh, C. Mitochondrial dysfunction is an early indicator of doxorubicin-induced apoptosis. *Biochim. Biophys. Acta* **2002**, *1588*, 94–101. [CrossRef]
131. Berthiaume, J.; Wallace, K.B. Adriamycin-induced oxidative mitochondrial cardiotoxicity. *Cell Biol. Toxicol.* **2007**, *23*, 15–25. [CrossRef]
132. Barth, E.; Stämmler, G.; Speiser, B.; Schaper, J. Ultrastructural quantitation of mitochondria and myofilaments in cardiac muscle from 10 different animal species including man. *J. Mol. Cell Cardiol.* **1992**, *24*, 669–681. [CrossRef] [PubMed]
133. Chen, X.; Sun, H.; Hu, J.; Han, X.; Liu, H.; Hu, Y. Transferrin gated mesoporous silica nanoparticles for redox-responsive and targeted drug delivery. *Colloids Surf. B Biointerfaces* **2017**, *152*, 77–84. [CrossRef]
134. Thomas, H.; Coley, H.M. Overcoming multidrug resistance in cancer: An update on the clinical strategy of inhibiting p-glycoprotein. *Cancer Control.* **2003**, *10*, 159–165. [CrossRef] [PubMed]
135. Fox, E.; Bates, S.E. Tariquidar (XR9576): A P-glycoprotein drug efflux pump inhibitor. *Expert Rev. Anticancer Ther.* **2007**, *7*, 447–459. [CrossRef] [PubMed]
136. Meerum Terwogt, J.M.; Malingré, M.M.; Beijnen, J.H.; ten Bokkel Huinink, W.W.; Rosing, H.; Koopman, F.J.; van Tellingen, O.; Swart, M.; Schellens, J.H. Coadministration of oral cyclosporin A enables oral therapy with paclitaxel. *Clin. Cancer Res.* **1999**, *5*, 3379–3384.
137. Malingre, M.; Beijnen, J.; Rosing, H.; Koopman, F.; Jewell, R.; Paul, E.; Huinink, W.; Schellens, J. Co-administration of GF120918 significantly increases the systemic exposure to oral paclitaxel in cancer patients. *Br. J. Cancer* **2001**, *84*, 42–47. [CrossRef]
138. Herben, V.; Rosing, H.; Huinink, W.; Van Zomeren, D.; Batchelor, D.; Doyle, E.; Beusenberg, F.; Beijnen, J.; Schellens, J. Oral topotecan: Bioavailability and effect of food co-administration. *Br. J. Cancer* **1999**, *80*, 1380–1386. [CrossRef]
139. Kruijtzer, C.; Beijnen, J.; Rosing, H.; ten Bokkel Huinink, W.; Schot, M.; Jewell, R.; Paul, E.; Schellens, J. Increased oral bioavailability of topotecan in combination with the breast cancer resistance protein and P-glycoprotein inhibitor GF120918. *J. Clin. Oncol.* **2002**, *20*, 2943–2950. [CrossRef]
140. Kuppens, I.E.; Witteveen, E.O.; Jewell, R.C.; Radema, S.A.; Paul, E.M.; Mangum, S.G.; Beijnen, J.H.; Voest, E.E.; Schellens, J.H. A phase I, randomized, open-label, parallel-cohort, dose-finding study of elacridar (GF120918) and oral topotecan in cancer patients. *Clin. Cancer Res.* **2007**, *13*, 3276–3285. [CrossRef]
141. Jackson, C.G.; Hung, T.; Segelov, E.; Barlow, P.; Prenen, H.; McLaren, B.; Hung, N.A.; Clarke, K.; Chao, T.Y.; Dai, M.S. Oral paclitaxel with encequidar compared to intravenous paclitaxel in patients with advanced cancer: A randomised crossover pharmacokinetic study. *Br. J. Clin. Pharmacol.* **2021**, *87*, 4670–4680. [CrossRef]
142. Kuppens, I.; Bosch, T.; Van Maanen, M.; Rosing, H.; Fitzpatrick, A.; Beijnen, J.; Schellens, J. Oral bioavailability of docetaxel in combination with OC144-093 (ONT-093). *Cancer Chemother. Pharmacol.* **2005**, *55*, 72–78. [CrossRef] [PubMed]
143. Rushing, D.A.; Raber, S.R.; Rodvold, K.A.; Piscitelli, S.C.; Plank, G.S.; Tewksbury, D.A. The effects of cyclosporine on the pharmacokinetics of doxorubicin in patients with small cell lung cancer. *Cancer* **1994**, *74*, 834–841. [CrossRef] [PubMed]
144. Giaccone, G.; Linn, S.C.; Welink, J.; Catimel, G.; Stieltjes, H.; Van der Vijgh, W.; Eeltink, C.; Vermorken, J.B.; Pinedo, H.M. A dose-finding and pharmacokinetic study of reversal of multidrug resistance with SDZ PSC 833 in combination with doxorubicin in patients with solid tumors. *Clin. Cancer Res.* **1997**, *3*, 2005–2015. [PubMed]
145. Onafuye, H.; Pieper, S.; Mulac, D.; Cinatl, J., Jr.; Wass, M.N.; Langer, K.; Michaelis, M. Doxorubicin-loaded human serum albumin nanoparticles overcome transporter-mediated drug resistance in drug-adapted cancer cells. *Beilstein J. Nanotechnol.* **2019**, *10*, 1707–1715. [CrossRef]
146. Nielsen, R.B.; Holm, R.; Pijpers, I.; Snoeys, J.; Nielsen, U.G.; Nielsen, C.U. Oral etoposide and zosuquidar bioavailability in rats: Effect of co-administration and in vitro-in vivo correlation of P-glycoprotein inhibition. *Int. J. Pharm. X* **2021**, *3*, 100089. [CrossRef]
147. Morschhauser, F.; Zinzani, P.L.; Burgess, M.; Sloots, L.; Bouafia, F.; Dumontet, C. Phase I/II trial of a P-glycoprotein inhibitor, Zosuquidar. 3HCl trihydrochloride (LY335979), given orally in combination with the CHOP regimen in patients with non-Hodgkin's lymphoma. *Leuk. Lymphoma* **2007**, *48*, 708–715. [CrossRef]
148. Toffoli, G.; Corona, G.; Basso, B.; Boiocchi, M. Pharmacokinetic optimisation of treatment with oral etoposide. *Clin. Pharmacokinet* **2004**, *43*, 441–466. [CrossRef]
149. Chen, M.-C.; Mi, F.-L.; Liao, Z.-X.; Hsiao, C.-W.; Sonaje, K.; Chung, M.-F.; Hsu, L.-W.; Sung, H.-W. Recent advances in chitosan-based nanoparticles for oral delivery of macromolecules. *Adv. Drug Deliv. Rev.* **2013**, *65*, 865–879. [CrossRef]
150. Sung, H.-W.; Sonaje, K.; Liao, Z.-X.; Hsu, L.-W.; Chuang, E.-Y. pH-responsive nanoparticles shelled with chitosan for oral delivery of insulin: From mechanism to therapeutic applications. *Acc. Chem. Res.* **2012**, *45*, 619–629. [CrossRef]
151. Hu, F.-Q.; Liu, L.-N.; Du, Y.-Z.; Yuan, H. Synthesis and antitumor activity of doxorubicin conjugated stearic acid-g-chitosan oligosaccharide polymeric micelles. *Biomaterials* **2009**, *30*, 6955–6963. [CrossRef]

152. Yang, Y.; Chen, Y.; Li, D.; Lin, S.; Chen, H.; Wu, W.; Zhang, W. Linolenic acid conjugated chitosan micelles for improving the oral absorption of doxorubicin via fatty acid transporter. *Carbohydr. Polym.* **2023**, *300*, 120233. [CrossRef]
153. Wang, J.; Li, L.; Du, Y.; Sun, J.; Han, X.; Luo, C.; Ai, X.; Zhang, Q.; Wang, Y.; Fu, Q.; et al. Improved oral absorption of doxorubicin by amphiphilic copolymer of lysine-linked ditocopherol polyethylene glycol 2000 succinate: In vitro characterization and in vivo evaluation. *Mol. Pharm.* **2015**, *12*, 463–473. [CrossRef] [PubMed]
154. Wang, J.; Sun, J.; Chen, Q.; Gao, Y.; Li, L.; Li, H.; Leng, D.; Wang, Y.; Sun, Y.; Jing, Y.; et al. Star-shape copolymer of lysine-linked di-tocopherol polyethylene glycol 2000 succinate for doxorubicin delivery with reversal of multidrug resistance. *Biomaterials* **2012**, *33*, 6877–6888. [CrossRef] [PubMed]
155. Kumbham, S.; Paul, M.; Itoo, A.; Ghosh, B.; Biswas, S. Oleanolic acid-conjugated human serum albumin nanoparticles encapsulating doxorubicin as synergistic combination chemotherapy in oropharyngeal carcinoma and melanoma. *Int. J. Pharm.* **2022**, *614*, 121479. [CrossRef]
156. Sarfraz, M.; Afzal, A.; Raza, S.M.; Bashir, S.; Madni, A.; Khan, M.W.; Ma, X.; Xiang, G. Liposomal co-delivered oleanolic acid attenuates doxorubicin-induced multi-organ toxicity in hepatocellular carcinoma. *Oncotarget* **2017**, *8*, 47136–47153. [CrossRef]
157. Kalaria, D.R.; Sharma, G.; Beniwal, V.; Ravi Kumar, M.N. Design of biodegradable nanoparticles for oral delivery of doxorubicin: In vivo pharmacokinetics and toxicity studies in rats. *Pharm. Res.* **2009**, *26*, 492–501. [CrossRef] [PubMed]
158. Astete, C.E.; Sabliov, C.M. Synthesis and characterization of PLGA nanoparticles. *J. Biomater. Sci. Polym. Ed.* **2006**, *17*, 247–289. [CrossRef] [PubMed]
159. Hussain, N.; Jaitley, V.; Florence, A.T. Recent advances in the understanding of uptake of microparticulates across the gastrointestinal lymphatics. *Adv. Drug Deliv. Rev.* **2001**, *50*, 107–142. [CrossRef]
160. Nguyen, T.T.; Duong, V.A.; Maeng, H.J. Pharmaceutical formulations with P-glycoprotein Inhibitory effect as promising approaches for enhancing oral drug absorption and bioavailability. *Pharmaceutics* **2021**, *13*, 1103. [CrossRef]
161. Choi, M.-K.; Lee, J.; Song, I.-S. Pharmacokinetic modulation of substrate drugs via the inhibition of drug-metabolizing enzymes and transporters using pharmaceutical excipients. *J. Pharm. Investig.* **2023**, *53*, 1–18. [CrossRef]
162. Maksimenko, O.; Malinovskaya, J.; Shipulo, E.; Osipova, N.; Razzhivina, V.; Arantseva, D.; Yarovaya, O.; Mostovaya, U.; Khalansky, A.; Fedoseeva, V.; et al. Doxorubicin-loaded PLGA nanoparticles for the chemotherapy of glioblastoma: Towards the pharmaceutical development. *Int. J. Pharm.* **2019**, *572*, 118733. [CrossRef]
163. Pereverzeva, E.; Treschalin, I.; Treschalin, M.; Arantseva, D.; Ermolenko, Y.; Kumskova, N.; Maksimenko, O.; Balabanyan, V.; Kreuter, J.; Gelperina, S. Toxicological study of doxorubicin-loaded PLGA nanoparticles for the treatment of glioblastoma. *Int. J. Pharm.* **2019**, *554*, 161–178. [CrossRef]
164. Cao, D.; Zhang, X.; Akabar, M.D.; Luo, Y.; Wu, H.; Ke, X.; Ci, T. Liposomal doxorubicin loaded PLGA-PEG-PLGA based thermogel for sustained local drug delivery for the treatment of breast cancer. *Artif. Cells Nanomed. Biotechnol.* **2019**, *47*, 181–191. [CrossRef] [PubMed]
165. Jain, A.K.; Swarnakar, N.K.; Das, M.; Godugu, C.; Singh, R.P.; Rao, P.R.; Jain, S. Augmented anticancer efficacy of doxorubicin-loaded polymeric nanoparticles after oral administration in a breast cancer induced animal model. *Mol. Pharm.* **2011**, *8*, 1140–1151. [CrossRef] [PubMed]
166. Hu, S.; Yang, Z.; Wang, S.; Wang, L.; He, Q.; Tang, H.; Ji, P.; Chen, T. Zwitterionic polydopamine modified nanoparticles as an efficient nanoplatform to overcome both the mucus and epithelial barriers. *Chem. Eng. J.* **2022**, *428*, 132107. [CrossRef]
167. Ahmad, N.; Ahmad, R.; Alam, M.A.; Ahmad, F.J. Enhancement of oral bioavailability of doxorubicin through surface modified biodegradable polymeric nanoparticles. *Chem. Cent. J.* **2018**, *12*, 65. [CrossRef]
168. Ahmad, N.; Ahmad, R.; Alam, M.A.; Ahmad, F.J.; Amir, M.; Pottoo, F.H.; Sarafroz, M.; Jafar, M.; Umar, K. Daunorubicin oral bioavailability enhancement by surface coated natural biodegradable macromolecule chitosan based polymeric nanoparticles. *Int. J. Biol. Macromol.* **2019**, *128*, 825–838. [CrossRef]
169. Khdair, A.; Hamad, I.; Alkhatib, H.; Bustanji, Y.; Mohammad, M.; Tayem, R.; Aiedeh, K. Modified-chitosan nanoparticles: Novel drug delivery systems improve oral bioavailability of doxorubicin. *Eur. J. Pharm. Sci.* **2016**, *93*, 38–44. [CrossRef]
170. Sun, M.; Li, D.; Wang, X.; He, L.; Lv, X.; Xu, Y.; Tang, R. Intestine-penetrating, pH-sensitive and double-layered nanoparticles for oral delivery of doxorubicin with reduced toxicity. *J. Mater. Chem. B* **2019**, *7*, 3692–3703. [CrossRef]
171. Głąb, T.K.; Boratyński, J. Potential of Casein as a Carrier for Biologically Active Agents. *Top. Curr. Chem.* **2017**, *375*, 71. [CrossRef]
172. Rehan, F.; Emranul Karim, M.; Ahemad, N.; Farooq Shaikh, M.; Gupta, M.; Gan, S.H.; Chowdhury, E.H. A comparative evaluation of anti-tumor activity following oral and intravenous delivery of doxorubicin in a xenograft model of breast tumor. *J. Pharm. Investig.* **2022**, *52*, 787–804. [CrossRef]
173. Feng, C.; Li, J.; Mu, Y.; Kong, M.; Li, Y.; Raja, M.A.; Cheng, X.J.; Liu, Y.; Chen, X.G. Multilayer micro-dispersing system as oral carriers for co-delivery of doxorubicin hydrochloride and P-gp inhibitor. *Int. J. Biol. Macromol.* **2017**, *94*, 170–180. [CrossRef]
174. Benezra, M.; Penate-Medina, O.; Zanzonico, P.B.; Schaer, D.; Ow, H.; Burns, A.; DeStanchina, E.; Longo, V.; Herz, E.; Iyer, S.; et al. Multimodal silica nanoparticles are effective cancer-targeted probes in a model of human melanoma. *J. Clin. Investig.* **2011**, *121*, 2768–2780. [CrossRef]
175. Zheng, N.; Li, J.; Xu, C.; Xu, L.; Li, S.; Xu, L. Mesoporous silica nanorods for improved oral drug absorption. *Artif. Cells Nanomed. Biotechnol.* **2018**, *46*, 1132–1140. [CrossRef]

176. Wang, Y.; Sun, Y.; Wang, J.; Yang, Y.; Li, Y.; Yuan, Y.; Liu, C. Charge-Reversal APTES-Modified Mesoporous Silica Nanoparticles with High Drug Loading and Release Controllability. *ACS Appl. Mater. Interfaces* **2016**, *8*, 17166–17175. [CrossRef]
177. Han, N.; Wang, Y.; Bai, J.; Liu, J.; Wang, Y.; Gao, Y.; Jiang, T.; Kang, W.; Wang, S. Facile synthesis of the lipid bilayer coated mesoporous silica nanocomposites and their application in drug delivery. *Microporous and Mesoporous Materials* **2016**, *219*, 209–218. [CrossRef]
178. Zhao, Q.; Liu, J.; Zhu, W.; Sun, C.; Di, D.; Zhang, Y.; Wang, P.; Wang, Z.; Wang, S. Dual-stimuli responsive hyaluronic acid-conjugated mesoporous silica for targeted delivery to CD44-overexpressing cancer cells. *Acta Biomater.* **2015**, *23*, 147–156. [CrossRef] [PubMed]
179. Bekaroğlu, G.M.; İşçi, S. Raw and Purified Clay Minerals for Drug Delivery Applications. *ACS Omega* **2022**, *7*, 38825–38831. [CrossRef] [PubMed]
180. Gerami, S.E.; Pourmadadi, M.; Fatoorehchi, H.; Yazdian, F.; Rashedi, H.; Nigjeh, M.N. Preparation of pH-sensitive chitosan/polyvinylpyrrolidone/α-Fe2O3 nanocomposite for drug delivery application: Emphasis on ameliorating restrictions. *Int. J. Biol. Macromol.* **2021**, *173*, 409–420. [CrossRef]
181. Rahmani, E.; Pourmadadi, M.; Ghorbanian, S.A.; Yazdian, F.; Rashedi, H.; Navaee, M. Preparation of a pH-responsive chitosan-montmorillonite-nitrogen-doped carbon quantum dots nanocarrier for attenuating doxorubicin limitations in cancer therapy. *Eng. Life Sci.* **2022**, *22*, 634–649. [CrossRef] [PubMed]
182. Liao, J.; Qian, Y.; Sun, Z.; Wang, J.; Zhang, Q.; Zheng, Q.; Wei, S.; Liu, N.; Yang, H. In Vitro Binding and Release Mechanisms of Doxorubicin from Nanoclays. *J. Phys. Chem. Lett.* **2022**, *13*, 8429–8435. [CrossRef] [PubMed]
183. Huang, H.-J.; Huang, S.-Y.; Wang, T.-H.; Lin, T.-Y.; Huang, N.-C.; Shih, O.; Jeng, U.S.; Chu, C.-Y.; Chiang, W.-H. Clay nanosheets simultaneously intercalated and stabilized by PEGylated chitosan as drug delivery vehicles for cancer chemotherapy. *Carbohydr. Polym.* **2023**, *302*, 120390. [CrossRef] [PubMed]

Disclaimer/Publisher's Note: The statements, opinions and data contained in all publications are solely those of the individual author(s) and contributor(s) and not of MDPI and/or the editor(s). MDPI and/or the editor(s) disclaim responsibility for any injury to people or property resulting from any ideas, methods, instructions or products referred to in the content.

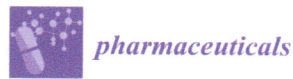

Review

The Therapeutic Potential of Novel Carnosine Formulations: Perspectives for Drug Development

Angela Bonaccorso [1,2,†], Anna Privitera [1,3,†], Margherita Grasso [4], Sonya Salamone [1], Claudia Carbone [1,2], Rosario Pignatello [1,2], Teresa Musumeci [1,2], Filippo Caraci [1,4,‡] and Giuseppe Caruso [1,4,*,‡]

1. Department of Drug and Health Sciences, University of Catania, 95125 Catania, Italy
2. NANOMED–Research Centre for Nanomedicine and Pharmaceutical Nanotechnology, University of Catania, 95125 Catania, Italy
3. Department of Biomedical and Biotechnological Sciences, University of Catania, 95123 Catania, Italy
4. Unit of Neuropharmacology and Translational Neurosciences, Oasi Research Institute-IRCCS, 94018 Troina, Italy
* Correspondence: giuseppe.caruso2@unict.it; Tel.: +39-095-7385036
† Consider that the first two should be regarded as joint First Authors.
‡ Consider that the last two should be regarded as joint Last Authors.

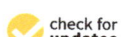

Citation: Bonaccorso, A.; Privitera, A.; Grasso, M.; Salamone, S.; Carbone, C.; Pignatello, R.; Musumeci, T.; Caraci, F.; Caruso, G. The Therapeutic Potential of Novel Carnosine Formulations: Perspectives for Drug Development. *Pharmaceuticals* 2023, 16, 778. https://doi.org/10.3390/ph16060778

Academic Editors: Silviya Petrova Zustiak and Era Jain

Received: 11 April 2023
Revised: 12 May 2023
Accepted: 16 May 2023
Published: 23 May 2023

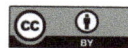

Copyright: © 2023 by the authors. Licensee MDPI, Basel, Switzerland. This article is an open access article distributed under the terms and conditions of the Creative Commons Attribution (CC BY) license (https://creativecommons.org/licenses/by/4.0/).

Abstract: Carnosine (beta-alanyl-L-histidine) is an endogenous dipeptide synthesized via the activity of the ATP-dependent enzyme carnosine synthetase 1 and can be found at a very high concentration in tissues with a high metabolic rate, including muscles (up to 20 mM) and brain (up to 5 mM). Because of its well-demonstrated multimodal pharmacodynamic profile, which includes anti-aggregant, antioxidant, and anti-inflammatory activities, as well as its ability to modulate the energy metabolism status in immune cells, this dipeptide has been investigated in numerous experimental models of diseases, including Alzheimer's disease, and at a clinical level. The main limit for the therapeutic use of carnosine is related to its rapid hydrolysis exerted by carnosinases, especially at the plasma level, reason why the development of new strategies, including the chemical modification of carnosine or its vehiculation into innovative drug delivery systems (DDS), aiming at increasing its bioavailability and/or at facilitating the site-specific transport to different tissues, is of utmost importance. In the present review, after a description of carnosine structure, biological activities, administration routes, and metabolism, we focused on different DDS, including vesicular systems and metallic nanoparticles, as well as on possible chemical derivatization strategies related to carnosine. In particular, a basic description of the DDS employed or the derivatization/conjugation applied to obtain carnosine formulations, followed by the possible mechanism of action, is given. To the best of our knowledge, this is the first review that includes all the new formulations of carnosine (DDS and derivatives), allowing a decrease or complete prevention of the hydrolysis of this dipeptide exerted by carnosinases, the simultaneous blood–brain barrier crossing, the maintenance or enhancement of carnosine biological activity, and the site-specific transport to different tissues, which then offers perspectives for the development of new drugs.

Keywords: carnosine; drug development; drug delivery; derivatives; conjugates; vesicular systems; nanoparticles

1. Introduction

The dipeptide carnosine (beta-alanyl-L-histidine) was discovered more than 100 years ago during a study carried out by Gulewitsch and Amiradžibi, both working at the Laboratorium der Universität Charkow (Ukraine), in which a meat extract was analyzed [1]. At the end of the analysis, different unknown nitrogen-containing compounds, including carnosine, were obtained. Based on the sample analyzed (minced meat), the molecule was named "carnosine", coming from the Latin *caro, carnis* (meat).

The synthesis of carnosine starting from β-alanine and L-histidine is related to the activity of the enzyme carnosine synthetase 1 (CARNS1). Carnosine is physiologically present in different mammalian tissues, with the highest tissue concentrations (millimolar order) observed in cardiac and skeletal muscles as well as at the central nervous system (CNS) level [1].

Carnosine possesses a well-known multimodal mechanism of action, including anti-aggregant, anti-inflammatory, and antioxidant properties [2–5], and has also shown the ability to enhance both antioxidant machinery [6] and energy metabolism [7–9] in different cell types, reasons why researchers have been encouraged to investigate its therapeutic potential in numerous multifactorial disorders such as Alzheimer's disease [10–12], depression [13,14], and Parkinson's disease [15,16].

In spite of high expectations, an important limit for carnosine therapeutic application is the reduction of its bioavailability due to degradation. Indeed, carnosine is cleaved by two human carnosinases, the serum-circulating carnosine dipeptidase 1 (CNDP1) and the cytosolic carnosine dipeptidase 2 (CNDP2), which is known to strongly reduce the bioavailability of carnosine [17,18]. For this reason, during the last two decades, different research groups have been working on the development of new approaches (e.g., drug delivery systems (DDS)) and new pharmacological formulations of carnosine in order to protect carnosine against carnosinases' degradation, then improving its bioavailability, and/or its ability to reach a specific target [19]. Based on the above, it also becomes clear the substantial heterogeneity regarding the route of carnosine administration in in vivo preclinical studies, where the oral administration through drinking water and the intraperitoneal (i.p.) injection represent the most widely employed [18]. One administration route that is attracting a lot of attention is the intranasal one [20], a route that might bypass the blood–brain barrier (BBB) and the first-pass metabolism [21,22]. Alternative and innovative approaches able to increase carnosine delivery include the use of vesicular (nanoliposomes, niosomes, and polymerosomes) and nanoparticulate systems. Nanovesicle systems are commonly used in the prognosis, diagnosis, and treatment of premalignant gastrointestinal tumors [23], while exosomes, cell-derived nanovesicles with a diameter ranging from 30 to 150 nm, have been considered in cancer therapy [24]. Niosomal formulations can be coupled to specific ligands able to be recognized by the BBB transporters [25]. Recently, nanoformulations, including nanovesicles, solid-lipid nanoparticles (NPs), nanoemulsions, and polymeric NPs, have shown promising results in the improvement of both efficacy and bioavailability of molecules of interest, as observed in the case of vitamin E [26]. Nanocapsules, composed of an inner liquid core and surrounded by a polymeric wall, are considered excellent carriers for a wide range of active pharmaceutical molecules [27], while nanoparticulate systems offer, among many, the advantage of improving the oral bioavailability of hydrophobic drugs [28].

The aim of this study was to explore the therapeutic potential of novel carnosine formulations and the perspectives for drug development, providing a narrative and critical analysis of the existing literature. We specifically focused on vesicular and nanoparticulate systems as well as on derivatives/conjugates able to increase carnosine activities, its stability to carnosinases, and/or facilitate the site-specific transport to different tissues.

2. Carnosine Structure, Biological Activities, Administration Routes, and Metabolism

As previously mentioned, carnosine is a dipeptide composed of β-alanine and L-histidine that are joined by CARNS1 enzyme (EC 6.3.2.11) [29,30] (Figure 1A,D).

With regards to the origin of the two amino acids forming carnosine, it is very different. In fact, β-alanine is synthesized at the liver level, primarily through uracil and thymine degradation [31], while L-histidine is an essential amino acid, thus not synthesized de novo in humans, that has to be ingested through the diet [32]. It is worth mentioning that, in mammals, β-alanine is used essentially for carnosine synthesis, while the remaining part is subjected to different metabolic pathways, including degradation and transamination.

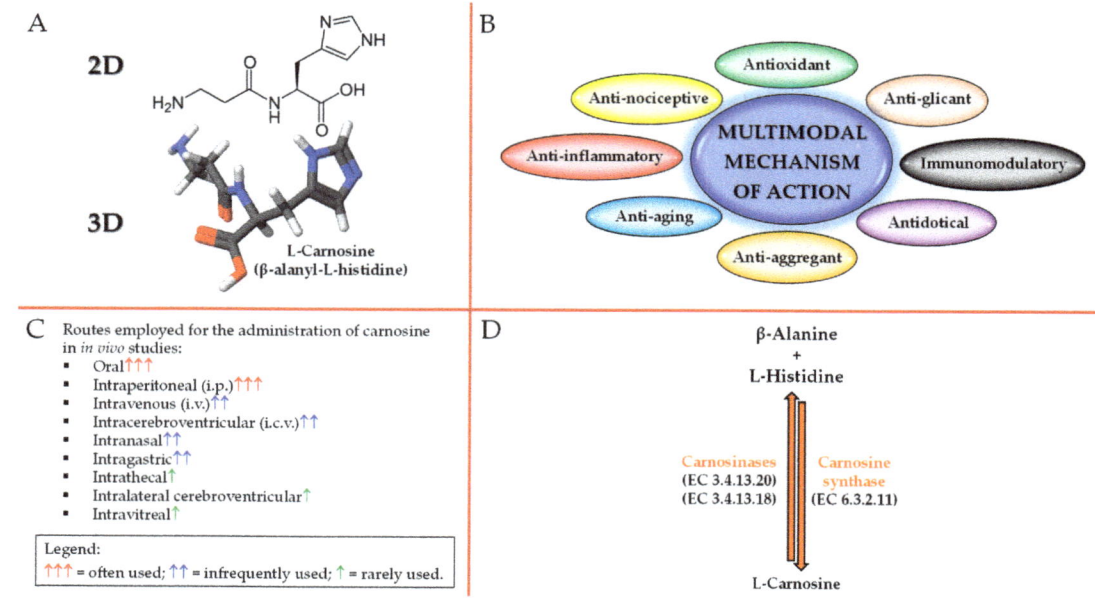

Figure 1. Schematic illustration of carnosine: (**A**) 2D and 3D structure, (**B**) biological activities, (**C**) administration routes, and (**D**) metabolism.

Carnosine is able to exert numerous biological and physiological roles. In fact, this naturally occurring dipeptide possesses a multimodal mechanism of action (Figure 1B). It is important to underline that despite its "preferential" localization (skeletal/cardiac muscles and brain), carnosine has shown the ability to exert biological activities in numerous and very different tissues. Since approximately 99% of carnosine can be found in muscle tissue [2], numerous studies have investigated the physiological activities of this dipeptide in muscles as well as the athletic benefits coming from its (or β-alanine precursor) supplementation. In addition to the well-demonstrated activities at muscle level, where carnosine has shown to favor muscle lactic acid detoxification and act as intramyocellular mobile buffer [33], also improving cytoplasmic Ca^{2+}-H^+ exchange/handling [34] and muscle contraction [35], mechanical work production (the so called "Severin's phenomenon") [36], muscle relaxation rates, as well as endurance exercise [37–43], carnosine can modulate energy metabolism in macrophages and microglia by restoring and/or enhancing the basal conditions (e.g., high-energy triphosphates and nicotinic coenzymes) [7–9,44], act as a neurotransmitter [45], regulate the activity of stem cells [46], modulate glucose metabolism, increasing fasting insulin levels and insulin resistance in non-diabetic overweight and obese individuals [47], enhance the degradation and/or scavenging of nitric oxide (NO) and related species [48–50], promote wound healing [51], exert anti-glycan and anti-aging activities [52,53], regulate osmotic pressure [54], modulate glutamate transport and production/metabolism at brain level [55], and interact with and chelate transition metals [56,57].

As described above, carnosine possesses several activities, but numerous research studies are still investigating its "additional" physiological roles. In this regard, in vivo studies employing transgenic models have been carried out. As recently described by Eckhardt and collaborators, mice knock-out (KO) for CARNS1 are characterized by reduced olfactory sensitivity [58]; in particular, the authors demonstrated that the absence of carnosine does not impair olfactory function in young CARNS1$^{-/-}$ mice, but does in aging CARNS1$^{-/-}$ mice, while there was an age-dependent decline in the number of olfactory receptor neurons in CARNS1$^{-/-}$ that was not observed in wild-type mice, suggesting that carnosine is not essential for information processing in the olfactory signaling but plays a role in the long-term protection of olfactory receptor neurons. In a different study conducted by Wang-Eckhardt et al., the absence of carnosine synthesis does not significantly modulate the carbonylation of proteins, and the same applies to the formation of advanced lipoxidation end products in different tissues/organs such as muscles and brain [59].

Despite the above-described multitude of activities, the therapeutic potential of carnosine is often mitigated by its massive degradation into its constituting amino acids exerted by CNDP1 (EC 3.4.13.20; sieric) and CNDP2 (EC 3.4.13.18; cytosolic) enzymes [42–44] (Figure 1D), both part of the M20 metalloprotease family. In greater detail, CNDP1 specifically degrades carnosine and its GABA analog (homocarnosine) [42], while CNDP2, a non-specific dipeptidase ubiquitously expressed in human tissues, degrades carnosine as well as other dipeptides, but instead, it is not able to degrade homocarnosine [43]. As a consequence of what described above, with the aim to deliver carnosine to different districts/tissues, also trying to protect it from enzyme degradation, researchers have employed a wide range of administration routes including oral, i.p., intravenous (i.v.), intracerebroventricular (i.c.v.), intranasal, intragastric, intrathecal, intralateral cerebroventricular, and intravitreal [18] (Figure 1C).

3. Drug Delivery Systems

The term "drug delivery system" (DDS) refers to a formulation that enables the introduction of a therapeutic or diagnostic molecule in the body and improves its effectiveness and safety by controlling the rate, time, and site of drug release after administration [60].

The first generation of DDS entered the market in the early 1950s and consisted of pharmaceutical formulations able to prolong drug activity and reduce dosing frequency [61]. DDS belonging to the "macroscopic scale era" (1950–1980) promoted drug release through dissolution, diffusion, osmosis, and ion exchange-based mechanisms, to produce systems that exhibited zero-order release rates, thus ensuring a constant drug plasma concentration (i.e., ophthalmic insert). The second generation of DDS (1980–2010) included both micro- (~1980s) and nano-sized (~1990–2000s) DDS as well as "smart" DDS technologies, the latter referring to systems developed to enable drug delivery in response to external stimuli, such as pH or temperature changes. This second generation is known as the "micro- and nano-scale era" and includes different DDS designed to promote a sustained and site-specific drug release (i.e., PEGylated DDS). The third generation of DDS (2010–present), defined as the "nanoscale era", is based on DDS modulation to overcome physico-chemical and biological barriers. Active targeting has become a major focus (i.e., DDS targeted by monoclonal antibodies or cell membrane receptor ligands [62]) as well as understanding how they behave in vivo. Drug delivery research collects systems with different properties that can be classified based on their structure and composition into three main categories: vesicular (i.e., liposomes, niosomes, transferosomes, ethosomes, phytosomes, and polymerosomes), particulates (i.e., lipidic, polymeric and metallic NPs, nanogel, and nanocrystals), and supramolecular (i.e., cyclodextrins, micro-conjugates, bio-conjugates) systems. All these systems present different features and benefits (Figure 2), because the physico-chemical and pharmacokinetic properties of the entrapped drug are temporarily masked by those of the carrier.

The selection of DDS is strictly related to the properties of the molecule that has to be delivered to the target site, as well as to the selected route of administration.

To date, the literature suggests that since 2000 different types of DDS have been designed to deliver carnosine [19]. In the following paragraph, an overview of the general features of DDS currently exploited for carnosine delivery has been detailed, while in Table 1, their main advantages and limitations were reported.

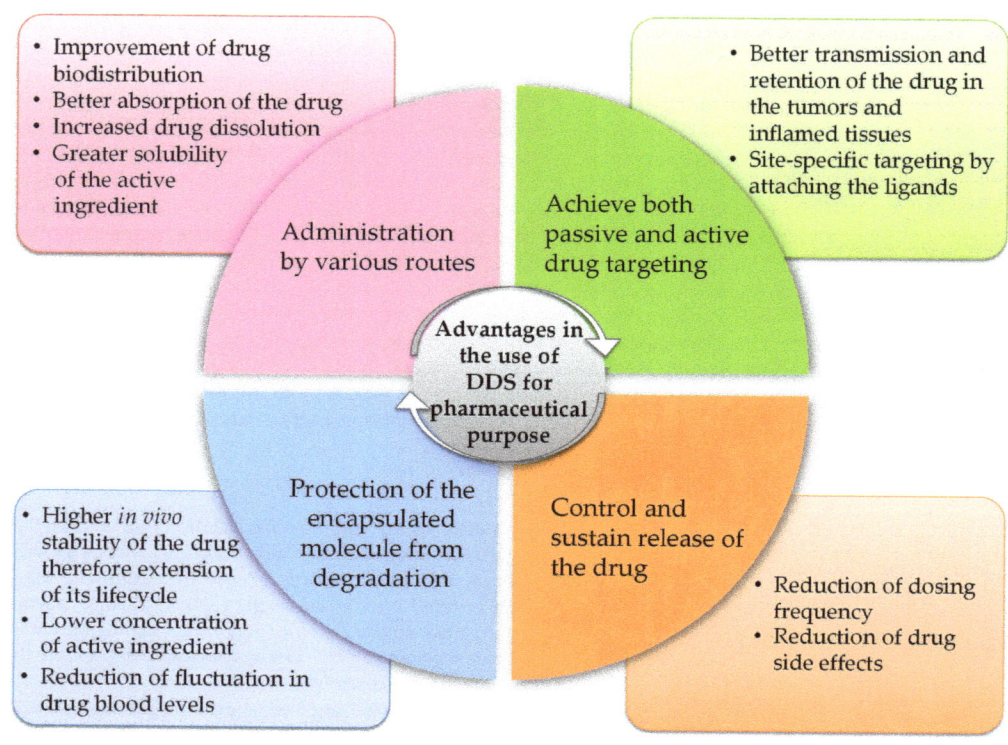

Figure 2. Advantages in the use of DDS for pharmaceutical purposes.

Table 1. Main advantages and limitations of vesicular systems, metallic NPs, and drug–conjugate derivatives.

		Advantages	Limitations
Vesicular Systems	Liposome	Made of natural ingredients; Biodegradable and biocompatible; Similarity to biomembrane.	Physical instability during storage; Susceptible to oxidation; Rigid liposomes remain confined to the stratum corneum.
	Elastic Liposome	Highly deforming ability and flexibility ensure deeper skin penetration and biomembrane crossing ability.	On prolonged storage, due to increased elasticity and flexibility, it tends to be less stable and lose the entrapped drug, which complicates the scaling process.
	Niosome	Chemical stability.	Lower biocompatibility.
	Phytosome	Enhancement of pharmacokinetic and pharmacodynamic properties of herbal-originated polyphenolic compounds; Improves skin absorption of phytoconstituents; Better stability of incorporated compounds owing to the chemical interaction.	Despite the easy scale-up production of phytosomes, the high pH sensitivity of some components could limit the large-scale synthesis of such formulations and should be considered during the manufacturing.
	Polymerosome	More stable than liposomes; Allows greater control of chemical and structural properties; Can be used to obtain controlled release kinetics by stimuli-response triggers.	In case of charged polymers, the self-assembled polymersome could induce stronger immune response and therefore be less tolerable for medical applications.

Table 1. Cont.

	Advantages	Limitations
Metallic NPs	Multiple shapes; Conductivity; Localized surface plasmon resonance; Ability to direct uptake through external magnetic stimulation.	Chemical contaminants from synthesis can cause toxicity issues.
Drug-conjugate derivatives	Increased compound half-life; Increased target specificity; Increase drug stability.	Modification can reduce the potency, especially for small peptides and proteins; Any covalent modification of peptides or proteins presents a potential risk of increased immunogenicity.

3.1. Vesicular Systems: From Liposomes to Polymerosomes

Vesicular systems are highly ordered assemblies comprising one or multiple concentric bilayers formulated as an outcome of the self-assembling of amphiphilic molecules in water.

Various types of vesicular systems, such as liposomes, polymerosomes, elastosomes, niosomes, and phytosomes can be included in this category of DDS [63,64] (Figure 3).

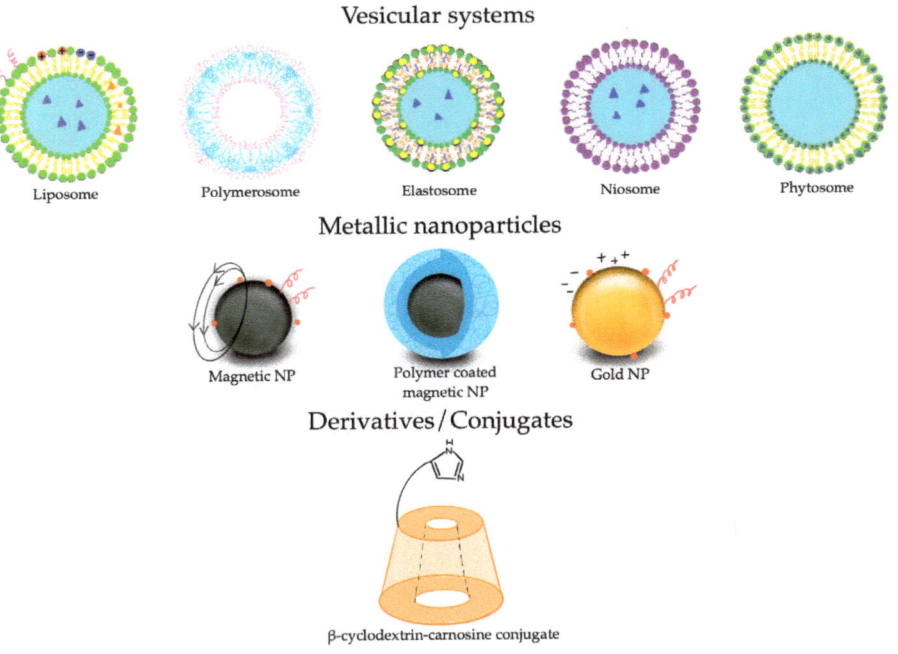

Figure 3. Some of the DDS used for pharmaceutical purposes.

Their applications can be found in different fields such as dermatology, immunology, eye disorders, brain targeting, infective diseases, and tumor therapy, and they have also been considered as vaccine adjuvant [65]. Liposomes belong to this DDS class and can be described as spherical vesicles in which one or more lipid bilayer(s) entraps an aqueous volume, formed by self-assembly of amphiphilic lipid molecules, with the polar head groups oriented to the inner and the non-polar chains outer aqueous phase. Their major components are usually phospholipids, with or without cholesterol, mimicking the physiological composition of biomembranes [66]. The most noteworthy advantages of liposomes are represented by their biocompatibility and safety due to their resemblance to biomembranes. The organized structure of liposomes offers the ability to load and deliver molecules with different solubility, with hydrophilic molecules placed into the aqueous core, hydrophobic molecules into the lipid layers, and amphiphilic molecules at the water/lipid bilayer interface [67]. According to the structure of the lipid bilayers of the vesicles, liposomes are commonly classified into unilamellar (ULV, all size range), multilamellar (MLV, >500 nm), and multivesicular (MVV, >1000 nm) vesicles (Figure 4).

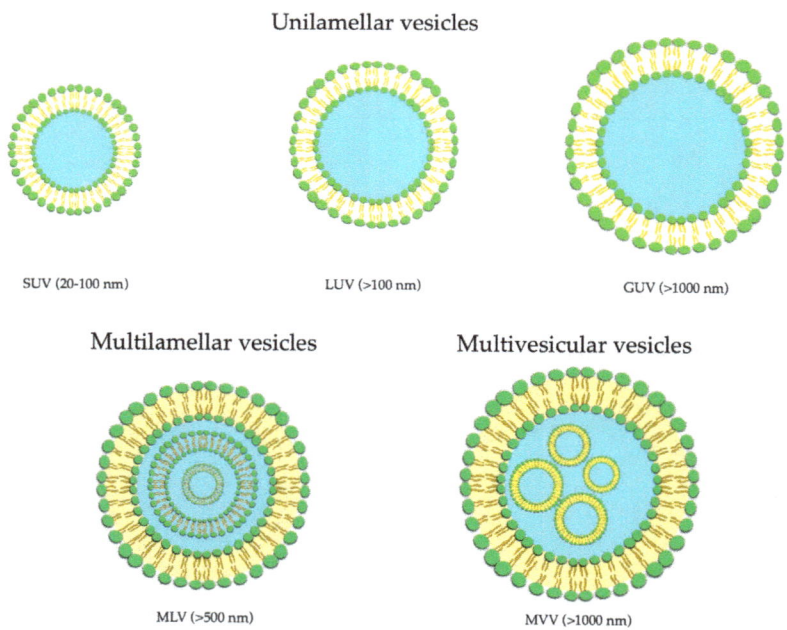

Figure 4. Classification of liposomes: unilamellar (ULV), multilamellar (MLV), and multivesicular (MVV) vesicles.

Based on vesicles size, ULV can be furtherly divided into three classes named small unilamellar vesicles (SUV, 20–100 nm), large unilamellar vesicles (LUV, >100 nm), and giant unilamellar vesicles (GUV, >1000 nm) (Figure 4). ULV is characterized by the presence of a single phospholipid bilayer that can encapsulate hydrophilic molecules, while MLV presents two or more concentric lipid bilayers characterized by an onion-like structure that can hold lipophilic compounds [68]. It is possible to modify the liposomal surfaces by conjugation to polymers and/or ligands to provide special properties such as active targeting to specific sites.

Liposomes whose size does not exceed the scale of 100 nm are called nanoliposomes. Elastic liposomes (EL) are vesicles characterized by flexibility, deformability, or ultradeformability. ELs were introduced in 1992 by Cevc and Blume as an alternative to conventional liposomes to facilitate drug passage across the stratum corneum of the skin [69].

Compared to conventional liposomes, it was found that ELs exert greater biomembrane crossing capabilities, including BBB, due to their small size and elastic nature [70].

ELs were first developed as novel and transdermal DDS; indeed, their elasticity enables them to cross membrane pores smaller than their own size by incorporating edge activators (surfactants) into lipid bilayers. Sodium cholate, Span 80, or Tween 80 were employed as surfactants [70]. The enhanced permeability of EL is due to their ability to act as carriers and penetrant agents. Surprisingly, ELs can penetrate the skin without disintegration [71].

During the last decades, different types of molecules (i.e., thermolabile proteins, acid-labile drugs, enzyme-susceptible, highly lipophilic, hydrophilic, photosensitive drugs, and high-molecular-weight molecules) have been encapsulated within EL for different applications [72–74]. Altamimi et al. designed EL for luteolin transdermal delivery for breast cancer therapy, demonstrating that the deformable vesicular carrier enhanced permeation parameters across rat skin, exhibiting a concentration-dependent MCF-7 cells inhibition and improving cellular internalization as compared with pure drug solution [75]. Montanari et al. [76] exploited ultradeformable liposomes activated by sunlight for the treatment of *Leishmania braziliensis* infections, demonstrating that the transcutaneous penetration of zinc phthalocyanine was about 10 times higher when encapsulated in ultradeformable liposomes compared to conventional liposomes, having a homogeneous distribution throughout the stratum corneum [77].

Niosomes are surfactant-based nanometric vesicles with advantageous characteristics compared to conventional liposomes. Niosomes are formed by non-ionic surfactants via self-assembly in an aqueous solution [78]. The use of non-ionic surfactants as membrane-forming constituents instead of phospholipids overcomes many of the disadvantages associated with liposomes, such as chemical instability, predisposition of phospholipids to oxidation, necessity of special handling, and storage conditions. Furthermore, their specific structure, composed of an inner aqueous compartment surrounded by a hydrophobic membrane, allows the incorporation and codelivery of hydrophobic and hydrophilic molecules. However, niosomes show some disadvantages, such as greater irritability compared to liposomes and lower biocompatibility than phospholipids due to the presence of surfactants [79]. Niosomes first emerged in the field of cosmetics by researchers from L'Oréal (Clichy, France) in the 1970s and 1980s. Since then, niosomes have been extensively investigated and are now attracting extensive attention as a vesicle delivery system for multiple applications in different fields, including pharmaceutical, cosmetic, and food sciences, leading to a large number of publications and patents [80–82].

Phytosomes, also called phyto-phospholipid complexes, are vesicular systems formed by the interaction between the hydrophilic parts of phospholipids and the phyto-active components, resulting in the formation of hydrogen bonds between them. The hydroxyl groups of polyphenols, or phytochemicals, produced by plants form hydrogen bonds with nitrate and phosphate groups of phospholipids. Phytosomes have a different structure compared to liposomes since the active ingredient is not located inside the hydrophilic cavity or within the layers of membranes, like in liposomes, but it is part of the membrane itself [83]. The chemical bonding ensures the stability of phytosomes and enhances the encapsulation efficiency of the bioactive compounds, generally at a stoichiometric molar ratio of 1:1 or 1:2 (phospholipids/phytochemicals) [84].

The lipid bilayer of the phytosomes helps contact-facilitated drug delivery in which there is a lipid–lipid interaction between the carrier and the cell membrane, leading to the diffusion of the bioactive compounds into the cell. The rate of release is slower than liposomes due to the association of the drug with the phosphatidyl head [85].

The first phytosomes were developed by Indena company (Milan, Italy) in the late 1980s, which aimed to increase the bioavailability of phytochemicals by complexing them to phospholipids [86]. Different phytosomes are available in the market (sylibin, ginkgo, cartaegus, and centella), and many others are currently under investigation in clinical trials, as detailed in a very interesting recently published review by Alharbi et al. [86].

The biological activities related to phytosomes are heterogeneous and involve different districts such as cardiovascular, central and peripheral nervous, gastrointestinal, genitourinary, immune, integumentary, musculoskeletal, and respiratory systems. For example, Panda and Naik investigated the cardioprotective activity of a combined treatment of *Ginkgo biloba* phytosomes and *Ocimum sanctum* extract in isoproterenol-induced myocardial necrosis in rats, showing an evident cardioprotective effect [87].

Polymerosomes are artificial vesicles enclosing an aqueous cavity formed by the self-assembly of amphiphilic natural or synthetic copolymers. Polymers are chemical compounds consisting of many repeating subunits called monomers and exist as chains or in branched form. Block copolymers are macromolecules that contain different adjacent blocks of chemically distinct monomers. Block copolymers contain both hydrophilic and hydrophobic blocks that possess amphiphilic properties [88]. Polymerosomes can have a size in the order of nanometric or micrometric scale, depending on the preparation method used, the amphiphilicity of polymers themselves, or external factors such as extrusion or sonication process during their synthesis. Polymerosomes have higher stability than liposomes and can be used to obtain more controlled release kinetics, also in a stimuli-response manner. The release of the drug can be triggered by several different factors, such as pH, temperature, redox potential, light, magnetic field, or instability of the system [89]. Polymerosomes can be loaded with hydrophilic, hydrophobic, or amphiphilic compounds, which makes them very attractive vesicles for various applications in drug delivery.

Use of polymersomes for drug delivery and targeting requires several steps that consists in the synthesis of amphiphilic block-copolymers, assembly of block-copolymers to form vesicles, and in some cases can include targeting of the vesicles by conjugation of specifically binding moieties, and strategies for controlling the release of drugs from polymersomes by the use of internal or external stimuli (hyperthermia and magnetic field-induced release, ultrasound-induced release, light-induced release, voltage-induced release) [90].

Polymersomes can also be designed for other purposes. These include the encapsulation of diagnostic markers, enzymes, or other reactive molecules (nanoreactors and artificial cells). Liu et al. investigated the use of polymersomes as a targeted contrasting agent for magnetic resonance imaging (MRI). The authors prepared folate-tagged poly(L-glutamic acid)-block-poly(ε-caprolactone) vesicles and subsequently formed superparamagnetic iron oxide (Fe_3O_4) NPs in their hydrophilic crowns. These superparamagnetic polymersomes successfully contrasted transplanted HeLa tumors in mice [91].

3.2. Metallic Nanoparticles

Metallic NPs represent an emerging category of DDS with a wide range of potential applications in biotechnology, targeted drug delivery, gene delivery, and diagnostic imaging. In 1857, Faraday first investigated the existence of metallic NPs in solution [92]. In 1908, Mie gave a quantitative explanation of their color [93]. Nowadays, these nanosystems can be prepared and modified with various chemical functional groups, which allows them to bind with antibodies, ligands, and/or drugs (Figure 5).

These systems can be made of pure metals (e.g., gold, platinum, silver, titanium, zinc, cerium, iron, and thallium) or their compounds (e.g., oxides, hydroxides, sulfides, phosphates, fluorides, and chlorides) [94].

During the last five decades, magnetic Fe_3O_4 NPs (MNPs) have been highly investigated mainly due to their optical, thermal, and magnetic properties, along with the fact that they can be manipulated with an external magnetic field. Among eight forms of Fe_3O_4, magnetite NPs are one of the most representative MNPs, having unique catalytic, biological, and magnetic properties such as the superparamagnetic ones. Superparamagnetic NPs only exhibit size-dependent magnetic features when exposed to an external magnetic field, while bulk magnetic particulates retain these features even without an external magnetic field [94].

The physico-chemical features of MNPs strongly depend on their size and shape; these features, along with coating molecules type and surface charge, influence pharmacokinetics and pharmacodynamics after in vivo administration [95]. In order to avoid the elimination by the mononuclear phagocytic system after MNPs administration [95] and to enhance their stability in vivo, different coating agents have been considered. The surface coating of MNPs drives their intracellular trafficking and degradation in endolysosomes, as well as dictating other cellular outcomes. Coating molecules into the MNPs surface can be useful to avoid their opsonization and to reduce their aggregation and agglomeration that impair the interaction with the cellular compartment. Several coating agents have been evaluated, for example, inorganic compounds, such as silica, that can enhance MNPs biocompatibility and stability, while metal conjugation of Fe_3O_4 with gold gives multifunctionality.

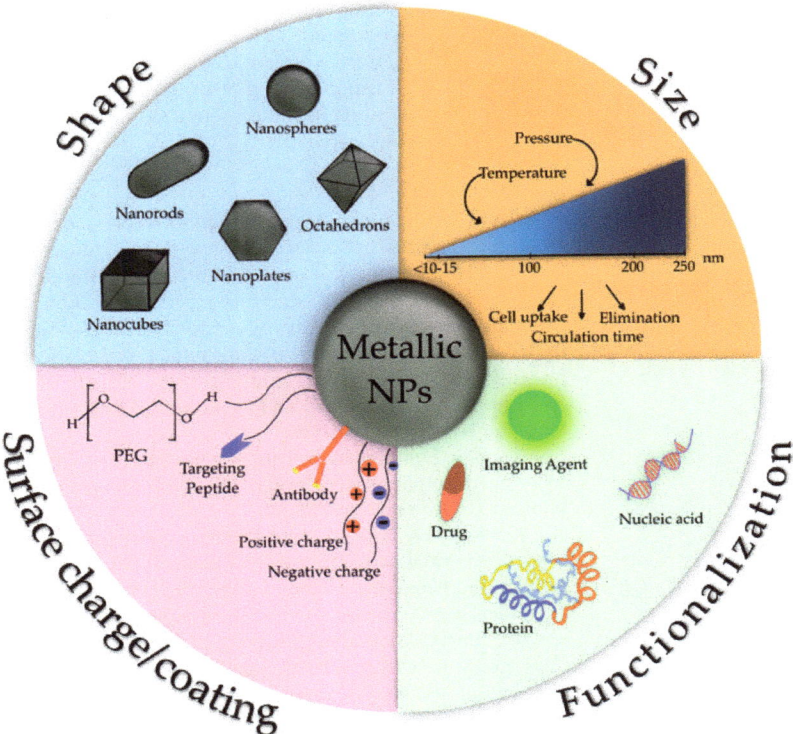

Figure 5. Characteristics of metallic NPs.

Organic compounds such as polyethylene glycol (PEG) and derivatives prevent plasma proteins adsorption onto MNPs surface, avoiding their uptake; other synthetic polymers like poly (D,L-lactide-co-glycolic) acid-based (PLGA) may also be used for other purposes. Polymer-functionalized MNPs have improved stability due to the increased repulsion, which provides an equilibrium of the magnetic and attractive forces. The functional groups of coating compounds, such as hydroxyl, carboxylic, or amine groups, offer MNPs the possibility to bind drugs, proteins, or biomolecules, providing reactive sites on the surface of MNPs potentially useful for the attachment of therapeutic agents [95].

Among metallic NPs, gold NPs (AuNPs) have piqued great interest due to their many advantages, such as the simplicity of synthesizing NPs with different shapes (i.e., rod-like, spherical, and cage-like) and tunable size, which confers optical and electrical properties. Additional characteristics of AuNPs are the net negative surface charge that allows the functionalization with biomolecules such as targeting ligands, the biocompatibility, and their surface effect, including macroscopic quantum tunneling effect and the presence of surface plasmon resonance bands [96]. Recent studies have shown that AuNPs not only can infiltrate the blood vessels but also enter inside the organelles, suggesting they can be employed as effective drug carriers. Small molecules, peptides, oligonucleotides, and DNA can be conjugated with AuNPs, obtaining an efficient release of these payloads via internal or external stimuli [97]. It has also been reported that encapsulating drugs or peptides into AuNPs can improve their bioavailability and biocompatibility [98].

AuNPs are increasingly actively employed for therapeutic reasons. Accumulation of AuNPs in the tumor is highlighted by the modification in the color of the tumor, which appears as a bright red color (typical of colloidal gold and its aggregates) [99]. Interestingly, it has been reported that AuNPs have favorable impacts on plant growth and development and have been recommended for use in a variety of agricultural crops, as well as in the germination of seeds from endangered plant species [100]. Arora et al. demonstrated that spraying AuNPs at concentrations of 10 and 25 mg/L on *Brassica juncea* plants can increase the quantity of chlorophyll and present a viable alternative to genetically modified crops for ensuring food security [101].

3.3. Derivative Conjugates

Compared to the majority of small molecules, peptides demonstrate short blood half-life due to their susceptibility to enzyme cleavage and rapid renal clearance [101]. Several strategies have been widely used to improve the chemical and physical stability of peptides and their pharmacokinetics and pharmacodynamics.

One of the most effective ways to prevent the degradation is to engineer analogs from dextrorotatory (D)-amino acids; in fact, these latter show improved stability among proteases [102]. However, it is important to consider the effects that such modifications could have on the overall secondary structure of the peptide, which risks losing the correct binding geometry to its target.

Backbone modifications [103], cyclization [104], lipidation [105], introduction of differently sized polymers [106], and conjugation represent additional strategies employed to improve peptide properties.

Conjugation of peptides with other peptides, small molecules, or biomolecules represents an essential tool in biomedical research. It can be used to promote cellular uptake or receptor-mediated drug delivery and/or to extend the peptide half-life in the bloodstream.

It has been reported that attaching moieties capable of increasing the size of peptides and/or altering their charge has the potential to successfully extend its blood half-life. Conjugates used in peptide therapeutics can either be non-biological molecules such as PEG or biological molecules such as sugars, proteins, or lipids. Increasing the molecular weight of peptides allows them to evade kidney filtration; otherwise, attaching a conjugate that is negatively charged helps to avoid renal clearance [107]. Conjugates that stabilize the structure of the therapeutic peptide can help to escape enzymatic degradation.

Conjugation is useful to facilitate site-specific transport to different tissues. It has been shown that animal lectins and galectins are important mediators in inflammatory diseases in recognition processes; it has prompted to synthesize glycoconjugates of small molecules or peptides, such as carnosine, with small sugars including glucose, lactose, or trehalose, to be specifically bound to a selected lectin [108].

Peptide-drug conjugates (PDCs) are a class of targeted therapeutics for cancer treatment, which can also be used as successful diagnostic tools in various scanning techniques by including radionuclides in their structure. PDCs consist of a homing peptide, which is chosen depending on its specific targeting properties, a cleavable or non-cleavable linker, and a cytotoxic payload [109].

Conjugation of a peptide with drugs can be further used to improve the effectiveness and reduce the side effects of the drug. Kulikova et al. formulated a synthetic derivative of acetylsalicylic acid and carnosine to take advantage of the superoxide scavenging and antiplatelet activities of carnosine to limit the adverse effects of the acetylsalicylic acid in the gastrointestinal tract [110].

In Figure 6, examples of other carnosine derivatives were depicted, while their detailed synthesis and applications can be found in the next section.

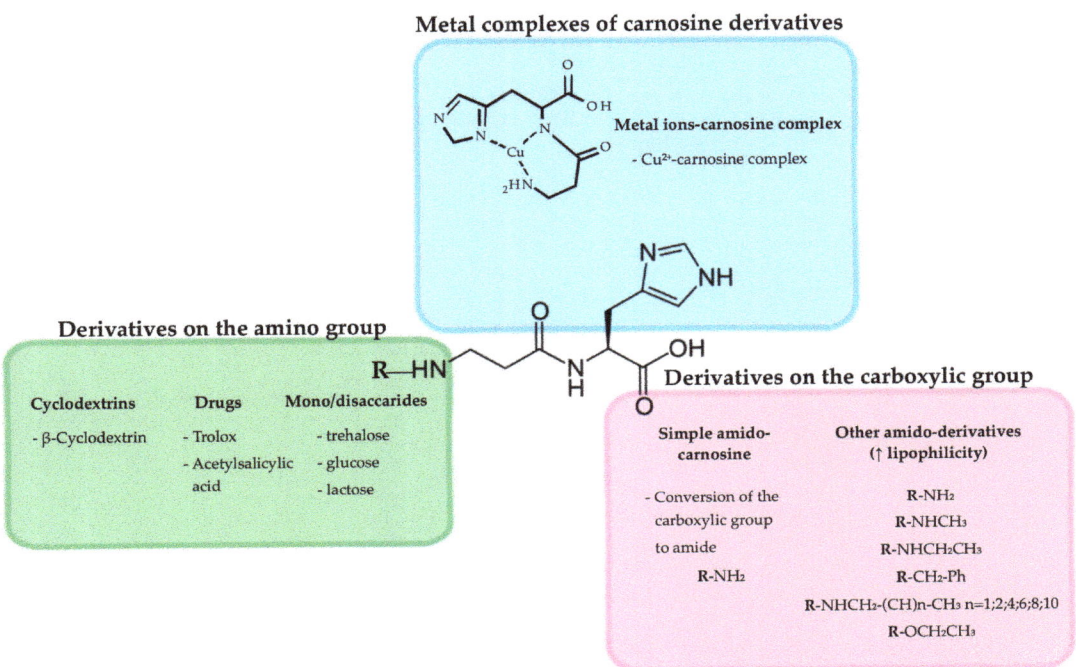

Figure 6. Graphical representation of potential carnosine derivatives.

4. Increasing Carnosine Bioavailability through DDS and/or Chemical Modifications

As previously mentioned, the therapeutic potential of carnosine is reduced as a consequence of its low stability/bioavailability due to CNDP1 and CNDP2 activity, metabolizing the dipeptide into its two constituting amino acids at sieric and intracellular levels, respectively. Because of that, different researchers have been working on the development of new approaches or new formulations trying to improve carnosine bioavailability as well as target selectivity (via DDS). One of the approaches considered was the use of selective inhibitors of carnosinases, as in the case of carnostatine (SAN9812) [111]. This protease-directed small-molecule was able to inhibit CNDP1 activity in human serum as well as in serum obtained from transgenic mice-overexpressing human CNDP1. In the same study, the authors were able to demonstrate that the simultaneous administration of carnosine and SAN9812 significantly increased the levels of carnosine in both plasma and kidney (up to 100-fold vs. treatment-naïve CNDP1-overexpressing mice). The ability of reduced glutathione (GSH), N-acetylcysteine, and cysteine to inhibit CNDP1 activity has also been considered. As shown by Peters and collaborators, these molecules have a dose-dependent effect in decreasing the efficiency of a recombinant CNDP1, also normalizing the increased activity of this peptidase in renal tissue samples obtained from diabetic mice [112]. Further investigations allowed to demonstrate that the inhibition of CNDP1 was allosteric.

As recently described by Grasso et al. [19], alternative and innovative approaches aiming at increasing carnosine bioavailability and/or its delivery consider the use of carnosine derivatives, vesicular systems, or nanoparticulate systems (Table 2), all described in detail in the next sub-sections.

Table 2. New vesicular system-based formulations of carnosine.

Formulation Name	Basic Description	Mode of Action	Ref.
Nanoliposomes	Carnosine incorporated into nanoliposomes could represent an innovative approach to overcoming the issues related to the direct application of this antioxidant peptide in food.	▪ Increased encapsulation efficiency	[113]
Liposomes	Liposomes are nanosized vesicles with a spherical shape that can be produced starting from natural or synthetic phospholipids. Encapsulation of antioxidants into liposomes has been shown to improve their therapeutic potential against oxidant-induced tissue injuries, facilitating intracellular delivery and extending the retention time of incorporated agents inside the cell.	▪ Reduced oxidative stress and inflammation	[114]
Elastic liposomes	EL encapsulated with carnosine represent a promising strategy to enhance the transport into the brain, protecting the dipeptide against enzymatic hydrolysis.	▪ Exerted neuroprotection	[115]
Niosome derivatized with lipoyl-carnosine	Niosomes are nanovesicles coupled to specific ligands selectively recognized by transporters expressed on the BBB that could promote the delivery of drugs (e.g., carnosine) at brain level.	▪ Drug delivery for simultaneous BBB crossing ▪ Reduced oxidative stress	[25]
Niosome	Carnosine-encapsulated niosomes represent a powerful drug delivery tool allowing it to reach specific organs such as the brain.	▪ Decreased oxidative stress and inflammation (AGEs and AOPP) ▪ Anti-aggregation (BSA)	[116,117]
Proniosome	Proniosomes are non-hydrated niosomes, which, upon hydration, form niosomes characterized by physical stability that overcome some problems presented by other vesicular systems, such as leaking, fusion, and aggregation.	▪ Increased bioavailability	[117]
Polymerosome	Polymersomes are synthetic vesicles formed through the self-assembly of amphiphilic co-polymers in aqueous conditions. Carnosine encapsulated in polymersomes could exert an enhanced neuroprotective potential.	▪ Exhibited remarkable neuroprotective effects with a dose of carnosine 3 orders of magnitude lower than free carnosine ▪ Reduced aggregation in the brain (LRP-1 target)	[118]
Phytosome	Carnosine loaded into lipid-based phytosomes represent an alternative for the prodrug N-acetyl-carnosine as a novel delivery system to the lens.	▪ Increased corneal permeation	[119]
Nanophytosome	Nanophytosomes represent one of the novel nanocarriers that could provide potent applications in both food and pharmaceutical fields. A novel nanophytosomal formulation obtained by physical mixture of two compounds, carnosine and Aloe vera, has shown a synergic effect in counteracting cell toxicity.	▪ Decreased oxidative stress and toxicity ▪ Increased proangiogenic activity (i.e., HIF-1α, VEGFA, bFGF, KDR, and Ang II genes)	[120]

4.1. Vesicular Systems

Different vesicular systems vehiculating carnosine, including nanoliposomes, liposomes, niosomes, proniosomes, polymerosomes, phytosomes, and nanophytosomes, have been investigated (Table 2).

Maherani et al. studied how lipid composition can influence the physico-chemical properties of nanoliposomes encapsulating carnosine [113]. In order to increase the encapsulation efficiency of carnosine, nanoliposomes were prepared considering the effects of 1,2-dioleoyl-sn-glycero-3-phosphocholine (DOPC), 1,2-dipalmitoyl-sn-glycero-3-phosphocholine (DPPC), and 1-palmitoyl-2-oleoyl-sn-glycero-3-phosphocholine (POPC) on vesicles' size, zeta potential, phase transition temperature, and fluidity, with DOPC and DPPC providing the best results in terms of size and encapsulation efficiency.

Anti-inflammatory and antioxidant effects of liposomal and non-liposomal carnosine in adjuvant arthritis were compared by Slovák et al. [114]. Both forms were able to decrease plasmatic levels of interleukin (IL)-1β, matrix metalloproteinase-9, and monocyte chemoattractant protein-1 (MCP-1), but only liposomal carnosine significantly reduced the levels of MCP-1. Of note, liposomal carnosine was more effective in counteracting oxidative stress in plasma as well as in decreasing the mRNA expression of inducible NO synthase in cartilage tissue compared to free carnosine. Neuroprotective effects of carnosine-loaded EL, prepared by extrusion method using egg phosphatidylcholine (phospholipid) and Tween 80 (edge activator), have instead been shown in a cerebral ischemia rat model [115]. Carnosine-loaded EL, having elasticity two-fold higher compared to conventional liposomes, was characterized by nanometric particle size close to 100 nm and homogeneous distribution, also showing a polydispersity index below 0.1. The elasticity of CAR-ELs was 2-fold higher than that of conventional liposomes.

A lipoic acid-based transient receptor potential ankyrin type-1 antagonist, obtained by condensing carnosine with lipoic acid, has been encapsulated into niosomes for brain targeting [25]. In a different study, carnosine and carnosine-loaded niosomes were investigated to evaluate their activities, including the ability to inhibit bovine serum albumin (BSA) aggregation [116]. Carnosine-loaded niosomes were demonstrated to be an efficient drug delivery platform for simultaneous BBB crossing along with the ability to reduce oxidative stress, measured in terms of advanced glycation end-products (AGEs) and advanced oxidation protein products formation, inflammation, and BSA aggregation [25,116,117].

Kim et al. have encapsulated carnosine in lipoprotein receptor-related protein-1 (LRP-1)-targeted functionalized polymersomes and investigated their effects in an in vivo ischemic stroke rat model [118]. Carnosine-loaded polymersomes reduced the aggregation of LRP-1 at the brain level and exhibited remarkable neuroprotective effects despite a dose of carnosine three orders of magnitude lower than the free form.

A study published in 2016 describes carnosine-loaded phytosomes as an alternative to the prodrug N-acetyl-carnosine as a novel delivery system to the lens [119]. It is worth mentioning that, as observed by analyzing ex vivo transcorneal permeation parameters, carnosine-loaded phytosomes showed significantly controlled corneal permeation without changes in primary human corneal cell viability. The same study showed the ability of these formulations to inhibit the brunescence of porcine lenses incubated in a high-glucose medium, indicating the potential for delaying changes that underlie cataractogenesis.

Recently, Darvishi and collaborators demonstrated the synergic effect of dual delivery of carnosine and aloe vera into nanophytosomes in enhancing the protective activity against methylglyoxal-induced angiogenesis impairment in human umbilical vein endothelial cells (HUVECs) [120]. Carnosine/aloe vera-loaded nanophytosomes decreased the toxicity induced by methylglyoxal in HUVEC cells and showed improved free radical scavenging potency and NO synthesizing capacity; these effects were paralleled by enhanced proangiogenic activity as showed by the increased expression of hypoxia-inducible factor 1-alpha (HIF-1α), vascular endothelial growth factor A (VEGFA), basic fibroblast growth factor (bFGF), kinase insert domain receptor (KDR), and Angiotensin II (Ang II) genes.

4.2. Nanoparticles

The use of MNPs coated with carnosine has been considered to obtain both a higher stability of the colloidal suspension and an enhanced therapeutic effect of carnosine [121] (Table 3).

Table 3. New metallic nanoparticle-based formulations of carnosine.

Formulation Name	Basic Description	Mode of Action	Ref.
Fe_3O_4	Carnosine-coated Fe_3O_4 NPs have been prepared via co-precipitation of Fe_3O_4 in the presence of carnosine. They are commonly used because of their superparamagnetic properties allowing potential applications in many fields.	■ Enhanced ac conductivity	[122]
Fe_3O_4 NPs/poly(lactic-co-glycolic acid) (PLGA) polymer-loaded dexamethasone functionalized with carnosine	PLGA functionalized Fe_3O_4 NPs with carnosine peptide composite loaded with dexamethasone represent suitable drug delivery carriers for biomedical applications able to improve the therapeutic efficiency of carnosine.	■ Drug delivery for simultaneous BBB crossing	[123]
Magnetic	Carnosine-coated MNPs were developed to enhance the chemotherapeutic activity of this dipeptide.	■ Enhanced toxicity ■ Improved physicochemical properties	[121] [124]
AuNPs/biotin	A new carnosine derivative with biotin was synthesized and structurally characterized. The binding affinity of the new molecular entity to avidin and streptavidin was exploited to functionalize avidin- and streptavidin-AuNPs with the carnosine–biotin conjugate.	■ Chelating activity (Cu^{2+} and Zn^{2+}) ■ Biotin-like affinity for avidin and streptavidin	[125]
AuNPs/N-acetyl-carnosine	NPs loaded with N-acetyl-carnosine were synthesized, characterized, and tested for cataract treatment. The AuNPs were biofabricated and characterized by using *Coccinia grandis* bark extract.	■ Increased biocompatibility and bioavailability of drug ■ Reduced toxicity	[126]
Poly (lactic-co-glycolic acid) microbeads	The Fe_3O_4 NPs have been encapsulated, along with carnosine, inside porous poly(lactic-co-glycolic acid) microbeads. These new drug-delivery vesicles have the potential to pave the way towards the safe and triggered release of onsite drug delivery as part of a theragnostic treatment for cancer.	■ Increased bioavailability of drug ■ Enhanced intracellular uptake	[127]

Carnosine-coated Fe_3O_4 NPs, obtained through the co-precipitation of Fe_3O_4 in the presence of the dipeptide, have been considered for different applications, including cell separation, diagnosis, and targeted drug delivery for cancer therapy [122]. In a different study, carnosine functionalized Fe_3O_4 NPs loaded with dexamethasone were studied as a possible drug delivery platform for simultaneous BBB crossing [123]. The authors investigated the possible cytotoxic effects to obtain information regarding their biocompatibility in drug delivery in the context of brain damage. The efficacy of BBB carriers was demonstrated and the drug release study for ischemic stroke treatment was presented.

Stimuli-responsive MNPs coated with carnosine have been synthetized and tested, both in vitro and in vivo, for breast cancer therapy [121]. The new formulation was characterized by colloidal stability and the absence of agglomeration issues. When tested in vitro on human breast cancer cells, carnosine-coated MNPs displayed a higher cytotoxic activity compared to free carnosine. Promising results were also obtained in vivo, where carnosine-coated MNPs were able to significantly reduce the size of the tumor without inducing systemic toxicity. The authors were also able to demonstrate an enhanced anti-angiogenic activity of the new formulation. Recently, Khramtsov et al. carried out a research study in which they synthesized nanoclusters of magnetic iron-carbon NPs coated with different proteins, analyzed their physico-chemical properties, and used nanoclusters conjugated with recombinant protein G from *Streptococcus* sp. as labels in a nuclear magnetic resonance immunoassay of IgG against the tetanus vaccine [124]. All four protein coatings (BSA, casein, and gelatins A and B) provided the nanoclusters with long-term storage stability, paralleled by good stability in physiological media and high relaxivity.

A new formulation of carnosine with biotin (BioCar), resistant to the degrading activity of carnosinases in human plasma, was made and structurally characterized by Bellia et al., with the main aim to take advantage of the avidin-biotin technology allowing for the selective delivery of biotinylated agents [125]. In this study, the binding affinity to avidin and streptavidin was used for the functionalization of avidin- and streptavidin- AuNPs with BioCar.

The synthesis, characterization, and cytotoxic effects of AuNPs and their loading with N-acetyl-carnosine for the treatment of cataract has also been performed [126]. The encapsulation of N-acetyl-carnosine into AuNPs significantly increased both biocompatibility and bioavailability without toxic effects when tested on fibroblast cells.

The ability of carnosine to inhibit the proliferation of glioblastoma U87 cancer cells and then to reduce the risk of metastasis has been recently demonstrated by Habra et al. [128]. The same authors have also investigated the controlled release of carnosine from poly(lactic-co-glycolic acid) beads using nanomechanical magnetic triggers [127]. The possibility of obtaining a safe and triggered release of onsite drug delivery of these new drug-delivery vesicles as part of a theragnostic treatment for glioblastoma was also proposed.

PEGylated liquisomes have been proposed as a novel combined passive targeting nanoplatform of carnosine for breast cancer [129]. These formulations were able to protect carnosine from degradation in vivo, prolonging its release and enhancing its anti-cancer activity (% tumor growth, VEGF, cyclin D1, and caspase-3 tissue levels) compared to free carnosine.

4.3. Derivatives/Conjugates

During the last two decades, different derivatization strategies aiming at increasing carnosine activity and its stability to carnosinases (e.g., derivatized with sulfamido pseudopeptides [130]), representing an important limit for the therapeutic use of this molecule [17], have been considered (Table 4).

Table 4. New carnosine formulations obtained by derivatization/conjugation.

Formulation Name	Basic Description	Mode of Action	Ref.
Derivatized with β-cyclodextrins	β-cyclodextrin is a heptasaccharide derived from glucose. Ciclodextrins are particularly used in pharmaceutical science for their ability to include and/or stabilize drugs. Glycoconjugate derivatives obtained by functionalization with carnosine in different positions of the sugar or the cyclodextrin are widely used because of their decreased susceptibility to degradation by carnosinases.	■ Antioxidant activity at concentrations 10–20 times lower than that reported for other synthetic derivatives	[131–133]
		■ Cu^{2+} modulation of carnosine derivative oligomeric species formation	[134]
N-acetylcarnosine	N-acetyl-carnosine is obtained by the addition of an acetyl group to carnosine structure, which makes the dipeptide more resistant to the degradation exerted by carnosinases.	■ Decreased oxidative stress and DNA damage	[135]
		■ Reduced oxidative stress and lipid peroxidation ■ Anti-aging	[136]
		■ Reduced oxidative stress ■ Reduced glycation process and AGEs formation	[137]
		■ Decreased oxidative stress and lipid peroxidation ■ Inhibition of UVB Erythema	[110]

Table 4. Cont.

Formulation Name	Basic Description	Mode of Action	Ref.
Derivatized by acylation with palmitoyl chain	Palmitic acid is a fatty acid with a 16-carbon chain. This compound is commonly used as a structure-directing agent to induce the fibrillization of carnosine. Its long lipid chains are able to drive self-assembly due to amphiphilicity, showing restricted dynamics and/or crystallization.	▪ Improved self-assembly into nanotapes	[138]
Derivatized by acylation with benzoic acid	Benzoic acid is a compound comprising a benzene ring core carrying a carboxylic acid substituent. N-(4-n-tetradecyloxybenzoyl)-L-carnosine represents a carnosine-based amphiphilic hydrogelator that efficiently gelates water and exhibits salt, pH, and thermoresponsive gelation properties.	▪ Increased amphiphilic hydrogelation	[139]
Histidine-based derivatives	Novel histidine-based complexing surfactants containing trifunctional moduli (peptidic/hydrophilic/hydrophobic). It is possible to establish various links between the different parts, allowing the modulation of the lipophilic/hydrophilic balance and obtaining amphiphilic compounds with complexing properties and surfactive or gelator properties.	▪ Improved self-assembling and complexing processes ▪ Increased amphiphilic hydrogelation	[140]
Lipoilcarnosine	Lipoic acid is an organosulfur compound derived from caprylic acid. Lipoilcarnosine is a conjugated molecule obtained by coupling α-lipoic acid to carnosine.	▪ Reduced oxidative stress and toxicity	[141]
Derivatized with trolox	Trolox (6-hydroxy-2,5,7,8-tetramethylchroman-2-carboxylic acid) is a water-soluble analog of vitamin E. (S)-trolox-L-carnosine (STC) and (R)-trolox-L-carnosine (RTC) represent novel derivatives of carnosine synthesized by N-acylation of carnosine with (S)- and (R)-trolox, respectively.	▪ Decreased oxidative stress	[142]
Derivatized with vitamin E-carnosine (VECAR)	VECAR is a novel heterodimer of α-tocopherol (vitamin E) and carnosine that was designed by using 13-carbon phytyl-chain to link carnosine to Trolox at the C2 carbon position, maintaining the antioxidant activities of the two components.	▪ Reduced oxidative stress	[143]
Derivatized with acetylsalicylic acid	Acetylsalicylic acid is a nonsteroidal anti-inflammatory drug (NSAID) used to reduce pain, fever, and/or inflammation and as an antithrombotic. Salicyl-carnosine was synthesized by condensation of acetylsalicylic acid and carnosine. Its properties are particularly promising for the potential development of new anti-inflammatory and antithrombotic drugs.	▪ Reduced oxidative stress ▪ Antiplatelet activity ▪ Protected the gastric mucosa against the formation of ulcerative stomach lesions (anti-ulcer activity)	[110]

Table 4. Cont.

Formulation Name	Basic Description	Mode of Action	Ref.
Derivatized with trehalose	Trehalose is a sugar consisting of two molecules of glucose. The glyco-conjugate trehalose-carnosine (TrCar), differently from carnosine, is not hydrolyzed by human carnosinases. Particular attention has been paid to the characterization of the Cu^{2+} binding features of TrCar.	■ Inhibited Aβ aggregation and glycation process ■ Decreased oxidative stress and toxicity ■ Modulation of Cu^{2+} activity ■ Activated tyrosine kinase cascade pathways ■ Induced the expression of BDNF and VEGF	[144] [145]
Derivatized with hyaluronic acid	Hyaluronic acid is a linear glycosaminoglycan, an anionic, gel-like polymer, found in the extracellular matrix of epithelial and connective tissues. A derivative obtained from hyaluronic acid and carnosine was considered a pharmacological approach to cure and/or prevent the onset of neurodegenerative disorders.	■ Inhibited aggregation of Aβ42 and toxicity	[146]
Carnosinol	A derivative of carnosine with high oral bioavailability because of its resistance to carnosinases. Carnosinol displayed a suitable ADMET (absorption, distribution, metabolism, excretion, and toxicity) profile and the greatest potency and selectivity toward α,β-unsaturated aldehydes.	■ Reduced oxidative stress and metabolic disorders	[147]
Amide derivatives	New family of amide derivatives that are not significantly hydrolyzed by carnosinases. In these derivatives, the sugar moiety can act as a recognition element.	■ Regulated metal homeostasis ■ Reduced oxidative stress (protect LDL from oxidation catalyzed by Cu^{2+} ion) ■ Exerted neuroprotection (protect primary mouse hippocampal neurons against HNE-induced death)	[108] [148]
Carnosine analogues containing NO-donor substructures	Carnosine analogs containing NO-donor substructures of which the physico-chemical characterization and preliminary pharmacological profile were carried out. These analogs are characterized by higher resistance to carnosinases' degradation.	■ Reduced oxidative stress (protect LDL from oxidation catalyzed by Cu^{2+} ion and HNE scavenging) ■ Exerted neuroprotection	[149]
Derivatized with sulfamido pseudopeptides	These compounds, characterized by the presence of a sulfonamido junction, present several interesting aspects which relate to the biological relevance of taurine and the stability toward enzymatic hydrolysis. The high polar character and the sulfur tetrahedral structure make these compounds suitable for the design of tight-binding enzyme inhibitors.	■ Inhibition of carnosinases' activity	[130]
FL-926-16	A novel, rationally designed carnosine peptidomimetic with a favorable pharmacokinetic profile, which might be suitable for testing in human subjects.	■ Reduced inflammation and oxidative stress (NLRP3 inflammasome and AGEs) ■ Anti-apoptotic	[150]

For example, the use of cyclodextrins (CDs) to synthesize carnosine derivatives has been exploited to enhance carnosine activity, with the ability of CDs to scavenge hydroxyl radicals being synergic with the antioxidant activity of carnosine [132]. The amino group of the β-alanine or the carboxyl group of the histidine can be both derivatized to obtain therapeutic carnosinase-resistant molecules. The addition of conjugates can confer a steric shielding effect against proteases and peptidases.

Several carnosine derivatives with saccharides, such as β-CD and trehalose, have been synthesized [108] (a graphic representation of β-CD-carnosine conjugate is depicted in Figure 3).

Different carnosine derivatives with β-CD have been synthesized and structurally characterized, but only a few of them have been tested in biological systems. More than 20 years ago, Vecchio et al. described the synthesis and conformation of β-CDs functionalized with enantiomers of Boc-carnosine [131], suggesting that the CD could represent a stabilizer and a carrier of the dipeptide. The authors further suggested that the moiety of carnosine, as well as the Boc group, may make β-CD-carnosine derivatives far more efficient artificial chaperones compared to free CDs because of the occurring hydrogen bond interactions. Numerous preclinical studies have shown that carnosine and its analog homocarnosine (beta-aminobutyril-L-histidine) are able to scavenge reactive oxygen species. In a study by Amorini et al., the synthesis and antioxidant activity of new homocarnosine β-CD conjugates were described [132]. β-CD-carnosine derivatives demonstrated a higher ability to inhibit the Cu^{2+}-driven low-density lipoprotein (LDL) oxidation compared to homocarnosine derivatives. An additional study related to this topic considered the synthesis of β-CD-carnosine derivatives and their hydroxyl radical scavenger ability [133]. By using pulse-radiolysis, it was shown that the new derivatives of carnosine considered are excellent scavengers of hydroxyl radical, with the activity coming from both the glucose moieties of the macrocycle and the formation of the stable imidazole-centered radical. The ability of β-CD-carnosine derivatives to interact with Cu^{2+} as well as that of this transition metal ion to induce the formation of supramolecular assemblies (β-CD-carnosine oligomeric species up to hexamer) have also been demonstrated [134]. Despite these promising results obtained by using cell-free systems, it remains to elucidate their therapeutic properties in biological systems such as cells in the absence or in the presence of pro-oxidant stimuli.

With regards to trehalose–carnosine conjugates, recently, the ionophore ability of a trehalose conjugate to activate tyrosine kinase cascade pathways and assist copper signal in triggering brain-derived neurotrophic factor (BDNF) and VEGF activation in PC12 cells has been proved [145]. In a different study, trehalose–carnosine conjugates ability to inhibit amyloid-β (Aβ) aggregation, tune Cu^{2+} activity, also decreasing the toxic effects exerted by acrolein has been described [144]. The newly synthesized glyco-conjugate (TrCar2) was resistant to human carnosinase hydrolysis, quenched acrolein and their Cu^{2+} complexes, showed superoxide dismutase (SOD)-like activity, and inhibited both self- and metal-induced Aβ aggregation. As for the latter activity, it has also been demonstrated for hyaluronan-carnosine conjugates [146]. These derivatives showed an inhibitory activity higher than the parent compounds, with an effect proportional to the loading of carnosine. Of note, hyaluronan–carnosine conjugates were also able to dissolve the amyloid fibrils and reduce Aβ-induced toxicity in undifferentiated SH-SY5Y cells. Numerous studies have been devoted to the investigation of N-acetyl-carnosine activity and, in particular, its ability to counteract oxidative stress [135–137]. This ability was also paralleled by decreased DNA damage [135], decreased lipid peroxidation [136], or reduced glycation process and AGEs formation [137]. The inhibition of AGEs has been proved in vivo by FL-926-16, a novel bioavailable carnosinase-resistant carnosine derivative [150]. This derivative also demonstrated the ability to prevent the onset and to block the progression of diabetic nephropathy in *db/db* mice by quenching reactive carbonyl species, thus reducing the accumulation of their protein adducts and the related inflammatory response (including the NLRP3 inflammasome).

Additional derivatives of carnosine able to significantly counteract oxidative stress phenomena are represented by carnosine derivatized with Trolox [142], vitamin E (VECAR) [143], or acetylsalicylic acid [110] as well as lipoilcarnosine [141], carnosine analogs containing NO-donor substructures [149], and amide derivatives [148]. The latter derivatives have also been shown to be able to regulate metal homeostasis [108]. Another study carried out by Anderson et al. described the pharmacological effects of carnosinol, a derivative of carnosine characterized by high oral bioavailability, in a model of diet-induced obesity and metabolic syndrome [147]. Carnosinol decreased the formation of 4-hydroxynonenal (HNE) adducts in both liver and skeletal muscle in a concentration-dependent manner, also counteracting other alterations, including inflammation and insulin resistance.

Improved self-assembling and complexing processes, along with increased amphiphilic hydrogelation, have been described for histidine-based derivatives inspired by carnosine [140]. Improved self-assembling was also demonstrated for carnosine derivatized by acylation with palmitoyl chain [138], while enhanced amphiphilic hydrogelation, including the ability to efficiently gelate water, was observed in the case of carnosine derivatized by acylation with benzoic acid [139].

5. Conclusions and Future Perspectives

Drug development is currently focused on the identification of novel carnosine formulations able to improve its efficacy and stability, finally increasing its therapeutic potential in humans. Nowadays, the use of innovative DDS and/or the chemical modifications of carnosine led to the development of formulations allowing to decrease, or in the best scenario, completely prevent its hydrolysis by carnosinases, the simultaneous BBB crossing, to maintain or enhance carnosine biological activity, as well as the site-specific transport to different tissues. Despite these promising results, further studies carried out both in cells challenged with specific pro-oxidant/pro-inflammatory stimuli and in animal models of systemic and neurodegenerative disorders are needed to translate these findings to clinical practice.

Author Contributions: Conceptualization, G.C. and F.C.; writing—original draft preparation, A.B., A.P., M.G., S.S. and G.C.; writing—review and editing, A.B., A.P., M.G., S.S., C.C., R.P., T.M., F.C. and G.C.; supervision, G.C. All authors have read and agreed to the published version of the manuscript.

Funding: G.C. and A.B. are researchers at the University of Catania within the EU-funded PON REACT project (Azione IV.4—"Dottorati e contratti di ricerca su tematiche dell'innovazione", nuovo Asse IV del PON Ricerca e Innovazione 2014–2020 "Istruzione e ricerca per il recupero—REACT—EU"; Progetti "Identificazione e validazione di nuovi target farmacologici nella malattia di Alzheimer attraverso l'utilizzo della microfluidica" (G.C.) and "Approcci terapeutici innovativi per il targeting cerebrale di farmaci e materiale genico" (A.B.); CUP E65F21002640005). This research was partially funded by Ricerca di Ateneo 2020–2022, Piano di incentivi per la ricerca (PIA.CE.RI.), Linea di intervento 2; Naso, Nanomedicina e Neuroterapie: Le 3 N per il target cerebrale di molecole bioattive (3 N-ORACLE), progetto interdipartimentale, CUP 57722172124, to T.M., and by the Italian Ministry of Health Research Program, RC2022-24, to G.C.

Institutional Review Board Statement: Not applicable.

Informed Consent Statement: Not applicable.

Data Availability Statement: Data sharing not applicable.

Acknowledgments: A.P. would like to thank the International Ph.D. Program in Neuroscience at the University of Catania (Italy).

Conflicts of Interest: The authors declare no conflict of interest.

References

1. Gulewitsch, W.; Amiradžibi, S. Ueber das carnosin, eine neue organische base des fleischextractes. *Ber. Dtsch. Chem. Ges.* **1900**, *33*, 1902–1903. [CrossRef]
2. Boldyrev, A.A.; Aldini, G.; Derave, W. Physiology and pathophysiology of carnosine. *Physiol. Rev.* **2013**, *93*, 1803–1845. [CrossRef] [PubMed]
3. Caruso, G.; Caraci, F.; Jolivet, R.B. Pivotal role of carnosine in the modulation of brain cells activity: Multimodal mechanism of action and therapeutic potential in neurodegenerative disorders. *Prog. Neurobiol.* **2019**, *175*, 35–53. [CrossRef] [PubMed]
4. Caruso, G.; Fresta, C.G.; Musso, N.; Giambirtone, M.; Grasso, M.; Spampinato, S.F.; Merlo, S.; Drago, F.; Lazzarino, G.; Sortino, M.A.; et al. Carnosine prevents aβ-induced oxidative stress and inflammation in microglial cells: A key role of tgf-β1. *Cells* **2019**, *8*, 64. [CrossRef] [PubMed]
5. Fleisher-Berkovich, S.; Abramovitch-Dahan, C.; Ben-Shabat, S.; Apte, R.; Beit-Yannai, E. Inhibitory effect of carnosine and n-acetyl carnosine on lps-induced microglial oxidative stress and inflammation. *Peptides* **2009**, *30*, 1306–1312. [CrossRef]
6. Caruso, G.; Privitera, A.; Antunes, B.M.; Lazzarino, G.; Lunte, S.M.; Aldini, G.; Caraci, F. The therapeutic potential of carnosine as an antidote against drug-induced cardiotoxicity and neurotoxicity: Focus on nrf2 pathway. *Molecules* **2022**, *27*, 4452. [CrossRef] [PubMed]
7. Fresta, C.G.; Fidilio, A.; Lazzarino, G.; Musso, N.; Grasso, M.; Merlo, S.; Amorini, A.M.; Bucolo, C.; Tavazzi, B.; Lazzarino, G.; et al. Modulation of pro-oxidant and pro-inflammatory activities of m1 macrophages by the natural dipeptide carnosine. *Int. J. Mol. Sci.* **2020**, *21*, 776. [CrossRef]
8. Caruso, G.; Fresta, C.G.; Fidilio, A.; O'Donnell, F.; Musso, N.; Lazzarino, G.; Grasso, M.; Amorini, A.M.; Tascedda, F.; Bucolo, C.; et al. Carnosine decreases pma-induced oxidative stress and inflammation in murine macrophages. *Antioxidants* **2019**, *8*, 281. [CrossRef]
9. Caruso, G.; Privitera, A.; Saab, M.W.; Musso, N.; Maugeri, S.; Fidilio, A.; Privitera, A.P.; Pittalà, A.; Jolivet, R.B.; Lanzanò, L.; et al. Characterization of carnosine effect on human microglial cells under basal conditions. *Biomedicines* **2023**, *11*, 474. [CrossRef]
10. Agostinho, P.; Cunha, R.A.; Oliveira, C. Neuroinflammation, oxidative stress and the pathogenesis of alzheimer's disease. *Curr. Pharm. Des.* **2010**, *16*, 2766–2778. [CrossRef]
11. Caruso, G.; Grasso, M.; Fidilio, A.; Torrisi, S.A.; Musso, N.; Geraci, F.; Tropea, M.R.; Privitera, A.; Tascedda, F.; Puzzo, D.; et al. Antioxidant activity of fluoxetine and vortioxetine in a non-transgenic animal model of alzheimer's disease. *Front. Pharmacol.* **2021**, *12*, 809541. [CrossRef]
12. Caruso, G.; Spampinato, S.F.; Cardaci, V.; Caraci, F.; Sortino, M.A.; Merlo, S. B-amyloid and oxidative stress: Perspectives in drug development. *Curr. Pharm. Des.* **2019**, *25*, 4771–4781. [CrossRef] [PubMed]
13. Araminia, B.; Shalbafan, M.; Mortezaei, A.; Shirazi, E.; Ghaffari, S.; Sahebolzamani, E.; Mortazavi, S.H.; Shariati, B.; Ardebili, M.E.; Aqamolaei, A.; et al. L-carnosine combination therapy for major depressive disorder: A randomized, double-blind, placebo-controlled trial. *J. Affect. Disord.* **2020**, *267*, 131–136. [CrossRef] [PubMed]
14. Caruso, G.; Benatti, C.; Blom, J.M.C.; Caraci, F.; Tascedda, F. The many faces of mitochondrial dysfunction in depression: From pathology to treatment. *Front. Pharmacol.* **2019**, *10*, 995. [CrossRef]
15. Hald, A.; Lotharius, J. Oxidative stress and inflammation in parkinson's disease: Is there a causal link? *Exp. Neurol.* **2005**, *193*, 279–290. [CrossRef] [PubMed]
16. Niranjan, R. The role of inflammatory and oxidative stress mechanisms in the pathogenesis of parkinson's disease: Focus on astrocytes. *Mol. Neurobiol.* **2014**, *49*, 28–38. [CrossRef]
17. Bellia, F.; Vecchio, G.; Rizzarelli, E. Carnosinases, their substrates and diseases. *Molecules* **2014**, *19*, 2299–2329. [CrossRef] [PubMed]
18. Caruso, G. Unveiling the hidden therapeutic potential of carnosine, a molecule with a multimodal mechanism of action: A position paper. *Molecules* **2022**, *27*, 3303. [CrossRef]
19. Grasso, M.; Caruso, G.; Godos, J.; Bonaccorso, A.; Carbone, C.; Castellano, S.; Currenti, W.; Grosso, G.; Musumeci, T.; Caraci, F. Improving cognition with nutraceuticals targeting tgf-β1 signaling. *Antioxidants* **2021**, *10*, 1075. [CrossRef]
20. Aldawsari, H.M.; Badr-Eldin, S.M.; Assiri, N.Y.; Alhakamy, N.A.; Privitera, A.; Caraci, F.; Caruso, G. Surface-tailoring of emulsomes for boosting brain delivery of vinpocetine via intranasal route: In vitro optimization and in vivo pharmacokinetic assessment. *Drug Deliv.* **2022**, *29*, 2671–2684. [CrossRef]
21. Bermúdez, M.L.; Skelton, M.R.; Genter, M.B. Intranasal carnosine attenuates transcriptomic alterations and improves mitochondrial function in the thy1-asyn mouse model of parkinson's disease. *Mol. Genet. Metab.* **2018**, *125*, 305–313. [CrossRef] [PubMed]
22. Musumeci, T.; Bonaccorso, A.; Puglisi, G. Epilepsy disease and nose-to-brain delivery of polymeric nanoparticles: An overview. *Pharmaceutics* **2019**, *11*, 118. [CrossRef] [PubMed]
23. Huang, Y.; Deng, X.; Liang, J. Review of the application of nanovesicles and the human interstitial fluid in gastrointestinal premalignant lesion detection, diagnosis, prognosis and therapy. *Int. J. Nanomed.* **2019**, *14*, 9469–9482. [CrossRef] [PubMed]
24. Liu, J.; Ren, L.; Li, S.; Li, W.; Zheng, X.; Yang, Y.; Fu, W.; Yi, J.; Wang, J.; Du, G. The biology, function, and applications of exosomes in cancer. *Acta Pharm. Sin. B* **2021**, *11*, 2783–2797. [CrossRef] [PubMed]
25. Maestrelli, F.; Landucci, E.; De Luca, E.; Nerli, G.; Bergonzi, M.C.; Piazzini, V.; Pellegrini-Giampietro, D.E.; Gullo, F.; Becchetti, A.; Tadini-Buoninsegni, F.; et al. Niosomal formulation of a lipoyl-carnosine derivative targeting trpa1 channels in brain. *Pharmaceutics* **2019**, *11*, 669. [CrossRef]

26. Mohd Zaffarin, A.S.; Ng, S.F.; Ng, M.H.; Hassan, H.; Alias, E. Pharmacology and pharmacokinetics of vitamin e: Nanoformulations to enhance bioavailability. *Int. J. Nanomed.* **2020**, *15*, 9961–9974. [CrossRef] [PubMed]
27. Erdoğar, N.; Akkın, S.; Bilensoy, E. Nanocapsules for drug delivery: An updated review of the last decade. *Recent Pat. Drug Deliv. Formul.* **2018**, *12*, 252–266. [CrossRef]
28. Laffleur, F.; Keckeis, V. Advances in drug delivery systems: Work in progress still needed? *Int. J. Pharm.* **2020**, *590*, 119912. [CrossRef]
29. Miao, J.; Li, F.; Zhang, M.; Zhou, C.; Ren, W.; Hu, X.; Li, N.; Lei, L. Carnosine synthase 1 contributes to interferon gamma-induced arginine depletion via mitogen-activated protein kinase 11 signaling in bovine mammary epithelial cells. *J. Interferon Cytokine Res.* **2022**, *42*, 501–512. [CrossRef]
30. Kwiatkowski, S.; Kiersztan, A.; Drozak, J. Biosynthesis of carnosine and related dipeptides in vertebrates. *Curr. Protein Pept. Sci.* **2018**, *19*, 771–789. [CrossRef]
31. Parthasarathy, A.; Savka, M.A.; Hudson, A.O. The synthesis and role of β-alanine in plants. *Front. Plant Sci.* **2019**, *10*, 921. [CrossRef] [PubMed]
32. Holeček, M. Histidine in health and disease: Metabolism, physiological importance, and use as a supplement. *Nutrients* **2020**, *12*, 848. [CrossRef]
33. Junge, W.; McLaughlin, S. The role of fixed and mobile buffers in the kinetics of proton movement. *Biochim. Biophys. Acta (BBA)-Bioenerg.* **1987**, *890*, 1–5. [CrossRef]
34. Swietach, P.; Youm, J.B.; Saegusa, N.; Leem, C.H.; Spitzer, K.W.; Vaughan-Jones, R.D. Coupled ca^{2+}/h+ transport by cytoplasmic buffers regulates local ca^{2+} and h+ ion signaling. *Proc. Natl. Acad. Sci. USA* **2013**, *110*, E2064–E2073. [CrossRef] [PubMed]
35. Dutka, T.L.; Lamboley, C.R.; McKenna, M.J.; Murphy, R.M.; Lamb, G.D. Effects of carnosine on contractile apparatus ca^{2+} sensitivity and sarcoplasmic reticulum ca^{2+} release in human skeletal muscle fibers. *J. Appl. Physiol.* **2012**, *112*, 728–736. [CrossRef]
36. Severin, S.E.; Kirzon, M.V.; Kaftanova, T.M. Effect of carnosine and anserine on action of isolated frog muscles. *Dokl. Akad. Nauk SSSR* **1953**, *91*, 691–694.
37. Sale, C.; Artioli, G.G.; Gualano, B.; Saunders, B.; Hobson, R.M.; Harris, R.C. Carnosine: From exercise performance to health. *Amino Acids* **2013**, *44*, 1477–1491. [CrossRef]
38. Boldyrev, A.A.; Petukhov, V.B. Localization of carnosine effect on the fatigued muscle preparation. *Gen. Pharmacol.* **1978**, *9*, 17–20. [CrossRef]
39. Brisola, G.M.P.; de Souza Malta, E.; Santiago, P.R.P.; Vieira, L.H.P.; Zagatto, A.M. B-alanine supplementation's improvement of high-intensity game activities in water polo. *Int. J. Sport. Physiol. Perform.* **2018**, *13*, 1208–1214. [CrossRef]
40. de Andrade Kratz, C.; de Salles Painelli, V.; de Andrade Nemezio, K.M.; da Silva, R.P.; Franchini, E.; Zagatto, A.M.; Gualano, B.; Artioli, G.G. Beta-alanine supplementation enhances judo-related performance in highly-trained athletes. *J. Sci. Med. Sport* **2017**, *20*, 403–408. [CrossRef]
41. Furst, T.; Massaro, A.; Miller, C.; Williams, B.T.; LaMacchia, Z.M.; Horvath, P.J. B-alanine supplementation increased physical performance and improved executive function following endurance exercise in middle aged individuals. *J. Int. Soc. Sport. Nutr.* **2018**, *15*, 32. [CrossRef] [PubMed]
42. Glenn, J.M.; Smith, K.; Moyen, N.E.; Binns, A.; Gray, M. Effects of acute beta-alanine supplementation on anaerobic performance in trained female cyclists. *J. Nutr. Sci. Vitaminol.* **2015**, *61*, 161–166. [CrossRef]
43. Culbertson, J.Y.; Kreider, R.B.; Greenwood, M.; Cooke, M. Effects of beta-alanine on muscle carnosine and exercise performance: A review of the current literature. *Nutrients* **2010**, *2*, 75–98. [CrossRef] [PubMed]
44. Privitera, A.; Cardaci, V.; Weerasekara, D.; Saab, M.W.; Diolosà, L.; Fidilio, A.; Jolivet, R.B.; Lazzarino, G.; Amorini, A.M.; Camarda, M. Microfluidic/hplc combination to study carnosine protective activity on challenged human microglia: Focus on oxidative stress and energy metabolism. *Front. Pharmacol.* **2023**, *14*, 667. [CrossRef] [PubMed]
45. Tiedje, K.; Stevens, K.; Barnes, S.; Weaver, D. B-alanine as a small molecule neurotransmitter. *Neurochem. Int.* **2010**, *57*, 177–188. [CrossRef] [PubMed]
46. Mal'tseva, V.V.; Sergienko, V.V.; Stvolinskii, S.L. The effect of carnosine on hematopoietic stem cell activity in irradiated animals. *Biokhimiia* **1992**, *57*, 1378–1382.
47. de Courten, B.; Jakubova, M.; de Courten, M.P.; Kukurova, I.J.; Vallova, S.; Krumpolec, P.; Valkovic, L.; Kurdiova, T.; Garzon, D.; Barbaresi, S.; et al. Effects of carnosine supplementation on glucose metabolism: Pilot clinical trial. *Obesity* **2016**, *24*, 1027–1034. [CrossRef]
48. Fresta, C.G.; Chakraborty, A.; Wijesinghe, M.B.; Amorini, A.M.; Lazzarino, G.; Lazzarino, G.; Tavazzi, B.; Lunte, S.M.; Caraci, F.; Dhar, P.; et al. Non-toxic engineered carbon nanodiamond concentrations induce oxidative/nitrosative stress, imbalance of energy metabolism, and mitochondrial dysfunction in microglial and alveolar basal epithelial cells. *Cell Death Dis.* **2018**, *9*, 245. [CrossRef]
49. Caruso, G.; Fresta, C.G.; Martinez-Becerra, F.; Antonio, L.; Johnson, R.T.; de Campos, R.P.S.; Siegel, J.M.; Wijesinghe, M.B.; Lazzarino, G.; Lunte, S.M. Carnosine modulates nitric oxide in stimulated murine raw 264.7 macrophages. *Mol. Cell. Biochem.* **2017**, *431*, 197–210. [CrossRef]
50. Caruso, G.; Benatti, C.; Musso, N.; Fresta, C.G.; Fidilio, A.; Spampinato, G.; Brunello, N.; Bucolo, C.; Drago, F.; Lunte, S.M.; et al. Carnosine protects macrophages against the toxicity of aβ1-42 oligomers by decreasing oxidative stress. *Biomedicines* **2021**, *9*, 477. [CrossRef]

51. Nagai, K.; Suda, T.; Kawasaki, K.; Mathuura, S. Action of carnosine and beta-alanine on wound healing. *Surgery* **1986**, *100*, 815–821. [PubMed]
52. Pepper, E.D.; Farrell, M.J.; Nord, G.; Finkel, S.E. Antiglycation effects of carnosine and other compounds on the long-term survival of escherichia coli. *Appl. Environ. Microbiol.* **2010**, *76*, 7925–7930. [CrossRef] [PubMed]
53. Boldyrev, A.A.; Gallant, S.C.; Sukhich, G.T. Carnosine, the protective, anti-aging peptide. *Biosci. Rep.* **1999**, *19*, 581–587. [CrossRef] [PubMed]
54. Abe, H. Role of histidine-related compounds as intracellular proton buffering constituents in vertebrate muscle. *Biochemistry* **2000**, *65*, 757–765.
55. Ouyang, L.; Tian, Y.; Bao, Y.; Xu, H.; Cheng, J.; Wang, B.; Shen, Y.; Chen, Z.; Lyu, J. Carnosine decreased neuronal cell death through targeting glutamate system and astrocyte mitochondrial bioenergetics in cultured neuron/astrocyte exposed to ogd/recovery. *Brain Res. Bull.* **2016**, *124*, 76–84. [CrossRef]
56. Hasanein, P.; Felegari, Z. Chelating effects of carnosine in ameliorating nickel-induced nephrotoxicity in rats. *Can. J. Physiol. Pharmacol.* **2017**, *95*, 1426–1432. [CrossRef]
57. Brown, C.E.; Antholine, W.E. Chelation chemistry of carnosine. Evidence that mixed complexes may occur in vivo. *J. Phys. Chem.* **1979**, *83*, 3314–3319. [CrossRef]
58. Wang-Eckhardt, L.; Bastian, A.; Bruegmann, T.; Sasse, P.; Eckhardt, M. Carnosine synthase deficiency is compatible with normal skeletal muscle and olfactory function but causes reduced olfactory sensitivity in aging mice. *J. Biol. Chem.* **2020**, *295*, 17100–17113. [CrossRef]
59. Wang-Eckhardt, L.; Becker, I.; Wang, Y.; Yuan, J.; Eckhardt, M. Absence of endogenous carnosine synthesis does not increase protein carbonylation and advanced lipoxidation end products in brain, kidney or muscle. *Amino Acids* **2022**, *54*, 1013–1023. [CrossRef]
60. Park, H.; Otte, A.; Park, K. Evolution of drug delivery systems: From 1950 to 2020 and beyond. *J. Control. Release* **2022**, *342*, 53–65. [CrossRef]
61. Park, K. Controlled drug delivery systems: Past forward and future back. *J. Control. Release* **2014**, *190*, 3–8. [CrossRef] [PubMed]
62. Benoit, D.S.; Overby, C.T.; Sims Jr, K.R.; Ackun-Farmmer, M.A. Drug delivery systems. In *Biomaterials Science*; Elsevier: Amsterdam, The Netherlands, 2020; pp. 1237–1266.
63. Witika, B.A.; Mweetwa, L.L.; Tshiamo, K.O.; Edler, K.; Matafwali, S.K.; Ntemi, P.V.; Chikukwa, M.T.; Makoni, P.A. Vesicular drug delivery for the treatment of topical disorders: Current and future perspectives. *J. Pharm. Pharmacol.* **2021**, *73*, 1427–1441. [CrossRef] [PubMed]
64. Alhakamy, N.A.; Badr-Eldin, S.M.; Fahmy, U.A.; Alruwaili, N.K.; Awan, Z.A.; Caruso, G.; Alfaleh, M.A.; Alaofi, A.L.; Arif, F.O.; Ahmed, O.A.A.; et al. Thymoquinone-loaded soy-phospholipid-based phytosomes exhibit anticancer potential against human lung cancer cells. *Pharmaceutics* **2020**, *12*, 761. [CrossRef] [PubMed]
65. Gangwar, M.; Singh, R.; Goel, R.; Nath, G. Recent advances in various emerging vesicular systems: An overview. *Asian Pac. J. Trop. Biomed.* **2012**, *2*, S1176–S1188. [CrossRef]
66. El Maghraby, G.M.; Williams, A.C. Vesicular systems for delivering conventional small organic molecules and larger macromolecules to and through human skin. *Expert Opin. Drug Deliv.* **2009**, *6*, 149–163. [CrossRef] [PubMed]
67. Guimarães, D.; Cavaco-Paulo, A.; Nogueira, E. Design of liposomes as drug delivery system for therapeutic applications. *Int. J. Pharm.* **2021**, *601*, 120571. [CrossRef]
68. Bondu, C.; Yen, F.T. Nanoliposomes, from food industry to nutraceuticals: Interests and uses. *Innov. Food Sci. Emerg. Technol.* **2022**, *81*, 103140. [CrossRef]
69. Hussain, A.; Singh, S.; Sharma, D.; Webster, T.J.; Shafaat, K.; Faruk, A. Elastic liposomes as novel carriers: Recent advances in drug delivery. *Int. J. Nanomed.* **2017**, *12*, 5087. [CrossRef]
70. Trotta, M.; Peira, E.; Debernardi, F.; Gallarate, M. Elastic liposomes for skin delivery of dipotassium glycyrrhizinate. *Int. J. Pharm.* **2002**, *241*, 319–327. [CrossRef]
71. El Maghraby, G.M.; Barry, B.W.; Williams, A. Liposomes and skin: From drug delivery to model membranes. *Eur. J. Pharm. Sci.* **2008**, *34*, 203–222. [CrossRef]
72. Chen, J.; Lu, W.-L.; Gu, W.; Lu, S.-S.; Chen, Z.-P.; Cai, B.-C. Skin permeation behavior of elastic liposomes: Role of formulation ingredients. *Expert Opin. Drug Deliv.* **2013**, *10*, 845–856. [CrossRef] [PubMed]
73. Mishra, D.; Dubey, V.; Asthana, A.; Saraf, D.; Jain, N. Elastic liposomes mediated transcutaneous immunization against hepatitis b. *Vaccine* **2006**, *24*, 4847–4855. [CrossRef] [PubMed]
74. Mishra, D.; Garg, M.; Dubey, V.; Jain, S.; Jain, N. Elastic liposomes mediated transdermal delivery of an anti-hypertensive agent: Propranolol hydrochloride. *J. Pharm. Sci.* **2007**, *96*, 145–155. [CrossRef] [PubMed]
75. Altamimi, M.A.; Hussain, A.; AlRajhi, M.; Alshehri, S.; Imam, S.S.; Qamar, W. Luteolin-loaded elastic liposomes for transdermal delivery to control breast cancer: In vitro and ex vivo evaluations. *Pharmaceuticals* **2021**, *14*, 1143. [CrossRef] [PubMed]
76. Montanari, J.; Maidana, C.; Esteva, M.I.; Salomon, C.; Morilla, M.J.; Romero, E.L. Sunlight triggered photodynamic ultradeformable liposomes against leishmania braziliensis are also leishmanicidal in the dark. *J. Control. Release* **2010**, *147*, 368–376. [CrossRef]
77. Souto, E.B.; Macedo, A.S.; Dias-Ferreira, J.; Cano, A.; Zielińska, A.; Matos, C.M. Elastic and ultradeformable liposomes for transdermal delivery of active pharmaceutical ingredients (apis). *Int. J. Mol. Sci.* **2021**, *22*, 9743. [CrossRef]

78. Du, X.; Huang, X.; Wang, L.; Mo, L.; Jing, H.; Bai, X.; Wang, H. Nanosized niosomes as effective delivery device to improve the stability and bioaccessibility of goat milk whey protein peptide. *Food Res. Int.* **2022**, *161*, 111729. [CrossRef]
79. Barani, M.; Sangiovanni, E.; Angarano, M.; Rajizadeh, M.A.; Mehrabani, M.; Piazza, S.; Gangadharappa, H.V.; Pardakhty, A.; Mehrbani, M.; Dell'Agli, M. Phytosomes as innovative delivery systems for phytochemicals: A comprehensive review of literature. *Int. J. Nanomed.* **2021**, *16*, 6983. [CrossRef]
80. Ge, X.; Wei, M.; He, S.; Yuan, W.-E. Advances of non-ionic surfactant vesicles (niosomes) and their application in drug delivery. *Pharmaceutics* **2019**, *11*, 55. [CrossRef]
81. Chen, S.; Hanning, S.; Falconer, J.; Locke, M.; Wen, J. Recent advances in non-ionic surfactant vesicles (niosomes): Fabrication, characterization, pharmaceutical and cosmetic applications. *Eur. J. Pharm. Biopharm.* **2019**, *144*, 18–39. [CrossRef]
82. Marianecci, C.; Di Marzio, L.; Rinaldi, F.; Celia, C.; Paolino, D.; Alhaique, F.; Esposito, S.; Carafa, M. Niosomes from 80s to present: The state of the art. *Adv. Colloid Interface Sci.* **2014**, *205*, 187–206. [CrossRef] [PubMed]
83. Hoque, M.; Agarwal, S.; Gupta, S.; Garg, S.; Syed, I.; Rupesh, A.; Mohapatra, N.; Bose, S.; Sarkar, P. Lipid nanostructures in food applications. *Innov. Food Sci. Emerg. Technol.* **2021**, 565–579.
84. Patel, J.; Patel, R.; Khambholja, K.; Patel, N. An overview of phytosomes as an advanced herbal drug delivery system. *Asian J. Pharm. Sci.* **2009**, *4*, 363–371.
85. Azeez, N.A.; Deepa, V.S.; Sivapriya, V. Phytosomes: Emergent promising nano vesicular drug delivery system for targeted tumor therapy. *Adv. Nat. Sci. Nanosci. Nanotechnol.* **2018**, *9*, 033001. [CrossRef]
86. Alharbi, W.S.; Almughem, F.A.; Almehmady, A.M.; Jarallah, S.J.; Alsharif, W.K.; Alzahrani, N.M.; Alshehri, A.A. Phytosomes as an emerging nanotechnology platform for the topical delivery of bioactive phytochemicals. *Pharmaceutics* **2021**, *13*, 1475. [CrossRef]
87. Panda, V.S.; Naik, S.R. Evaluation of cardioprotective activity of ginkgo biloba and ocimum sanctum in rodents. *Altern. Med. Rev.* **2009**, *14*, 161.
88. Zhang, X.-Y.; Zhang, P.-Y. Polymersomes in nanomedicine—A review. *Curr. Nanosci.* **2017**, *13*, 124–129. [CrossRef]
89. Lee, J.S.; Feijen, J. Polymersomes for drug delivery: Design, formation and characterization. *J. Control. Release* **2012**, *161*, 473–483. [CrossRef]
90. Meerovich, I.; Dash, A.K. Polymersomes for drug delivery and other biomedical applications. In *Materials for Biomedical Engineering*; Elsevier: Amsterdam, The Netherlands, 2019; pp. 269–309.
91. Liu, Q.; Song, L.; Chen, S.; Gao, J.; Zhao, P.; Du, J. A superparamagnetic polymersome with extremely high t2 relaxivity for mri and cancer-targeted drug delivery. *Biomaterials* **2017**, *114*, 23–33. [CrossRef]
92. Bayda, S.; Adeel, M.; Tuccinardi, T.; Cordani, M.; Rizzolio, F. The history of nanoscience and nanotechnology: From chemical–physical applications to nanomedicine. *Molecules* **2019**, *25*, 112. [CrossRef]
93. Harris, N.; Blaber, M.; Schatz, G. Optical properties of metal nanoparticles. *Encycl. Nanotechnol.* **2012**, *481*, 9751–9754.
94. Chandrakala, V.; Aruna, V.; Angajala, G. Review on metal nanoparticles as nanocarriers: Current challenges and perspectives in drug delivery systems. *Emergent Mater.* **2022**, *5*, 1593–1615. [CrossRef] [PubMed]
95. Nowak-Jary, J.; Machnicka, B. Pharmacokinetics of magnetic iron oxide nanoparticles for medical applications. *J. Nanobiotechnology* **2022**, *20*, 1–30. [CrossRef] [PubMed]
96. Kong, F.-Y.; Zhang, J.-W.; Li, R.-F.; Wang, Z.-X.; Wang, W.-J.; Wang, W. Unique roles of gold nanoparticles in drug delivery, targeting and imaging applications. *Molecules* **2017**, *22*, 1445. [CrossRef] [PubMed]
97. Martinkova, P.; Brtnicky, M.; Kynicky, J.; Pohanka, M. Iron oxide nanoparticles: Innovative tool in cancer diagnosis and therapy. *Adv. Healthc. Mater.* **2018**, *7*, 1700932. [CrossRef] [PubMed]
98. Amina, S.J.; Guo, B. A review on the synthesis and functionalization of gold nanoparticles as a drug delivery vehicle. *Int. J. Nanomed.* **2020**, *15*, 9823–9857. [CrossRef] [PubMed]
99. Daraee, H.; Eatemadi, A.; Abbasi, E.; Fekri Aval, S.; Kouhi, M.; Akbarzadeh, A. Application of gold nanoparticles in biomedical and drug delivery. *Artif. Cells Nanomed. Biotechnol.* **2016**, *44*, 410–422. [CrossRef]
100. Hammami, I.; Alabdallah, N.M. Gold nanoparticles: Synthesis properties and applications. *J. King Saud Univ.-Sci.* **2021**, *33*, 101560. [CrossRef]
101. Arora, S.; Sharma, P.; Kumar, S.; Nayan, R.; Khanna, P.K.; Zaidi, M.G.H. Gold-nanoparticle induced enhancement in growth and seed yield of Brassica juncea. Plant growth regulation. *Plant Growth Regul.* **2012**, *66*, 303–310. [CrossRef]
102. Garton, M.; Nim, S.; Stone, T.A.; Wang, K.E.; Deber, C.M.; Kim, P.M. Method to generate highly stable d-amino acid analogs of bioactive helical peptides using a mirror image of the entire pdb. *Proc. Natl. Acad. Sci. USA* **2018**, *115*, 1505–1510. [CrossRef]
103. Liu, A.; Krushnamurthy, P.; Subramanya, K.; Mitchell, D.A.; Mahanta, N. Enzymatic thioamidation of peptide backbones. In *Methods in Enzymology*; Elsevier: Amsterdam, The Netherlands, 2021; Volume 656, pp. 459–494.
104. Bartling, C.R.O.; Alexopoulou, F.; Kuschert, S.; Chin, Y.K.; Jia, X.; Sereikaite, V.; Özcelik, D.; Jensen, T.M.; Jain, P.; Nygaard, M.M.; et al. Comprehensive peptide cyclization examination yields optimized app scaffolds with improved affinity toward mint2. *J. Med. Chem.* **2023**, *66*, 3045–3057. [CrossRef] [PubMed]
105. Armas, F.; Di Stasi, A.; Mardirossian, M.; Romani, A.A.; Benincasa, M.; Scocchi, M. Effects of lipidation on a proline-rich antibacterial peptide. *Int. J. Mol. Sci.* **2021**, *22*, 7959. [CrossRef] [PubMed]

106. Moreira Brito, J.C.; Carvalho, L.R.; Neves de Souza, A.; Carneiro, G.; Magalhães, P.P.; Farias, L.M.; Guimarães, N.R.; Verly, R.M.; Resende, J.M.; Elena de Lima, M. Pegylation of the antimicrobial peptide lyetx i-b maintains structure-related biological properties and improves selectivity. *Front. Mol. Biosci.* **2022**, *9*, 1001508. [CrossRef] [PubMed]
107. Wijesinghe, A.; Kumari, S.; Booth, V. Conjugates for use in peptide therapeutics: A systematic review and meta-analysis. *PLoS ONE* **2022**, *17*, e0255753. [CrossRef]
108. Lanza, V.; Bellia, F.; D'Agata, R.; Grasso, G.; Rizzarelli, E.; Vecchio, G. New glycoside derivatives of carnosine and analogs resistant to carnosinase hydrolysis: Synthesis and characterization of their copper(ii) complexes. *J. Inorg. Biochem.* **2011**, *105*, 181–188. [CrossRef]
109. Cooper, B.M.; Iegre, J.; DH, O.D.; Ölwegård Halvarsson, M.; Spring, D.R. Peptides as a platform for targeted therapeutics for cancer: Peptide-drug conjugates (pdcs). *Chem. Soc. Rev.* **2021**, *50*, 1480–1494. [CrossRef]
110. Kulikova, O.I.; Stvolinsky, S.L.; Migulin, V.A.; Andreeva, L.A.; Nagaev, I.Y.; Lopacheva, O.M.; Kulichenkova, K.N.; Lopachev, A.V.; Trubitsina, I.E.; Fedorova, T.N. A new derivative of acetylsalicylic acid and carnosine: Synthesis, physical and chemical properties, biological activity. *DARU J. Pharm. Sci.* **2020**, *28*, 119–130. [CrossRef]
111. Qiu, J.; Hauske, S.J.; Zhang, S.; Rodriguez-Niño, A.; Albrecht, T.; Pastene, D.O.; van den Born, J.; van Goor, H.; Ruf, S.; Kohlmann, M.; et al. Identification and characterisation of carnostatine (san9812), a potent and selective carnosinase (cn1) inhibitor with in vivo activity. *Amino Acids* **2019**, *51*, 7–16. [CrossRef]
112. Peters, V.; Schmitt, C.P.; Weigand, T.; Klingbeil, K.; Thiel, C.; van den Berg, A.; Calabrese, V.; Nawroth, P.; Fleming, T.; Forsberg, E.; et al. Allosteric inhibition of carnosinase (cn1) by inducing a conformational shift. *J. Enzym. Inhib. Med. Chem.* **2017**, *32*, 1102–1110. [CrossRef]
113. Maherani, B.; Arab-Tehrany, E.; Kheirolomoom, A.; Cleymand, F.; Linder, M. Influence of lipid composition on physicochemical properties of nanoliposomes encapsulating natural dipeptide antioxidant l-carnosine. *Food Chem.* **2012**, *134*, 632–640. [CrossRef]
114. Slovák, L.; Poništ, S.; Fedorova, T.; Logvinenko, A.; Levacheva, I.; Samsonova, O.; Bakowsky, U.; Pašková, L'.; Čavojský, T.; Tsiklauri, L.; et al. Evaluation of liposomal carnosine in adjuvant arthritis. *Gen. Physiol. Biophys.* **2017**, *36*, 471–479. [CrossRef] [PubMed]
115. Zeb, A.; Cha, J.-H.; Noh, A.R.; Qureshi, O.S.; Kim, K.-W.; Choe, Y.-H.; Shin, D.; Shah, F.A.; Majid, A.; Bae, O.-N. Neuroprotective effects of carnosine-loaded elastic liposomes in cerebral ischemia rat model. *J. Pharm. Investig.* **2020**, *50*, 373–381. [CrossRef]
116. Moulahoum, H.; Sanli, S.; Timur, S.; Zihnioglu, F. Potential effect of carnosine encapsulated niosomes in bovine serum albumin modifications. *Int. J. Biol. Macromol.* **2019**, *137*, 583–591. [CrossRef] [PubMed]
117. Lundie, M.M. Formulation and Topical Delivery of Niosomes and Proniosomes Containing Carnosine. Ph.D. Thesis, Potchefstroom Campus, North-West University (South Africa), Potchefstroom, South Africa, 2016.
118. Kim, E.-S.; Kim, D.; Nyberg, S.; Poma, A.; Cecchin, D.; Jain, S.A.; Kim, K.-A.; Shin, Y.-J.; Kim, E.-H.; Kim, M. Lrp-1 functionalized polymersomes enhance the efficacy of carnosine in experimental stroke. *Sci. Rep.* **2020**, *10*, 699. [CrossRef] [PubMed]
119. Abdelkader, H.; Longman, M.R.; Alany, R.G.; Pierscionek, B. Phytosome-hyaluronic acid systems for ocular delivery of l-carnosine. *Int. J. Nanomed.* **2016**, *11*, 2815. [CrossRef]
120. Darvishi, B.; Dinarvand, R.; Mohammadpour, H.; Kamarul, T.; Sharifi, A.M. Dual l-carnosine/aloe vera nanophytosomes with synergistically enhanced protective effects against methylglyoxal-induced angiogenesis impairment. *Mol. Pharm.* **2021**, *18*, 3302–3325. [CrossRef]
121. Farid, R.M.; Gaafar, P.M.E.; Hazzah, H.A.; Helmy, M.W.; Abdallah, O.Y. Chemotherapeutic potential of l-carnosine from stimuli-responsive magnetic nanoparticles against breast cancer model. *Nanomedicine* **2020**, *15*, 891–911. [CrossRef]
122. Durmus, Z.; Kavas, H.; Baykal, A.; Sozeri, H.; Alpsoy, L.; Çelik, S.; Toprak, M. Synthesis and characterization of l-carnosine coated iron oxide nanoparticles. *J. Alloy. Compd.* **2011**, *509*, 2555–2561. [CrossRef]
123. Lu, X.; Zhang, Y.; Wang, L.; Li, G.; Gao, J.; Wang, Y. Development of l-carnosine functionalized iron oxide nanoparticles loaded with dexamethasone for simultaneous therapeutic potential of blood brain barrier crossing and ischemic stroke treatment. *Drug Deliv.* **2021**, *28*, 380–389. [CrossRef]
124. Khramtsov, P.; Barkina, I.; Kropaneva, M.; Bochkova, M.; Timganova, V.; Nechaev, A.; Byzov, I.; Zamorina, S.; Yermakov, A.; Rayev, M. Magnetic nanoclusters coated with albumin, casein, and gelatin: Size tuning, relaxivity, stability, protein corona, and application in nuclear magnetic resonance immunoassay. *Nanomaterials* **2019**, *9*, 1345. [CrossRef]
125. Bellia, F.; Oliveri, V.; Rizzarelli, E.; Vecchio, G. New derivative of carnosine for nanoparticle assemblies. *Eur. J. Med. Chem.* **2013**, *70*, 225–232. [CrossRef] [PubMed]
126. Wang, Y.; Xia, R.; Hu, H.; Peng, T. Biosynthesis, characterization and cytotoxicity of gold nanoparticles and their loading with n-acetylcarnosine for cataract treatment. *J. Photochem. Photobiol. B Biol.* **2018**, *187*, 180–183. [CrossRef] [PubMed]
127. Habra, K.; Morris, R.H.; McArdle, S.E.B.; Cave, G.W.V. Controlled release of carnosine from poly(lactic-co-glycolic acid) beads using nanomechanical magnetic trigger towards the treatment of glioblastoma. *Nanoscale Adv.* **2022**, *4*, 2242–2249. [CrossRef]
128. Habra, K.; McArdle, S.E.B.; Morris, R.H.; Cave, G.W.V. Synthesis and functionalisation of superparamagnetic nano-rods towards the treatment of glioblastoma brain tumours. *Nanomaterials* **2021**, *11*, 2157. [CrossRef] [PubMed]
129. Gaafar, P.M.E.; El-Salamouni, N.S.; Farid, R.M.; Hazzah, H.A.; Helmy, M.W.; Abdallah, O.Y. Pegylated liquisomes: A novel combined passive targeting nanoplatform of l-carnosine for breast cancer. *Int. J. Pharm.* **2021**, *602*, 120666. [CrossRef] [PubMed]
130. Calcagni, A.; Ciattini, P.G.; Di Stefano, A.; Duprè, S.; Luisi, G.; Pinnen, F.; Rossi, D.; Spirito, A. Ψ (so2nh) transition state isosteres of peptides. Synthesis and bioactivity of sulfonamido pseudopeptides related to carnosine. *Il Farm.* **1999**, *54*, 673–677. [CrossRef]

131. Vecchio, G.; La Mendola, D.; Rizzarelli, E. The synthesis and conformation of β-cyclodextrins functionalized with enantiomers of boc-carnosine. *J. Supramol. Chem.* **2001**, *1*, 87–95. [CrossRef]
132. Amorini, A.M.; Bellia, F.; Di Pietro, V.; Giardina, B.; La Mendola, D.; Lazzarino, G.; Sortino, S.; Tavazzi, B.; Rizzarelli, E.; Vecchio, G. Synthesis and antioxidant activity of new homocarnosine beta-cyclodextrin conjugates. *Eur. J. Med. Chem.* **2007**, *42*, 910–920. [CrossRef]
133. La Mendola, D.; Sortino, S.; Vecchio, G.; Rizzarelli, E. Synthesis of new carnosine derivatives of β-cyclodextrin and their hydroxyl radical scavenger ability. *Helv. Chim. Acta* **2002**, *85*, 1633–1643. [CrossRef]
134. Mineo, P.; Vitalini, D.; La Mendola, D.; Rizzarelli, E.; Scamporrino, E.; Vecchio, G. Coordination features of difunctionalized β-cyclodextrins with carnosine: Esi-ms and spectroscopic investigations on 6a, 6d-di-(β-alanyl-l-histidine)-6a, 6d-dideoxy-β-cyclodextrin and 6a, 6c-di-(β-alanyl-l-histidine)-6a, 6c-dideoxy-β-cyclodextrin and their copper (ii) complexes. *J. Inorg. Biochem.* **2004**, *98*, 254–265.
135. Babizhayev, M.A.; Deyev, A.I.; Yermakova, V.N.; Semiletov, Y.A.; Davydova, N.G.; Kurysheva, N.I.; Zhukotskii, A.V.; Goldman, I.M. N-acetylcarnosine, a natural histidine-containing dipeptide, as a potent ophthalmic drug in treatment of human cataracts. *Peptides* **2001**, *22*, 979–994. [CrossRef] [PubMed]
136. Babizhayev, M.A. Biological activities of the natural imidazole-containing peptidomimetics n-acetylcarnosine, carcinine and l-carnosine in ophthalmic and skin care products. *Life Sci.* **2006**, *78*, 2343–2357. [CrossRef] [PubMed]
137. Babizhayev, M.A.; Guiotto, A.; Kasus-Jacobi, A. N-acetylcarnosine and histidyl-hydrazide are potent agents for multitargeted ophthalmic therapy of senile cataracts and diabetic ocular complications. *J. Drug Target.* **2009**, *17*, 36–63. [CrossRef] [PubMed]
138. Castelletto, V.; Cheng, G.; Stain, C.; Connon, C.J.; Hamley, I.W. Self-assembly of a peptide amphiphile containing l-carnosine and its mixtures with a multilamellar vesicle forming lipid. *Langmuir* **2012**, *28*, 11599–11608. [CrossRef]
139. Pal, A.; Shrivastava, S.; Dey, J. Salt, ph and thermoresponsive supramolecular hydrogel of n-(4-n-tetradecyloxybenzoyl)-l-carnosine. *Chem. Commun.* **2009**, *45*, 6997–6999. [CrossRef]
140. Gizzi, P.; Pasc, A.; Dupuy, N.; Parant, S.; Henry, B.; Gérardin, C. *Molecular Tailored Histidine-Based Complexing Surfactants: From Micelles to Hydrogels*; Wiley Online Library: Hoboken, NJ, USA, 2009.
141. Stvolinsky, S.; Antonova, N.; Kulikova, O.; Lopachev, A.; Abaimov, D.; Al-Baidani, I.; Lopacheva, O.; Fedorova, T.; Kaplun, A.; Sorokoumova, G. Lipoilcarnosine: Synthesis, study of physico-chemical and antioxidant properties, biological activity. *Biomeditsinskaia Khimiia* **2018**, *64*, 268–275. [CrossRef]
142. Stvolinsky, S.; Bulygina, E.; Fedorova, T.; Meguro, K.; Sato, T.; Tyulina, O.; Abe, H.; Boldyrev, A. Biological activity of novel synthetic derivatives of carnosine. *Cell. Mol. Neurobiol.* **2010**, *30*, 395–404. [CrossRef]
143. Astete, C.E.; Songe Meador, D.; Spivak, D.; Sabliov, C. Synthesis of vitamin e-carnosine (vecar): New antioxidant molecule with potential application in atherosclerosis. *Synth. Commun.* **2013**, *43*, 1299–1313. [CrossRef]
144. Grasso, G.I.; Bellia, F.; Arena, G.; Satriano, C.; Vecchio, G.; Rizzarelli, E. Multitarget trehalose-carnosine conjugates inhibit aβ aggregation, tune copper(ii) activity and decrease acrolein toxicity. *Eur. J. Med. Chem.* **2017**, *135*, 447–457. [CrossRef]
145. Naletova, I.; Greco, V.; Sciuto, S.; Attanasio, F.; Rizzarelli, E. Ionophore ability of carnosine and its trehalose conjugate assists copper signal in triggering brain-derived neurotrophic factor and vascular endothelial growth factor activation in vitro. *Int. J. Mol. Sci.* **2021**, *22*, 13504. [CrossRef]
146. Greco, V.; Naletova, I.; Ahmed, I.M.M.; Vaccaro, S.; Messina, L.; La Mendola, D.; Bellia, F.; Sciuto, S.; Satriano, C.; Rizzarelli, E. Hyaluronan-carnosine conjugates inhibit aβ aggregation and toxicity. *Sci. Rep.* **2020**, *10*, 15998. [CrossRef] [PubMed]
147. Anderson, E.J.; Vistoli, G.; Katunga, L.A.; Funai, K.; Regazzoni, L.; Monroe, T.B.; Gilardoni, E.; Cannizzaro, L.; Colzani, M.; De Maddis, D. A carnosine analog mitigates metabolic disorders of obesity by reducing carbonyl stress. *J. Clin. Investig.* **2018**, *128*, 5280–5293. [CrossRef] [PubMed]
148. Bertinaria, M.; Rolando, B.; Giorgis, M.; Montanaro, G.; Guglielmo, S.; Buonsanti, M.F.; Carabelli, V.; Gavello, D.; Daniele, P.G.; Fruttero, R. Synthesis, physicochemical characterization, and biological activities of new carnosine derivatives stable in human serum as potential neuroprotective agents. *J. Med. Chem.* **2011**, *54*, 611–621. [CrossRef]
149. Bertinaria, M.; Rolando, B.; Giorgis, M.; Montanaro, G.; Marini, E.; Collino, M.; Benetti, E.; Daniele, P.G.; Fruttero, R.; Gasco, A. Carnosine analogues containing no-donor substructures: Synthesis, physico-chemical characterization and preliminary pharmacological profile. *Eur. J. Med. Chem.* **2012**, *54*, 103–112. [CrossRef] [PubMed]
150. Iacobini, C.; Menini, S.; Blasetti Fantauzzi, C.; Pesce, C.M.; Giaccari, A.; Salomone, E.; Lapolla, A.; Orioli, M.; Aldini, G.; Pugliese, G. Fl-926-16, a novel bioavailable carnosinase-resistant carnosine derivative, prevents onset and stops progression of diabetic nephropathy in db/db mice. *Br. J. Pharmacol.* **2018**, *175*, 53–66. [CrossRef]

Disclaimer/Publisher's Note: The statements, opinions and data contained in all publications are solely those of the individual author(s) and contributor(s) and not of MDPI and/or the editor(s). MDPI and/or the editor(s) disclaim responsibility for any injury to people or property resulting from any ideas, methods, instructions or products referred to in the content.

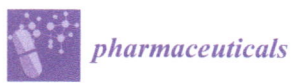

Review

Drug Delivery Strategies and Nanozyme Technologies to Overcome Limitations for Targeting Oxidative Stress in Osteoarthritis

Jessica Lee Aldrich, Arjun Panicker, Robert Ovalle, Jr. and Blanka Sharma *

J. Crayton Pruitt Family Department of Biomedical Engineering, University of Florida, Gainesville, FL 32611, USA; jessica.aldrich@ufl.edu (J.L.A.)
* Correspondence: blanka.sharma@bme.ufl.edu; Tel.: +1-352-273-9329

Abstract: Oxidative stress is an important, but elusive, therapeutic target for osteoarthritis (OA). Antioxidant strategies that target oxidative stress through the elimination of reactive oxygen species (ROS) have been widely evaluated for OA but are limited by the physiological characteristics of the joint. Current hallmarks in antioxidant treatment strategies include poor bioavailability, poor stability, and poor retention in the joint. For example, oral intake of exogenous antioxidants has limited access to the joint space, and intra-articular injections require frequent dosing to provide therapeutic effects. Advancements in ROS-scavenging nanomaterials, also known as nanozymes, leverage bioactive material properties to improve delivery and retention. Material properties of nanozymes can be tuned to overcome physiological barriers in the knee. However, the clinical application of these nanozymes is still limited, and studies to understand their utility in treating OA are still in their infancy. The objective of this review is to evaluate current antioxidant treatment strategies and the development of nanozymes as a potential alternative to conventional small molecules and enzymes.

Keywords: nanozyme; osteoarthritis; reactive oxygen species; antioxidant; oxidative stress

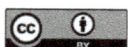

Citation: Aldrich, J.L.; Panicker, A.; Ovalle, R., Jr.; Sharma, B. Drug Delivery Strategies and Nanozyme Technologies to Overcome Limitations for Targeting Oxidative Stress in Osteoarthritis. *Pharmaceuticals* **2023**, *16*, 1044. https://doi.org/10.3390/ph16071044

Academic Editors: Qian Chen, Silviya Petrova Zustiak and Era Jain

Received: 21 April 2023
Revised: 26 June 2023
Accepted: 12 July 2023
Published: 23 July 2023

Copyright: © 2023 by the authors. Licensee MDPI, Basel, Switzerland. This article is an open access article distributed under the terms and conditions of the Creative Commons Attribution (CC BY) license (https://creativecommons.org/licenses/by/4.0/).

1. Introduction

Osteoarthritis (OA) is a degenerative disease of the whole joint, characterized by cartilage loss and crosstalk with the bone, synovium, tendon, and nervous system [1–3]. Despite decades of efforts, there are no commercially available disease-modifying osteoarthritic drugs (DMOADS). Disease modification refers to the slowing or mitigation of structural changes to the joint, such as cartilage protection, in concert with improvements in pain and joint function. The current standard of care for OA is palliative management until disease severity dictates the need for a total joint replacement. This results in nearly 800,000 total knee arthroplasties each year in the United States [4]. As the average age of patients diagnosed with OA decreases due to traumatic knee injuries (post-traumatic osteoarthritis, PTOA) from sports, accidents, or military service, joint replacement is not a reasonable option. It is necessary to further understand the barriers to treating osteoarthritis and engineer therapeutic strategies to protect against disease progression.

Oxidative stress is a key driver in OA pathogenesis, resulting from the overproduction of reactive oxygen species (ROS) in the joint. The development of oxidative stress, either following a traumatic joint injury or due to aging-related joint changes, creates a negative signaling cascade which includes mitochondrial dysfunction, cartilage breakdown, synovial inflammation, and other downstream effects that are known contributors to OA [5]. While not the only contributing factor in the development of OA, oxidative stress is a strong candidate for therapeutic intervention. Oxidative stress occurs when there is an imbalance between the production of ROS and antioxidants within the joint [6,7]. Antioxidant enzymes are critical for scavenging excess ROS and maintaining redox balance—when these endogenous enzymes are overwhelmed, oxidative stress ensues, followed by oxidation of macromolecules and adverse secondary signaling [6,7]. There are currently no approved methods for mitigating oxidative stress in OA, though it remains an important disease target.

The objective of this review is to identify and discuss current applications of ROS-scavenging nanomaterials, or nanozymes, to target oxidative stress in OA joints. This includes evaluating the limitations of current antioxidant-based therapies and the potential benefits of engineered material strategies. While treatment strategies for OA have been widely discussed and reviewed, this is the first comprehensive analysis of nanozyme technologies specifically for use in knee OA.

Important Considerations for Nanomaterial Delivery

Nanomedicine has been widely used in applications ranging from cancer [8], neurological disorders [8], and vaccine development [9], to name a few. Nanomaterials have been developing rapidly, owing to their potential use as both treatment tools and diagnostic tools [10,11]. These types of therapies can be engineered for targeted, site-specific delivery, delayed/controlled release, and novel, patient-specific treatments. In many clinical applications, nanomaterials have served as key enabling technologies for improving bioavailability and stability of small molecule drugs, proteins, and nucleic acids, though challenges with site-specific targeting often remain.

The use of nanomaterials to overcome the limitations specific to treating OA has been a rapidly advancing area of research and there have been many advancements in the field. It is becoming increasingly recognized that delivery of therapeutics to specific cells and tissues and in response to specific disease stimuli may be important. This also requires consideration of the unique transport barriers to overcome as well as disease-related mechanisms to leverage. For example, leveraging electrostatic interactions between a negatively charged cartilage matrix and a positively charged nanomaterial may improve cartilage targeting and retention [12–14]. Alternatively, stimuli-sensitive nanomaterials may be designed to respond to changes in enzyme function, pH, temperature, and endogenous oxygen levels and provide a targeted therapeutic approach, thereby improving efficacy and decreasing off-target adverse effects [15]. These are just a few of the many considerations necessary in designing nanomaterials to treat OA. A variety of other biomaterials engineered for intraarticular delivery include micelles [16], dendrimers [17], liposomes, and many others, have been thoroughly reviewed [18]. We point the reader to reviews focused on nanomaterial engineering for targeted delivery to the joint [14,19–23]. This review will focus on the emerging application of nanozymes as a potential treatment for OA.

2. Understanding Antioxidant Strategies

The role of oxidative stress on disease progression in OA has been widely reviewed and characterized [5,24–27]. Subsequently, several exogenous antioxidants and antioxidant-like strategies have been studied for use as OA therapies [28–30]. The application of antioxidant-based therapies is an effort to maintain the necessary redox balance for healthy cell signaling without causing negative downstream effects.

The relationship between ROS and antioxidants, in both function and location, is complex and interconnected. Cells must maintain a normal level of ROS to complete necessary cell signaling pathways, a complete loss of ROS may be just as detrimental to joint health as an overabundance [31]. It is also necessary to consider intra and extracellular locations of ROS and antioxidants. ROS targeting strategies will only be as effective as their ability to reach the necessary compartments where the ROS are produced; without this connection there may be a mismatch between the therapy location and the target.

Specifically in OA, prolonged ROS overproduction that outpaces endogenous antioxidant function is detrimental to joint health. This overproduction may be caused by abnormal mechanical stimuli, increased inflammation, and mitochondrial dysfunction [32]. Mitochondrial dysfunction, for example, is a known hallmark of intracellular ROS overproduction and could be one key target for slowing disease progression; however, it may require antioxidant treatments tailored for mitochondrial targeting [33]. Alternatively, regulating the NF-κB signaling pathway or the NOX4 signaling pathway whose components may be found in the cytosol or inner mitochondrial membrane, respectively, may be other compartment-specific targets for antioxidant treatment in OA [34,35]. The numerous locations and interconnected nature of ROS/antioxidant relationships yield a variety of targets for antioxidant-based treatment.

Reactive oxygen species implicated in OA include oxygen radicals (O_2^-, OH^-) and nonradical, oxygen-containing reactive agents (H_2O_2, O_2, O_3, etc.) (Figure 1) [7,36]. Hydrogen peroxide (H_2O_2) is abundantly produced in OA and can cross the cell membrane, and thus is present in both intra- and extracellular microenvironments. H_2O_2 is a product of several antioxidant enzymes (superoxide dismutase (SOD) and NADPH oxidase (NOX)) and reacts with transition metals to yield a hydroxyl radical (-OH) [36]. In addition to the direct formation of radicals, H_2O_2 overproduction can disrupt the NF-κB signaling pathway and stimulate pro-inflammatory cytokines and chemokines that lead to cartilage degeneration [34,37]. Superoxide radicals (O_2^-) and nitric oxide radicals (NO) are present within the cell and react together to form peroxynitrite, a potentially cytotoxic ROS [38]. Superoxide anions are predominantly produced in the mitochondria and can be mediated by the mitochondrial electron transport chain [7]. These anions contribute to the production of H_2O_2 following a reaction with SOD. Hydroxyl radicals are present within a defined cellular compartment and can be produced by a reaction between O_2^- and H_2O_2 or following a Fenton reaction [39]. The Fenton reaction is an oxidation process that causes the production of hydroxyl radicals from hydrogen peroxide and iron [40].

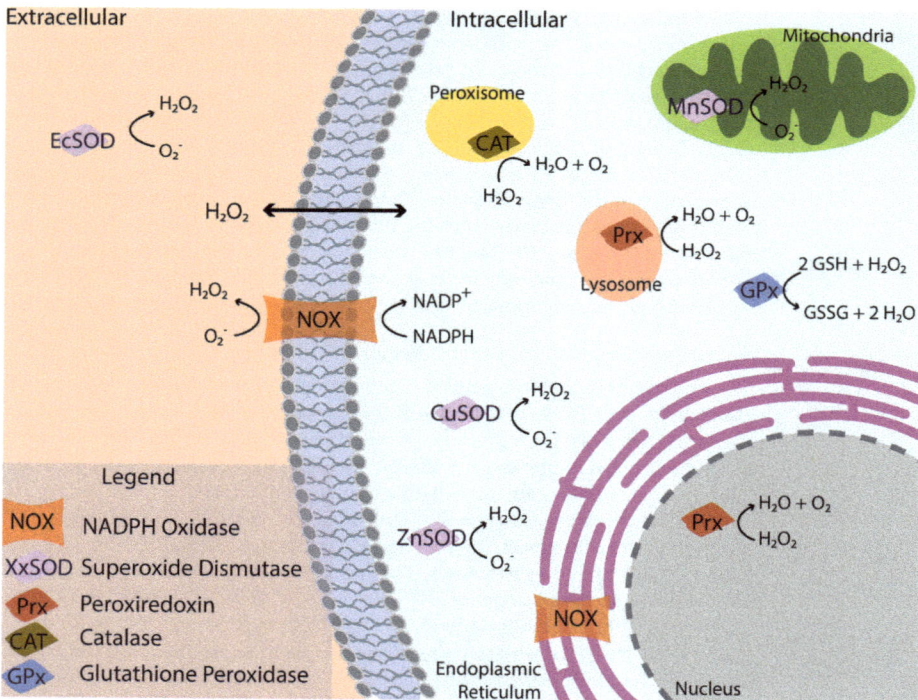

Figure 1. Key enzyme functions in the cartilage microenvironment that scavenge and produce ROS critical for intracellular signaling and chondrocyte function. Enzymatic functions occurring in both intra and extracellular regions validate the need to understand where treatments localize, to fully understand and evaluate therapeutic efficacy.

Glutathione, another key player in the antioxidant system, is predominantly reduced via glutathione peroxidase (GPX) in the cytosol and is retained within the cell, though GPX can be found in all cellular compartments. Similarly, specific forms of superoxide dismutase (SOD) are found in the extracellular space (EcSOD) while others can be found in the mitochondria (MnSOD) or the cytosol (ZnSOD, CuSOD). The different types of SOD use different transition metals as cofactors in the generation of H_2O_2 from oxygen radicals. The complexity and inter-connected nature of ROS generation has been well described in other reviews [38,39].

Antioxidant enzymes are predominantly found intracellularly; however, extracellular enzyme function is important in regulating cell–cell communication. These enzymes target specific ROS based on their location, as described above, and their mechanism of action. Transition metal ions, including iron and copper, are also found in the extracellular space and can produce H_2O_2 in the presence of OH^- [36] but they have also been shown to produce additional hydroxyl radicals [41]. Iron, specifically, may participate in the Fenton reaction, producing hydroxide and a hydroxyl radical when reacted with H_2O_2. Other intracellular antioxidants include GPX and peroxiredoxins. Peroxiredoxins (PRX), specifically in OA tissues, can be found within the mitochondria, nucleus, lysosomes, and cytosol [42]. PRXs protect against oxidative stress by reducing hydroperoxide and peroxynitrite. They have also been shown to play a role in the development of age-related OA [32,43]. GPX disposes of H_2O_2 through the oxidation of reduced glutathione (GSH) to oxidized glutathione (GSSG) is essential for maintaining redox homeostasis [7,44].

This vast network of enzymes, ROS, and cell functions makes it necessary to understand the timing and location of ROS overproduction, as it relates to developing oxidative stress. If antioxidant-like treatments cannot reach the site(s) of ROS generation, then the treatment cannot perform its intended function, thereby limiting therapeutic efficacy. Interestingly, few antioxidant-based therapies evaluate or address the issue of cellular and subcellular localization. Antioxidant strategies that consider and control ROS levels in different cellular and extracellular compartments may be necessary to achieve therapeutic success.

3. Current Antioxidant Strategies

Targeting oxidative stress is a promising treatment strategy for OA and other diseases caused by disruptions in redox signaling. In OA, translation of these therapies has been limited due to poor bioavailability and poor retention in the joint space. Current research has predominantly focused on oral intake of vitamins or nutraceuticals, but this approach is limited by poor stability and bioavailability to the joint [45]. Intra-articular injections of small molecules have similar limitations due to physical barriers in the joint. Targeting ROS production in the cartilage is difficult because the tissue is avascular and has a dense extracellular matrix (ECM), creating a unique transport barrier. The underlying subchondral bone, which exhibits abnormal remodeling during OA progression, is also challenging to access via the joint space [46]. Tissue localization of therapies can be hindered by rapid drug clearance through the synovial fluid via blood vessels in the synovium, thereby limiting the retention of treatments in the joint space. Once inside the joint, barriers to intracellular localization pose an additional challenge. Physiological barriers in the OA joint limit the effectiveness of several routes of administration for promising OA therapies. The addition of engineered multi-enzymatic treatment systems are a promising strategy to overcome these limitations.

Advances in the development of antioxidant mimicking biomaterial systems may overcome limitations of current therapeutic treatments. These challenges point to the reality, as described by Halliwell, that which ROS, how much, and the precise molecular target are key factors to consider in the development of therapies to tackle imbalance in any of these species [47]. In addition, further advancements in redox biology are necessary to measure ROS in vitro and in vivo are currently being developed. A critical limitation in this space is the inability to accurately, and sensitively, measure ROS produced within the system [39,48,49]. Due to the short half-lives of most ROS, they can be difficult to measure in vitro and in vivo. Although H_2O_2 is one of the most stable ROS, and is commonly produced in oxidative stress environments, it often requires sophisticated probes [49,50] or must be present in high quantities to be measured. This, along with challenges in targeting other ROS that are overproduced in OA, showcases a need for innovative strategies.

3.1. Overview of the Antioxidants Used for Osteoarthritis Therapy

Endogenous antioxidant enzymes are the most efficient mechanism to manage oxidative stress within the joint. However, in oxidative stress conditions, the supplementation with exogenous antioxidants, their mimics, and activators may be needed to restore redox balance and mitigate downstream disease pathways. Current antioxidant therapies under investigation include small molecules such as resveratrol, curcumin, and vitamins C, D, and E (Table 1). While promising, each of these antioxidants has unique challenges that limit their therapeutic efficacy.

3.1.1. Vitamins, Minerals, and Flavonoids

Natural, food-based compounds have been widely cited as a possible therapeutic strategy for treating OA [51]. Specifically, vitamins C, D, and E have been evaluated through clinical trials and other elements found in trace quantities through the body are becoming more popular. Vitamins C (L-ascorbic acid) and E (α-tocopherol) neutralize free radicals in aqueous phases and lipid membranes, respectively, but do so less efficiently relative to endogenous antioxidant enzymes. Vitamin C provides an electron to neutralize free radicals and is known to produce the semidehydroascorbate radical that is responsible for limiting the production of additional free radicals produced by endogenous enzymes [36]. Vitamin C is known to play a crucial role in promoting musculoskeletal development and is a cofactor for enzymes necessary for collagen matrix synthesis [7]. In a comprehensive review of vitamin C as an OA therapy, Dunlap et al. found conflicting results for preclinical and clinical trials of vitamin C supplementation. While the therapeutic effects of vitamin C supplementation are unclear, there is a consensus that overdosing vitamin C is detrimental to both the development and progression of OA [52]. In comparison, vitamins D and E, both membrane-bound antioxidants, have been investigated as potential OA therapeutics. Vitamin E has shown promising chondroprotective effects in rodent models of OA. However, Vitamin D, which is known for its role in regulating bone metabolism, is more well known for contributing to OA progression when it is deficient in the body [53–56]. Vitamin D supplementation has shown conflicting results on joint structure and OA-related pain [53,57]. Like vitamins C and E, oral supplements of vitamin D may not produce a disease-modifying effect. Additionally, most studies that involve oral super dosing of vitamins have had less than promising results in human studies [47].

Zinc, an essential nutrient for enzymatic functions and immune support, has been identified as another potential treatment for OA. Supplementation of zinc could block inflammation-induced oxidative stress [58]. The antioxidant-like function of zinc centers around the activation of Nrf2 which provides support for enzymes including SOD, GPX, and heme oxygenase-1. It may protect against oxidative stress and support the function of critical enzymes that maintain redox balance. In a rodent model of inflammatory OA, a daily supplement of 1.6 mg/kg/day of zinc was sufficient to decrease OA pathogenesis, specifically protecting cartilage structure, compared to a non-treated group. Dietary supplements, however, do have key limitations that inhibit their clinical translation. Specifically for zinc, it has been found that increasing doses does not increase therapeutic efficacy, and there is the potential for acute toxicity if overdosed.

Quercetin, a flavonoid found in fruits and vegetables, has recently been studied as an alternative therapeutic for treating oxidative-stress-induced endoplasmic reticulum stress (ER stress). A known contributor to OA progression, ER stress plays a role in regulating chondrocyte apoptosis and cartilage degeneration [59]. Quercetin has chondroprotective effects including suppression of chondrocyte apoptosis and regulating SIRT1 (a key player in the biological response to oxidative stress). Through in vivo evaluation of quercetin given via intraperitoneal (IP) injection, it has been found that the compound attenuates cartilage degradation through activation of SIRT1 and AMPK [60,61].

Although the addition of supplemental antioxidants has been evaluated for several years, results surrounding disease modification are scarce and most therapies have stalled in pre-clinical models. As pure compounds, these strategies are ineffective for treating OA. However, the addition of adequate delivery vehicles may support their translation from pre-clinical models to clinical trials and commercial availability.

3.1.2. Resveratrol

Resveratrol is one of the most cited nutraceuticals for use in OA owing to its anti-inflammatory effects through inhibition of NF-κB [62,63]. Resveratrol produces antioxidant effects by scavenging free radicals [64]. It has also been suggested that resveratrol may compete with coenzyme Q to decrease ROS generation from the oxidative chain complex, scavenge O_2^- radicals from mitochondria, and may inhibit lipid-peroxidation-induced byproducts from the Fenton reaction [65]. There is also evidence that resveratrol can maintain homeostatic levels of GSH in vitro [66]. Though these results in chondrocytes have yet to be confirmed, it is evident that the antioxidant functions of resveratrol require intracellular localization.

Resveratrol is predominantly administered via oral and injectable routes of delivery, with varying success in preclinical models [67]. Most therapies utilize free resveratrol that has not been encapsulated or integrated with other components [68–71]. Free drug treatments require injections as often as daily for 2 to 3 weeks [70,71] to maintain therapeutic levels within the joint. Currently, there is no evidence to support therapeutic residence within chondrocytes using these methods. And, while these dosing schemes may be effective in pre-clinical models, the translational ability of these therapies is limited due to the high dosing frequency and potential challenges with patient compliance.

A limitation of free resveratrol is the risk of conformational change of the drug when exposed to microenvironments in the body. When studied in vitro, polyphenols such as resveratrol are dissolved in organic solvents before use, due to their low water solubility [72]. Organic solvents can artificially increase chondrocyte permeability and thereby increase the intracellular uptake of the polyphenol which does not recapitulate the joint space.

To address some of these limitations, there have been advances in encapsulating or complexing resveratrol with biomaterials for improved drug delivery. For example, Cui et al. have coupled resveratrol with an oxidized cellulose aerogel (RLTA) creating a sustained release profile for the resveratrol [73,74]. The sustained release lasted for 5 h with a release of 40% total resveratrol encapsulated [74]. Application of the RLTA decreased inflammatory factors (IL-6, TNF-α) in an exercise-induced rodent model of OA. However, in vitro release and intracellular localization should be evaluated to advance this aerogel system.

Alternatively, lipid-core nanocapsules (LNC) with a polycaprolactone biodegradable shell have been tested for combination resveratrol and curcumin delivery [72]. Co-encapsulation techniques such as the LNCs are a promising technique to deliver polyphenols that traditionally have limited stability profiles [75]. Resveratrol could be released for up to 24 h surpassing the retention time in other free drug models. As with the prior system, cellular and in vivo models with the LNCs will be necessary to further understand their efficacy as a therapeutic delivery system.

In several aspects these strategies provide an improvement in free-drug methods of delivery. However, the LNC co-encapsulation system has not been used with chondrocytes or OA based applications [75]. The RLTA treatment, administered via oral gavage, showed promising effects on IL-6 and TNF-α expression [73]. This work indicates a potential for oral therapy, but further characterization is necessary to understand how it may be providing a disease modifying result.

3.1.3. Curcumin

Derived from turmeric, curcumin has been referred to as the "spice" for mitigating joint inflammation [76]. Curcumin is known to suppress the function of the NF-κB signal transduction pathway which can inhibit the cellular inflammatory response. It has also been shown to inhibit apoptosis by interrupting the expression of p38 and c-Jun N-terminal kinase (JNK). Lastly, curcumin acts as a free radical and H_2O_2 scavenger through H-atom donation from a phenolic group on the compound [77]. Therapeutic effects with curcumin may result from both intra and extracellular ROS scavenging, as it decreases general H_2O_2 production that may occur in both locations. Its effects on intra and extracellular ROS may enhance the therapeutic potential of curcumin and provide opportunities for various delivery vehicles or routes to be considered.

Curcumin is limited by poor joint bioavailability, with oral dosing leading to bioavailability only as high as 1% [78]. However, oral supplementation remains the primary method of treatment evaluated for curcumin in OA.

Similar to resveratrol, coupling the therapeutic effects of curcumin with materials to enhance bioavailability has expanded the therapeutic potential of this nutraceutical. For example, silk fibroin nanoparticles (SFN) loaded with curcumin improved ROS scavenging properties of curcumin, as measured by DPPH free radical scavenging in an acellular model, compared to free-drug. They also decreased the activity of markers connected with increased inflammation (RANTES, IL-6, NO) [79]. The SFNs created a controlled release of curcumin for as long as 24 h, which may overcome joint retention challenges. Further in vivo evaluation is necessary to determine if overcoming the limitation of joint retention is enough to make the therapeutic clinically viable, depending on the route of administration. The fact that the LNCs described previously improved curcumin release to 72 h supports efforts to apply sustained release systems to nutraceutical use [75].

Alternatively, a prodrug strategy, amphiphilic curcumin polymer micelles (ACP), using an acid-activatable curcumin polymer, has been developed to improve curcumin bioavailability in the joint. Kang et al. integrated curcumin with a polymer backbone such that the polymer can self-assemble into micelles in acidic environments [80]. The pH-responsive nature of the micelles creates a theranostic approach that can have both disease detection and therapeutic capabilities. In a neutral environment, the micelles are characterized by fluorescent quenching; however, in an acidic environment, the micelles dissociate, allowing the fluorescent particles to be visualized and the curcumin to be released in the joint. The ACP micelles, when given via an intra-muscular injection in an inflammatory model of OA, suppressed IL-1β and TNF-α expression and showed potential for cartilage protection. Micelles were injected every 3 days for a period of 28 days, and while the compounding anti-inflammatory effects may be beneficial in decreasing cartilage breakdown, it does not appear to overcome the barrier of therapeutic retention in the joint.

Curcumin has long been evaluated as an approach to decrease oxidative stress and reduce inflammation through antioxidant functions that may support intra and extracellular management of ROS production [79]. Like resveratrol and other vitamin treatments, implementing the right delivery system for the desired route of administration will be necessary to advance and implement curcumin as a prescribed treatment for OA.

3.1.4. Exogenous Enzymes

Given their efficient ROS-scavenging properties, the delivery of exogenous antioxidant enzymes has been explored for the treatment of OA. Exogenous enzymes, specifically catalase and SOD, have been injected into the joint with varying success.

The addition of exogenous SOD has been discussed since the 1980s, ranging from applications with liposomes or microinjections to intra-articular or systemic injections of the enzyme alone [81]. Some well-known challenges in using exogenous SOD to scavenge ROS include the inability of SOD to enter cells, its inability to survive unchanged in the GI tract, and that the byproducts of SOD must be less toxic than the superoxide that is broken down in the reaction to be effective as a therapeutic. Early results of SOD injection used 2–16 mg SOD injected on a weekly or biweekly basis and showed improvements in patient reported pain and joint function. However, radiographic evidence of joint structure remained unchanged based on the therapeutic treatment, indicating that the effect was only on the short-term inflammatory aspects of the disease. In studies with higher dosages of SOD (16 and 32 mg) given weekly for 3 weeks via IA injection, there was a reduction in OA symptoms for up to 3 months [82]. Limitations of using free enzymes may be overcome by loading SOD into nanoparticle systems. However, many of these systems exhibit poor enzyme loading, decreased enzymatic function after release, or enzyme inactivation following conjugation [83–85].

More recently, a polymersome made of amphiphilic synthetic coblock polymers was used in a pre-clinical model of OA [86]. Loaded with SOD, these nanoparticles were designed to breakdown superoxide radicals. When given via IA injection, SOD-NPs were retained in the joint for up to 4 weeks following a DMM surgery, an improvement on the retention time of most injectable therapies. Gui et al. found that the SOD-NPs localized to the synovium in vivo and that they decreased the ROS production in vitro [86]. This recent advancement in the use of SOD with a nanoparticle system shows that the application of exogenous enzymes may still be a viable option if paired with a suitable carrier.

Though less commonly evaluated, catalase is another endogenous enzyme that could be used as a therapeutic agent for slowing the development of oxidative stress. Free catalase is limited by a short half-life within the joint [87]. Previous studies have attempted to overcome this limitation by PEG-conjugating the enzyme to improve biostability [88,89]. In a rodent model of OA, intra-articular injection of cationized catalase was retained in the joint and mitigated inflammation [90]. However, the addition of non-cationized exogenous catalase did not influence disease progression. This work also points to H_2O_2 concentration as the rate-limiting factor to catalase function. This dose-dependent relationship should be considered in future work with enzyme mimicking nanomaterials; however, it is rarely discussed in the current literature. Recent efforts to utilize catalase as a treatment for OA have focused on applications in rheumatoid arthritis [91]. Unfortunately, beyond challenges of joint stability and bioavailability, exogenous enzymes can be expensive and complex to produce, making translation into the clinic challenging [92].

3.1.5. Superoxide Dismutase Mimics and Activators

SOD plays a significant role in redox homeostasis and the development of oxidative stress. In a homeostatic environment, SOD catalyzes the conversion of O_2^- into oxygen and H_2O_2. Through this, SOD decreases one type of ROS, O_2^-, by creating another which can be more readily broken down—H_2O_2. To support endogenous SOD function, treatments that mimic SOD function or contribute to increased production of SOD have been developed and tested in pre-clinical models. SOD mimics have been studied across a variety of medical fields [91] with some applications in orthopedic research [93–95].

Manganese porphyrin has been used as a synthetic SOD mimic that scavenges O_2^- in environments with oxidative stress. Manganese porphyrin has grown in clinical relevance as a potential cancer therapeutic [90,96] and is understood to protect against mitochondrial damage related to oxidative stress [97]. Although not yet used in OA models, manganese porphyrin has been studied on intervertebral disc cells to mitigate oxidative stress in degenerative disc disease [98]. When encapsulated in a chondroitin sulfate microparticle system, there was a sustained release of manganese over 3 months. Even more promisingly, the microparticles were taken up by nucleus pulposus cells. Further study into their SOD-mimicking functions and the potential for intracellular SOD function will be necessary to advance this therapy. Success in the disc model is promising and may be translatable into OA models.

Another small molecule, BNTA (N-[2-bromo-4-(phenylsulfonyl)-3-thienyl]-2-chlorobenzamide), induces SOD expression and superoxide anion elimination [93]. The application of BNTA in vitro has been found to significantly increase extracellular SOD (EcSOD or SOD3) function and facilitate ECM production in OA chondrocytes, OA cartilage explants, and in a rodent model of OA. The application of BNTA following an ACLT (anterior cruciate ligament-transection) surgery resulted in decreased OA related joint changes compared to a vehicle control based on histological results. Similar to other injectable therapies, one key limitation in the application of BNTA as a DMOAD is the need to deliver an IA injection two times per week for a sustained duration (4 or 8 weeks, in this example) to see the desired effects.

Mitigation of extracellular ROS could play a role in interrupting disease-related intercellular signaling within the extracellular matrix. BNTA has a unique ability to enhance the function of EcSOD, which could play a role in downstream ROS production and cellular signaling cascades. Both manganese porphyrin and BNTA showcase the importance of supporting enzyme function in both the intra- and extra-cellular microenvironment. They further advance the idea that therapies with cell-specific and compartment-specific targeting may be necessary to prevent or slow oxidative stress effectively, to produce disease-modifying effects.

Table 1. A sampling of antioxidant therapeutics used for the treatment of OA across clinical and pre-clinical models.

		Antioxidant Therapies Used in OA			
Therapeutic	Antioxidant Effect	Treatment Method	Disease Model	Effects	Citation
Resveratrol	↑ Intracellular SOD	50 mg/kg 3 days/week for 8 weeks	MIA-induced OA, male Wistar rats	↓ inflammatory cytokine expression, ↑ NRF2 expression, ↓ NF-κB	Wei 2018 [68]
Curcumin	↑ Phosphorylation and DNA binding activity of NRF2, free radical scavenger	Varied oral dosing regimens	Human OA patients, clinical trials	↓ NF-κB, ↓ chondrocyte apoptosis, ↓ oxidative stress	Chin 2016 [76]
Manganese porphyrin	SOD mimic, scavenges O_2^-, activates NRF2	BuOE MPs @ 100 μg/mL	Human nucleus pulposus cells	↓ radiation-induced oxidative damages, ↓ inflammation by blocking NF-κB activation	Lee 2022 [98]
BNTA	SOD mimic, ↑ SOD3, and ↓ O_2^-	IA injection of BNTA, 100 μL at 0.015, 0.15, 1.5 mg/kg 2×/week for 4/8 weeks	ACLT-induced OA, male Sprague Dawley rats	↑ expression of ECM components, ↑ cartilage ECM synthesis, ↓ inflammatory mediators	Shi 2019 [95]
Vitamin C	Scavenges free oxygen radicals	Varied oral dosing regimens	Human OA patients, clinical trials	↓ chondrocyte apoptosis, ↓ production of pro-inflammatory markers, overdose can be detrimental	Dunlap 2021 [52]
Zinc	↓ ROS production, ↑ GSH by MIA	1.6–8.0 mg zinc/kg/day via gavage for 2 weeks	MIA-induced OA, male Wistar rats	↓ arthritic progression, ↓ proteoglycan loss, ↓ IL-1β levels, ↑ antioxidative capacity	Huang 2018 [58]
Quercetin	↓ ER stress, ↑ SIRT1 and AMPK	50–100 mg/kg quercetin via IP injection daily for 12 weeks	MMT-induced OA, male Sprague Dawley rats	↓ chondrocyte apoptosis, ↓ cartilage degeneration	Feng 2019 [60]

Abbreviations: MIA—monoiodoacetate; ACLT—anterior cruciate ligament transection; MMT—medial meniscus transection.

3.2. Overview of Delivery Methods Used for Osteoarthritis Therapy

Although we are always told that taking vitamins and eating fruit were the tricks to increasing antioxidant levels in our bodies, the limited stability and absorption of antioxidants moving through the digestive system hinder their efficacy in diseases such as

OA. Beyond ingesting these therapies, clinical trials have evaluated topical treatments with limited success, and most pre-clinical models have settled on high dose rates of therapies via frequent intraarticular (IA) injection. The route of administration for antioxidant-based therapies is a key consideration in their efficacy.

3.2.1. Oral Delivery

Ingestible antioxidants, such as resveratrol and curcumin, are the most common antioxidant strategies. Oral therapies can be implemented as a lifestyle choice or may be prescribed after disease diagnosis based on pain or radiographic evidence of OA. Unfortunately, these are often implemented after disease onset and may have limited efficacy on protecting the joint from further damage. Although popular in clinical trials for nutraceutical-based approaches, oral delivery can be associated with gastrointestinal (GI) complications or negative side effects [99]. Oral supplements may also have limited bioavailability and may be inactivated through the metabolic process. Drug delivery strategies for antioxidants must overcome formulation barriers, including low solubility and low stability, and biological barriers, particularly short GI transit time, low permeability/absorption, and pre-systemic clearance.

Nutraceuticals are frequently given via oral supplementation through dietary changes [100]. For example, preclinical studies supplementing resveratrol in a high-fat diet with a mouse model of obesity-induced OA have shown joint structure recovery through histological evaluation and a reduction in chondrocyte apoptosis [101]. In a clinical trial, oral resveratrol administered once daily (500 mg) for 90 days increased serum levels of aggrecan which may suggest a protection or recovery of joint structure; however, there was no radiographic evidence of joint change [100]. However, serum levels of type II collagen, a necessary building block for cartilage, were unchanged. In another study, oral dosing of curcumin (500 mg 3x/day for 12 weeks) led to a reduction in OA-related pain [102]. Although promising, a critical limitation in translating oral applications of free-drug, beyond stability and bioavailability concerns, is patient compliance. There are no concerns about toxicity, but the dose rate may not be sustainable for long term treatment.

Oral delivery of vitamins C and E are another common home remedy that have been tested as a dietary supplement to slow or prevent joint breakdown. However, clinical trials have consistently shown no correlation between dietary changes with these vitamins and OA disease progression [54,103–105]. Willow bark extract, another supplement compound with aspirin-like anti-inflammatory and ROS-scavenging properties, has also been investigated for OA in preclinical models. In a rodent model of OA, this compound has been shown to improve cartilage health and reduce inflammatory mediators (TNF-α, IL-1β, and IL-6). However, in clinical trials, the results regarding pain management and disease-modifying effects have been mixed [106]. Currently, these antioxidants are available as over-the-counter supplements, but they have not been classified as DMOADs and are not considered a standard of care.

3.2.2. Topical Application

Topical applications of a therapeutic allow for targeted treatment at the site of pain and provide a patient centered approach, giving the patient control of applying the treatment. Most topical treatments include topical NSAIDs, which are often a first line of therapeutic treatment in age-related OA [107,108]. Topical application of NSAIDS, particularly diclofenac [109], for pain management have shown some benefit in early-stage OA [108]. However, this standard of treatment does not provide disease-modifying effects, specifically radiographic evidence of cartilage protection.

Curcumin nanoparticles (NPs) applied to the skin at the site of pain have been shown to improve joint retention with sustained therapeutic effects when compared to oral supplementation of free curcumin [110]. Curcumin nanoparticles applied topically to the joint were measurable in the infrapatellar fat pad within 3 h of application; however, they were not present after 6 h. The curcumin NPs were not visible in the cartilage or synovium, indicating that they did not travel beyond the fat pad. Histological results have shown improved cartilage pathology following the treatment, indicating that curcumin in the fat pad may have joint wide effects. The pain relief and cartilage protection from the in vivo model may be attributed to the suppression of inflammatory cytokines measured in vitro. However, further studies to confirm these effects may be necessary.

Though an interesting strategy, bioavailability to the joint is a key concern in the adoption of topical treatments. The mechanism by which therapies reach the desired joint tissue through the physical barriers, including the skin, musculature, and synovium, is currently unknown. Visible particle uptake in the fat pad is a promising step toward understanding these mechanisms in future work. If effective, topical strategies such as the curcumin nanoparticles may improve patient compliance.

3.2.3. Parenteral Therapies

Most pre-clinical models rely on injectable therapies to target a site-specific dose either indirectly (systemic injections) or directly into the joint space (intra-articular injections). This strategy avoids some of the limitations of other routes such as poor bioavailability and poor joint targeting.

Injectable Materials

The size and type of delivery vehicle and cargo are key considerations in the development of nano- and microparticles used for parenteral treatments. Microparticles, ranging from synthetic polymers to natural macromolecules, have been shown to improve drug stability and allow for the sustained release of drugs. Synthetic polymers, such as poly lactic-co-glycolic acid (PLGA), have been engineered into microspheres that can be loaded with a drug cargo [111]. These microspheres significantly prolong the residence time of drugs in the joint space and can have sustained release up to 3 months after injection [112,113]. Microparticles typically function as depot systems and are non-phagocytocable above 10 µm. Through diffusion and/or degradation, they release the therapy into the joint space over time, reducing the frequency of injections required. This may be useful for improving extracellular ROS scavenging or, if the released cargo can be taken up into cells, intracellular ROS scavenging.

On a smaller scale, nanoparticles made from natural macromolecules such as chitosan, hyaluronic acid (HA), polyester amides, and other peptides or from synthetic polymers and molecules, including hollow mesoporous silica nanoparticles, gold nanoparticles, nanocrystal polymer particles, and metal–organic frameworks have been evaluated as potential OA therapies [114]. Nanoparticle systems can protect the antioxidant until it is delivered intracellularly, which may improve drug targeting for intracellular oxidative stress. Both, microspheres and nanoparticles also improve drug bioavailability and stability, allow for better sustained and controlled release of the drug, and require lower dosages than free-drug treatments. Microparticle formulations for other OA drugs have been investigated clinically, but injectable, antioxidant-based treatments have not expanded beyond preclinical models [11]. Nano and micro scale particle systems may also be an effective strategy in oral or topical routes of administration and may protect the antioxidant from metabolism and improve bioavailability. Currently, most particle formulations are being investigated as IA injectable therapies in pre-clinical models.

Similar to polymeric encapsulation, liposomes have also been used to provide targeted delivery to specific cell types [115,116]. Liposomes are spheres enclosed by a lipid bilayer, mimicking the cell membrane and allowing for more effective uptake into cells. Liposomes may contribute to joint lubrication, which may also contribute to OA treatment by supporting the function of lubricin and the synovial fluid [117–121]. As a drug delivery vehicle, liposomes have been evaluated for delivering various types of drugs—mostly non-steroidal anti-inflammatory drugs (NSAIDs), cartilage matrix components, and nucleic acids for gene therapy [122–124]. However, liposomes loaded with antioxidants have recently been evaluated as a method to prevent oxidative stress in OA [125]. Gold nanoparticles with antioxidant functions have been loaded into surface-active phospholipid mimetic (DPPC) liposomes as a therapeutic for a rodent model of OA. Gold NPs are known to down regulate Cox-2, IL-1β and PGE-2, which are implicated in disease pathogenesis.

Injectable hydrogels are highly tunable and can also be used as a depot delivery system for therapeutics into the joint space [126]. Hydrogels for OA therapy have been investigated for their potential to deliver NSAIDS, hyaluronic acid, glycosaminoglycan, and antioxidant therapeutics. Injectable hydrogels with ROS-scavenging properties have been investigated as one solution for sustained release within the joint space. A hydrogel containing epigallocatechin-3-gallate (EGCG) has shown ROS-scavenging properties and protects against the upregulation of IL-1β [127,128]. Eicosapentaenoic acid, an antioxidant that scavenges free radicals [129], has been added to a gelatin-based hydrogel to evaluate its effects on slowing disease progression in a preclinical model of OA [130]. Creating a sustained release profile, on the order of weeks, this therapy is an improvement over most injectable therapies that are known to clear the joint within hours.

Injected therapeutics are typically cleared from the joint through lymphatic draining and in the capillaries that underlie the synovium. Fine tuning the drug delivery system to provide the right drug at a sufficient dose and time within the joint is important to consider when developing injectable therapies.

Injection Methods

Intraperitoneal (IP) injections provide a route of administration that bypasses metabolism in the digestive system and are often used in pre-clinical rodent models. Free curcumin administered via an IP injection has been shown to reduce the progression of OA by inhibiting apoptotic pathways and proinflammatory mediators and cytokines in rats (50–150 mg/kg) [131] and mice (50 μM) [132]. Although effective, these studies required high dose rates and had clear dose-dependent chondroprotective effects. Alternatively, acid-activatable micelles delivered via intramuscular injection may improve the bioavailability of curcumin [80]. Using a prodrug form of curcumin encapsulated in the micelle, the therapeutic could bypass physical barriers for intracellular delivery with a sustained drug release profile. When injected, these micelles improved chondroprotective effects compared to free drug while using a lower dose rate (2.5 mg/kg, 5 mg/kg, respectively). However, they are a promising strategy to utilize a common nutraceutical therapeutic in a delivery vehicle that can overcome traditional OA barriers. Systemic injections face similar challenges as other indirect routes of administration—due to the barriers associated with ensuring targeted therapies enter the joint to provide optimal antioxidant effects.

Intra-articular (IA) injections are the most direct method for targeted therapies to enter the joint space. They ensure the delivery of the therapeutic compound into the joint and may improve the bioavailability of the therapy while limiting the potential off-target effects. They also provide opportunities to improve stability, retention, and sustained-release characteristics using delivery vehicles loaded with antioxidant-based therapies. A critical limitation of IA injections is the need for frequent, high-dose injections (i.e., 2–5 times/week for the duration of the study) to obtain therapeutic benefit [114,133]. Frequent dosing schemes are the result of poor joint retention, with injected therapies often cleared from the joint within a few hours.

IA injections are a standard practice in pre-clinical models of OA, although strategies involving antioxidant-like or ROS-scavenging therapies have limited examples. Direct injection may overcome limitations of other routes of administration including bioavailability and retention challenges. However, there may still be concerns about rapid clearance and poor localization to specific target tissues within the joint space.

3.3. Engineering Strategies for a Biological Challenge

The studies reviewed so far highlight the potential for antioxidant therapies to treat OA; however, they require high dosing and frequent injections, which are problematic for preclinical-to-clinical translation. One emerging strategy involves the use of synthetic nanomaterials with inherent antioxidant properties. Often referred to as "nanozymes," these materials demonstrate ROS-scavenging kinetics that approach that of endogenous antioxidant enzymes, while being able to address the issues of stability, bioavailability, and cost of delivering exogenous antioxidant enzymes [134,135]. These new strategies have been widely used in energy transfer and environmental engineering applications [136], and have recently demonstrated potential to provide a multi-enzyme-mimicking approach in biomedical applications, including OA treatment.

4. Biomaterial Strategies as Antioxidant Mimics to Treat OA

Nanozymes are a class of biomaterials that are characterized by their ability to display enzyme-like characteristics [134,137,138]. These biomaterials have grown in prevalence since the early 2000s; however, their exact definition is still up for debate.

In the context of this work, we evaluate nanomaterials with at least one known enzyme-mimicking function. One limitation in evaluating and characterizing nanozymes is that the mechanism of action for the enzyme-mimicking function may not be fully understood. Further exploration of these novel materials may shed light on these comparisons; however in this case we will consider any enzyme-like activity to be worth discussing in this context.

Nanozymes have emerged as an enzyme-mimicking solution to the high cost and poor stability of endogenous enzymes. Biomaterials as enzyme-mimics can be broadly characterized by their specific enzyme function: catalase (CAT), SOD, peroxidase, and oxidase mimics [139,140]. Medical interest in nanozymes has been increasing [135,141,142], for example, with cobalt ferrite nanozymes [143] and single-atom manganese oxide [144] used in cancer applications [142]. They have also been used in applications for treating inflammatory bowel disease [145] and as biosensing platforms [137,146]. While nanozymes and their derivatives can be found widely in the literature, direct applications of antioxidant-mimicking therapies for osteoarthritis are limited (Table 2). Manganese dioxide and ceria oxide, used alone or in concert with other strategies are the most cited nanozyme strategies for OA applications.

Table 2. Nanozyme therapies currently being investigated as ROS scavenging treatments for OA.

Nanozymes in OA					
Nanozyme	Antioxidant Function	Treatment Method	Disease Model	Effects	Citation
HA-CeO$_2$	SOD Mimic, ↓ H$_2$O$_2$ concentration	Coincubation with 0.2 g/mL CeO$_2$ NPs for 1–3 days	0.3 mM H$_2$O$_2$ for 30 min. on bovine chondrocytes	↓ cartilage degeneration, ↓ chondrocyte apoptosis, ↑ H$_2$O$_2$ scavenging	Lin 2020 [147]
Nanoceria (nCe)	SOD Mimic	30 μL 250–2000 μg/mL nCe injected into synovial joint cavity	CFA-induced TMJ OA, male Sprague Dawley rats	↓ cellular apoptosis, ↓ catabolic proteins and pro-inflammatory cytokines (IL-1β/TNFα), ↑ polarization of M2 macrophages, ↑ anti-inflammatory cytokines (IL-10) and chondrogenic glycoproteins	Dashnyam 2021 [148]
MnO$_2$	Scavenges H$_2$O$_2$, catalase mimic	20 μL 5 mg/mL via IA injection	Healthy male Lewis rats	↓ loss of glycosaminoglycans, ↓nitric oxide, ↓ H$_2$O$_2$	Kumar 2019 [149]
MnO$_2$	Scavenges H$_2$O$_2$, catalase mimic	0–200 μg/mL	Murine insulinoma cells (BTC3)	↓ oxidative stress, mimics SOD and CAT, ↓ cell death	Tootoonchi 2017 [150]

Table 2. Cont.

Nanozyme	Antioxidant Function	Treatment Method	Disease Model	Effects	Citation
		Nanozymes in OA			
H-MnO$_2$	Scavenges H$_2$O$_2$	0.2 mL 30 μg/mL H-MnO2, 3x/week, 4 weeks, via IA injection	DMM-induced OA, female C57BL/6 mice	↓ cartilage degeneration, ↓ subchondral bone remodeling, ↓ inflammatory cytokines (IL6, IL1β, TNFα)	Chen 2021 [151]
HA/PRP/BM hydrogel	ROS scavenging	1.5 mg/mL HA/PRP/BM hydrogel, single injection 3 days after MIA induction	MIA-induced OA, Sprague Dawley rats	↓ cartilage degeneration, ↓ subchondral bone remodeling	Zhou 2022 [152]
WY-CMC-MnOx	↓ oxidative stress	100 μL 2.5 mg/kg MnOx, every 2 weeks for 6 weeks via IA injection	DMM-induced OA, male Sprague Dawley rats	Theranostic agent, ↑ chondrogenesis, ↓ cartilage degeneration	Lin 2022 [153]
Hollow Prussian-blue nanozymes (HPBzymes)	Scavenges H$_2$O$_2$, OH$^-$, OOH	0.36–3.6 μg/mL HPBzyme injection 1x/week, for 4 weeks post surgery	MMT-induced OA, male Sprague Dawley rats	↓ IL1B, ↓ Rac1-ROS-NFκB signaling pathway	Hou 2021 [154]
Hollow manganese Prussian-blue nanozymes (HMPBzymes)	Catalyzes H$_2$O$_2$ into O$_2$, ↓ HIF-1α expression, ↓ ROS levels	80 ug/mL HMPBzyme 1x/week for 4 weeks	MIA-induced OA, male Sprague Dawley rats	↓ inflammation, polarizes macrophages from M1 to M2	Xiong 2022 [155]
Gold Nanoparticles with Hyaluronic Acid (GNPs + HA)	↑ NRF2 to induce signaling of genes that encode antioxidants	2.5 mg/L GNP +/− 0.9% HA injection every 15 days for 90 days	Median meniscectomy induced OA, male Wistar rats	↑ NRF2, ↓ inflammation, ↓ cartilage degeneration	Filho 2021 [156]
AuNPs	↓ ROS production	30 ug/kg AuNPs +/− Diacerin (50 mg/kg) via oral route using a stomach tube weekly for 5 weeks	MIA-induced OA, female Sprague Dawley rats	Preserved GPX and SOD function in kidney and liver, ↓ cartilage degeneration, ↓ DNA fragmentation	Abdel-Aziz 2021 [157]

Abbreviations: CFA—complete Freund's Adjuvent; TMJ—temporomandibular joint; DMM—destabilization of medial meniscus; MIA—monoiodoacetate; MMT—medial meniscus transection.

Some benefits and considerations for nanozymes include the potential for compartment-specific uptake, as with other therapies discussed here, which may be important in mitigating the oxidative stress. Prolonged extracellular retention may also have therapeutic benefits, given the relatively fewer endogenous mechanisms in the EC space. The possibility to engineer nanomaterial properties to direct their tissue and cell localization and antioxidant functions is an advantage over conventional antioxidant systems. Additionally, multi-enzyme mimicry may provide therapeutic benefits that are not specific to a single target, which could be advantageous in OA.

4.1. Metal Oxides

Metal oxide nanoparticles are the most commonly studied nanozyme for OA [48]. Metal oxides are highly tunable, can be combined with a variety of other treatments, and are cost-effective to produce. It is expected that the smaller the particle size, the stronger the enzymatic activity and the more readily they can be taken up within the cell [55]. Metal oxide NPs smaller than 8 nm may enter the cell via direct diffusion [48]. Larger metal oxide NPs may enter the cell through endocytic mechanisms, such as clathrin or caveolin-mediated endocytosis, after adhering to the cell membrane.

Despite the innate benefits of using metal oxide nanozymes, some common limitations must also be addressed. Depending on the specific metal oxide structure and composition, there may be concerns of intracellular toxicity or inactivity of the therapeutic based on the cellular compartment to which they localize. Metal oxides may generate additional free radicals, for example, through the Fenton reaction where partially or fully oxidized nanoparticle systems may generate additional ROS [158]. Iron- and cerium-based NPs have been known participate in this reaction and develop additional free radicals, potentially limiting their efficacy.

Common metal oxides include cerium oxide (CeO_2) [159], manganese oxide (MnO) [149,160,161], magnesium oxide [162], and zinc oxide [58,162].

4.1.1. Cerium Oxide

Cerium oxide NPs, also known as ceria oxide or nanoceria, can have SOD-, CAT-, oxidase-, and peroxidase-mimicking activities depending on their formulation [163–166]. Ceria nanoparticles have been shown to scavenge H_2O_2 in vitro [147], provide chondroprotection in vivo [148], and ameliorate inflammation in models of rheumatoid arthritis [166]. Cerium oxide nanoparticles produce their enzyme mimicking effects while fluctuating their valance states between Ce^{3+} and Ce^{4+} [164]. The NPs exhibit more SOD-like activity during the conversion from Ce^{3+} to Ce^{4+} and have more CAT-like activity when converting from Ce^{4+} to Ce^{3+} [48]. Size also plays a critical role in their oxidative function, with smaller nanoparticles exhibiting stronger SOD-like effects than larger particle systems [164].

In a rodent model of temporomandibular joint (TMJ) osteoarthritis, nanoceria (nCe) preserved cartilage and subchondral bone structures [148]. Three days after the induction of TMJ OA, nanoceria particles were injected into the joint cavity and effects were observed after 10 days. A single injection of 20 nm particles ranging from 100–2000 μg/mL appeared to preserve cartilage and subchondral bone structure. Dashnyam et al. also found that the nCe supported macrophage polarization toward the M2, or anti-inflammatory, phenotype by suppressing the pro-inflammatory effects of the disease. They also exhibited ROS-scavenging effects in a model of chondrocytes exposed to H_2O_2 followed by treatment with nCe. The measurements for ROS production and scavenging focused on changes in intracellular ROS; while there was no determination that the nCe were taken up by the cells, the decrease in ROS is indicative of effective antioxidant functions. The advancement of a single-dose therapeutic is a promising improvement compared to other direct injection strategies that require consistent dosing to show a therapeutic effect. Future applications of this therapy may be dependent on the duration of the therapeutic effect, but the inhibition of ROS production may be enough to create a sustained effect. Other joints affected by OA, specifically the knee, may need further evaluation to determine whether the barriers within the joint inhibit the function of nCe.

When used in combination with HA, cerium oxide nanoparticles improved therapeutic efficacy and may be a viable strategy for improving the application of other well-known therapeutic agents that are limited by bioavailability and targeting strategy challenges [147]. The interaction between the HA and CeO_2 NPs, as well as their location within the cell, are currently unknown. However, when used in combination, they protect Col1A1 expression in the presence of H_2O_2, a downstream effect of oxidative stress. The system also protects against characteristic loss of proteoglycan when exposed to H_2O_2.

The predominant function of cerium oxide NPs relies on their ability to target intracellular ROS, therefore requiring them to be designed for intracellular localization. However, cerium oxide is non-degradable and drug clearance may be a critical limitation in implementing this nanosystem as an OA therapeutic [167]. Evaluation of nanoparticle localization, as well as the safety and efficacy of these therapies are necessary steps to advance cerium oxide as a potential OA strategy.

4.1.2. Manganese Oxide

Manganese oxide has been used in biomedical and environmental applications [48]. It has been shown that various formulations of MnO have the potential to mimic peroxidase, SOD, and CAT functions [150,160]. There is also some evidence that MnO nanozymes may improve neuropathic pain responses in rodent models of OA [168]. The structure of manganese oxide nanosystems affects the catalytic activity and stability/degradation rates of the material [169]. This structure–function relationship is important for understanding MnO material function and its relevance in treating OA; however, it has not been widely studied.

Manganese is an essential nutrient that is necessary for biological functions [170]. It acts as a cofactor for a variety of enzymes including arginase, glutamine synthase, and MnSOD. The byproducts of Mn based nanoparticles create Mn ions that support the function of these enzymes and may improve mitochondrial functions to scavenge ROS production. The potential overabundance of intracellular Mn needs to be mitigated, as too much may cause further mitochondrial dysfunction and oxidative stress. Additionally, there is some risk of Mn toxicity, specifically in the brain [171]. However, this risk is likely minimal due to the low dose used in most studies of manganese oxide treatments for OA.

Manganese oxide NPs are characterized by their ability to catalyze the breakdown of H_2O_2 into water and oxygen, providing SOD-, peroxidase-, and potentially, catalase-like functions in vitro. PEG-stabilized MnO_2 has been used as a stand-alone therapeutic treatment [149] to scavenge H_2O_2 and decrease inflammatory markers relevant to osteoarthritis. Kumar et al. engineered MnO_2 NPs with a cationic zeta potential and size of less than 13 nm to leverage electrostatic interactions and integrate with the dense extracellular matrix [149]. It is expected that the MnO_2 NPs are also small enough to be taken up intracellularly and may be able to scavenge H_2O_2 produced within the cell, though this has yet to be reported. They have also shown chondroprotective effects in cartilage explants, with a decrease in glycosaminoglycan loss and nitric oxide production following IL-1β stimulation. Via cartilage targeting, these NPs have also shown improved joint retention on the order of days. Combining antioxidant effects with chondroprotection and increased joint retention make MnO_2 NPs a promising therapeutic for OA treatment. Additional evaluation of in vivo effects will be necessary to further the application of this nanozyme therapy.

Chen et al. utilized a hollow-MnO_2 (h-MnO_2) that may protect against cartilage damage in a surgical model of OA. In this model, h-MnO_2 NPs decreased the presence of inflammatory mediators (IL-1β, IL6) in serum and may prevent joint remodeling [151]. Similar to Kumar et al. [149,151], the h-MnO_2 NPs were coated with poly(allylamine) hydrochloride (PAH) to functionalize the surface of the hollow MnO_2 NPs [151]. In mice, 30 µg/mL h-MnO_2 NPs given 3x/week for 4 weeks showed protection of the cartilage and joint structure with a surgical model of OA. This dosing scheme is consistent with the high dose rates found with other injectable-based therapies which may, like the others, be a limitation for the long-term application of this therapy. The results suggest that the h-MnO_2 protected against characteristic cartilage breakdown and bone remodeling consistent with the DMM model and is a promising option for future work.

Other methods utilizing MnO_2 as a therapeutic have leveraged combination treatment strategies. Zhou et al. fabricated an MnO_2 nanozyme-encapsulated hydrogel by dispersing bovine serum albumin (BSA)-MnO_2 nanoparticles in a hyaluronic acid/platelet rich plasma (PRP) gel network [152]. This conglomerate is intended to provide multi-functional support to cartilage. MnO_2 NPs, as previously discussed, can slow the development of oxidative stress through CAT- and SOD-like functions. The MnO_2 NPs specifically target H_2O_2 but may have broader antioxidative effects that can be leveraged in this system. Additionally, PRP promotes chondrocyte proliferation and has been widely used as a potential treatment for joint injuries that allows for patient-specific treatment. The multifunctional properties of this hydrogel system are aimed at targeting specific challenges in treating the OA joint: sustained release of the therapy for up to 3 days, decreasing ROS production in the presence of the hydrogel, and providing structural protection to the joint following an in vivo inflammatory response. Overcoming some of the limitations of a single nanozyme treatment, this hydrogel also utilizes components found naturally within the joint. As with many of the other therapies discussed here, there is a need to do further research on the behavioral effects of this therapy and a need to better understand intracellular mechanisms of action to fully understand how the therapy is protecting the joint.

Carboxymethyl-chitosan-assisted MnO_x (WY-CMC-MnOx) nanoparticles leverage the theranostic properties of MnO nanozymes in combination with a cartilage-targeting peptide as a treatment for the early stages of osteoarthritis [153]. Manganese oxide is a known potential contrast agent and has been used as a theranostic agent in tumor-based cancers [172]. Early diagnosis of OA through MR imaging may provide additional opportunities to interfere with the negative feedback loop of oxidative stress that promotes OA pathogenesis [153], and is a practical application of MnO_x for orthopedics. Lin et al. found that the WY-CMC-MnO_x particles improved MR imaging of cartilage lesions, owing to their small size and cartilage targeting properties. In models with mesenchymal stem cells, the WY-CMC-MnO_x promoted chondrogenesis and protected against cartilage breakdown in vivo. Complexing components with chondroprotective or therapeutic effects may provide an advantage for treating OA by improving retention in the joint without re-engineering the basic material properties of the therapy.

Presently, there are only four known applications of Mn-based particle systems for managing oxidative stress production in OA. However, outside of the OA field, research has evaluated encapsulated MnO_2 [173] and MnO_2 used to decorate the surface of larger particle systems [174] as techniques to scavenge ROS from oxidative stress environments. Both particle systems were developed at the micro-particle scale and may have limited ability to translate as an OA therapy but showcase the versatility of MnO_2 as a possible treatment for oxidative stress. As a transition metal conjugate, MnO_2 may provide therapeutic effects both intra and extracellularly, catalyzing the breakdown of H_2O_2 into water and oxygen through CAT-mimicking functions or by decomposing H_2O_2 into OH^- if the Mn^{2+} ion dissociates from the particle in the extracellular matrix [36]. Further understanding of the intracellular localization of these therapies will be necessary to understand their full therapeutic potential.

4.1.3. Iron Oxides

Iron oxide nanomaterials have a broad range of functions owing to the combination of superparamagnetic functions and enzyme-mimicking functions. Iron oxide particles, referred to as IONzymes, have the potential to act as a theranostic nanozyme [141]. Ferromagnetic nanoparticles (Fe_3O_4) possess peroxidase-like activity, behaving like horseradish peroxidase (HRP) [175], and catalyzing the oxidation of standard peroxidase substrates such as TMB and DAB. Additionally, the magnetic properties of Fe_3O_4 provide opportunities to capture the particles after use. IONzymes follow Michaelis–Menten kinetics, and both Fe_2O_3 and Fe_3O_4 have been reported to have peroxidase- and catalase-like functions. Gold-coated, superparamagnetic iron oxide nanoparticles leverage the properties of both IONzymes and gold, thereby acting as a multi-functional treatment strategy. These nanoparticles decreased inflammation in a collagenase-induced model of OA [176]. By leveraging these characteristics, further described by Gao 2007, iron oxide nanomaterials have therapeutic potential as a nanozyme for the treatment and detection of osteoarthritis [175]. However, iron-based materials may contribute to the production of additional ROS through the Fenton reaction, which may limit their therapeutic efficacy. Iron-oxide-based nanomaterials have been used broadly in the OA field as a mechanism to label and track cell and treatment movement in vitro and in pre-clinical models [177–181]. However, these studies do not address the potential enzyme functions of this material. Future work with other iron oxide systems may reveal additional multi-functional treatment systems effective for treating OA.

4.1.4. Additional Metal Oxides

There is an interest in evaluating a broad spectrum of biocompatible metals as potential nanozymes due to their promise as a treatment for oxidative stress. To date, biological evaluation has been conducted for silver-, aluminum-, cadmium-, copper-, magnesium-, titanium-, vanadium-, tungsten-, and zinc-based oxide particle systems [162].

Zhang et al. conducted a proteome-wide assessment of oxidative stress responses to metal oxide nanoparticles with human macrophages. Macrophages are critical immune cells in OA progression that contribute to the inflammatory state of the joint. They evaluated 11 different nanoparticles, including ceria-based NPs which have been previously discussed. From these 11 particles, there was a correlation between the level of proteome change, the induction of ROS-responsive proteins, and the eventual cytotoxic outcome following particle exposure. Taken from their results, it may be beneficial to evaluate the ROS-scavenging properties of metal oxides with low toxicity and minimal proteome change, such as MgO or SiO_2, in a model of osteoarthritis. Additionally, this work showed that ceria oxide nanoparticles may also be useful in treating oxidative stress without causing off-target downstream effects. Luo et al. propose the potential use of magnesium oxide nanoparticles, due to their therapeutic potential as an ROS-scavenging agent [182], and zinc oxide due to its ability to inhibit gene expression of inflammatory markers and the effects of exogenous zinc [58]. While the list of promising therapeutics is continuing to evolve, only a few metal oxide nanozymes have been evaluated for the treatment of osteoarthritis, lagging behind the implementation and evaluation of nanozymes in other applications.

4.2. Prussian Blue Nanozymes

Prussian blue nanozymes are another advancement in engineered nanosystems with catalytic functions. Prussian blue is a versatile and biocompatible material known for its distinct blue color [183]. The compound, $Fe_4[Fe(CN)_6]_3$, derives many of its properties from charge transfers through across Fe atoms and has been cited as a potential theranostic in biomedical applications. With a variety of uses in medicine, Prussian blue is best known for its function as an antidote for cesium and thallium poisoning [184]. Approved by the US Food and Drug Administration, Prussian blue nanozymes are known to have robust antioxidative-mimicking properties. Specifically, they leverage electron transport properties to exhibit peroxidase-, catalase-, SOD-, and other ROS-scavenging functions. Prussian blue nanozymes are highly tunable, with sizes ranging from ultrasmall (~3.4 nm) to >100 nm in hydrodynamic diameter based on the synthesis method. They are cost-effective to produce and do not generate additional free radicals typically found in other iron-based particle systems through the Fenton reaction. Because these particle systems can be engineered with a variety of different catalytic properties, it will be important to assess their compartment-specific localization within cells and their ability to be endocytosed in order to understand which ROS are being targeted and how the therapeutic effect is being achieved.

Hollow Prussian blue nanozymes (HPBzymes) are one formulation that has been engineered for use in osteoarthritis [154]. HPBzymes were designed with a mesoporous structure to increase the specific surface area, with a size of 78 nm and a zeta potential of 1.85 mV. The pores of the mesoporous surface area range from 2–5 nm and have improved the reactions between HPBzymes and the substrates within the OA microenvironment. In vitro models have showcased the potential therapeutic effects of the HPBzymes, catalyzing the breakdown of OH^-, OOH, and H_2O_2. In a rat MMT model of OA, the application of the HPBzymes (1x/week for 4 weeks) significantly reduced the structural effects of the MMT surgery (via histological analysis). Immunofluorescence has also shown a decrease in the expression of iNOS and COX-2. A high dose of HPBzymes (3.6 µg/mL) was more effective than a low dose (0.36 µg/mL). And, with injections 1x/week the use of the HPBzymes may be an improvement over many other injectable therapies given more frequently. Compartment-specific localization may still need to be addressed with this nanosystem, in large part due to their size and neutral charge.

Another Prussian-blue-based system leverages a pH-responsive, biodegradable structure (HMPBzymes) [155]. The HMPBzymes measure 210 nm in hydrodynamic diameter with a zeta potential of −20 mV and are readily taken up by bone-marrow-derived macrophages, indicating the likelihood of ROS scavenging from within the cell. Macrophages have also shown the ability to polarize from an M1, proinflammatory, phenotype to an M2, anti-inflammatory, phenotype. This may indicate a shift in the joint microenvironment to promote a decrease in inflammatory cytokines and other downstream mediators of oxidative stress. A key contribution of this particle system is the ability to inhibit hypoxia as measured by the suppression of HIF-1α and the generation of oxygen in vitro. When given via IA injection following an inflammatory model of OA, weekly injections of the HMPBzymes have been shown to significantly improve joint structure. The HMPBzymes were also retained within the joint space for at least 7 days, protecting against a complete loss of therapeutic effects between injections. This advancement is important in overcoming the limitations of joint retention and sustained therapeutic effects. And, as one of few studies focused on macrophage function in OA, this work has shown the ability to have a therapeutic effect on joint structure without targeting cartilage.

Various forms of HPBzymes have been widely studied for use in other disease conditions such as ischemic stroke [185], inflammatory bowel disease [186], neurological decline [187], osteoporosis [188], and cancer [189]. Their advancement across a broad range of fields is a valuable step toward the application of HPBzymes in clinical trials and their potential availability in the future.

4.3. Gold-Based Nanozymes

Gold-based, micro- and nano-scale therapies are another therapeutic intervention that has have been tested in OA applications, but they are more commonly utilized in rheumatoid arthritis applications [190–192]. Gold-based nanotherapies used in OA applications range from biologic carriers [193], a use as miRNA biomarkers [194], as a standalone therapy [157,195], and being integrated with iron oxide nanoparticles to combine antioxidant functions [176]. Despite their wide use, little is known about the antioxidant properties of gold-based therapies. Some studies suggest that gold-based treatments have peroxidase-mimicking functions which can help downregulate pro-inflammatory responses [196], or that they may support the production and function of catalase [197]. However, most studies do not discuss the potential antioxidant properties of this biomaterial. The translation of gold NPs into clinical settings is, in part, limited by issues of aggregation in the kidneys, liver, and spleen [198,199], and they have been shown to induce the formation of ROS, thereby having the opposite effect to we would expect [200]. These negative side effects have yet to be evaluated in OA applications, but are important to consider with the development of this treatment as a potential OA therapy. As the antioxidant effects of gold NPs have not been widely accepted, only a few of the current applications of these therapies to OA have been evaluated here.

As a potential OA therapeutic, gold NPs offer several benefits including a high degree of tunability, and they are easy to combine with other biologic components. Filho et al. synthesized a 20-nm gold NP (GNP) that was given in combination with HA (0.9%) via IA injection in Wistar rats, following an MMT surgical procedure [156]. They found that the combination of GNPs and HA protected cartilage structure and decreased the pro-inflammatory cytokines. The GNP + HA treatment also decreased the effects of oxidative stress including nitrite and myeloperoxidase production, to name a few. It is expected that the GNPs improved integration of the HA therapy with the local joint environment. In terms of antioxidant function, this system was found to support the activation of NRF2, which activates KEAP1, leading to an increased production of antioxidants. However, the details of this pathway are uncertain. This is a promising therapeutic approach combining a nanozyme material with a commonly used adjuvant therapy, and future work may support its translation into a clinical setting.

Similarly, Abdel-Aziz et al. used a similar gold nanoparticle (AuNP) with a small size (20 nm) and positive charge but coupled its application with Diacerein [157]. Diacerein is an anthraquinone derivative that inhibits IL-1β and has been recommended by the European League Against Rheumatism since the early 2000s [201]. Although typically used as an RA treatment, Diacerein used in combination with the AuNPs had promising effects related to slowing the progression of OA [157]. When given orally, the AuNPs + Diacerein improved oxidative stress markers, decreased DNA fragmentation, and protected cartilage structure more effectively compared to the MIA-induced OA controls. These results also indicated that the AuNPs were safe for use and did not have toxicity concerns commonly attributed to gold-based therapies. Interestingly, this is one of two studies highlighted in this review that utilized female rodents, which speaks to the need to evaluate sex as a biological variable in OA therapies. Further evaluation of the function of these therapies and a deeper understanding of their ROS functions will be necessary to further this application.

There may be promise in furthering our understanding and use of gold-based nanomaterials for OA. However, a deep evaluation of their antioxidant-like properties will be necessary to advance their application as a nanozyme in any field.

4.4. Single-Atom Nanozymes

Single-atom catalysts have been developed with a variety of different metal active sites to create catalytically active nanomaterials [144,202]. An SAzyme with a Cl-Cu-N_4 active center has been designed with identical geometric and electronic structures as naturally occurring SOD [202]. These SAzymes were designed to scavenge O_2^- radicals and were able to degrade H_2O_2 in a catalase-mimicking function. The aggregation of SAzymes in chondrocytes has been shown to decrease the levels of intracellular ROS. This suggests that the SAzymes can enter chondrocytes and support endogenous enzyme function. In vivo, these effects were consistent as the SAzymes protected against cartilage breakdown following an ACLT model of OA. While further investigation of this therapy is necessary, it remains a promising and novel approach to enzyme-mimicking strategies that may overcome many of the limitations of current therapies.

4.5. Additional Considerations in the Development of Nanozyme Technologies

There is a significant number of considerations when designing nanomaterials as treatments or delivery vehicles for OA. The nanozymes presented here have only been evaluated in vitro and in rodent preclinical models (Table 2). However, molecular transport at these scales may not translate at larger scales, such as with large animal models or humans. Transport properties change with increasing cartilage thickness [13,14,203,204], meaning that therapies developed to target cartilage may encounter differences in tissue retention as the thickness increases. Once in the cartilage, if the nanomaterial is intended to target intracellular localization to chondrocytes, transport through the cartilage ECM, the pericellular matrix [205,206], and the cell membrane should be taken into account [19,207,208]. Upon entry into the joint, nanomaterials will develop a protein corona, a protein coat that attaches the material surface which can influence nanomaterial interactions with cells and tissues [196,209,210]. These considerations, as well as the proper delivery method and route of administration, may change depending on the specific location of interest. Numerous reviews on these nanoparticle characteristics and others necessary for joint delivery have been published [19–21,99,210].

In addition, nanomaterial fate and byproducts should be considered in the design and application of nanozymes. As ROS production differs intra- and extracellularly, nanozyme function should be matched with its intended location within the joint. Nanomaterial systems too large to passively cross cell membranes may be endocytosed and degraded in lysosomes or trafficked/exocytosed from the cell. Alternatively, systems that bypass these fates and remain in the cytosol could impact intracellular ROS either in the cytosol, mitochondria, or the nucleus. Over time, byproducts of these materials may produce neutral species or additional free radicals. While the exact byproducts are not known for all nanozymes, it is important to consider how they may affect the system and could further exacerbate the imbalance of antioxidants to ROS. Similar to discussions on nanomaterial transport, nanozyme fate may differ between pre-clinical rodent models of OA and clinical studies due to the scale of cartilage structure.

Endogenous enzymes are the most efficient mechanism for scavenging ROS and maintaining redox balance in the joint. The rate at which enzyme-mimicking strategies are deployed in the joint and the amount of therapeutic benefit is also important to consider in their design and implementation. Augmenting endogenous enzymes, the addition of synthetic nanomaterials (or nanozymes), could support enzymatic function without disrupting cell function. Although most of our focus has been on the intracellular effects of nanozymes, the actual location of most nanozymes after delivery has not been widely studied. Future work evaluating the intracellular localization and antioxidant pathways of nanozymes will be critical in advancing their efficacy.

5. Conclusions

At the time of writing, a literature search for 'Nanozymes' and 'Osteoarthritis' results in 11 results from as early as 2020. While nanozymes may be widely used in other applications, their use in orthopedics is in its infancy. Early adopters to the development and use of these materials may be on the forefront of a potential technology that could improve our ability to target oxidative stress in OA, and consequently improve treatment for the disease. However, a common limitation of the therapies discussed here is the limited understanding of how the antioxidant mechanisms work, and for how long. As this field develops, it will be critical to consider and understand the ROS target for which these nanozyme systems are developed and how their antioxidant functions improve therapeutic efficacy.

Nanozymes may play a role in the continued development of other cutting-edge therapies, specifically for personalized medicine and gene therapy applications. Characteristics of nanozymes, similar to other nanomaterials, can be tailored through simple biomaterial and synthesis changes. Nanozymes can also be loaded into scaffolds or gels to provide additional benefits in inflammatory tissues. This flexibility and the enzyme functions of nanozymes make them a compelling tool for more advanced applications. Future work with gene therapy and tissue-engineered materials may leverage these properties.

The development of nanozymes specifically for OA is still in its infancy. This class of therapies may overcome the limitations of traditional treatments that have often stalled following pre-clinical evaluation. Many of the challenges in developing DMOADs, such as the ability to identify and treat the disease before cartilage loss, will continue to be a challenge for these nanomaterials. However, engineering a treatment system that mimics endogenous functions is a promising gateway to further advancements in the OA field. It is possible that additional therapies and formulations of nanozymes will become a key focus for treating OA over the next several years.

Author Contributions: Conceptualization, J.L.A.; writing—original draft preparation, J.L.A., A.P. and R.O.J.; writing—review and editing, J.L.A. and B.S., visualization, J.L.A.; funding acquisition, B.S. All authors have read and agreed to the published version of the manuscript.

Funding: This research was funded by the National Institute of Health, National Institute on Arthritis and Musculoskeletal and Skin Diseases, Awards R01AR080687 and R01AR071335.

Institutional Review Board Statement: Not applicable.

Informed Consent Statement: Not applicable.

Data Availability Statement: Data is contained within the article.

Acknowledgments: All authors and funding sources have been acknowledged.

Conflicts of Interest: The authors declare no conflict of interest.

Abbreviations

ACLT	Anterior cruciate ligament transection
ACP	Amphiphilic curcumin polymer micelles
AuNP	Gold nanoparticles
BNTA	(N-[2-bromo-4-(phenylsulfonyl)-3-thienyl]-2-chlorobenzamide)
BSA	Bovine serum albumin
CAT	Catalase

CeO$_2$	Cerium oxide
CFA	Complete Freund's adjuvant
DMM	Destabilization of medial meniscus
DMOAD	Disease-modifying osteoarthritis drug
ECM	Extracellular matrix
ER	Endoplasmic reticulum
GI	Gastrointestinal
GNP	Gold nanoparticles
GPX	Glutathione peroxidase
GSH	Glutathione
GSSG	Oxidized glutathione
h-MnO$_2$	Hollow manganese dioxide
H$_2$O$_2$	Hydrogen peroxide
HA	Hyaluronic acid
HPBzymes	Hollow Prussian blue nanozymes
HRP	Horse radish peroxidase
IA	Intra-articular
IP	Intraperitoneal
LNC	Lipid core nanocapsules
M2	Macrophage
MIA	Mono-iodoacetate
MMT	Medial meniscus transection
MnO$_2$	Manganese dioxide
nCe	Nanoceria
NO	Nitric oxide
NOX	NADPH-oxidase
NP	Nanoparticle
NSAID	Nonsteroidal anti-inflammatory drug
OA	Osteoarthritis
PAH	Poly(allylamine) hydrochloride
PEG	Polyethylene glycol
PLGA	Poly-lactic co glycolic acid
PRP	Platelet-rich plasma
PRX	Peroxidredoxin
PTOA	Post-traumatic osteoarthritis
RLTA	Oxidized cellulose aerogel
ROS	Reactive oxygen species
SAzymes	Single-atom nanozymes
SFN	Silk fibroin nanoparticle
SOD	Superoxide dismutase
TMJ	Temporomandibular joint

References

1. Loeser, R.F.; Goldring, S.R.; Scanzello, C.R.; Goldring, M.B. Osteoarthritis: A disease of the joint as an organ. *Arthritis Rheum.* **2012**, *64*, 1697–1707. [CrossRef] [PubMed]
2. Xia, B.; Chen, D.; Zhang, J.; Hu, S.; Jin, H.; Tong, P. Osteoarthritis Pathogenesis: A Review of Molecular Mechanisms. *Calcif. Tissue Int.* **2014**, *95*, 495–505. [CrossRef] [PubMed]
3. Vincent, T.L.; Alliston, T.; Kapoor, M.; Loeser, R.F.; Troeberg, L.; Little, C.B. Osteoarthritis Pathophysiology. *Clin. Geriatr. Med.* **2022**, *38*, 193–219. [CrossRef]
4. Weinstein, A.M.; Rome, B.N.; Reichmann, W.M.; Collins, J.E.; Burbine, S.A.; Thornhill, T.S.; Wright, J.; Katz, J.N.; Losina, E. Estimating the burden of total knee replacement in the United States. *J. Bone Jt. Surg.* **2013**, *95*, 385. [CrossRef] [PubMed]
5. Zahan, O.M.; Serban, O.; Gherman, C.; Fodor, D. The evaluation of oxidative stress in osteoarthritis. *Med. Pharm. Rep.* **2020**, *93*, 12–22. [CrossRef] [PubMed]
6. Tudorachi, N.B.; Totu, E.E.; Fifere, A.; Ardeleanu, V.; Mocanu, V.; Mircea, C.; Isildak, I.; Smilkov, K.; Carausu, E. The implication of reactive oxygen species and antioxidants in knee osteoarthritis. *Antioxidants* **2021**, *10*, 985. [CrossRef]
7. Birben, E.; Sahiner, U.M.; Sackesen, C.; Erzurum, S.; Kalayci, O. Oxidative stress and antioxidant defense. *World Allergy Organ. J.* **2012**, *5*, 9. [CrossRef]

8. Jagaran, K.; Singh, M. Nanomedicine for Neurodegenerative Disorders: Focus on Alzheimer's and Parkinson's Diseases. *Int. J. Mol. Sci.* **2021**, *22*, 9082. [CrossRef]
9. Uchida, S.; Perche, F.; Pichon, C.; Cabral, H. Nanomedicine-Based Approaches for mRNA Delivery. *Mol. Pharm.* **2020**, *17*, 3654–3684. [CrossRef] [PubMed]
10. Contera, S.; Bernardino de la Serna, J.; Tetley, T.D. Biotechnology, nanotechnology and medicine. *Emerg. Top. Life Sci.* **2020**, *4*, 551–554. [CrossRef] [PubMed]
11. Patra, J.K.; Das, G.; Fraceto, L.F.; Campos, E.; Rodriguez-Torres, M.; Acosta-Torres, L.; Diaz-Torres, L.; Grillo, R.; Swamy, M.; Sharma, S.; et al. Nano based drug delivery systems: Recent developments and future prospects. *J. Nanobiotechnol.* **2018**, *16*, 71. [CrossRef]
12. Bajpayee, A.G.; Grodzinsky, A.J. Cartilage-targeting drug delivery: Can electrostatic interactions help? *Nat. Rev. Rheumatol.* **2017**, *13*, 183–193. [CrossRef]
13. Vedadghavami, A.; Mehta, S.; Bajpayee, A.G. Characterization of Intra-Cartilage Transport Properties of Cationic Peptide Carriers. *J. Vis. Exp.* **2020**, *162*, e61340. [CrossRef]
14. Mehta, S.; He, T.; Bajpayee, A.G. Recent advances in targeted drug delivery for treatment of osteoarthritis. *Curr. Opin. Rheumatol.* **2021**, *33*, 94–109. [CrossRef]
15. Wang, Z.; Wang, S.; Wang, K.; Wu, X.; Tu, C.; Gao, C. Stimuli-Sensitive Nanotherapies for the Treatment of Osteoarthritis. *Macromol. Biosci.* **2021**, *21*, 2100280. [CrossRef]
16. Na, H.S.; Woo, J.S.; Kim, J.H.; Lee, J.S.; Um, I.G.; Cho, K.; Kim, G.H.; Cho, M.; Chung, S.J.; Park, S. Coenzyme Q10 encapsulated in micelles ameliorates osteoarthritis by inhibiting inflammatory cell death. *PLoS ONE* **2022**, *17*, e0270351. [CrossRef] [PubMed]
17. Geiger, B.C.; Wang, S.; Padera, R.F.; Grodzinsky, A.J.; Hammond, P.T. Cartilage-penetrating nanocarriers improve delivery and efficacy of growth factor treatment of osteoarthritis. *Sci. Transl. Med.* **2018**, *10*, eaat8800. [CrossRef]
18. Kou, L.; Xiao, S.; Sun, R.; Bao, S.; Yao, Q.; Chen, R. Biomaterial-engineered intra-articular drug delivery systems for osteoarthritis therapy. *Drug Deliv.* **2019**, *26*, 870–885. [CrossRef]
19. Mao, L.; Wu, W.; Wang, M.; Guo, J.; Li, H.; Zhang, S.; Xu, J.; Zuo, J. Targeted treatment for osteoarthritis: Drugs and delivery system. *Drug Deliv.* **2021**, *28*, 1861–1876. [CrossRef] [PubMed]
20. Brown, S.; Kumar, S.; Sharma, B. Intra-articular targeting of nanomaterials for the treatment of osteoarthritis. *Acta Biomater.* **2019**, *93*, 239–257. [CrossRef]
21. Brown, S.; Pistiner, J.; Adjei, I.M.; Sharma, B. Nanoparticle Properties for Delivery to Cartilage: The Implications of Disease State, Synovial Fluid, and Off-Target Uptake. *Mol. Pharm.* **2019**, *16*, 469–479. [CrossRef]
22. Kumar, S.; Sharma, B. Leveraging Electrostatic Interactions for Drug Delivery to the Joint. *Bioelectricity* **2020**, *2*, 82–100. [CrossRef]
23. Younas, A.; Gu, H.; Zhao, Y.; Zhang, N. Novel approaches of the nanotechnology-based drug delivery systems for knee joint injuries: A review. *Int. J. Pharm.* **2021**, *608*, 121051. [CrossRef]
24. Lepetsos, P.; Papavassiliou, A.G. ROS/oxidative stress signaling in osteoarthritis. *Biochim. Biophys. Acta Mol. Basis Dis.* **2016**, *1862*, 576–591. [CrossRef]
25. Loeser, R.F. The Role of Aging in the Development of Osteoarthritis. *Trans. Am. Clin. Climatol. Assoc.* **2017**, *128*, 44–54.
26. Maneesh, M.; Jayalekshmi, H.; Suma, T.; Chatterjee, S.; Chakrabarti, A.; Singh, T.A. Evidence for oxidative stress in osteoarthritis. *Indian J. Clin. Biochem.* **2005**, *20*, 129–130. [CrossRef]
27. Ansari, M.Y.; Ahmad, N.; Haqqi, T.M. Oxidative stress and inflammation in osteoarthritis pathogenesis: Role of polyphenols. *Biomed. Pharmacother.* **2020**, *129*, 110452. [CrossRef] [PubMed]
28. Mobasheri, A.; Biesalski, H.K.; Shakibaei, M.; Henrotin, Y. Antioxidants and Osteoarthritis. In *Systems Biology of Free Radicals and Antioxidants*; Springer: Berlin/Heidelberg, Germany, 2014; pp. 2997–3026. [CrossRef]
29. Rosenbaum, C.C.; O'Mathúna, D.P.; Chavez, M.; Shields, K. Antioxidants and antiinflammatory dietary supplements for osteoarthritis and rheumatoid arthritis. *Altern. Ther. Health Med.* **2010**, *16*, 32–40.
30. Henrotin, Y.; Kurz, B. Antioxidant to Treat Osteoarthritis: Dream or Reality? *Curr. Drug Targets* **2007**, *8*, 347–357. [CrossRef] [PubMed]
31. D'Autréaux, B.; Toledano, M.B. ROS as signalling molecules: Mechanisms that generate specificity in ROS homeostasis. *Nat. Rev. Mol. Cell Biol.* **2007**, *8*, 813–824. [CrossRef] [PubMed]
32. Loeser, R.F.; Collins, J.A.; Diekman, B.O. Ageing and the pathogenesis of osteoarthritis. *Nat. Rev. Rheumatol.* **2016**, *12*, 412–420. [CrossRef]
33. López-Otín, C.; Blasco, M.A.; Partridge, L.; Serrano, M.; Kroemer, G. The hallmarks of aging. *Cell* **2013**, *153*, 1194–1217. [CrossRef] [PubMed]
34. Arra, M.; Swarnkar, G.; Ke, K.; Otero, J.; Ying, J.; Duan, X.; Maruyama, T.; Rai, M.; O'Keefe, R.; Mbalaviele, G.; et al. LDHA-mediated ROS generation in chondrocytes is a potential therapeutic target for osteoarthritis. *Nat. Commun.* **2020**, *11*, 3427. [CrossRef] [PubMed]
35. Wegner, A.M.; Campos, N.R.; Robbins, M.A.; Haddad, A.; Cunningham, H.; Yik, J.; Christiansen, B.; Haudenschild, D. Acute Changes in NADPH Oxidase 4 in Early Post-Traumatic Osteoarthritis. *J. Orthop. Res.* **2019**, *37*, 2429–2436. [CrossRef]
36. Halliwell, B.; Murcia, M.A.; Chirico, S.; Aruoma, O.I. Free Radicals and Antioxidants in Food and In Vivo: What They Do and How They Work. *Crit. Rev. Food Sci. Nutr.* **1995**, *35*, 7–20. [CrossRef] [PubMed]

37. Rigoglou, S.; Papavassiliou, A.G. The NF-κB signalling pathway in osteoarthritis. *Int. J. Biochem. Cell Biol.* **2013**, *45*, 2580–2584. [CrossRef]
38. Murphy, M.P.; Bayir, H.; Belousov, V.; Change, C.; Davies, K.; Davies, M.; Dick, T.; Finkel, T.; Forman, H.; Janssen-Heininger, Y.; et al. Guidelines for measuring reactive oxygen species and oxidative damage in cells and in vivo. *Nat. Metab.* **2022**, *4*, 651–662. [CrossRef] [PubMed]
39. Yang, B.; Chen, Y.; Shi, J. Reactive oxygen species (ROS)-based nanomedicine. *Chem. Rev.* **2019**, *119*, 4881–4985. [CrossRef]
40. Winterbourn, C.C. Toxicity of iron and hydrogen peroxide: The Fenton reaction. *Toxicol. Lett.* **1995**, *82–83*, 969–974. [CrossRef]
41. Rodrigo-Moreno, A.; Poschenrieder, C.; Shabala, S. Transition metals: A double edge sward in ROS generation and signaling. *Plant Signal Behav.* **2013**, *8*, e23425. [CrossRef]
42. Rhee, S.G.; Kil, I.S. Multiple functions and regulation of mammalian peroxiredoxins. *Annu. Rev. Biochem.* **2017**, *86*, 749–775. [CrossRef] [PubMed]
43. Bolduc, J.A.; Collins, J.A.; Loeser, R.F. Reactive oxygen species, aging and articular cartilage homeostasis. *Free Radic. Biol. Med.* **2019**, *132*, 73–82. [CrossRef] [PubMed]
44. Kwon, S.; Ko, H.; You, D.G.; Kataoka, K.; Park, J.H. Nanomedicines for Reactive Oxygen Species Mediated Approach: An Emerging Paradigm for Cancer Treatment. *Acc. Chem. Res.* **2019**, *52*, 1771–1782. [CrossRef]
45. Pérez-Lozano, M.L.; Cesaro, A.; Mazor, M.; Esteve, E.; Beretina-Raboin, S.; Best, T.; Lespessailles, E.; Toumi, H. Emerging Natural-Product-Based Treatments for the Management of Osteoarthritis. *Antioxidants* **2021**, *10*, 265. [CrossRef] [PubMed]
46. Chen, Y.; Wu, X.; Li, J.; Jiang, Y.; Xu, K.; Su, J. Bone-Targeted Nanoparticle Drug Delivery System: An Emerging Strategy for Bone-Related Disease. *Front. Pharmacol.* **2022**, *13*, 909408. [CrossRef]
47. Halliwell, B. Reactive oxygen species (ROS), oxygen radicals and antioxidants: Where are we now, where is the field going and where should we go? *Biochem. Biophys. Res. Commun.* **2022**, *633*, 17–19. [CrossRef]
48. Luo, J.; Zhang, Y.; Zhu, S.; Tong, Y.; Ji, L.; Zhang, W.; Zhang, Q.; Bi, Q. The application prospect of metal/metal oxide nanoparticles in the treatment of osteoarthritis. *Naunyn Schmiedebergs Arch. Pharmacol.* **2021**, *394*, 1991–2002. [CrossRef]
49. Rodrigues, J.V.; Gomes, C.M. Enhanced superoxide and hydrogen peroxide detection in biological assays. *Free Radic. Biol. Med.* **2010**, *49*, 61–66. [CrossRef]
50. Ye, S.; Hu, J.J.; Zhao, Q.A.; Yang, D. Fluorescent probes for in vitro and in vivo quantification of hydrogen peroxide. *Chem. Sci.* **2020**, *11*, 11989–11997. [CrossRef]
51. Castrogiovanni, P.; Trovato, F.M.; Loreto, C.; Nsir, H.; Szychlinska, M.A.; Musumeci, G. Nutraceutical supplements in the management and prevention of osteoarthritis. *Int. J. Mol. Sci.* **2016**, *17*, 2042. [CrossRef]
52. Dunlap, B.; Patterson, G.T.; Kumar, S.; Vyavahare, S.; Mishra, S.; Isales, C.; Fulzele, S. Vitamin C supplementation for the treatment of osteoarthritis: Perspectives on the past, present, and future. *Ther. Adv. Chronic Dis.* **2021**, *12*, 20406223211047026. [CrossRef] [PubMed]
53. Tagliaferri, S.; Porri, D.; De Giuseppe, R.; Manuelli, M.; Alessio, F.; Cena, H. The controversial role of vitamin D as an antioxidant: Results from randomised controlled trials. *Nutr. Res. Rev.* **2019**, *32*, 99–105. [CrossRef] [PubMed]
54. McAlindon, T.; LaValley, M.; Schneider, E.; Nuite, M.; Lee, J.Y.; Price, L.L.; Lo, G.; Dawson-Hughes, B. Effect of vitamin D supplementation on progression of knee pain and cartilage volume loss in patients with symptomatic osteoarthritis: A randomized controlled trial. *JAMA* **2013**, *309*, 155–162. [CrossRef]
55. Wang, E.W.; Siu, P.M.; Pang, M.Y.; Woo, J.; Collins, A.R.; Benzie, I.F.F. Vitamin D deficiency, oxidative stress and antioxidant status: Only weak association seen in the absence of advanced age, obesity or pre-existing disease. *Br. J. Nutr.* **2017**, *118*, 11–16. [CrossRef] [PubMed]
56. Mabey, T.; Honsawek, S. Role of Vitamin D in Osteoarthritis: Molecular, Cellular, and Clinical Perspectives. *Int. J. Endocrinol.* **2015**, *2015*, 383918. [CrossRef] [PubMed]
57. Garfinkel, R.J.; Dilisio, M.F.; Agrawal, D.K. Vitamin D and Its Effects on Articular Cartilage and Osteoarthritis. *Orthop. J. Sports Med.* **2017**, *5*, 232596711771137. [CrossRef]
58. Huang, T.C.; Chang, W.T.; Hu, Y.C.; Hsieh, B.; Cheng, H.; Yen, J.; Chiu, P.; Chang, K. Zinc protects articular chondrocytes through changes in Nrf2-mediated antioxidants, cytokines and matrix metalloproteinases. *Nutrients* **2018**, *10*, 471. [CrossRef] [PubMed]
59. Hughes, A.; Oxford, A.E.; Tawara, K.; Jorcyk, C.L.; Oxford, J.T. Endoplasmic reticulum stress and unfolded protein response in cartilage pathophysiology; contributing factors to apoptosis and osteoarthritis. *Int. J. Mol. Sci.* **2017**, *18*, 665. [CrossRef]
60. Feng, K.; Chen, Z.; Pengcheng, L.; Zhang, S.; Wang, X. Quercetin attenuates oxidative stress-induced apoptosis via SIRT1/AMPK-mediated inhibition of ER stress in rat chondrocytes and prevents the progression of osteoarthritis in a rat model. *J. Cell Physiol.* **2019**, *234*, 18192–18205. [CrossRef]
61. Wang, X.P.; Xie, W.P.; Bi, Y.F.; Wang, B.A.; Song, H.B.; Wang, S.L.; Bi, R.X. Quercetin suppresses apoptosis of chondrocytes induced by IL-1β via inactivation of p38 MAPK signaling pathway. *Exp. Ther. Med.* **2021**, *21*, 468. [CrossRef]
62. Deng, Z.; Li, Y.; Liu, H.; Xiao, S.; Li, L.; Tian, J.; Cheng, C.; Zhang, G.; Zhang, F. The role of sirtuin 1 and its activator, resveratrol in osteoarthritis. *Biosci. Rep.* **2019**, *39*, BSR20190189. [CrossRef]
63. Nguyen, C.; Savouret, J.F.; Widerak, M.; Corvol, M.T.; Rannou, F. Resveratrol, potential therapeutic interest in joint disorders: A critical narrative review. *Nutrients* **2017**, *9*, 45. [CrossRef]
64. Alarcón De La Lastra, C.; Villegas, I. Resveratrol as an antioxidant and pro-oxidant agent: Mechanisms and clinical implications. *Biochem. Soc. Trans.* **2007**, *35*, 1156–1160. [CrossRef]

65. Zini, R.; Morin, C.; Bertelli, A.; Bertelli, A.A.E.; Tillement, J.P. Effects of resveratrol on the rat brain respiratory chain. *Drugs Under Exp. Clin. Res.* **1999**, *25*, 87–97.
66. Yen, G.C.; Der Duh, P.; Lin, C.W. Effects of resveratrol and 4-hexylresorcinol on hydrogen peroxide-induced oxidative DNA damage in human lymphocytes. *Free Radic. Res.* **2003**, *37*, 509–514. [CrossRef]
67. Yang, S.; Sun, M.; Zhang, X. Protective Effect of Resveratrol on Knee Osteoarthritis and its Molecular Mechanisms: A Recent Review in Preclinical and Clinical Trials. *Front. Pharmacol.* **2022**, *13*, 921003. [CrossRef] [PubMed]
68. Wei, Y.; Jia, J.; Jin, X.; Tong, W.; Tian, H. Resveratrol ameliorates inflammatory damage and protects against osteoarthritis in a rat model of osteoarthritis. *Mol. Med. Rep.* **2018**, *17*, 1493–1498. [CrossRef] [PubMed]
69. Elmali, N.; Baysal, O.; Harma, A.; Esenkaya, I.; Mizrak, B. Effects of resveratrol in inflammatory arthritis. *Inflammation* **2007**, *30*, 52–58. [CrossRef] [PubMed]
70. Elmali, N.; Esenkaya, I.; Harma, A.; Ertem, K.; Turkoz, Y.; Mizrak, B. Effect of resveratrol in experimental osteoarthritis in rabbits. *Inflamm. Res.* **2005**, *54*, 158–162. [CrossRef]
71. Wang, J.; Gao, J.S.; Chen, J.W.; Li, F.; Tian, J. Effect of resveratrol on cartilage protection and apoptosis inhibition in experimental osteoarthritis of rabbit. *Rheumatol. Int.* **2012**, *32*, 1541–1548. [CrossRef]
72. Kann, B.; Spengler, C.; Coradini, K.; Rigo, L.A.; Bennink, M.L.; Jacobs, K.; Offerhause, H.L.; Beck, R.C.R.; Windbergs, M. Intracellular Delivery of Poorly Soluble Polyphenols: Elucidating the Interplay of Self-Assembling Nanocarriers and Human Chondrocytes. *Anal. Chem.* **2016**, *88*, 7014–7022. [CrossRef]
73. Cui, N.; Xu, Z.; Zhao, X.; Yuan, M.; Pan, L.; Lu, T.; Du, A.; Zin, L. In Vivo Effect of Resveratrol-Cellulose Aerogel Drug Delivery System to Relieve Inflammation on Sports Osteoarthritis. *Gels* **2022**, *8*, 544. [CrossRef]
74. Qin, L.; Zhao, X.; He, Y.; Wang, H.; Wei, H.; Zhu, Q.; Zhang, T.; Qin, Y.; Du, A. Preparation, characterization, and in vitro evaluation of resveratrol-loaded cellulose aerogel. *Materials* **2020**, *13*, 1624. [CrossRef]
75. Coradini, K.; Lima, F.O.; Oliveira, C.M.; Chaves, P.S.; Athayde, M.L.; Carvalho, L.M.; Beck, R.C.R. Co-encapsulation of resveratrol and curcumin in lipid-core nanocapsules improves their in vitro antioxidant effects. *Eur. J. Pharm. Biopharm.* **2014**, *88*, 178–185. [CrossRef]
76. Chin, K.Y. The spice for joint inflammation: Anti-inflammatory role of curcumin in treating osteoarthritis. *Drug Des. Devel Ther.* **2016**, *10*, 3029–3042. [CrossRef] [PubMed]
77. Ak, T.; Gülçin, I. Antioxidant and radical scavenging properties of curcumin. *Chem. Biol. Interact.* **2008**, *174*, 27–37. [CrossRef]
78. Yang, K.Y.; Lin, L.C.; Tseng, T.Y.; Wang, S.C.; Tsai, T.H. Oral bioavailability of curcumin in rat and the herbal analysis from Curcuma longa L. by LC-MS/MS. *J. Chromatogr. B Anal. Technol. Biomed. Life Sci.* **2007**, *853*, 183–189. [CrossRef] [PubMed]
79. Crivelli, B.; Bari, E.; Perteghella, S.; Catenacci, L.; Sorrenti, M.; Mocchi, M.; Farago, S.; Tripodo, G.; Prina-Mello, A.; Torre, M.L. Silk fibroin nanoparticles for celecoxib and curcumin delivery: ROS-scavenging and anti-inflammatory activities in an in vitro model of osteoarthritis. *Eur. J. Pharm. Biopharm.* **2019**, *137*, 37–45. [CrossRef] [PubMed]
80. Kang, C.; Jung, E.; Hyeon, H.; Seon, S.; Lee, D. Acid-activatable polymeric curcumin nanoparticles as therapeutic agents for osteoarthritis. *Nanomedicine* **2020**, *23*, 102104. [CrossRef] [PubMed]
81. Flohé, L. Superoxide dismutase for therapeutic use: Clinical experience, dead ends and hopes. *Mol. Cell. Biochem.* **1988**, *84*, 123–131. [CrossRef] [PubMed]
82. McIlwain, H.; Silverfield, J.C.; Cheatum, D.E.; Poiley, J.; Taborn, J.; Ignaczak, T.; Multz, C.V. Intra-articular orgotein in osteoarthritis of the knee: A placebo-controlled efficacy, safety, and dosage comparison. *Am. J. Med.* **1989**, *87*, 295–300. [CrossRef]
83. Mao, G.D.; Poznansky, M.J. Electron spin resonance study on the permeability of superoxide radicals in lipid bilayers and biological membranes. *FEBS Lett.* **1992**, *305*, 233–236. [CrossRef]
84. Ghitman, J.; Biru, E.I.; Stan, R.; Iovu, H. Review of hybrid PLGA nanoparticles: Future of smart drug delivery and theranostics medicine. *Mater. Des.* **2020**, *193*, 108805. [CrossRef]
85. Sah, E.; Sah, H. Recent Trends in Preparation of Poly(lactide-*co*-glycolide) Nanoparticles by Mixing Polymeric Organic Solution with Antisolvent. *J. Nanomater.* **2015**, *2015*, 794601. [CrossRef]
86. Gui, T.; Luo, L.; Chhay, B.; Zhong, L.; Wei, Y.; Yao, L.; Yu, W.; Li, J.; Nelson, C.L.; Tsourkas, A.; et al. Superoxide dismutase-loaded porous polymersomes as highly efficient antioxidant nanoparticles targeting synovium for osteoarthritis therapy. *Biomaterials* **2022**, *283*, 121437. [CrossRef]
87. Greenwald, R.A. Superoxide dismutase and catalase as therapeutic agents for human diseases a critical review. *Free Radic. Biol. Med.* **1990**, *8*, 201–209. [CrossRef]
88. Ashcraft, K.A.; Boss, M.K.; Tovmasyan, A.; Choudhury, K.R.; Fontanella, A.N.; Young, K.H.; Palmer, G.M.; Birer, S.R.; Landon, C.D.; Park, W.; et al. Novel manganese-porphyrin superoxide dismutase-mimetic widens the therapeutic margin in a preclinical head and neck cancer model. *Int. J. Radiat. Oncol. Biol. Phys.* **2015**, *93*, 892–900. [CrossRef]
89. Xu, Q.; Zhan, G.; Zhang, Z.; Yong, T.; Yang, X.; Gan, L. Manganese porphyrin-based metal-organic framework for synergistic sonodynamic therapy and ferroptosis in hypoxic tumors. *Theranostics* **2021**, *11*, 1937–1952. [CrossRef]
90. Schalkwijk, J.; van den Berg, W.B.; van de Putte, L.B.; Joosten, L.A.; van den Bersselaar, L. Cationization of catalase, peroxidase, and superoxide dismutase. Effect of improved intraarticular retention on experimental arthritis in mice. *J. Clin. Investig.* **1985**, *76*, 198–205. [CrossRef]
91. Batinić-Haberle, I.; Rebouças, J.S.; Spasojević, I. Superoxide dismutase mimics: Chemistry, pharmacology, and therapeutic potential. *Antioxid. Redox Signal.* **2010**, *13*, 877–918. [CrossRef]

92. Cioni, P.; Gabellieri, E.; Campanini, B.; Bettati, S.; Raboni, S. Use of Exogenous Enzymes in Human Therapy: Approved Drugs and Potential Applications. *Curr. Med. Chem.* **2022**, *29*, 411–452. [CrossRef] [PubMed]
93. Cernanec, J.M.; Weinberg, J.B.; Batinic-Haberle, I.; Guilak, F.; Fermor, B. Influence of oxygen tension on interleukin 1-induced peroxynitrite formation and matrix turnover in articular cartilage. *J. Rheumatol.* **2007**, *34*, 401–407. [PubMed]
94. Yudoh, K.; Shishido, K.; Murayama, H.; Yano, M.; Masubayashi, K.; Takada, H.; Nakamura, H.; Masuko, K.; Kato, T.; Nishioka, K. Water-soluble C60 fullerene prevents degeneration of articular cartilage in osteoarthritis via down-regulation of chondrocyte catabolic activity and inhibition of cartilage degeneration during disease development. *Arthritis Rheum.* **2007**, *56*, 3307–3318. [CrossRef]
95. Shi, Y.; Hu, X.; Cheng, J.; Zhang, X.; Zhao, F.; Shi, W.; Ren, B.; Yu, H.; Yang, P.; Li, Z.; et al. A small molecule promotes cartilage extracellular matrix generation and inhibits osteoarthritis development. *Nat. Commun.* **2019**, *10*, 1914. [CrossRef] [PubMed]
96. Chen, M.; Daddy JC, K.A.; Su, Z.; Guissi, N.E.I.; Xiao, Y.; Zong, L.; Ping, Q. Folate Receptor-Targeting and Reactive Oxygen Species-Responsive Liposomal Formulation of Methotrexate for Treatment of Rheumatoid Arthritis. *Pharmaceutics* **2019**, *11*, 582. [CrossRef]
97. Saba, H.; Batinic-Haberle, I.; Munusamy, S.; Mitchell, T.; Lichti, C.; Megyesi, J.; MacMillan-Crow, L.A. Manganese porphyrin reduces renal injury and mitochondrial damage during ischemia/reperfusion. *Free Radic. Biol. Med.* **2007**, *42*, 1571–1578. [CrossRef]
98. Lee, F.S.; Ney, K.E.; Richardson, A.N.; Oberley-Deegan, R.E.; Wachs, R.A. Encapsulation of Manganese Porphyrin in Chondroitin Sulfate-A Microparticles for Long Term Reactive Oxygen Species Scavenging. *Cell. Mol. Bioeng.* **2022**, *15*, 391–407. [CrossRef]
99. Holyoak, D.T.; Tian, Y.F.; van der Meulen, M.C.H.; Singh, A. Osteoarthritis: Pathology, Mouse Models, and Nanoparticle Injectable Systems for Targeted Treatment. *Ann. Biomed. Eng.* **2016**, *44*, 2062–2075. [CrossRef]
100. Marouf, B.H. Effect of Resveratrol on Serum Levels of Type II Collagen and Aggrecan in Patients with Knee Osteoarthritis: A Pilot Clinical Study. *BioMed Res. Int.* **2021**, *2021*, 3668568. [CrossRef]
101. Gu, H.; Li, K.; Li, X.; Yu, X.; Wang, W.; Ding, L.; Liu, L. Oral resveratrol prevents osteoarthritis progression in C57BL/6J mice fed a High-Fat Diet. *Nutrients* **2016**, *8*, 233. [CrossRef] [PubMed]
102. Haroyan, A.; Mukuchyan, V.; Mkrtchyan, N.; Minasyan, N.; Gasparyan, S.; Sargsyan, A.; Narimanyan, M.; Hovhannisyan, A. Efficacy and safety of curcumin and its combination with boswellic acid in osteoarthritis: A comparative, randomized, double-blind, placebo-controlled study. *BMC Complement. Altern. Med.* **2018**, *18*, 7. [CrossRef]
103. Canter, P.H.; Wider, B.; Ernst, E. The antioxidant vitamins A, C, E and selenium in the treatment of arthritis: A systematic review of randomized clinical trials. *Rheumatology* **2007**, *46*, 1223–1233. [CrossRef] [PubMed]
104. McAlindon, T.E.; Jacques, P.; Zhang, Y.; Hannan, M.T.; Aliabadi, P.; Weissman, B.; Rush, D.; Levy, D.; Felson, D.T. Do antioxidant micronutrients protect against the development and progression of knee osteoarthritis? *Arthritis Rheum.* **1996**, *39*, 648–656. [CrossRef] [PubMed]
105. Messina, O.D.; Vidal Wilman, M.; Vidal Neira, L.F. Nutrition, osteoarthritis and cartilage metabolism. *Aging Clin. Exp. Res.* **2019**, *31*, 807–813. [CrossRef] [PubMed]
106. Biegert, C.; Wagner, I.; Lüdtke, R.; Kotter, I.; Lohmuller, C.; Gunaydin, I.; Taxis, K.; Heide, L. Efficacy and safety of willow bark extract in the treatment of osteoarthritis and rheumatoid arthritis: Results of 2 randomized double-blind controlled trials. *J. Rheumatol.* **2004**, *31*, 2121–2130.
107. Altman, R.D.; Barthel, H.R. Topical therapies for osteoarthritis. *Drugs* **2011**, *71*, 1259–1279. [CrossRef]
108. Rodriguez-Merchan, E.C. Topical therapies for knee osteoarthritis. *Postgrad. Med.* **2018**, *130*, 607–612. [CrossRef]
109. Peniston, J.H.; Gold, M.S.; Alwine, L.K. An open-label, long-term safety and tolerability trial of diclofenac sodium 1% gel in patients with knee osteoarthritis. *Phys. Sportsmed.* **2011**, *39*, 31–38. [CrossRef]
110. Zhang, Z.; Leong, D.J.; Xu, L.; He, Z.; Wang, A.; Navati, M.; Kim, S.J.; Hirsh, D.M.; Hardin, J.A.; Cobelli, N.J.; et al. Curcumin slows osteoarthritis progression and relieves osteoarthritis-associated pain symptoms in a post-traumatic osteoarthritis mouse model. *Arthritis Res. Ther.* **2016**, *18*, 128. [CrossRef]
111. Gambaro, F.M.; Ummarino, A.; Andón, F.T.; Ronzoni, F.; Di Matteo, B.; Kon, E. Drug delivery systems for the treatment of knee osteoarthritis: A systematic review of in vivo studies. *Int. J. Mol. Sci.* **2021**, *22*, 9137. [CrossRef]
112. Zhang, X.; Shi, Y.; Zhang, Z.; Yang, Z.; Huang, G. Intra-articular delivery of tetramethylpyrazine microspheres with enhanced articular cavity retention for treating osteoarthritis. *Asian J. Pharm. Sci.* **2018**, *13*, 229–238. [CrossRef]
113. Pak, J.; Lee, J.H.; Park, K.S.; Jeong, B.C.; Lee, S.H. Regeneration of cartilage in human knee osteoarthritis with autologous adipose tissue-derived stem cells and autologous extracellular matrix. *Biores Open Access* **2016**, *5*, 192–200. [CrossRef] [PubMed]
114. Cao, Y.; Ma, Y.; Tao, Y.; Lin, W.; Wang, P. Intra-articular drug delivery for osteoarthritis treatment. *Pharmaceutics* **2021**, *13*, 2166. [CrossRef] [PubMed]
115. Johny, J.; Sreedhar, S.; Aiswarya, P.R.; Mohan, A.B.; Kavya, A.S. Liposome assisted drug delivery—A review. *World J. Adv. Res. Rev.* **2021**, *12*, 594–601. [CrossRef]
116. Sercombe, L.; Veerati, T.; Moheimani, F.; Wu, S.Y.; Sood, A.K.; Hua, S. Advances and challenges of liposome assisted drug delivery. *Front. Pharmacol.* **2015**, *6*, 286. [CrossRef]
117. Maudens, P.; Jordan, O.; Allémann, E. Recent advances in intra-articular drug delivery systems for osteoarthritis therapy. *Drug Discov. Today* **2018**, *23*, 1761–1775. [CrossRef]

118. Seror, J.; Zhu, L.; Goldberg, R.; Day, A.J.; Klein, J. Supramolecular synergy in the boundary lubrication of synovial joints. *Nat. Commun.* **2015**, *6*, 6497. [CrossRef] [PubMed]
119. Gaisinskaya-Kipnis, A.; Klein, J. Normal and Frictional Interactions between Liposome-Bearing Biomacromolecular Bilayers. *Biomacromolecules* **2016**, *17*, 2591–2602. [CrossRef]
120. Lei, Y.; Wang, Y.; Shen, J.; Cai, Z.; Zhao, C.; Chen, H.; Luo, X.; Hu, N.; Cui, W.; Huang, W. Injectable hydrogel microspheres with self-renewable hydration layers alleviate osteoarthritis. *Sci. Adv.* **2022**, *8*, eabl6449. [CrossRef]
121. Wathier, M.; Lakin, B.A.; Cooper, B.G.; Bansal, P.N.; Bendele, A.M.; Entezari, V.; Suzuki, H.; Snyder, B.D.; Grinstaff, M.W. A synthetic polymeric biolubricant imparts chondroprotection in a rat meniscal tear model. *Biomaterials* **2018**, *182*, 13–20. [CrossRef]
122. Ji, X.; Yan, Y.; Sun, T.; Zhang, Q.; Wang, Y.; Zhang, M.; Zhang, H.; Zhao, X. Glucosamine sulphate-loaded distearoyl phosphocholine liposomes for osteoarthritis treatment: Combination of sustained drug release and improved lubrication. *Biomater. Sci.* **2019**, *7*, 2716–2728. [CrossRef]
123. He, K.; Huang, X.; Shan, R.; Yang, X.; Song, R.; Xie, F.; Huang, G. Intra-articular Injection of Lornoxicam and MicroRNA-140 Co-loaded Cationic Liposomes Enhanced the Therapeutic Treatment of Experimental Osteoarthritis. *AAPS PharmSciTech* **2022**, *23*, 9. [CrossRef] [PubMed]
124. Liang, Y.; Xu, X.; Xu, L.; Iqbal, Z.; Ouyang, K.; Zhang, H.; Wen, C.; Duan, L.; Xia, J. Chondrocyte-specific genomic editing enabled by hybrid exosomes for osteoarthritis treatment. *Theranostics* **2022**, *12*, 4866–4878. [CrossRef] [PubMed]
125. Sarkar, A.; Carvalho, E.; D'Souza, A.A.; Banerjee, R. Liposome-encapsulated fish oil protein-tagged gold nanoparticles for intra-articular therapy in osteoarthritis. *Nanomedicine* **2019**, *14*, 871–887. [CrossRef] [PubMed]
126. He, Z.; Wang, B.; Hu, C.; Zhao, J. An overview of hydrogel-based intra-articular drug delivery for the treatment of osteoarthritis. *Colloids Surf. B Biointerfaces* **2017**, *154*, 33–39. [CrossRef]
127. Wang, S.; Qiu, Y.; Qu, L.; Wang, Q.; Zhou, Q. Hydrogels for Treatment of Different Degrees of Osteoarthritis. *Front. Bioeng. Biotechnol.* **2022**, *10*, 858656. [CrossRef]
128. Jin, Y.; Koh, R.H.; Kim, S.H.; Kim, K.M.; Park, G.K.; Hwang, N.S. Injectable anti-inflammatory hyaluronic acid hydrogel for osteoarthritic cartilage repair. *Mater. Sci. Eng. C* **2020**, *115*, 111096. [CrossRef]
129. de Viteri, M.S.; Hernandez, M.; Bilbao-Malavé, V.; Fernandez-Robredo, P.; Gonzalez-Zamora, J.; Garcia-Garcia, L.; Ispizua, N.; Recalde, S.; Garcia-Layana, A. A higher proportion of eicosapentaenoic acid (EPA) when combined with docosahexaenoic acid (DHA) in omega-3 dietary supplements provides higher antioxidant effects in human retinal cells. *Antioxidants* **2020**, *9*, 828. [CrossRef]
130. Tsubosaka, M.; Kihara, S.; Hayashi, S.; Nagata, J.; Kuwarhara, T.; Fujita, M.; Kikuchi, K.; Takashima, Y.; Kamenaga, T.; Kuroda, Y.; et al. Gelatin hydrogels with eicosapentaenoic acid can prevent osteoarthritis progression in vivo in a mouse model. *J. Orthop. Res.* **2020**, *38*, 2157–2169. [CrossRef]
131. Feng, K.; Ge, Y.; Chen, Z.; Li, X.; Liu, Z.; Li, X.; Li, H.; Tang, T.; Yang, F.; Wang, X. Curcumin Inhibits the PERK-eIF2 α-CHOP Pathway through Promoting SIRT1 Expression in Oxidative Stress-induced Rat Chondrocytes and Ameliorates Osteoarthritis Progression in a Rat Model. *Oxid. Med. Cell Longev.* **2019**, *2019*, 8574386. [CrossRef]
132. Sun, Y.; Liu, W.; Zhang, H.; Li, H.; Liu, J.; Zhang, F.; Jiang, T.; Jinag, S. Curcumin Prevents Osteoarthritis by Inhibiting the Activation of Inflammasome NLRP3. *J. Interferon Cytokine Res.* **2017**, *37*, 449–455. [CrossRef]
133. Huang, H.; Lou, Z.; Zheng, S.; Wu, J.; Yao, Q.; Chen, R.; Kou, L.; Chen, D. Intra-articular drug delivery systems for osteoarthritis therapy: Shifting from sustained release to enhancing penetration into cartilage. *Drug Deliv.* **2022**, *29*, 767–791. [CrossRef] [PubMed]
134. Zandieh, M.; Liu, J. Nanozymes: Definition, Activity, and Mechanisms. *Adv. Mater.* **2023**, 2211041. [CrossRef] [PubMed]
135. Jiang, D.; Ni, D.; Rosenkrans, Z.T.; Huang, P.; Yan, X.; Cai, W. Nanozyme: New horizons for responsive biomedical applications. *Chem. Soc. Rev.* **2019**, *48*, 3683–3704. [CrossRef] [PubMed]
136. Singh, R.; Umapathi, A.; Patel, G.; Patra, C.; Malik, U.; Bhargava, S.K.; Daima, H.K. Nanozyme-based pollutant sensing and environmental treatment: Trends, challenges, and perspectives. *Sci. Total Environ.* **2023**, *854*, 158771. [CrossRef]
137. Mangalsana, H.; Mohanty, A.; Vernekar, A.A. Rise of supramolecular nanozymes: Next-generation peroxidase enzyme-mimetic materials. In *Supramolecular Coordination Complexes*; Elsevier: Amsterdam, The Netherlands, 2023; pp. 329–387. [CrossRef]
138. Robert, A.; Meunier, B. How to Define a Nanozyme. *ACS Nano* **2022**, *16*, 6956–6959. [CrossRef]
139. Wu, J.; Wang, X.; Wang, Q.; Lou, Z.; Li, S.; Zhu, Y.; Zin, L.; Wei, H. Nanomaterials with enzyme-like characteristics (nanozymes): Next-generation artificial enzymes (II). *Chem. Soc. Rev.* **2019**, *48*, 1004–1076. [CrossRef]
140. Wei, H.; Wang, E. Nanomaterials with enzyme-like characteristics (nanozymes): Next-generation artificial enzymes. *Chem. Soc. Rev.* **2013**, *42*, 6060–6093. [CrossRef]
141. Gao, L.; Fan, K.; Yan, X. Iron oxide nanozyme: A multifunctional enzyme mimetic for biomedical applications. *Theranostics* **2017**, *7*, 3207–3227. [CrossRef]
142. Wang, H.; Cui, Z.; Wang, X.; Sun, S.; Zhang, D.; Fu, C. Therapeutic Applications of Nanozymes in Chronic Inflammatory Diseases. *BioMed Res. Int.* **2021**, *2021*, 9980127. [CrossRef]
143. Chang, J.; Qin, X.; Li, S.; He, F.; Gai, S.; Ding, H.; Yang, P. Combining Cobalt Ferrite Nanozymes with a Natural Enzyme to Reshape the Tumor Microenvironment for Boosted Cascade Enzyme-Like Activities. *ACS Appl. Mater. Interfaces* **2022**, *14*, 45217–45228. [CrossRef]

144. Ye, J.; Lv, W.; Li, C.; Liu, X.; Yang, X.; Zhang, J.; Wang, C.; Xu, J.; Jin, G.; Li, B.; et al. Tumor Response and NIR-II Photonic Thermal Co-Enhanced Catalytic Therapy Based on Single-Atom Manganese Nanozyme. *Adv. Funct. Mater.* **2022**, *32*, 2206157. [CrossRef]
145. Li, M.; Liu, J.; Shi, L.; Zhou, C.; Zou, M.; Fu, D.; Yuan, Y.; Yao, C.; Zhang, L.; Zin, S.; et al. Gold nanoparticles-embedded ceria with enhanced antioxidant activities for treating inflammatory bowel disease. *Bioact. Mater.* **2023**, *25*, 95–106. [CrossRef]
146. Wang, Q.; Lv, L.; Chi, W.; Bai, Y.; Gao, W.; Zhu, P.; Yu, J. Porphyrin-Based Covalent Organic Frameworks with Donor-Acceptor Structure for Enhanced Peroxidase-like Activity as a Colorimetric Biosensing Platform. *Biosensors* **2023**, *13*, 188. [CrossRef]
147. Lin, Y.W.; Fang, C.H.; Meng, F.Q.; Ke, C.J.; Lin, F.H. Hyaluronic acid loaded with cerium oxide nanoparticles as antioxidant in hydrogen peroxide induced chondrocytes injury: An in vitro osteoarthritis model. *Molecules* **2020**, *25*, 4407. [CrossRef]
148. Dashnyam, K.; Lee, J.H.; Singh, R.K.; Yoon, J.Y.; Lee, J.H.; Jin, G.; Kim, H. Optimally dosed nanoceria attenuates osteoarthritic degeneration of joint cartilage and subchondral bone. *Chem. Eng. J.* **2021**, *422*, 130066. [CrossRef]
149. Kumar, S.; Adjei, I.M.; Brown, S.B.; Liseth, O.; Sharma, B. Manganese dioxide nanoparticles protect cartilage from inflammation-induced oxidative stress. *Biomaterials* **2019**, *224*, 119467. [CrossRef] [PubMed]
150. Tootoonchi, M.H.; Hashempour, M.; Blackwelder, P.L.; Fraker, C.A. Manganese oxide particles as cytoprotective, oxygen generating agents. *Acta Biomater.* **2017**, *59*, 327–337. [CrossRef] [PubMed]
151. Chen, L.; Tiwari, S.R.; Zhang, Y.; Zhang, J.; Sun, Y. Facile Synthesis of Hollow MnO_2 Nanoparticles for Reactive Oxygen Species Scavenging in Osteoarthritis. *ACS Biomater. Sci. Eng.* **2021**, *7*, 1686–1692. [CrossRef]
152. Zhou, T.; Ran, J.; Xu, P.; Shen, L.; He, Y.; Ye, J.; Wu, L.; Gao, C. A hyaluronic acid/platelet-rich plasma hydrogel containing $MnO2$ nanozymes efficiently alleviates osteoarthritis in vivo. *Carbohydr. Polym.* **2022**, *292*, 119667. [CrossRef]
153. Lin, T.; Zhao, Y.; Chen, J.; Wu, C.; Li, Z.; Cao, Y.; Lu, R.; Zhang, J.; Zhao, C.; Lu, Y. Carboxymethyl chitosan-assisted MnOx nanoparticles: Synthesis, characterization, detection and cartilage repair in early osteoarthritis. *Carbohydr. Polym.* **2022**, *294*, 119821. [CrossRef] [PubMed]
154. Hou, W.; Ye, C.; Chen, M.; Goa, W.; Xie, X.; Uw, J.; Zhang, K.; Zhang, W.; Zheng, Y.; Cai, X. Excavating bioactivities of nanozyme to remodel microenvironment for protecting chondrocytes and delaying osteoarthritis. *Bioact. Mater.* **2021**, *6*, 2439–2451. [CrossRef] [PubMed]
155. Xiong, H.; Zhao, Y.; Xu, Q.; Xie, X.; Wu, J.; Hu, B.; Chen, S.; Cai, X.; Zheng, Y.; Fan, C. Biodegradable Hollow-Structured Nanozymes Modulate Phenotypic Polarization of Macrophages and Relieve Hypoxia for Treatment of Osteoarthritis. *Small* **2022**, *18*, 2439–2451. [CrossRef] [PubMed]
156. Filho, M.C.B.; Santos Haupenthal, D.P.; Zaccaron, R.P.; Silveira, B.D.B.; Casagrande, L.D.R.; Lupselo, F.S.; Alves, N.; Mariano, S.D.S.; Bomfim, F.R.C.D.; Andrade, T.A.M.D.; et al. Intra-articular treatment with hyaluronic acid associated with gold nanoparticles in a mechanical osteoarthritis model in Wistar rats. *J. Orthop. Res.* **2021**, *39*, 2546–2555. [CrossRef] [PubMed]
157. Abdel-Aziz, M.A.; Ahmed, H.M.S.; El-Nekeety, A.A.; Sharaf, H.A.; Abdel-Aziem, S.H.; Abdel-Wahhab, M.A. Biosynthesis of gold nanoparticles for the treatment of osteoarthritis alone or in combination with Diacerein® in a rat model. *Inflammopharmacology* **2021**, *29*, 705–719. [CrossRef]
158. Tournebize, J.; Sapin-Minet, A.; Bartosz, G.; Leroy, P.; Boudier, A. Pitfalls of assays devoted to evaluation of oxidative stress induced by inorganic nanoparticles. *Talanta* **2013**, *116*, 753–763. [CrossRef]
159. Li, H.; Xia, P.; Pan, S.; Qi, Z.; Fu, C.; Yu, Z.; Kong, W.; Chang, Y.; Wang, K.; Wu, D.; et al. The advances of ceria nanoparticles for biomedical applications in orthopaedics. *Int. J. Nanomed.* **2020**, *15*, 7199–7214. [CrossRef]
160. Singh, N.; Geethika, M.; Eswarappa, S.M.; Mugesh, G. Manganese-Based Nanozymes: Multienzyme Redox Activity and Effect on the Nitric Oxide Produced by Endothelial Nitric Oxide Synthase. *Chem. A Eur. J.* **2018**, *24*, 8393–8403. [CrossRef]
161. Bizeau, J.; Tapeinos, C.; Marella, C.; Larrañaga, A.; Pandit, A. Synthesis and characterization of hyaluronic acid coated manganese dioxide microparticles that act as ROS scavengers. *Colloids Surf. B Biointerfaces* **2017**, *159*, 30–38. [CrossRef]
162. Zhang, T.; Gaffrey, M.J.; Thomas, D.G.; Weber, T.J.; Hess, B.M.; Weitz, K.K.; Piehowski, P.D.; Petyuk, V.A.; Moore, R.J.; Qian, W.J.; et al. A proteome-wide assessment of the oxidative stress paradigm for metal and metal-oxide nanomaterials in human macrophages. *NanoImpact* **2020**, *17*, 100194. [CrossRef]
163. Ponnurangam, S.; O'Connell, G.D.; Chernyshova, I.V.; Wood, K.; Hung, C.T.H.; Somasundaran, P. Beneficial effects of cerium oxide nanoparticles in development of chondrocyte-seeded hydrogel constructs and cellular response to interleukin insults. *Tissue Eng. Part A* **2014**, *20*, 2908–2919. [CrossRef] [PubMed]
164. Zheng, Q.; Fang, Y.; Zeng, L.; Li, X.; Chen, H.; Song, H.; Huang, J.; Shi, S. Cytocompatible cerium oxide-mediated antioxidative stress in inhibiting ocular inflammation-Associated corneal neovascularization. *J. Mater. Chem. B* **2019**, *7*, 6759–6769. [CrossRef] [PubMed]
165. Adebayo, O.A.; Akinloye, O.; Adaramoye, O.A. Cerium Oxide Nanoparticles Attenuate Oxidative Stress and Inflammation in the Liver of Diethylnitrosamine-Treated Mice. *Biol. Trace Elem. Res.* **2020**, *193*, 214–225. [CrossRef] [PubMed]
166. Dhall, A.; Self, W. Cerium oxide nanoparticles: A brief review of their synthesis methods and biomedical applications. *Antioxidants* **2018**, *7*, 97. [CrossRef] [PubMed]
167. Xu, C.; Qu, X. Cerium oxide nanoparticle: A remarkably versatile rare earth nanomaterial for biological applications. *NPG Asia Mater.* **2014**, *6*, e90. [CrossRef]
168. Kuthati, Y.; Busa, P.; Davuluri, V.N.G.; Wong, C.S. Manganese oxide nanozymes ameliorate mechanical allodynia in a rat model of partial sciatic nerve-transection induced neuropathic pain. *Int. J. Nanomed.* **2019**, *14*, 10105–10117. [CrossRef]

169. Ghosh, S.K. Diversity in the Family of Manganese Oxides at the Nanoscale: From Fundamentals to Applications. *ACS Omega* **2020**, *5*, 25493–25504. [CrossRef]
170. Leach, R.M.; Lilburn, M.S. Manganese metabolism and its function. *World Rev. Nutr. Diet.* **1978**, *32*, 123–134. [CrossRef]
171. Takeda, A. Manganese action in brain function. *Brain Res. Rev.* **2003**, *41*, 79–87. [CrossRef]
172. Hao, Y.; Wang, L.; Zhang, B.; Zhao, H.; Niu, M.; Hu, Y.; Zheng, C.; Zhang, H.; Chang, J.; Zhang, Z.; et al. Multifunctional nanosheets based on folic acid modified manganese oxide for tumor-targeting theranostic application. *Nanotechnology* **2015**, *27*, 025101. [CrossRef]
173. Marin, E.; Tapeinos, C.; Lauciello, S.; Ciofani, G.; Sarasua, J.R.; Larrañaga, A. Encapsulation of manganese dioxide nanoparticles into layer-by-layer polymer capsules for the fabrication of antioxidant microreactors. *Mater. Sci. Eng. C* **2020**, *117*, 111349. [CrossRef]
174. Tapeinos, C.; Larrañaga, A.; Sarasua, J.R.; Pandit, A. Functionalised collagen spheres reduce H_2O_2 mediated apoptosis by scavenging overexpressed ROS. *Nanomedicine* **2018**, *14*, 2397–2405. [CrossRef] [PubMed]
175. Gao, L.; Zhuang, J.; Nie, L.; Zhang, J.; Zhang, Y.; Gu, N.; Wang, T.; Feng, J.; Yang, D.; Perrett, S.; et al. Intrinsic peroxidase-like activity of ferromagnetic nanoparticles. *Nat. Nanotechnol.* **2007**, *2*, 577–583. [CrossRef] [PubMed]
176. Carneiro, M.F.H.; Machado, A.R.T.; Antunes, L.M.G.; Souza, T.E.; Freitas, V.A.; Oliveria, L.C.A.; Rodrigues, J.L.; Pereira, M.C.; Barbosa, F., Jr. Gold-Coated Superparamagnetic Iron Oxide Nanoparticles Attenuate Collagen-Induced Arthritis after Magnetic Targeting. *Biol. Trace Elem. Res.* **2020**, *194*, 502–513. [CrossRef] [PubMed]
177. Xie, M.; Luo, S.; Li, Y.; Lu, L.; Deng, C.; Cheng, Y.; Yin, F. Intra-articular tracking of adipose-derived stem cells by chitosan-conjugated iron oxide nanoparticles in a rat osteoarthritis model. *RSC Adv.* **2019**, *9*, 12010–12019. [CrossRef] [PubMed]
178. Delling, U.; Brehm, W.; Metzger, M.; Ludewig, E.; Winter, K.; Jülke, H. In Vivo Tracking and Fate of Intra-Articularly Injected Superparamagnetic Iron Oxide Particle-Labeled Multipotent Stromal Cells in an Ovine Model of Osteoarthritis. *Cell Transplant.* **2015**, *24*, 2379–2390. [CrossRef]
179. Zhang, M.; Hu, W.; Cai, C.; Wu, Y.; Li, J.; Dong, S. Advanced application of stimuli-responsive drug delivery system for inflammatory arthritis treatment. *Mater. Today Bio* **2022**, *14*, 100223. [CrossRef]
180. Farrell, E.; Wielopolski, P.; Pavljasevic, P.; Kops, N.; Weinans, H.; Bernsen, M.R.; van Osch, G.J.V.M. Cell labelling with superparamagnetic iron oxide has no effect on chondrocyte behaviour. *Osteoarthr. Cartil.* **2009**, *17*, 961–967. [CrossRef]
181. Ajayi, T.O.; Liu, S.; Rosen, C.; Rinaldi-Ramos, C.M.; Allen, K.D.; Sharma, B. Application of magnetic particle imaging to evaluate nanoparticle fate in rodent joints. *J. Control. Release* **2023**, *356*, 347–359. [CrossRef]
182. Moeini-Nodeh, S.; Rahimifard, M.; Baeeri, M.; Abdollahi, M. Functional Improvement in Rats' Pancreatic Islets Using Magnesium Oxide Nanoparticles Through Antiapoptotic and Antioxidant Pathways. *Biol. Trace Elem. Res.* **2017**, *175*, 146–155. [CrossRef]
183. Busquets, M.A.; Estelrich, J. Prussian blue nanoparticles: Synthesis, surface modification, and biomedical applications. *Drug Discov. Today* **2020**, *25*, 1431–1443. [CrossRef] [PubMed]
184. Estelrich, J.; Busquets, M.A. Prussian blue: A nanozyme with versatile catalytic properties. *Int. J. Mol. Sci.* **2021**, *22*, 5993. [CrossRef] [PubMed]
185. Zhang, K.; Tu, M.; Gao, W.; Cai, X.; Song, F.; Chen, Z.; Zhang, Q.; Wang, J.; Jin, C.; Shi, J.; et al. Hollow Prussian Blue Nanozymes Drive Neuroprotection against Ischemic Stroke via Attenuating Oxidative Stress, Counteracting Inflammation, and Suppressing Cell Apoptosis. *Nano Lett.* **2019**, *19*, 2812–2823. [CrossRef] [PubMed]
186. Zhao, J.; Gao, W.; Cai, X.; Xu, J.; Zou, D.; Li, Z.; Hu, B.; Zheng, Y. Nanozyme-mediated catalytic nanotherapy for inflammatory bowel disease. *Theranostics* **2019**, *9*, 2843–2855. [CrossRef]
187. Cai, X.; Zhang, K.; Xie, X.; Zhu, Z.; Feng, J.; Jin, Z.; Zhang, H.; Tian, M.; Chen, H. Self-assembly hollow manganese Prussian white nanocapsules attenuate Tau-related neuropathology and cognitive decline. *Biomaterials* **2020**, *231*, 119678. [CrossRef]
188. Ye, C.; Zhang, W.; Zhao, Y.; Zhang, J.; Hou, W.; Chen, M.; Lu, J.; Wu, J.; He, R.; Gao, Y.; et al. Prussian Blue Nanozyme Normalizes Microenvironment to Delay Osteoporosis. *Adv. Healthc. Mater.* **2022**, *11*, 2200787. [CrossRef]
189. Shen, W.; Han, G.; Yu, L.; Yang, S.; Li, X.; Zhang, W.; Pei, P. Combined Prussian Blue Nanozyme Carriers Improve Photodynamic Therapy and Effective Interruption of Tumor Metastasis. *Int. J. Nanomed.* **2022**, *17*, 1397–1408. [CrossRef]
190. Costa Lima, S.A.; Reis, S. Temperature-responsive polymeric nanospheres containing methotrexate and gold nanoparticles: A multi-drug system for theranostic in rheumatoid arthritis. *Colloids Surf. B Biointerfaces* **2015**, *133*, 378–387. [CrossRef]
191. Thakor, A.S.; Jokerst, J.; Zavaleta, C.; Massoud, T.F.; Gambhir, S.S. Gold Nanoparticles: A Revival in Precious Metal Administration to Patients. *Nano Lett.* **2011**, *11*, 4029–4036. [CrossRef]
192. Balfourier, A.; Kolosnjaj-Tabi, J.; Luciani, N.; Carn, F.; Gazeau, F. Gold-based therapy: From past to present. *Proc. Natl. Acad. Sci. USA* **2020**, *117*, 22639–22648. [CrossRef]
193. Dwivedi, P.; Nayak, V.; Kowshik, M. Role of gold nanoparticles as drug delivery vehicles for chondroitin sulfate in the treatment of osteoarthritis. *Biotechnol. Prog.* **2015**, *31*, 1416–1422. [CrossRef] [PubMed]
194. Pitou, M.; Papi, R.M.; Tzavellas, A.N.; Choli-Papadopoulou, T. ssDNA-Modified Gold Nanoparticles as a Tool to Detect miRNA Biomarkers in Osteoarthritis. *ACS Omega* **2023**, *8*, 7529–7535. [CrossRef] [PubMed]
195. Rasmussen, S.; Kjær Petersen, K.; Kristiansen, M.K.; Skallerup, J.; Aboo, C.; Thomsen, M.E.; Skjoldemose, E.; Jorgensen, N.K.; Stensballe, A.; Arendt-Nielsen, L. Gold micro-particles for knee osteoarthritis. *Eur. J. Pain* **2022**, *26*, 811–824. [CrossRef]
196. Kumawat, M.; Madhyastha, H.; Umapathi, A.; Singh, M.; Revaprasadu, N.; Daima, H.K. Surface Engineered Peroxidase-Mimicking Gold Nanoparticles to Subside Cell Inflammation. *Langmuir* **2022**, *38*, 1877–1887. [CrossRef]

197. Kirdaite, G.; Leonaviciene, L.; Bradunaite, R.; Vasiliauskas, A.; Rudys, R.; Ramanaviciene, A.; Mackiewicz, Z. Antioxidant effects of gold nanoparticles on early stage of collagen-induced arthritis in rats. *Res. Vet. Sci.* **2019**, *124*, 32–37. [CrossRef]
198. Daems, N.; Penninckx, S.; Nelissen, I.; Hoecke, K.V.; Cardinaels, T.; Baatout, S.; Michiels, C.; Lucas, S.; Aerts, A. Gold nanoparticles affect the antioxidant status in selected normal human cells. *Int. J. Nanomed.* **2019**, *14*, 4991–5015. [CrossRef] [PubMed]
199. Chen, Y.S.; Hung, Y.C.; Liau, I.; Huang, G.S. Assessment of the In Vivo Toxicity of Gold Nanoparticles. *Nanoscale Res. Lett.* **2009**, *4*, 858. [CrossRef]
200. Li, J.J.; Hartono, D.; Ong, C.N.; Bay, B.H.; Yung, L.Y.L. Autophagy and oxidative stress associated with gold nanoparticles. *Biomaterials* **2010**, *31*, 5996–6003. [CrossRef]
201. Kongtharvonskul, J.; Anothaisintawee, T.; McEvoy, M.; Attia, J.; Woratanarat, P.; Thakkinstian, A. Efficacy and safety of glucosamine, diacerein, and NSAIDs in osteoarthritis knee: A systematic review and network meta-analysis. *Eur. J. Med. Res.* **2015**, *20*, 24. [CrossRef] [PubMed]
202. Zhong, J.; Yang, X.; Gao, S.; Luo, J.; Xiang, J.; Li, G.; Liang, Y.; Tang, L.; Qian, C.; Zhou, J.; et al. Geometric and Electronic Structure-Matched Superoxide Dismutase-Like and Catalase-Like Sequential Single-Atom Nanozymes for Osteoarthritis Recession. *Adv. Funct. Mater.* **2023**, *33*, 2209399. [CrossRef]
203. DiDomenico, C.D.; Lintz, M.; Bonassar, L.J. Molecular transport in articular cartilage—What have we learned from the past 50 years? *Nat. Rev. Rheumatol.* **2018**, *14*, 393–403. [CrossRef]
204. Pouran, B.; Arbabi, V.; Bajpayee, A.G.; van Tiel, J.; Toyras, J.; Jurvelin, J.S.; Malda, J.; Zadpoor, A.A.; Weinans, H. Multi-scale imaging techniques to investigate solute transport across articular cartilage. *J. Biomech.* **2018**, *78*, 10–20. [CrossRef]
205. Xu, R.; Xiong, B.; Zhou, R.; Shen, H.; Yeung, E.S.; He, Y. Pericellular matrix plays an active role in retention and cellular uptake of large-sized nanoparticles. *Anal. Bioanal. Chem.* **2014**, *406*, 5031–5037. [CrossRef]
206. Guilak, F.; Nims, R.J.; Dicks, A.; Wu, C.L.; Meulenbelt, I. Osteoarthritis as a disease of the cartilage pericellular matrix. *Matrix Biol.* **2018**, *71–72*, 40–50. [CrossRef]
207. Xu, X.L.; Xue, Y.; Ding, J.Y.; Zhu, Z.H.; Wu, X.C.; Song, Y.J.; Cao, Y.L.; Tang, L.G.; Ding, D.F.; Xu, J.G. Nanodevices for deep cartilage penetration. *Acta Biomater.* **2022**, *154*, 23–48. [CrossRef] [PubMed]
208. Rampado, R.; Crotti, S.; Caliceti, P.; Pucciarelli, S.; Agostini, M. Recent Advances in Understanding the Protein Corona of Nanoparticles and in the Formulation of "Stealthy" Nanomaterials. *Front. Bioeng. Biotechnol.* **2020**, *8*, 166. [CrossRef] [PubMed]
209. von Mentzer, U.; Selldén, T.; Råberg, L.; Erensoy, G.; Hultgård Ekwall, A.K.; Stubelius, A. Synovial fluid profile dictates nanoparticle uptake into cartilage—Implications of the protein corona for novel arthritis treatments. *Osteoarthr. Cartil.* **2022**, *30*, 1356–1364. [CrossRef] [PubMed]
210. Hodgkinson, T.; Kelly, D.C.; Curtin, C.M.; O'Brien, F.J. Mechanosignalling in cartilage: An emerging target for the treatment of osteoarthritis. *Nat. Rev. Rheumatol.* **2022**, *18*, 67–84. [CrossRef] [PubMed]

Disclaimer/Publisher's Note: The statements, opinions and data contained in all publications are solely those of the individual author(s) and contributor(s) and not of MDPI and/or the editor(s). MDPI and/or the editor(s) disclaim responsibility for any injury to people or property resulting from any ideas, methods, instructions or products referred to in the content.

MDPI
St. Alban-Anlage 66
4052 Basel
Switzerland
www.mdpi.com

Pharmaceuticals Editorial Office
E-mail: pharmaceuticals@mdpi.com
www.mdpi.com/journal/pharmaceuticals

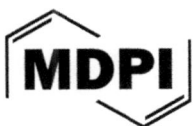

Disclaimer/Publisher's Note: The statements, opinions and data contained in all publications are solely those of the individual author(s) and contributor(s) and not of MDPI and/or the editor(s). MDPI and/or the editor(s) disclaim responsibility for any injury to people or property resulting from any ideas, methods, instructions or products referred to in the content.

www.ingramcontent.com/pod-product-compliance
Lightning Source LLC
LaVergne TN
LVHW070203100526
838202LV00015B/1989